Lippincott's
state board examination review for nurses

Contributors

MARION CARPENEDO CZUBIAK,
R.N., M.S.
Instructor in Nursing, Los Angeles Valley
College, Van Nuys, California

CAROLYN M. BOLTER FELLER,
R.N., M.S.N
Assistant Professor, College of Nursing,
Arizona State University, Tempe, Arizona

BARBARA BATES HINDMAN,
R.N., M.N.
Instructor, College of Nursing, Arizona
State University, Tempe, Arizona

SHANNON E. PERRY, R.N., M.S.
Formerly Instructor, College of Nursing,
Arizona State University, Tempe, Arizona

DANIEL W. TETTING, R.N., M.S.N.
Associate Chief, Nursing Service for
Education, Veteran's Administration
Hospital, Ann Arbor, Michigan

MARJORIE SNODGRASS
VANDERLINDEN, R.N., M.S.N.
Assistant Professor, College of Nursing,
Arizona State University, Tempe, Arizona

Reviewers

KAY MILLER FORD, R.N., M.S.
Perinatal Nurse Coordinator, St. Francis
Hospital, Peoria, Illinois

ZEE ROBB, R.N., M.S.
Instructor, School of Nursing, University
of Texas at Arlington, Fort Worth, Texas

DEBORAH JANE SPEEGLE,
R.N., M.S.N.
Clinical Nurse Specialist, Division of
Pediatric Nephrology, University of Texas
Medical Branch, Galveston, Texas

BARBARA A. TEBBITT, R.N., M.S.
Coordinator, Nursing Resources,
Department of Nursing Service,
University of Minnesota Hospitals and
Clinics, Minneapolis, Minnesota

Lippincott's state board examination review for nurses

LuVerne Wolff Lewis, R.N., M.A.
Formerly Consultant, College of Nursing,
Arizona State University, Tempe, Arizona;
Research Associate, Institute of Research and
Service in Nursing Education, Teachers College
Columbia University, New York

J. B. LIPPINCOTT COMPANY
PHILADELPHIA
New York / San Jose / Toronto

Copyright © 1978 by J. B. Lippincott Company

This book is fully protected by copyright and,
with the exception of brief excerpts for review,
no part of it may be reproduced in any form by
print, photoprint, microfilm, or by any other
means without the written permission of the
publishers.

Distributed in Great Britain by
Blackwell Scientific Publications
London   Oxford   Edinburgh

ISBN 0-397-54214-3

Library of Congress Catalog Card Number 77-27368

Printed in the United States of America

2 4 6 8 9 7 5 3 1

Library of Congress Cataloging in Publication Data

Lewis, LuVerne Wolff.
Lippincott State board examination review for
nurses.

Bibliography: p. 738
1. Nursing—Examinations, questions, etc.
I. Title. II. Title: State board examination
review for nurses. [DNLM: 1. Nursing—Examination questions. WY18 L674L]
RT55.L48   610.73'076   77-27368
ISBN 0-397-54214-3

preface

Many persons recommend that the best way to prepare for an examination is to study regularly during the entire period when a particular course of study is offered. While this is good advice, it is the rare person who approaches an examination without feeling a need for a period of concentrated review. This appears to be especially true of those who are required to write a licensure examination before being able to practice in the profession of their choice.

This book was prepared primarily for review purposes for persons preparing to write the registered nurse licensure examinations. The examinations are presently used in the 50 states, Washington, D.C., the Virgin Islands, and Guam. Students graduated from baccalaureate, diploma, and associate degree programs in nursing, whether educated in the United States or elsewhere, are required to take the same examinations for licensure purposes.

Each State Board of Nursing is legally charged with the responsibility of determining an individual's competency to practice nursing. Representatives from the State Boards of Nursing make up the Council of State Boards of Nursing of the American Nurses' Association. The registered nurse licensure examinations, called the State Board Test Pool Examinations, are prepared under the guidance of this Council. The items are written by faculty members who teach in various types of educational programs for nursing. The Department of Evaluation Services of the National League for Nursing is authorized to act as the testing service.

A committee of the ANA Council of State Boards of Nursing prepares a blueprint consisting of agreed-upon abilities that are considered essential for nurses to have in giving safe and effective care. The committee also indicates the percentage of items to be used in the licensure examinations for testing each ability. The blueprint prepared by that committee was used to prepare the examinations presented in this book.

The items in this book were constructed so that they closely resemble the type used in the State Board Test Pool Examination. They are objective and, except in a few instances, offer four alternatives from which to select the best or correct answer. The items test not only specific facts but also the ability to apply knowledge in situations requiring judgment and decision-making when giving patient care.

Answer sheets similar to those used for the licensure examinations as well as for most other objective-type tests, are provided. Correct answers with their rationales are given at the end of each examination. References most commonly used for validating correct responses are given beginning on page 738.

Contributors and reviewers who assisted with the preparation of this book were selected for their expertise in the various clinical areas in nursing. An effort was made to select people with different educational and work experiences in order to help prevent, as much as possible, testing regional policies and practices.

The examinations presented here can be used effectively for purposes other than reviewing for the registered nurse licensure examinations. For example, the examinations offer a good review for various types of achievement examinations. They can also be used to prepare for challenge examinations that some schools now use to exempt certain students from selected areas of study. For the inactive nurse who wishes to return to practice and for the practicing nurse too, this book presents excellent material for review and for self-appraisal. Faculty members will find the tests useful for developing new insights and ideas for teaching purposes. Also, the examinations may serve as a guide for constructing tests for classroom purposes.

Certain policies are observed in this book for consistency and clarity:

• The word *patient* is used to refer to persons receiving services from health personnel.

• Feminine pronouns are used when referring to the nurse; male pronouns are used when referring to the physician. This has been done for convenience with no slight intended to the increasing ranks of male graduates in nursing and of female graduates in medicine.

• It is recognized that some nurses, especially those working in psychiatric nursing, prefer calling patients by their first names when the practice appears to strengthen a positive nurse/patient relationship. However, in this book, the title, Mr., is used when referring to men; the title, Ms., is used when referring to women. Given names are used for children and teenage patients.

• The word *sign* is used to describe observations made by health personnel; the word *symptom* is used to describe observations reported by patients.

• Generic names of drugs are used; common brand or trade names are given in parentheses following the generic names when they first appear in a situation.

The ultimate purpose of this book will have been well met when its use results in quality care for persons who require the services of a nurse.

contents

introduction 1

medical nursing 9

surgical nursing   163

obstetric nursing   341

nursing of children   470

psychiatric nursing 601

introduction

Evaluation techniques have been used since the beginning of time for everything from choosing a mate to determining the strength of an adversary. The art of measurement has become more sophisticated through the years as evaluation continues to play a major role in everyone's life.

This book, intended for review purposes, presents five examinations. They are similar to those used to evaluate nursing competency of candidates for registered nurse licensure. The names of the examinations and the number of test items are as follows:

Name of examination	Approximate number of items in licensure examination	Number of items in this book
Medical Nursing	120	609
Surgical Nursing	120	608
Obstetric Nursing	90	456
Nursing of Children	90	456
Psychiatric Nursing	90	439

No examination is capable of testing all knowledge related to a particular course of study. Therefore, every test samples material relevant to the objectives being measured. Although considerably longer than the State Board Test Pool Examination, the examinations in this book represent a sampling of knowledge considered important for competent nursing care.

use of patient situations

Most of the test items are presented in patient situations; that is, a patient is described and a group of items pertaining to that patient follows. Some items which appear last in the examinations are of a general nature. Both patient situations and some general items are used in the licensure examinations and also in many other types of tests.

While patient situations which nurses commonly encounter are presented, you may find some situations with which you have had little or no experience. This offers you an opportunity to apply facts and principles to new or unfamiliar situations. Also, unfamiliar situations will help call your attention to areas in which further study may be indicated.

Many patients have conditions that may not be directly related to their present reason for seeking health care. For example, a patient who requires the surgical removal of a diseased organ may also have diabetes mellitus. Or, a patient who hãs suffered a heart attack may have glaucoma. Nursing is based on the philosophy that patients—not diseases—require care. It is hoped that the manner in which situations are presented will help you focus on the patient and his needs rather than on specific disease entities.

The patient situations are not necessarily complete; that is, some situations consider only part of the patient's total needs for care. To have included all pertinent care for every patient would have resulted in extensive redundancy in many instances.

As is true in many other examinations, the tests here have integrated the basic natural and social sciences, nutrition and diet therapy, pharmacology and therapeutics, fundamentals of nursing, communicable diseases, legal and ethical considerations, and the like. As you study the examinations, you will find that each patient situation includes items that test your knowledge of these basic underlying sciences as applied to a particular patient.

Some people prefer reading an entire situation with its items very rapidly before studying each item more carefully. This is a matter of individual preference. However, if the test you are writing must be completed within a specific period, this practice may leave you with insufficient time to complete the entire examination. The licensure examinations are scheduled to be written within a specific time. The time is considered sufficient for completing entire examinations but does not allow for excessive reading and rereading.

the item: the stem and the options

Most objective-type items consist of two parts: the stem and the options. The stem presents the problem. It may be stated in the form of a question or as an incomplete sentence. The options present alternatives from which you are asked to select the correct answer.

All items in this book are objective. You are given four options, except in a few instances when there are three options. In every item, you are asked to select the *one best* or *correct answer*. Below are two examples of items. In the first, the stem is stated as a question; in the second, the stem is in the form of an incomplete sentence.

EXAMPLE 1.

Which chamber of the heart normally receives oxygenated blood
    from the pulmonary veins?
1. The left atrium.
2. The right atrium.
3. The left ventricle.
4. The right ventricle.

                                Option 1 is the correct answer.

EXAMPLE 2.

The name of the bone in the thigh is the
1. tibia.
2. femur.
3. fibula.
4. humerus.

                                Option 2 is the correct answer.

There may be times when you believe the options do not include what you think is the best possible response in a particular situation. Nevertheless, you are still asked to select one best answer. In such instances, it is helpful to remember that you should select the best answer from the presented options even though, in your opinion, the best possible choice may not have been stated.

Be sure to read the stem carefully! Watch for key words, such as best, least, usually, rarely, highest, lowest, primarily, contraindicated, and the like. When key words are overlooked, there is often no basis for selecting a correct response. Also, do not read anything into the stem. Use only the information you are given. It is suggested that you read the stem carefully, identify the specific problem it presents, try to state the correct answer in your mind, and proceed to read the options for a correct response.

In many instances, it may be relatively quick and easy to rule out one or two of the options as being incorrect. Then, concentrate on the remaining two or three options. Narrowing your choices by eliminating the obviously wrong options tends to sharpen your thinking by focusing attention on those options you have identified as being reasonably correct.

If you find a particular item difficult, make a note of it but continue with the examination. Once you have completed the entire test, go back and spend time studying difficult items more thoroughly.

scoring an examination by correcting for guessing

You may wonder if it is a good idea to make a guess when you are uncertain of the correct answer to an item. Many examinations, including the State Board Test Pool Examination, are corrected for guessing when they are scored. The most common formula used for correcting for guessing is as follows:

$$\text{Score} = R - \frac{W}{n-1}$$

when

R is the number of items answered correctly;
W is the number of items answered incorrectly; and
n is the number of options in the item.

Assume a test had 60 items and you answered all items. You had 48 correct responses. Each item had four options from which to choose a correct answer. Using the above formula, your final score would be determined as follows:

$$\text{Score} = 48 - \frac{12}{4-1} = 48 - \frac{12}{3} = 48 - 4 = 44$$

As you will note, you were penalized $\frac{1}{3}$ of a point for every incorrect response.

Now assume that of the 60 items in the examination, you were unsure of the correct response for 12. You took an "educated guess" on six items and answered three of them correctly and three incorrectly. You chose not to answer the remaining six items since you had no good basis for selecting a correct response. You selected the correct response for the 48 other items. Using the formula given above, your final score would be determined as follows:

$$\text{Score} = 51 - \frac{3}{4-1} = 51 - \frac{3}{3} = 51 - 1 = 50$$

As you see, you were still penalized ⅓ of a point for every incorrect response. However, when you did not answer an item, you neither received nor lost credit for it.

These examples illustrate that, when a test score is corrected for guessing, it is better to omit answering items when you are completely unfamiliar with knowledge they test rather than to take "wild guesses." On the other hand, it is helpful to use an "educated guess" when you select an option based on related knowledge you have.

preparing for and taking an examination

Be sure to follow instructions concerning examinations you are required to write for completing application forms, submitting fees, and the like. Allow sufficient time for such requirements.

Have sufficient rest and a good night's sleep before the examination. A tired person has more difficulty concentrating and tends to become more tense and confused than the rested person.

Plan some diversion in each day's activities before an examination. This is a healthful practice and helps relieve tensions and worries you may have.

Review for an examination as necessary in order to bring sound knowledge to the testing situation. It is probably of little help to "cram" the night before the examination. It may actually interfere. Since most examinations test integrated material presented over a period of time, it is possible that study the night before may result in remembering a few specific facts at the expense of remembering the total body of knowledge required to successfully complete the examination.

Eat a nourishing breakfast before the examination. Some exercise, such as a brisk walk, often helps one to relax before an examination.

Most examinations, including the licensure examinations, do not allow you to take books or notes to the test. Answer sheets are provided as well as pencils and scrap paper.

Carefully follow all instructions given to you at the time of the examination. This usually includes all identifying information requested concerning your name, address, and the like. Be aware of the amount of time you are given to complete the examination. Use the answer sheet exactly as you are instructed.

suggestions for using examinations in this book

The information and the suggestions just given concerning the preparation for taking of examinations apply when using this book for review purposes. Here are some additional suggestions:

• There are answer sheets provided for the examinations following each examination. Each sheet is marked so that it can be cut from the book when you write the examinations. Extra answer sheets are included, should you waste a sheet or wish to take the examination a second time. The answer sheets contain directions concerning their use.

• You will have defeated part of the reason for your review when you look at the answers prior to writing the examinations.

• Avoid searching for cues to correct answers among the items in this book. Concentrate on understanding the information being tested.

• Pace yourself occasionally when writing examinations in this book. For example, select 60 items and plan to answer them in about 90 minutes, using approximately 1½ minutes per item. If you are progressing well, slow your pace. But if you are falling behind, try to work faster. This type of practice helps prepare you for writing timed examinations.

• After you have completed an examination, refer to the section on Correct Answers and Rationales for that test. Make a check on your answer sheet next to items you failed to answer correctly. When you have completed checking your answer sheet, you can easily determine the number of items you answered incorrectly.

• Study the rationales given for each item. These rationales often contain information in addition to specific knowledge asked for in the item and, hence, will help you accomplish a more complete review. Use references given in this book, your own texts, and class notes for further review.

• For still additional reviewing, ask questions for all items, such as these:

Do you understand the knowledge upon which the item was based? Do you understand why each wrong option was incorrect?

Could you have answered the item correctly if the answer had been the stem and the stem had been stated as an option?

Is there additional information concerning the patient that was not sampled in these examinations but which is important, in your opinion, and may appear in the test for which you are reviewing?

● It is extremely unlikely that an item in this book will be identical to an item appearing in an examination you write, including the licensure examination. Therefore, place your emphasis on understanding the knowledge upon which items are based rather than trying to memorize correct answers.

preparing for examinations other than the licensure examinations

The suggestions just given apply when using this book to prepare for any test you may be required to write.

Assume you are preparing to write a medical nursing examination which, as the examination in this book does, has integrated the basic sciences. Reviewing only the medical nursing examination would be insufficient. The best policy would be to study the other four examinations also. Select those situations or items that test information that could logically appear in a medical nursing examination. For example, the Medical Nursing Examination in this book has one situation pertaining to a patient who has diabetes mellitus. However, there are also situations dealing with patients with diabetes mellitus in the Surgical Nursing, the Obstetric Nursing, and the Nursing of Children Examinations. Study all of these situations in order to complete a review of information concerning the care of a patient with diabetes mellitus.

As another example, items dealing with information that is usually considered to be gynecological nursing appear in the Medical Nursing, the Surgical Nursing, the Obstetric Nursing, and the Psychiatric Nursing Examinations. If you are preparing for an examination that includes gynecological nursing, be sure to review situations and items that are included in all four of these examinations.

The examinations in this book can be used for reviewing for achievement examinations in any of the basic social, physical, and biological sciences. Assume you are preparing to write an examination in anatomy and physiology. Use the five tests presented here but select those items in each patient situation that ask for knowledge related to anatomy and physiology for your review. The same procedure can be used if you are preparing for a test in one of the other sciences. The names of the examinations and a few items from each of them illustrate how anatomy and physiology can be reviewed:

Name of Examination	*Examples of Items Related to Knowledge of Anatomy and Physiology*
Medical Nursing	5, 6, 7, 34, 35, 36, 37, 38, and so on.
Surgical Nursing	4, 44, 55, 61, 69, 90, 91, 108, and so on.
Obstetric Nursing	1, 2, 3, 4, 5, 6, 7, 8, and so on.
Nursing of Children	38, 39, 46, 58, 91, 132, 150, 175, and so on.
Psychiatric Nursing	63, 107, 108, 215, 240, 298, 321, 373, and so on.

conclusion

A considerable body of knowledge pertaining to nursing has been sampled in the items presented in this book. When used in the manner just described, the book can be an invaluable tool to prepare for writing the registered nurse licensure examination as well as for other review purposes.

medical nursing

A nurse has been assigned to care for patients in a cardiac care unit. Items 1 through 40 pertain to knowledge that will help the nurse give her patients competent care.

Items 1 through 3 deal with the parts of a heartbeat that are illustrated in the figures below.

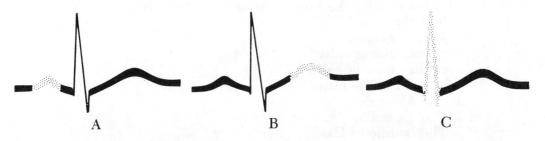

A   B   C

1. The dotted area of the electrocardiogram shown in Figure A is called the
   1. T wave.
   2. P wave.
   3. ST segment.
   4. QRS complex.
2. The dotted area of the electrocardiogram shown in Figure B is called the
   1. S wave.
   2. ST segment.
   3. PR interval.
   4. QRS interval.

3. The dotted area of the electrocardiogram shown in Figure C is called the
   1. Q wave.
   2. R wave.
   3. S wave.
   4. T wave.
4. What time interval is represented on each small square on the horizontal axis of electrocardiogram paper?
   1. 0.04 second.
   2. 0.2 second.
   3. 0.4 second.
   4. 0.5 second.
5. During normal heart activity, there is a slight delay of the electrical impulse at the atrioventricular node. This delay is important *primarily* in order that the
   1. sinoatrial node has sufficient time to recover.
   2. ventricles can be prepared to contract simultaneously.
   3. blood in the atria can be completely emptied into the ventricles.
   4. impulse to contract has time to travel throughout the Purkinje system.
6. The impulse for the heart to beat normally originates in the
   1. hypothalamus.
   2. jugular ganglia.
   3. preganglionic cells.
   4. cardiac muscle cells.
7. What area of the heart is called its pacemaker?
   1. The AV node.
   2. The SA node.
   3. The bundle of His.
   4. The Purkinje fibers.
8. The deflection on an electrocardiogram which is the result of an electrical impulse traveling through the atria is called the
   1. P wave.
   2. Q wave.
   3. S wave.
   4. T wave.
9. The deflection on an electrocardiogram that signifies recovery of electrical forces is called the
   1. T wave.
   2. ST segment.
   3. QRS complex.
   4. PR interval.

10. Which phenomenon is *not* ordinarily visible on an electrocar-
    diogram?
    1. Atrial depolarization.
    2. Atrial repolarization.
    3. Ventricular depolarization.
    4. Ventricular repolarization.

11. What is the approximate heart rate of the patient with the follow-
    ing electrocardiogram?

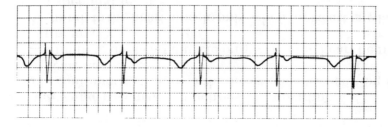

    1. 80 beats per minute.
    2. 90 beats per minute.
    3. 100 beats per minute.
    4. 110 beats per minute.

12. What rhythm abnormality is present in the following electrocar-
    diogram?

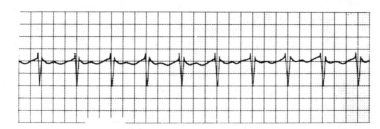

    1. Atrial flutter.
    2. Sinus arrhythmia.
    3. Sinus bradycardia.
    4. Ventricular tachycardia.

13. Which one of the following electrocardiogram findings would
    suggest that the patient *most likely* had a myocardial infarction
    some time ago?
    1. Prolonged P wave.
    2. Long, flat T wave.
    3. Elevated ST segment.
    4. Abnormally large Q wave.

14. Which one of the following electrocardiograms illustrates that the patient has a pacemaker?

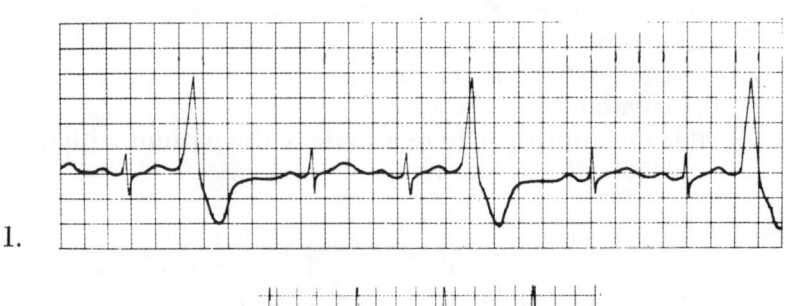

1.

2.

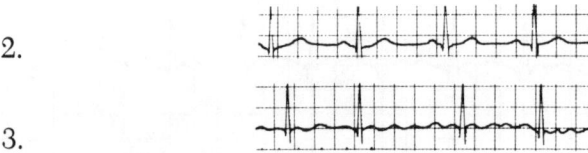

3.

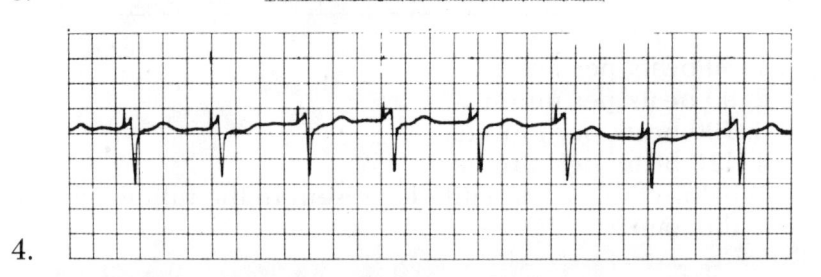

4.

15. A *demand* pacemaker functions by providing
    1. a continuous stimuli to the heart muscle resulting in a fixed heart rate.
    2. stimuli to the heart muscle only when the heart begins to beat irregularly.
    3. stimuli to the heart muscle only when the heart rate falls below a specified level.
    4. continuous stimuli to the heart muscle whenever ventricular fibrillation is present.
16. A hospitalized patient states he is afraid of his pacemaker. Which one of the following comments would be *most appropriate* for the nurse to make?
    1. "All patients have fears so you really need not worry."
    2. "Tell me more about what frightens you concerning your pacemaker."
    3. "There is no need to worry if you see your physician as regularly as he suggests."
    4. "Here is a manual you may read before I begin to teach you about your pacemaker."
17. A patient with a pacemaker has in his home the equipment listed

below. Many authorities teach that the item that is *most likely* to present a hazard to this patient, even when the pacemaker and the item are in good working order, is the
1. dehumidifier.
2. electric razor.
3. microwave range.
4. high fidelity record player.

18. The *characteristic* electrocardiogram finding of patients having premature atrial contractions (PAC) or paroxysmal atrial tachycardia (PAT) is that the
   1. P wave is deflected.
   2. T wave is premature.
   3. QRS complex is absent.
   4. ST interval is prolonged.

19. The impulse for the heartbeat of persons with PAC's or PAT's begins in the
   1. atria.
   2. ventricles.
   3. SA node.
   4. AV node.

20. When ventricular tachycardia is present, the atria and ventricles will characteristically beat
   1. simultaneously.
   2. very rapidly.
   3. independently of each other.
   4. at the same rate that the patient breathes.

21. When premature ventricular contractions (PVC's) are present, the stimulant for the heartbeat originates in the
   1. atria.
   2. SA node.
   3. AV node.
   4. ventricles.

22. Sinus tachycardia is considered to be present when the heart has reached the point of beating faster than
   1. 85 beats per minute.
   2. 90 beats per minute.
   3. 95 beats per minute.
   4. 100 beats per minute.

23. Cardioversion differs from electrical defibrillation in that cardioversion
   1. is always delivered on the P wave.
   2. is performed with one paddle only.
   3. has a synchronized electrical current.
   4. has a very high amount of watt-seconds.

24. To prevent the operator from receiving the shock instead of the

patient when electrical defibrillation is used, the operator
should
1. avoid touching the patient or his bed.
2. cover the paddles generously with electrode paste.
3. place the paddles so that the electrical wires are not crossed.
4. remove the paddles immediately after the shock has been
   administered.

25.   The figures below illustrate various placements of electrode
paddles on the patient's anterior chest wall.   Which one of the
figures depicts the *most common* placement of the paddles
when electrical defibrillation is used?

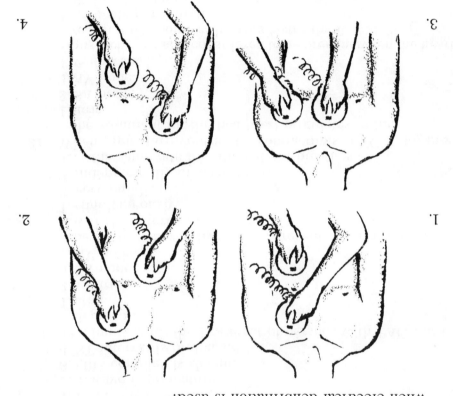

1.   2.

3.   4.

26.   A nurse caring for an alert, convalescing cardiac patient with a
pulse rate of approximately 72 per minute noted that the patient suddenly demonstrated the electrocardiogram shown on
page 15 on the monitor.
The *most likely* cause of the distortion is
1. the development of ventricular fibrillations.
2. a sudden increase in the patient's systolic blood pressure.

3. the patient's turning from side to side in bed while being made comfortable.
4. the patient's refusal to take a prescribed digitalis preparation 2 hours earlier.

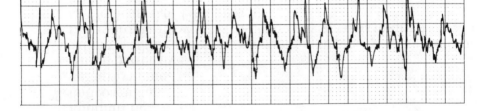

27. If it became apparent that there were U waves on one patient's electrocardiogram, the nurse should prepare to carry out orders that will help to correct the condition known as

1. hypercalcemia (calcium excess in the blood).
2. hyperkalemia (potassium excess in the blood).
3. hypocalcemia (calcium deficit in the blood).
4. hypokalemia (potassium deficit in the blood).

28. Which one of the following measures, all of which were prescribed for a patient with heart failure, is directed *primarily* toward decreasing the threat of emboli formation?

1. Giving digoxin (Lanoxin).
2. Restricting fluid intake.
3. Using elasticized stockings.
4. Allowing commode privileges.

29. Which one of the following drugs acts to slow conduction of impulses through the atrioventricular node?

1. Digitalis.
2. Nitroglycerin.
3. Quinidine hydrochloride.
4. Lidocaine hydrochloride.

30. Atropine sulfate affects the cardiovascular system by

1. blocking vagal responses.
2. stimulating cardioinhibitor cells in the medulla.
3. depressing synapse excitability in the hypothalamus.
4. diminishing sensitivity of chemoreceptors in the carotid bodies.

31. The drug metaraminol bitartrate (Aramine) is used *primarily* to increase a patient's

1. pulse rate.
2. clotting time.

32. The drug lidocaine hydrochloride (Xylocaine) is classified as a local anesthetic and as an
   1. antidiuretic.
   2. anticoagulant.
   3. antiarrhythmic.
   4. Antihypertensive.

33. A patient is taking a digitalis preparation regularly. The medication is ordinarily withheld and the physician is notified as soon as the heart rate falls below
   1. 80 beats per minute.
   2. 70 beats per minute.
   3. 60 beats per minute.
   4. 50 beats per minute.

34. Which one of the following electrolytes helps to release contrac- tile substances (actin and myosin) that are important for normal cardiac functioning?
   1. Sodium.
   2. Calcium.
   3. Chloride.
   4. Potassium.

35. When the body makes physiological demands on the heart, the message reaches the heart via the
   1. brain.
   2. craniospinal nerves.
   3. autonomic nervous system.
   4. chemoreceptors in the aortic arch.

36. What is the name of the tissue that forms the innermost wall of the heart?
   1. Epicardium.
   2. Myocardium.
   3. Pericardium.
   4. Endocardium.

37. The chamber of the heart that receives venous blood from body tissues is the
   1. left atrium.
   2. right atrium.
   3. left ventricle.
   4. right ventricle.

38. Which one of the following anatomical structures prevents blood from leaving the right ventricle and entering the right atrium?
   1. Bicuspid valve.
   2. Tricuspid valve.

3. Aortic semilunar valve.
4. Pulmonary semilunar valve.

39. A patient is being observed closely for cardiogenic shock. Which one of the following vital signs is most *characteristic* of cardiogenic shock?
1. Slow pulse rate.
2. Low blood pressure.
3. Subnormal temperature.
4. Slow respiratory rate.

40. It has been observed that, under the age of 50 years, approximately twice as many men as women suffer from atherosclerotic changes in coronary vessel walls. It is generally believed that this difference is due to women's having
1. higher blood levels of estrogen than men.
2. life styles with fewer stresses than men.
3. life styles with more activity and exercise than men.
4. diets that result in lower blood cholesterol levels than men.

Sixty-three-year-old Mr. Edward Brown was under the care of a physician who had prescribed digoxin (Lanoxin) 0.25 mg. daily for congestive heart failure. Mr. Brown stopped taking the digoxin when he began suffering from headaches, which he thought were being caused by the medication. Ten days later he was admitted to the hospital with a diagnosis of congestive heart failure with acute pulmonary edema. He was edematous, cyanotic, appeared distressed, and complained of feeling nauseated. His orders included oxygen therapy.

Items 41 through 67 pertain to this situation.

41. Statement A below is a correct statement. What is the relationship between statements A and B?
Statement A: Oxygen supports combustion.
Statement B: Humidity added to help Mr. Brown breathe while receiving oxygen therapy decreases the danger of fire.
1. Statement B is true; statement A explains or confirms statement B.
2. Statement B is true; statement A neither helps explain nor confirm statement B.
3. Statement B is false; statement A contradicts or indicates the falsity of statement B.
4. Statement B is false; statement A neither contradicts nor indicates the falsity of statement B.

42. Mr. Brown is ordered to have rotating tourniquets applied, the *primary* purpose being to help

43. When rotating tourniquets are used, each tourniquet is rotated so that the number of minutes the blood flow is decreased to any one extremity will be no longer than
    1. 15 minutes.
    2. 30 minutes.
    3. 45 minutes.
    4. 60 minutes.

44. During the procedure of rotating tourniquets, how many extremities should have compression applied at one time?
    1. One.
    2. Two.
    3. Three.
    4. Four.

45. Blood pressure cuffs are used as tourniquets for Mr. Brown. The *best* guide for determining the amount of inflation each cuff should have is that, in relation to the patient's blood pressure, inflation should be slightly
    1. above his systolic pressure.
    2. below his systolic pressure.
    3. below his diastolic pressure.
    4. above his diastolic pressure.

46. When the procedure of rotating tourniquets is completed for Mr. Brown, in which one of the following orders should the cuffs be removed?
    1. From the legs first, then the arms.
    2. From the arms first, then the legs.
    3. One at a time at 15-minute intervals.
    4. All at one time as quickly as possible.

47. In which one of the following positions in bed is Mr. Brown likely to be *most* comfortable?
    1. Semisitting (low Fowler's position).
    2. Lying on his right side (Sims's position).
    3. Sitting nearly upright (high Fowler's position).
    4. Lying on his back with his head somewhat lowered (Trendelenburg's position).

48. When using auscultation to listen to Mr. Brown's respirations, the nurse will *most likely* hear
    1. coarse rales.
    2. bubbling sounds.
    3. high-pitched wheezing tones.
    4. louder inspiratory sounds than expiratory sounds.

49. The physician orders Mr. Brown to have morphine sulfate sub-cutaneously shortly after admission. In this situation, the *most likely* reason for giving the medication is to reduce
    1. nausea.
    2. anxiety.
    3. blood pressure.
    4. bronchial secretions.

50. Mr. Brown is ordered to receive meralluride sodium (Mercuhy-drin), which is a mercurial diuretic. This type of diuretic is used *primarily* because it
    1. promotes the excretion of sodium.
    2. inhibits the production of aldosterone.
    3. increases the rate of glomerular filtration.
    4. inhibits the production of antidiuretic hormone (ADH).

51. Digoxin had been ordered for Mr. Brown because the drug helps to
    1. dilate coronary arteries.
    2. strengthen the heartbeat.
    3. decrease arrhythmias in the heart.
    4. decrease the electrical conductivity of the myocardium.

52. Which one of the following symptoms will Mr. Brown *most likely* notice when digitalis toxicity is occurring?
    1. Diarrhea.
    2. Loss of appetite.
    3. Skin rash.
    4. Light headedness.

53. Of the following signs, the one the nurse is *most likely* to notice first when Mr. Brown is developing digitalis toxicity is a
    1. heart murmur.
    2. slow pulse rate.
    3. slow respiratory rate.
    4. drop in blood pressure.

54. Which one of the following findings, if noted in Mr. Brown's blood examination, is *most likely* to increase his risk of devel-oping digitalis toxicity?
    1. Low sodium level.
    2. Low potassium level.
    3. High glucose level.
    4. High calcium level.

55. Mr. Brown is ordered to have chlorthalidone (Hygroton) after initial therapy with meralluride sodium was discontinued. A characteristic of chlorthalidone, in contrast to meralluride sodium, is that chlorthalidone
    1. can be taken by mouth.
    2. has long-lasting effects.

3. has few undesirable side effects.
4. rarely upsets electrolyte balance.

56. If the physician writes the following orders for Mr. Brown, which one is intended to help him evaluate the effectiveness of the diuretic therapy?
   1. Weigh the patient daily.
   2. Obtain blood pressure q.i.d.
   3. Determine arterial blood gases three times a week.
   4. Send urine specimen for routine analysis daily.

57. The *primary* reason for giving diuretics early in the day is to help
   1. decrease gastrointestinal irritation.
   2. retard the rapid absorption of the drug.
   3. excrete fluids accumulated during the night.
   4. prevent disturbances of rest during the night.

58. Mr. Brown will require careful skin care *primarily* because an edematous patient is prone to develop
   1. decubitus ulcers.
   2. itchy skin.
   3. electrolyte imbalance.
   4. distention of weakened veins.

59. Mr. Brown is ordered to have a diet with rigid sodium restriction. The daily *maximum* amount of sodium intake recommended by the American Heart Association is
   1. 0.5 Gm.
   2. 1.0 Gm.
   3. 2.0 Gm.
   4. 3.0 Gm.

60. Which one of the following foods is ordinarily allowed for a patient on a diet with rigid sodium restriction?
   1. Apples.
   2. Frozen peas.
   3. Hard cheeses.
   4. Luncheon meat.

61. Which one of the following foods is the *best* source of potassium?
   1. Tomatoes.
   2. Cheese.
   3. Bananas.
   4. Asparagus.

62. Which one of the following substances would be *contraindicated* for seasoning Mr. Brown's food?
   1. Wine.
   2. Herbs.
   3. Catsup.
   4. Lemon juice.

63. The symptom Mr. Brown *most likely* noticed when congestive
    heart failure began was
    1. loss of weight.
    2. slow heartbeat.
    3. nighttime voiding.
    4. shortness of breath.

64. Where does pathology *most often* begin when left-sided heart
    failure develops?
    1. The left atrium.
    2. The left ventricle.
    3. The pulmonary vein.
    4. The pulmonary artery.

65. Of the following signs, the one *most typical* of right-sided heart
    failure is an increase in
    1. urinary output.
    2. pulse pressure.
    3. valvular heart murmurs.
    4. central venous pressure.

66. The following diagnostic measures are often used to determine
    heart function.   Which one is noninvasive and, therefore, does
    not require the use of sterile technique?
    1. Echocardiography.
    2. Angiocardiography.
    3. Blood circulation time.
    4. Central venous pressure.

67. Investigations have shown that one very *common* reason pa-
    tients fail to take medications at home as directed is that they
    1. fear the dangers of overdosages.
    2. neglect to fill their prescriptions promptly.
    3. take the importance of accuracy lightly when taking medica-
       tions.
    4. fail to understand directions for taking their medications.

Sixty-year-old Ms. Myra Cone was admitted to the hospital with severe anterior chest pain that radiated to her shoulders
and arms.   Rales in both lower lobes of the lungs were noted.
The patient became very worried, frightened, and restless when
pain occurred.   Admission diagnosis was acute myocardial infarction.   The admission orders included the following:

Keep open IV with 5% dextrose in distilled water.
Cardiac diet.
Meperidine hydrochloride (Demerol) 100 mg. IM q 3 to 4 h. prn.

Furosemide (Lasix) 10 mg. PO stat.
Diazepam (Valium) 5 mg. PO as often as t.i.d., prn.

Items 68 through 101 relate to this situation.

68. The pain associated with Ms. Cone's illness is due to
1. overloaded ventricles.
2. impending circulatory collapse.
3. imbalances in extracellular electrolytes.
4. insufficient oxygen reaching heart muscle tissues.

69. During periods of pain, Ms. Cone's arterial blood pressure rises as high as 200 mm. Hg. Between attacks, it remains between 110 and 120 mm. Hg. It is *most likely* that the increase in arterial blood pressure during attacks of pain is due to
1. the patient's anxiety.
2. a poor oxygen supply to the heart.
3. excessive activity by the patient.
4. an accumulation of sodium ions in heart muscle tissues.

70. When Ms. Cone has an attack of pain, which one of the following actions should the nurse take *first*?
1. Give diazepam.
2. Give meperidine hydrochloride.
3. Increase the rate of administering intravenous fluids.
4. Order emergency laboratory work to determine level of oxygen tension (pO₂).

71. Keeping the intravenous open is ordered for Ms. Cone *primarily* in order to
1. help keep the patient well hydrated.
2. help keep the patient well nourished.
3. prevent the possibility of kidney failure.
4. be prepared to give intravenous drugs in an emergency.

72. A cardiac diet is characteristically low in
1. salt.
2. sugar.
3. potassium.
4. lactic acid.

73. Which one of the following signs/symptoms presented by Ms. Cone serves as the rationale for the physician's order for furosemide?
1. Pain.
2. Rales.
3. Anxiety.
4. Glycosuria.

74. Which two of the following laboratory findings are *most* characteristic of an acute myocardial infarction?

1. Blood pH level—7.38.
   Triglycerides—89 mg. per 100 ml.
2. Hemaglobin—14 Gm. per 100 ml.
   Sedimentation rate—15 mm. per 1 hr.
3. Blood cholesterol level—230 mg. per 100 ml.
   Arterial carbon dioxide tension (pCO_2)—40 mm. Hg.
4. Serum glutamic oxalacetic transaminase (SGOT)—225 units per ml.
   Serum creatine phosphokinase (CPK)—52 Sigma unit per ml.

75. Which one of the following drugs should the nurse have in readiness if Ms. Cone demonstrates signs of cardiogenic shock?
1. Morphine sulfate.
2. Calcium chloride.
3. Lidocaine hydrochloride.
4. Levarterenol bitartrate (Levophed).

76. If Ms. Cone develops a serious arrhythmia following the myocardial infarction, the arrhythmia is *most likely* to be
1. sinus tachycardia.
2. atrial fibrillation.
3. ventricular fibrillation.
4. paroxysmal atrial tachycardia (PAT).

77. If the nurse does not read the mercury at eye level when she takes Ms. Cone's blood pressure with a mercury manometer, there will be an error because of the phenomenon of
1. torque.
2. parallax.
3. ballistics.
4. depolarization.

78. The nurse notes that Ms. Cone's blood pressure had been recorded as 130/86/76 mm. Hg. What do the numbers 86 and 76 represent?
1. The numbers represent the points at which a muffled sound was heard on two consecutive readings.
2. The numbers represent the points at which the last distinct sound was heard on two consecutive readings.
3. The number 86 represents the point at which a muffled sound was first heard, and the number 76 represents the point at which the last distinct sound was heard.
4. The number 86 represents the point at which the last distinct sound was heard and the number 76 represents the point at which a muffled sound was heard.

79. Which one of the following statements *best* describes what diastolic blood pressure is?

1. It is the minimum pressure exerted on the walls of veins.
2. It is the minimum pressure exerted on the walls of the arteries.
3. It is the minimum pressure within the left ventricle.
4. It is the minimum pressure within the entire circulatory system.

80. The physician tells Ms. Cone to move her legs about freely and often while resting in bed. This type of exercise is recommended *primarily* in order to help
1. prepare the patient for ambulation.
2. prevent thrombophlebitis and blood clot formation.
3. stimulate the heart to beat with greater strength.
4. divert the patient's attention from her illness and anxiety.

81. After one attack of pain, the patient makes this comment to the nurse: "My husband died of a heart attack and I suppose I will too." Which one of the following questions would be the *most appropriate* response for the nurse to make?
1. "Are you thinking that you will not recover from this illness?"
2. "Would you like to tell me how you feel about what you just said?"
3. "Since you have a fine doctor, don't you think everything will be all right soon?"
4. "Would you agree with me that this would be a very unlikely and only a coincidental happening?"

82. Passive range-of-motion exercises are started for Ms. Cone. While the patient is lying on her back, the nurse straightens Ms. Cone's arm and then moves it upward so that it is resting alongside of her head. The shoulder motion accomplished by this maneuver is
1. pronation of the shoulder.
2. adduction of the shoulder.
3. extension of the shoulder.
4. abduction of the shoulder.

83. The nurse wishes to alternate placing Ms. Cone's forearm and hand in the supine and prone positions. Ms. Cone's hand will be pronated when it is held with the
1. palm facing upward.
2. palm facing downward.
3. hand closed into a fist.
4. hand in the hand-shaking position.

84. Which one of the following activities of daily living would be *contraindicated* for Ms. Cone?
1. Manicuring her fingernails.
2. Lying on her stomach for a back rub.
3. Using the commode for a bowel movement.

85. At midnight, the night nurse noted that Ms. Cone was sleeping; at 3 A.M., she is awake. She has not received a sedative which was prescribed on a prn basis nor is she accustomed to taking sedatives. Which one of the following nursing actions should receive the *lowest* priority in this situation?
    1. Administer the sedative.
    2. Give the patient a back rub.
    3. Offer the patient a bedpan.
    4. Change the patient's position in bed.

86. The nurse determines that Ms. Cone rarely sleeps more than 5 hours each night but takes a nap most mornings and afternoons. The nurse assesses Ms. Cone's sleeping habits as poor. Which one of the following statements *most accurately* describes the nurse's assessment?
    1. The assessment is incorrect; the total number of hours the patient sleeps in each 24-hour period is more important than when she sleeps.
    2. The assessment is incorrect; it has been found that sleeping for short periods usually is more healthful than sleeping for one long period in each 24-hour period.
    3. The assessment is correct; the total number of hours the patient is sleeping is insufficient for a person of her age.
    4. The assessment is correct; frequent short periods of sleeping interfere with the quality of sleep.

87. Which one of the following sensations normally reaches the *greatest depth* of unconsciousness during deep sleep?
    1. The sensation of pain.
    2. The sensation of touch.
    3. The sensation of hearing.
    4. The sensation of smelling.

88. Which one of the following statements *most accurately* describes the normal state of the body during the REM (rapid eye movement) stage of sleep?
    1. The person is in a stage of dreaming.
    2. The person is in a stage of deep sleep.
    3. The person's oxygen needs are at the lowest sleep-time average values.
    4. The person's blood pressure is at the lowest sleep-time average values.

89. Investigations have demonstrated that many drugs commonly used to produce sleep have the *disadvantage* of influencing normal sleep by
    1. stimulating the production of urine.

90. The night nurse caring for Ms. Cone is also responsible for three additional patients. Which one of the four patients is *most likely* to complain of nightmares?
1. Mr. Unger who has received chloral hydrate due to restlessness related to his alcoholism.
2. Ms. Cone who is not accustomed to taking hypnotics but took one as prescribed one evening shortly after admission.
3. Mr. Yeates who has been addicted to hypnotics for about a year but refused to take a hypnotic the evening he was admitted.
4. Ms. Long who has been taking hypnotics regularly for several months and continues to take them nightly during this period of hospitalization.

91. When persons are denied opportunities to dream while sleeping, they tend to develop signs of
1. anxiety
2. insomnia.
3. gastric hyperacidity.
4. involuntary muscular contractions.

92. Nursing care for Ms. Cone includes measures to prevent sensory deprivation while she is in the cardiac care unit. Which one of the following activities would be *least appropriate* for this patient?
1. Watching television.
2. Visiting with her daughter.
3. Reading her daily newspaper.
4. Moving to the adjoining patio in a wheelchair.

93. Of the following guides, the *best* one on which to base progression of activity for Ms. Cone is her
1. degree of edema.
2. degree of cyanosis.
3. amount of dyspnea.
4. amount of weight loss.

94. During the rehabilitation stage following her myocardial infarction, a reasonable schedule for returning to normal activity is prescribed for Ms. Cone *primarily* in order to allow the body sufficient time to
1. absorb the blood clot in the affected artery.
2. improve its resistance to endocardial diseases.
3. return to a state of normal electrolyte and fluid balance.
4. develop adequate collateral circulation to the affected heart muscle.

95. Ms. Cone indicated that she had smoked two packs of cigarettes

daily for about 30 years. Statement A below is a correct statement. What is the relationship between statements A and B?
Statement A: Any situation that repeatedly stimulates the secretion of epinephrine in the body tends to predispose the person to
atherosclerosis in the heart's blood vessels.
Statement B: It has been demonstrated that heavy cigarette
smokers tend to have more heart attacks than nonsmokers.
1. Statement B is true; statement A explains or confirms statement B.
2. Statement B is true; statement A neither helps to explain nor
   confirms statement B.
3. Statement B is false; statement A contradicts or indicates the
   falsity of statement B.
4. Statement B is false; statement A neither contradicts nor indicates the falsity of statement B.

96. If a patient displays behavior that is detrimental to his health,
    such as cigarette smoking, techniques of behavior modifica-
    tion may be used to help the patient change behavior. When
    new (adaptive) behavior replaces old (nonadaptive) behavior,
    the new behavior is *best* reinforced by
    1. explaining how the old behavior leads to ill health.
    2. withholding praise until the new behavior is well established.
    3. rewarding the patient whenever he performs acceptable be-
       havior.
    4. discussing the advantages for developing behavior that is
       healthful.

97. Ms. Cone's occlusion occurred in her left coronary artery. The
    anatomical structure from which this artery arises is
    1. the aorta.
    2. a pulmonary vein.
    3. the coronary sinus.
    4. the left ventricle.

98. Ms. Cone loses 3.2 kilograms of weight while hospitalized.
    How many pounds has she lost?
    1. Approximately 1½ pounds.
    2. Approximately 3 pounds.
    3. Approximately 5¼ pounds.
    4. Approximately 7 pounds.

99. Of the following factors related to daily living, the one which
    appears *most closely* linked to coronary artery disease is
    1. diet.
    2. climate.
    3. exercise.
    4. air pollution.

100. Which one of the following pathological changes occurs in the

walls of blood vessels when atherosclerosis is present?
1. Plaques on the tunica intima.
2. A thickening of the tunica externa.
3. Constriction of the vaso vasorum.
4. Calcium deposits on the tunica media.

101. Anxiety and stress related to daily living are often associated with coronary heart disease. However, certain amounts contribute to well-being *primarily* by helping to
1. prepare the body for restful sleep.
2. stimulate the body to develop adaptive behavior.
3. create a stimulus for normal brain cell activity.
4. produce stimuli for proper respiratory functioning.

While attending a church function, Mr. Ralph Bernard, a 67-year-old retired engineer, becomes dizzy and shortly thereafter loses consciousness, slumping to the ground. A nurse in the group comes forward to help him. The nurse notes that Mr. Bernard has a bounding, rapid pulse and labored respirations. She observes that his cheek puffs out on the right side of his face on expiration, and considers it likely that he has had a cerebrovascular accident (CVA).

Items 102 through 130 pertain to this situation.

102. Which one of the following measures should be included in the emergency care of an unconscious person who has had a possible CVA?
1. Turn the person on his weaker, affected side.
2. Move the person to a private, well-ventilated place.
3. Position the person on his stronger, unaffected side.
4. Keep the head of the person lower than the rest of his body.

103. Which one of the following symptoms is the *least typical* warning of an impending CVA?
1. Headache.
2. Drowsiness.
3. Incontinence.
4. Mental confusion.

104. Mr. Bernard is taken to the hospital by ambulance. A diagnosis of cerebrovascular accident and right hemiplegia is made and he is admitted for care. Hemiplegia is the paralysis of
1. one complete side of the body.
2. the part of the body below the neck.
3. the area of the body below the waist.
4. one side of the face and the opposite side of the body.

105. It is determined that Mr. Bernard has damage to the left side of

his brain. The damage makes understanding what others say difficult for the patient, although he is able to communicate through gestures. This type of aphasia is known as

1. global aphasia.
2. acoustic aphasia.
3. receptive aphasia.
4. expressive aphasia.

106. Which one of the following actions is *least helpful* when communicating with an aphasic patient?
1. Conversing in a slow manner.
2. Using gestures to accompany the spoken word.
3. Giving him directions on a one-at-a-time basis.
4. Speaking in a louder-than-normal tone of voice.

107. When Mr. Bernard's wife notes her husband's inability to respond verbally and his paralysis, she sobs and states in the patient's presence, "I shall probably have to send him to a nursing home if his condition is permanent." Which one of the following possible interventions by the nurse would demonstrate the *best* command of the situation?
1. Take Ms. Bernard to a private room to talk.
2. Offer Ms. Bernard a tissue and a cup of coffee.
3. Encourage Ms. Bernard to sit down in the room and talk more about her feelings.
4. Ask Ms. Bernard if she would like the nurse to call her physician for some sedation for her.

108. The nurse aligns Mr. Bernard's body properly, using a footboard, trochanter rolls, and pillows. One common orthopedic deformity patients with CVA tend to develop and which the nurse is trying to prevent by her actions is
1. plantar extension.
2. abduction of the arm.
3. external rotation of the hip.
4. internal rotation of the hip.

109. When helping Mr. Bernard with his pajama top, by which one of the following principles should the nurse be guided?
1. The affected arm is put into the sleeve first.
2. The unaffected arm is put into the sleeve first.
3. The sleeve is removed from the affected arm first.
4. The pajama top is slipped over the head first before removing the sleeve from either arm.

110. When a patient is immobilized, which one of the following areas of the body is *least likely* to develop pressure sores?
1. The occiput.
2. The scapulae.

111. The *earliest* sign of skin breakdown the nurse ordinarily observes is a skin area that is
1. dry.
2. cracking.
3. blanched.
4. reddened.

112. The nurse carries out range-of-joint-motion exercises on Mr.
Bernard during his bath. Which one of the following statements about range-of-motion exercises is *most accurate?*
1. They are best limited to one session daily.
2. They should be continued beyond the point of pain.
3. They may be performed by the nurse at her discretion.
4. They are easiest for the patient if done early in the day.

113. Mr. Bernard receives bishydroxycoumarin (Dicumarol) during
the acute stage of his illness. Which one of the following
conditions is a side effect of this drug that the nurse should
record and report?
1. Nausea.
2. Urticaria.
3. Epistaxis.
4. Diaphoresis.

114. For which one of the following reasons is the practice of taking
the temperature rectally sometimes *contraindicated* for patients who have had a CVA, especially after they have had a
cerebral hemorrhage?
1. It can induce convulsions.
2. It can injure the rectal mucosa.
3. It can raise the intracranial pressure.
4. It can cause peristaltic spasms of the lower colon.

115. Mr. Bernard demonstrates fear when he realizes how ill he is.
His fear will increase the work of the heart *primarily* by
stimulating the secretion of the hormone
1. insulin.
2. thyroxin.
3. epinephrine.
4. aldosterone.

116. Mr. Bernard is ordered to receive oxygen therapy. Which one of
the following measures should the nurse use before starting
the oxygen therapy?
1. Press on the patient's diaphragm to help him deep breathe.
2. Keep the patient's chin up and mouth cleared of secretions.

3. Position the patient comfortably and have him cough regularly.
4. Let the patient lie in a supine position with his arms and feet elevated.

117. Mr. Bernard has an irritated cornea for which he receives sterile eyedrops. To which one of the following causes is the patient's corneal irritation *most likely* due?
   1. The continuous glare of overhead lighting in his room.
   2. The careless shaking of linens near his face by the nurse.
   3. The trauma of the fall when he lost consciousness prior to hospitalization.
   4. The temporary loss of his blinking reflex in the eye of his affected side.

118. Mr. Bernard has difficulty swallowing food. Which one of the following approaches will the nurse find *most helpful* in aiding him to swallow?
   1. Stimulate his gag reflex.
   2. Place food on the back of his tongue.
   3. Have him practice blowing up balloons.
   4. Apply pressure to the affected side of his neck.

119. After several days of hospitalization, Mr. Bernard becomes aware of and discouraged by his physical handicaps. The nurse can *best* help him overcome a negative self-concept by showing an attitude of
   1. helpfulness with sympathy.
   2. concern with charitableness.
   3. direction while displaying firmness.
   4. encouragement while exhibiting patience.

120. When his condition becomes less critical, Mr. Bernard should be moved to a room that is
   1. near the nurses' station.
   2. equipped with all-electric beds.
   3. away from disturbing activities.
   4. occupied by more than one patient.

121. Mr. Bernard's family is concerned about his frequent "crying jags." If the nurse teaches family members to change the subject of conversation, or to snap their fingers at Mr. Bernard and say his name sharply when he cries, the *most likely* result would be that
   1. Mr. Bernard's feelings will be hurt.
   2. Mr. Bernard will become angry with his family.
   3. Mr. Bernard's crying behavior will be interrupted.
   4. Mr. Bernard will have fewer crying spells in the future.

122. As a result of his CVA, Mr. Bernard has blindness in half of his visual field. *Although* all of the following measures might be useful to reduce visual disability of the patient, which measure should be taught *primarily* as a *safety* precaution?
    1. Wear a patch over one of his eyes.
    2. Turn his head both left and right when ambulating.
    3. Lie in bed with his unaffected side toward the door.
    4. Place his personal articles on his side of awareness.

123. When walking in his room with assistance, the *least important* article Mr. Bernard should be advised to wear is
    1. an eye patch.
    2. a trouser belt.
    3. a sling on his affected arm.
    4. a pair of leather-soled shoes.

124. Mr. Bernard attends physical therapy daily. For which one of the following reasons should the patient with a CVA be provided with a practice setting in the rehabilitation unit that is similar to his home environment?
    1. His need to be catered to and pampered.
    2. His difficulty in generalizing the skills learned.
    3. His level of depression when he is assigned new tasks to do.
    4. His hostile reluctance to adapt himself to surroundings.

125. Which one of the following causes of a CVA *most often* results in hemiplegia?
    1. Cerebral embolism.
    2. Cerebral thrombosis.
    3. Cerebral hemorrhage.
    4. Cerebral arteriosclerosis.

126. In relation to prognosis, which one of the following vital sign patterns offers the *least* hope of recovery for a patient who has had a CVA?
    1. Low temperature, rapid pulse and respiratory rates.
    2. Elevated temperature, slow pulse and respiratory rates.
    3. Elevated temperature, rapid pulse and respiratory rates.
    4. Normal temperature, rapid pulse rate, slow respiratory rate.

127. Which one of the following disorders *best* identifies a pathological result that could develop if the nurse neglected oral hygiene for the unconscious patient?
    1. Chancres.
    2. Parotitis.
    3. Trench mouth.
    4. Aspiration pneumonia.

128. The recent stroke victim is often incontinent of urine. *All* of the following nursing measures are advisable to help overcome

incontinence *except*
1. restricting the patient's intake of fluids.
2. giving the bedpan to the patient after meals.
3. toileting the patient on a schedule of every 2 hours.
4. keeping the signal light accessible to the patient's unaffected hand.

129. Because of the likelihood of perceptual and visual defects, the food tray that will usually be the *most* appealing and conducive to frustration-free eating for the patient who has had a CVA is one set up with
1. a wide variety of foods to taste.
2. solid foods but no liquids to spill.
3. spoons but no knives or forks to handle.
4. a limited number of foods from which to choose.

130. Which one of the following types of cues is usually *most effective* in helping the patient with right-sided brain damage (left hemiplegia) and spatial-perceptual deficits to understand a message?
1. Pantomime.
2. Demonstration.
3. Verbal instruction.
4. Written corresponpondence.

A nurse was called to her neighbor's home when 61-year-old Mr. Carl Jones collapsed. The nurse's husband accompanied her. After a quick assessment of the patient, the nurse starts cardiopulmonary resuscitation with her husband as her assistant, while Mrs. Jones calls for an ambulance.
Items 131 through 146 relate to this situation.

131. Which one of the following statements describes an *error* in the procedure of cardiac compression?
1. The rescuer should be located at the victim's side.
2. The rescuer's shoulders should be directly above the victim's sternum.
3. The rescuer should use two hands when applying pressure on the victim's sternum.
4. The rescuer's elbow(s) should be slightly flexed when applying pressure on the victim's sternum.

132. The xiphoid process at the lower end of the sternum should *not* be deeply compressed when administering cardiopulmonary resuscitation because of the danger of lacerating the
1. lungs.
2. liver.

133. The nurse's husband administers artificial ventilation while the nurse administers cardiac compressions. When there are two rescuers, the recommended number of cardiac compressions per minute is
   1. 40.
   2. 50.
   3. 60.
   4. 70.

134. During mouth-to-mouth resuscitation of an adult, it is usually recommended that the number of complete respiratory cycles per minute should be
   1. 8.
   2. 12.
   3. 16.
   4. 20.

135. Approximately what percentage of oxygen will the patient receive when he is being resuscitated by mouth-to-mouth breathing?
   1. 11 percent.
   2. 16 percent.
   3. 21 percent.
   4. 26 percent.

136. Assuming all of the following arteries are accessible, the *most frequently* recommended site for obtaining the pulse rate in an adult while administering cardiopulmonary resuscitation is the
   1. radial artery.
   2. celiac artery.
   3. carotid artery.
   4. brachial artery.

137. The *most common* reason for the chest wall *not* rising during each inflation when giving cardiopulmonary resuscitation is that the
   1. airway is not clear.
   2. patient is beyond hope of resuscitating.
   3. inflations are being given at a too rapid rate.
   4. rescuer is using inadequate force to apply cardiac massage.

138. Mr. Jones, accompanied by his wife, is transported by ambulance to the hospital's emergency room where the admitting nurse quickly assesses the patient's condition. Of the following observations, the one *most often* recommended for determining the effectiveness of cardiopulmonary resuscitation is not-

ing whether or not the
1. pulse rate is normal.
2. mucous membranes are pink.
3. pupils are reacting to light.
4. systolic blood pressure is at least 80 mm. Hg.

139. When epinephrine (adrenalin) is given during cardiopulmonary resuscitation, it is administered *primarily* because of its ability to
1. dilate bronchioles.
2. constrict arterioles.
3. free glycogen from the liver.
4. enhance myocardial contractability.

140. By which route are drugs *most often* administered during cardiopulmonary resuscitation?
1. Intravenously.
2. Subcutaneously.
3. Instilled rectally.
4. Injected into heart muscle.

141. Of the following drugs, which one can the nurse anticipate will *very nearly always* be ordered for patients who require cardiopulmonary resuscitation?
1. Digitalis.
2. Atropine sulfate.
3. Sodium bicarbonate.
4. Lidocaine hydrochloride (Xylocaine).

142. When Mr. Jones regains consciousness, he asks the nurse if she thinks he will live. Which one of the following responses would be *best* for the nurse to make?
1. "Oh, yes. You have an excellent and very skilled doctor."
2. "We don't know yet but we certainly hope and pray you will live."
3. "You are very ill but we are here to help you in every way we can."
4. "You can help most if you try not to worry about whether you will live."

143. About 2 hours after Mr. Jones entered the emergency room, his blood pressure is 160/80 mm. Hg. The patient's pulse pressure is
1. ½.
2. 2.
3. 80.
4. 240.

144. Mr. Jones acts and appears very fearful as the various health personnel work about him. Which one of the following

courses of action is likely to give this patient the *most* support while life-saving measures are being carried out?

1. Occasionally hold his hand firmly.
2. Ask him if he knows why he is afraid.
3. Remind him that his wife is in the waiting room.
4. Tell him that he can help also by trying to relax.

145. For which one of the following patients is a precordial thump for cardiac arrest ordinarily *not* recommended?
1. A young child.
2. A patient with a pacemaker.
3. A patient over approximately 75 years of age.
4. A patient being monitored by an electrocardiograph.

146. If a nurse observes a hospitalized 63-year-old man having cardiac arrest, which one of the following actions should she take *first*?
1. Administer a precordial thump.
2. Sound the hospital's emergency call signal.
3. Attach electrocardiogram leads to the patient.
4. Assemble emergency equipment at the patient's bedside.

Ms. Maria Caselli, an alert 67 year old with diabetes mellitus, was discharged from the hospital one week ago. At that time a community health referral was made. The nurse was asked to reinforce the teaching that was done in the hospital. Ms. Caselli is taking phenformin (DBI) which is a biguanide. Items 147 through 174 pertain to this situation.

147. Phenformin lowers Ms. Caselli's level of blood glucose by
1. potentiating the action of insulin.
2. lowering the renal threshhold of glucose.
3. stimulating the pancreatic cells to release insulin.
4. chemically combining with glucose to render it inert.

148. Ms. Caselli complains to the nurse that her feet often feel cold. Which one of the following factors is *least likely* to be contributing to this sensation?
1. Wearing garters.
2. Smoking cigarettes.
3. Wearing low-heeled shoes.
4. Crossing legs when sitting.

149. In relation to the care of her feet, Ms. Caselli should be taught to avoid
1. going barefoot.
2. wearing hard-soled shoes.
3. applying polish to her toenails.
4. using bar detergent to wash her feet.

150. In relation to the care of her toenails, it is best for Ms. Caselli to avoid
   1. filing them with an emery board.
   2. cutting the corners of her nails.
   3. using a podiatrist to care for her nails.
   4. trimming them straight across the end of the nail.
151. After giving herself foot care, Ms. Caselli should be instructed to massage her feet gently with
   1. alcohol.
   2. cornstarch.
   3. bath powder.
   4. vegetable oil.
152. When Ms. Caselli asks the nurse to recommend something to remove corns from her toes, the nurse should advise her to
   1. apply a good corn plaster.
   2. consult her physician about removing corns.
   3. apply iodine to the corns before peeling them off.
   4. soak her feet in borax solution to peel off the corns.
153. To which one of the following diseases does Ms. Caselli's diabetes predispose her *most*?
   1. Arthritis.
   2. Osteoporosis.
   3. Otitis media.
   4. Atherosclerosis.
154. Ms. Caselli tells the nurse she cut her thumb while preparing a meal but, she says, "The cut isn't all that big." Which one of the following responses would be *most appropriate* for the nurse to make?
   1. "Let's call your doctor now."
   2. "For a diabetic, a cut is worthy of concern."
   3. "Don't worry about it. Just keep it clean and covered."
   4. "Nurses worry about things that don't bother other people."
155. Ms. Caselli was placed on a diet which permits her to have 190 Gm. of carbohydrate, 90 Gm. of fat, and 100 Gm. of protein. Approximately how many calories are contained in her diet?
   1. 1600 calories.
   2. 1800 calories.
   3. 2000 calories.
   4. 2200 calories.
156. Which one of the following foods would be an appropriate substitute in Ms. Caselli's diet for one small apple?
   1. One medium banana.
   2. One cup of pineapple.

3. One-half medium canteloupe.
4. One-half cup of orange juice.

157. Which one of the following foods would be considered an appropriate exchange for one slice of bread in Ms. Caselli's diet?
1. One-third cup of corn.
2. Eight saltine crackers.
3. One cup of cooked cereal.
4. One-fourth cup of ice cream.

158. Which one of the following foods is considered equivalent to one fat exchange?
1. One-half of a ripe avocado.
2. One tablespoon of mayonnaise.
3. One tablespoon of sour cream.
4. One slice of crisply dried bacon.

159. Which one of the following foods is equivalent to 1 ounce of lean meat?
1. One egg.
2. Two ounces of cheddar cheese.
3. One-half cup of cottage cheese.
4. One tablespoon of peanut butter.

160. All of the following foods are included in Ms. Caselli's diet. Which are especially rich in vitamin A content?
1. Cereals and breads.
2. Lean cuts of beef and veal.
3. Green and yellow vegetables.
4. Citrus fruits and tuberous vegetables.

161. Ms. Caselli says that, because of her Italian background, pasta products (spaghetti, macaroni, etc.) have been an important part of her diet.   Statement A below is a correct statement. What is the relationship between statements A and B?
Statement A: Body cells require adequate amounts of essential nutrients in order to function properly.
Statement B: Ms. Caselli should be taught how to use pasta products in her diet.
1. Statement B is true; statement A explains or confirms statement B.
2. Statement B is true; statement A neither helps explain nor confirm statement B.
3. Statement B is false; statement A contradicts or indicates the falsity of statement B.
4. Statement B is false; statement A neither contradicts nor indicates the falsity of statement B.

162. The nurse recommends moderate daily exercise for Ms. Caselli. In which one of the following ways does exercise affect the

physiological functioning of the body?

1. It helps to avoid hypoglycemia.
2. It stimulates an overproduction of insulin.
3. It decreases the renal threshhold for glucose.
4. It increases the utilization of carbohydrates.

163. For which one of the following patients, all of whom have diabetes mellitus, can the nurse anticipate that the physician is *most likely* to prescribe an oral hypoglycemic, such as the one prescribed for Ms. Caselli?

1. Mary, who is 10 years old and has had diabetes for 3 years.
2. Joe, who is 21 years old and a golf professional.
3. Mr. Hines, who is 32 years old and has had problems regulating his dosages of regular insulin.
4. Ms. Zedak, who is 67 years old and has just learned that she has diabetes.

164. Vascular changes that occur in the diabetic affect all organs of the body but have their most serious effects, in terms of danger to life, when they become prevalent in the

1. lungs.
2. liver.
3. kidneys.
4. pancreas.

165. Which one of the following eye problems is *least likely* to be related to a person's having diabetes mellitus?

1. Blindness.
2. Cataracts.
3. Astigmatism.
4. Blurred vision.

166. The retina of the eye is affected by vascular degeneration of the blood vessels more quickly than other body tissues because the retina has the

1. smallest arterioles.
2. thinnest cellular layer.
3. fewest number of blood vessels.
4. highest rate of oxygen consumption.

167. Carbohydrates are stored in the body in the form of

1. glucose.
2. lactose.
3. dextrose.
4. glycogen.

168. Ketone bodies in the bloodstream are the result of the incomplete oxidation of

1. fats.
2. minerals.

3. proteins.
4. carbohydrates.
169. Which one of the following ethnic groups tends to have the *lowest* incidence of diabetes mellitus?
   1. Jews.
   2. Blacks.
   3. Eskimos.
   4. Orientals.
170. Where in the kidney is glucose reabsorbed?
   1. Tubules.
   2. Glomeruli.
   3. Renal pelvis.
   4. Renal arterioles.
171. One of the functions of insulin is to
   1. decrease formation of glycogen.
   2. prevent excess fat storage in the liver.
   3. stimulate the kidneys to reabsorb glucose.
   4. stimulate the metabolism of carbohydrates.
172. Another patient with diabetes mellitus the community health nurse is caring for uses chlorpropamide (Diabinese) which is a sulfonylurea compound. The nurse should caution the patient against taking large amounts of aspirin because aspirin tends to
   1. depress the appetite.
   2. increase bleeding time.
   3. increase the hypoglycemic effects of a sulfonylurea compound.
   4. interfere with the hypoglycemic effects of a sulfonylurea compound.
173. In the patient with diabetes insipidus there is a faulty functioning of the
   1. thyroid gland.
   2. adrenal glands.
   3. pituitary gland.
   4. parathyroid glands.
174. The patient with diabetes insipidus characteristically complains of extreme
   1. hunger.
   2. thirst.
   3. fatigue.
   4. weight loss.

A nurse works for a group of urologists. Items 175

through 207 relate to knowledge that will help the nurse give urologic patients competent care.

175. Ms. Wolker is to have a cystoscopy. Which one of the following measures will add *most* to her comfort when the nurse positions her for cystoscopy?
1. Place the patient's arms on a pillow above her head.
2. Place padding on the stirrups under the patient's knees.
3. Place trochanter rolls along the sides of the patient's hips.
4. Place the patient's feet so that they are at right angles to her lower legs.

176. Which one of the following types of anesthesia should the nurse anticipate that the physician will *most likely* use when performing the cystoscopy?
1. Field block.
2. Local infiltration.
3. Surface anesthesia.
4. Central nerve block.

177. The physician ordered that Ms. Howe be catheterized for a urine specimen for culturing. The *most frequently* recommended method for sterilizing catheterization equipment is the use of
1. dry heat.
2. boiling water.
3. free-flowing steam.
4. steam under pressure.

178. The figures below and on page 42 relate to preparing for catheterization. Which one illustrates *poor* aseptic technique?

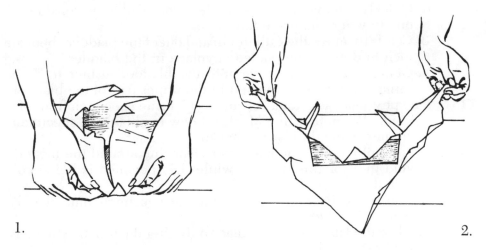

1.   2.

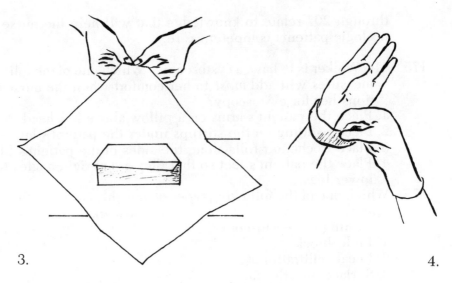

3.　　　　　　　　　　　　　　　　　　　4.

179. When lubricating the catheter before inserting it, the nurse should take precautions to *avoid*
1. lubricating more than the tip of the catheter.
2. contaminating her gloved hand with the lubricant.
3. plugging the eye of the catheter with the lubricant.
4. using so much lubricant that some may enter the bladder with the catheter.

180. If the urine stops flowing while Ms. Howe is being catheterized, which one of the following actions should the nurse take?
1. Slowly remove the catheter to drain urine that may be near the exit of the bladder.
2. Quickly remove the catheter since the bladder is considered empty when the urine flow stops.
3. Carefully move the catheter in and out of the bladder about an inch to drain urine pooled anyplace in the bladder.
4. Gently push the catheter into the bladder further to drain urine that may have pooled in the upper part of the bladder.

181. The physician asks for a "clean catch" urine specimen from Ms. Lind. When teaching Ms. Lind how to obtain the specimen, the nurse should instruct her to
1. void into a clean bedpan after cleansing around the meatus.
2. void in a forcible manner while the specimen is being collected.
3. stop the collection of urine for the specimen immediately before the bladder feels empty.
4. allow the labia to fall into place only after the urinary stream is well established.

182. Mr. Jones is to collect a "midstream" urine specimen. *All* of the following instructions apply when teaching Mr. Jones how to obtain the specimen *except*
   1. voiding directly into the sterile specimen container.
   2. discarding the first approximately 30 ml. of urine that is voided.
   3. stopping the collection of urine well before the bladder is empty.
   4. cleansing the urethral meatus directly after the specimen has been obtained.

183. After examining Mr. Jones's specimen, the laboratory reported the findings listed below. When assessing these findings, which one should the nurse consider to be the *least* significant?
   1. pH—5.9.
   2. Albumin—2+.
   3. Colony count—150,000 per ml.
   4. Sodium concentration—60 mEq. per L.

184. The physician orders that Ms. Kayer is to collect a 24-hour urine specimen: 10 A. M. Wednesday—10 A. M. Thursday. In relation to collecting specimens, the nurse should teach Ms. Kayer to
   1. discard urine voided at 10. A. M. on Wednesday and begin the specimen collection after that.
   2. begin the collection with urine voided at 10 A. M. on Wednesday.
   3. discard urine voided at 10 A. M. on Thursday and consider the specimen completed.
   4. discard only the urine voided upon arising Thursday morning during the 24-hour period.

185. Ms. Polter occasionally experiences poor bladder control. Which one of the following exercises is *most often* recommended to improve bladder control?
   1. Swimming at least once a day.
   2. Taking several short walks each day.
   3. Alternately contracting and relaxing the perineal muscles.
   4. Alternately contracting and relaxing the lower abdominal muscles.

186. Mr. Wyeth comes to the office to have his retention catheter changed. He complains of pain while the nurse is inflating the balloon after she has the new catheter in place. The *most likely* cause of the discomfort is that the balloon is
   1. in the urethra.
   2. near a ureteral orifice.

3. located too low inside the bladder.

4. overdistended within the bladder.

187. Which one of the following measures should the nurse teach Mr. Boeter who is suspected of having renal calculi?

1. Have him strain his urine.

2. Have him stay on bed rest for several days.

3. Have him limit his fluid intake for the next 48 hours.

4. Have him obtain urine specimens every 2 hours for the next 24-hour period.

188. The physician plans to do a phenolsulfonphthalein (PSP) test on Mr. Quiller who is 55 years old. The *primary* purpose of the test is to determine the amount of damage to the kidneys'

1. tubules.

2. calyces.

3. pelves.

4. glomeruli.

189. The *most frequently* used route for administering dye used in the PSP test is the

1. oral route.

2. intravenous route.

3. subcutaneous route.

4. intramuscular route.

190. Mr. Quiller is also to have an intravenous pyelogram (IVP) examination. The preparation for this examination ordinarily includes restricting the patient's

1. salt intake.

2. fluid intake.

3. use of tobacco.

4. physical activities.

191. Ms. Baxter is diagnosed as having cystitis. It is generally believed that most cases of cystitis are the result of

1. an infection elsewhere in the body.

2. congenital strictures in the urethra.

3. an ascending infection from the urethra.

4. a stasis of urine in the urinary bladder.

192. The nurse notes albumin in Ms. McCord's urine specimen. Ms. McCord, a department store sales person, collected the specimen at the end of her working day. Which one of the following procedures should the nurse observe when she checks another specimen for accuracy?

1. Catheterize the patient for a specimen immediately.

2. Have the patient obtain a "clean catch" specimen immediately.

3. Have the patient bring another specimen of urine collected at

the same time the next day.

4. Have the patient bring a specimen of urine which she voids immediately upon arising in the morning.

193. Mr. Avero, who stops at his physician's office before having his periodic hemodialysis treatment, expresses depression when he cries and shouts at the nurse, "I am no use to anyone. Why can't I just die and have it over with once and for all?" Which one of the following statements offers the nurse the *best* guide to understanding Mr. Avero's comment?

1. The patient's feelings are temporary and can be expected to subside as soon as accumulated wastes have been removed from his circulatory system.

2. The patient's feelings of depression most likely reflect a home situation in which family members are not offering sufficient emotional support.

3. The patient's feelings are an uncommon reaction to hemodialysis, and he is possibly suffering from a mental disturbance as well as his kidney disease.

4. The patient's feelings of depression are quite typical of someone suffering from tensions associated with long-term, expensive therapy for an incurable disease.

194. The *most commonly* used method for determining how much fluid the patient loses during hemodialysis is to compare findings, taken before and after the treatment, of the patient's

1. weight.
2. blood pressure.
3. ankle and waist measurements.
4. blood hematocrit and clotting time.

195. The medication of choice to counteract the effects of heparin administered to a patient having hemodialysis is

1. vitamin K.
2. quinidine sulfate.
3. protamine sulfate.
4. sodium bicarbonate.

196. Patients requiring hemodialysis became eligible for financial assistance when an amendment was added to a law that is commonly called the

1. Bolton Act.
2. Social Security Act.
3. Health Amendments Act.
4. Workmen's Compensation Act.

197. *All* of the following beverages contain a substance (other than water) that acts as a diuretic *except*

1. tea.

2. cocoa.
3. coffee.
4. root beer.
198. The urge to void is aroused when distention stimulates stretch
receptors in the
1. urethral orifices.
2. ureteral sphincter.
3. lower abdominal wall.
4. urinary bladder wall.
199. Urine is moved along the ureters by
1. cilia.
2. gravity.
3. peristaltic waves.
4. pressure differentials.
200. Reabsorption of substances needed by the body occurs in anatomical structure(s) in the kidneys called the
1. glomeruli.
2. capsule of Bowman.
3. convoluted tubules.
4. peritubular capillaries.
201. The reabsorption of water into the bloodstream from the kidneys
occurs by the process of
1. osmosis.
2. diffusion.
3. filtration.
4. active transport.
202. From which anatomical structure(s) in the body is the antidiuretic hormone (ADH) released?
1. Hypothalamus.
2. Pituitary gland.
3. Medulla oblongata.
4. Parathyroid glands.
203. When a patient becomes emotionally upset, which one of the
following substances can be expected to appear in the urine?
1. Serum.
2. Glucose.
3. Ketone bodies.
4. Microscopic casts.
204. Which one of the following substances is *not* normally found in
voided urine?
1. Ammonia.
2. Albumin.
3. Potassium.
4. Sodium chloride.

205. The organism *most often* responsible for urinary tract infection is the
    1. *Escherichia coli.*
    2. *Candida albicans.*
    3. *Staphylococcus aureus.*
    4. *Enterobacter aerogenes.*
206. Investigations have shown that the *most common* predisposing factor for chronic kidney diseases is a
    1. respiratory infection.
    2. hematological disorder.
    3. congenital malformation.
    4. circulatory disturbance.
207. Which one of the following methods is the *safest* one for destroying spores believed to be present on surgical instruments?
    1. Soaking them in formaldehyde.
    2. Placing them in boiling water.
    3. Exposing them to free-flowing steam.
    4. Placing them in steam under pressure.

Acutely ill Steve Olden, a 17-year-old high school basketball player, was admitted to the hospital with a diagnosis of acute glomerulonephritis.
Items 208 through 218 pertain to this situation.

208. While the nurse is obtaining Steve's history, Steve says he has voided "very little" during the previous 24 hours. The production of scanty amounts of urine is called
    1. anuria.
    2. dysuria.
    3. oliguria.
    4. enuresis.
209. Acute glomerulonephritis *most often* develops as a complication of an infection caused by the microorganism
    1. *Streptococcus aureus.*
    2. *Neisseria meningitidis.*
    3. *Haemophilus influenzae.*
    4. *Diplococcus pneumoniae.*
210. Steve's mouth is dry and his lips are crusted with mucus. Which one of the following preparations is *best* initially for cleansing his mouth?
    1. A jelly-type toothpaste.
    2. A mild white vinegar solution.
    3. Undiluted antiseptic mouthwash.
    4. Half-strength hydrogen peroxide.

211. The physician orders that Steve's fluid intake be restricted to 1000 ml. in each 24-hour period. Which one of the following fluids will help *most* to prevent excessive thirst?
1. Tap water.
2. Ice chips.
3. Hot bouillon or tea.
4. Lemonade or orangeade.

212. During the conference when Steve's history was obtained, Steve indicated that he had had "wet dreams" several times during the previous couple of weeks. This phenomenon is *most often* considered to be
1. a symptom of a sexual disorder.
2. a normal occurrence at the patient's age.
3. an early symptom of acute glomerulonephritis.
4. a positive sign that the patient is producing live sperm.

213. Steve's teacher tells the nurse, "I never worry about Steve. He always lands on his feet." This description of Steve's personality is characteristic of a person who
1. is of superior intelligence.
2. has an attitude of self-confidence.
3. has a poor relationship with his parents.
4. is from a family in the upper socioeconomic class.

214. Steve complains about the food served him in the hospital. He indicates he would like any of the four foods listed below. Which one would be *contraindicated* for him?
1. An ice cream sundae.
2. A piece of apple pie.
3. A serving of barbequed ribs.
4. A waffle with butter and maple syrup.

215. If all of the following diversional activities are available and not contraindicated for Steve, which one is he *most likely* to enjoy during his convalescence?
1. Playing chess with his father.
2. Watching television with a classmate.
3. Explaining the rules of basketball to a 10-year-old patient.
4. Having his mother share reading a mystery novel out loud with him.

216. *All* of the following developmental characteristics are commonly observed among persons of Steve's age *except*
1. moodiness.
2. submissiveness.
3. concern with personal appearance.
4. interest in members of the opposite sex.

217. Which one of the following statements *most accurately* describes normal human growth?
    1. The rate of growth varies among individuals.
    2. Growth does not normally follow a continuous pattern.
    3. Various parts of the body grow at about the same rate.
    4. There is no particular order in which normal growth occurs.
218. Which one of the following factors is the *most controversial* in relation to influences that affect one's personality?
    1. Heredity.
    2. Early habit training.
    3. Relationships with parents.
    4. Experiences during infancy.

Ms. Lois Janter was flown from a rural area to a metropolitan hospital. She was admitted with a diagnosis of acute renal failure. She hemorrhaged shortly after arrival 3 days ago.
Items 219 through 235 relate to this situation.

219. Ms. Janter was found to have an elevated blood urea nitrogen (BUN) level upon admission. Her BUN was elevated because of
    1. wasting of kidney cells.
    2. decreased metabolic rate.
    3. hemolysis of red blood cells.
    4. increased protein catabolism.
220. Laboratory findings indicate that Ms. Janter's potassium blood level is elevated. Her physician orders that she be given sodium polystyrene sulfonate (Kayexalate) in a retention enema. Ms. Janter is given the drug because of its ability to
    1. remove protein wastes of metabolism.
    2. release hydrogen ions for sodium ions.
    3. increase calcium absorption in the colon.
    4. exchange sodium for potassium ions in the colon.
221. When potassium intoxification is threatening, for which one of the following emergency situations should the nurse be prepared?
    1. Cardiac arrest.
    2. Pulmonary edema.
    3. Circulatory collapse.
    4. Recurring hemorrhaging.
222. High carbohydrate feedings are prescribed for Ms. Janter, the rationale being that they will
    1. act as a diuretic.

2. reduce demands on the liver.

3. help to maintain urine acidity.

4. offer a good source of calories.

223. A low protein diet is ordered for Ms. Janter. What is the rationale for giving her this type of diet?

1. Low protein intake minimizes protein breakdown.

2. Low protein intake helps reduce the metabolic rate.

3. Low protein intake minimizes sodium intoxification.

4. Low protein intake minimizes chances of developing pulmonary edema.

224. If the patient likes all of the following fruits, which one should be *avoided* in her diet?

1. Pears.

2. Apples.

3. Peaches.

4. Bananas.

225. A nursing assistant helps the nurse with Ms. Janter's care. If the nursing assistant is assigned to carry out all of the following procedures, which one should the nurse check with *special* care?

1. Obtaining the patient's temperature.

2. Recording the patient's intake and output.

3. Noting the amount of food the patient has eaten.

4. Cleansing the patient's skin and mucous membranes.

226. Peritoneal dialysis is ordered for Ms. Janter. Which one of the following procedures *must* be done before peritoneal dialysis is started?

1. Have x-ray examinations of the patient's abdomen.

2. Have the patient sign a permit for the procedure.

3. Notify the blood bank technician to have blood ready for transfusing.

4. Notify the patient's husband of the time when the procedure will be done.

227. One purpose for having Ms. Janter dialyzed is to remove excess extracellular fluid. To reach this goal, in relation to its concentration, the dialyzing solution for Ms. Janter should be

1. isotonic.

2. hypotonic.

3. hypertonic.

228. Which one of the following nursing measures will help *most* to promote drainage of the dialyzing solution?

1. Keep the patient flat in bed.

2. Turn the patient from side to side.

3. Elevate the height of the dialysate bottle.

4. Apply external pressure on the patient's lower abdomen.
229. The *best* rationale for using a warm dialyzing solution is that it helps to
    1. promote relaxation of abdominal muscles.
    2. decrease the risk of peritoneal infection.
    3. dilate the blood vessels in the peritoneum.
    4. prevent the body temperature from falling precipitously.
230. The morning after peritoneal dialysis is started, the night nurse reports on Ms. Janter's condition. Which one of the following descriptions would be *least helpful* in assisting the day nurse plan the patient's care?
    1. "The patient's fluid intake during the last 24-hour period was 600 ml.; her urinary output was 560 ml."
    2. "Yesterday morning at 6 A. M., the patient weighed 56.3 kg. (124.3 pounds); this morning she weighed 55.9 kg. (123.4 pounds)."
    3. "The patient was more lethargic tonight than last night. When awake, she responded slowly and seemed poorly oriented. The night before she was well oriented and responded to her name."
    4. "I gave the patient her prn medication for pain when she was awake during the night. She was complaining of a headache and said the medication relieved the headache for about an hour."
231. If Mr. Janter expresses anxiety concerning his wife's recovery, the nurse should explain that her prognosis is
    1. poor; it is the rare patient who survives a kidney ailment as serious as acute failure.
    2. fair; it is most likely that considerable permanent damage has occurred to the patient's kidneys.
    3. good in terms of living but poor in terms of the patient's illness recurring.
    4. very good; the kidneys have great ability to survive serious illness.
232. During her hospitalization, Ms. Janter, who is 24 years old, tries hard to do whatever is asked of her, and she shows obvious pleasure when the nurses praise her efforts. Which one of the following statements *best* describes Ms. Janter's behavior?
    1. The behavior is abnormal for a woman of her age.
    2. The behavior is much more typical of men than of women.
    3. The behavior is common for persons who wish to gain control of situations in which they feel helpless.
    4. The behavior can usually be expected when persons are attempting to meet their needs for self-esteem.

233. Ms. Janter's psychological need for feeling included in personal relationships while hospitalized is *most likely* to be met when the nurse takes actions to
1. relate to the patient in a way that shows her the nurse is interested in her.
2. encourage visitors to the greatest extent that hospital policy and the patient's condition allow.
3. assure the patient that the nurse has respect for and confidence in the patient's choice of physician.
4. be certain that the patient understands that the nurse will make decisions for her in relation to her nursing care.

234. While caring for Ms. Janter, techniques of medical asepsis are carefully observed. It is generally believed that *most* organisms are spread in health agencies by
1. patients admitted with unsuspected infections.
2. health practitioners whose hands are not clean.
3. dressings, cotton balls, and body discharges that are improperly discarded.
4. pillows, mattresses, and blankets that are improperly cleaned between patient uses.

235. Acute renal failure is due to
1. sclerosis of renal arteries.
2. bleeding into renal tissues.
3. inadequate renal circulation.
4. blood clots in the loops of Henle.

A nurse has been assigned to care for a group of patients receiving therapy to prevent or treat fluid and electrolyte imbalances.

Items 236 through 275 relate to knowledge that will help the nurse give her patients competent care.

Items 236 through 242 contain paired phrases marked A and B. Indicate as the correct answer the number

1 if A is normally larger than B.
2 if A is normally smaller than B.
3 if A and B are normally equal or very nearly equal.

236. A. HCO_3 in venous blood.
    B. HCO_3 in arterial blood.
237. A. pO_2 in venous blood.
    B. pO_2 in arterial blood.
238. A. pCO_2 in venous blood.
    B. pCO_2 in arterial blood.

239. A. Sodium cations in extracellular fluid.
     B. Sodium cations in intracellular fluid.
240. A. Total number of cations in extracellular fluid.
     B. Total number of anions in extracellular fluid.
241. A. Total number of cations in intracellular fluid.
     B. Total number of anions in intracellular fluid.
242. A. Potassium cations in extracellular fluid.
     B. Potassium cations in intracellular fluid.
243. Electrolytes move from cytoplasm through cell membranes by the process of
     1. osmosis.
     2. diffusion.
     3. filtration.
     4. active transport.
244. In addition to water taken into the body by fluids and food, the body receives water from
     1. humidity in inhaled air.
     2. metabolism of organic foodstuffs.
     3. moisture absorbed through skin pores.
     4. electrolytic activity of inorganic salts.
245. By which one of the following routes is the largest amount of water lost from the body?
     1. Skin.
     2. Lungs.
     3. Gastrointestinal tract.
246. Potassium excess or depletion in the body will produce signs that relate to potassium's effect on
     1. protein synthesis.
     2. cell membrane permeability.
     3. cartilage and bone tissues.
     4. cardiac and skeletal muscles.
247. The *most common* symptom of excessive sodium in the body is
     1. edema.
     2. thirst.
     3. tremors.
     4. diarrhea.
248. Which one of the following signs is *most typical* of a marked reduction in the plasma concentration of calcium?
     1. Anuria.
     2. Tetany.
     3. Absence of deep reflexes.
     4. Paralysis of skeletal muscles.
249. Which one of the following vitamins plays the most important role in calcium absorption in the body?

1. Vitamin A.
2. Vitamin B.
3. Vitamin C.
4. Vitamin D.

250. The electrolyte *most responsible* for the amount of aldosterone the body secretes is
   1. sodium.
   2. calcium.
   3. chloride.
   4. magnesium.

251. Which one of the following organs assumes the *greatest responsibility* for the body's potassium balance?
   1. Skin.
   2. Lungs.
   3. Kidneys.
   4. Gastrointestinal tract.

252. Of the following disorders, the one *most often* seen with careless or indiscriminate use of diuretics is
   1. nephrosis.
   2. hypokalemia.
   3. tubular necrosis.
   4. metabolic acidosis.

253. When respiratory acidosis is present, the body is trying to compensate when the kidneys excrete less than normal amounts of
   1. water.
   2. sodium.
   3. proteinates.
   4. bicarbonate.

254. Which one of the statements below describes the following equation most accurately?

$$CO_2 + H_2O \rightleftarrows H_2CO_3 \rightleftarrows H + HCO_3$$

   1. The carbon dioxide ion is a cation.
   2. Reactions in the equation are reversible.
   3. The equation illustrates impending alkalosis.
   4. The equation illustrates an acid-base imbalance.

255. Which one of the following blood examinations is generally considered *best* for judging whether pulmonary ventilation is within normal range?
   1. Determination of acidity/alkalinity(pH).
   2. Determination of the bicarbonate values (CHO_3).
   3. Determination of the partial pressure of oxygen (pO_2).

4. Determination of the partial pressure of carbon dioxide (pCO_2).

256. The pH of the blood is within normal range when the ratio of HCO_3 to CO_2 is approximately
   1. 1 to 1.
   2. 5 to 1.
   3. 10 to 1.
   4. 20 to 1.

257. Which one of the following blood findings is characteristic of metabolic acidosis?
   1. Increased bicarbonate content.
   2. Decreased bicarbonate content.
   3. Increased carbon dioxide content.
   4. Decreased carbon dioxide content.

258. A diabetic patient whose body is excreting large amounts of urine in order to rid itself of excess glucose is likely to develop an electrolyte imbalance as a result of a
   1. calcium excess.
   2. sodium deficit.
   3. protein deficit.
   4. carbonate excess.

Items 259 through 263 relate to a patient's arterial blood findings which are as follows:

pH—7.20.
pCO_2—40 mm. Hg.
HCO_3—13.5 mEq. per L.
B.E.——11.

Indicate as the correct answer the number

1 if the statement is supported by laboratory findings.
2 if the statement is not supported by laboratory findings.
3 if the statement is neither supported nor contradicted by laboratory findings.

259. The pCO_2 is lower than normal.
260. HCO_3 and B.E. are lower than normal.
261. The patient is in great need of oxygen.
262. Compensation for acidemia has just begun.
263. The patient is in a state of metabolic acidosis.

Items 264 through 267 pertain to a patient's laboratory findings and gas diffusion, as illustrated in the following diagram:

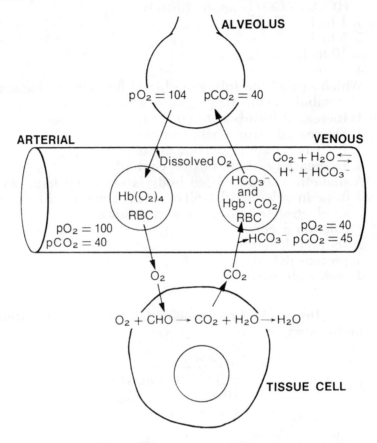

Indicate as the correct answer the number

1 if the statement is supported by the diagram.
2 if the statement is not supported by the diagram.
3 if the statement is neither supported nor contradicted by the diagram.

264. The patient's arterial, venous, and alveolar gas findings are essentially normal.
265. Carbon dioxide is incapable of combining with hemoglobin.
266. Carbonic acid dissociates into hydrogen and bicarbonate ions.
267. This patient is receiving oxygen therapy.
268. The nurse prepares to start intravenous therapy on one patient and notes that the patient has veins suitable for entry low on

his arm as well as in his anticubital area. Which one of the following statements offers the *best* reason for the nurse's choosing to enter a vein low on the patient's arm?

1. Damage to a vein high on the arm limits subsequent use of veins low on the arm.
2. Veins high on the arm tend to break and scar more easily than veins low on the arm.
3. It takes more pressure to introduce solution into veins high on the arm than into veins low on the arm.
4. The anticubital area should be reserved for emergencies and for use by laboratory technicians to obtain arterial blood samples.

269. Which one of the following measurements describes the gauge of a needle used for injection purposes?

1. The length of the bevel.
2. The length of the needle.
3. The diameter of the lumen.
4. The circumference of the hub.

270. In which area should the nurse start cleansing the skin over the vein into which she will inject an intravenous needle?

1. At the site of injection.
2. About an inch above the site of injection.
3. About an inch below the site of injection.
4. About an inch on either side of the site of injection.

271. It is generally recommended that the nurse hold her thumb on the patient's vein a short distance below the intended site of entry because her thumb will help to

1. keep the patient's vein well engorged with blood.
2. prevent the patient's vein from moving under the skin.
3. reduce the patient's sense of discomfort when the needle enters the skin.
4. steady the nurse's hand as she inserts the needle into the patient's vein.

272. Solutions normally enter a vein in the arm during intravenous therapy because the

1. force of gravity carries fluid into the vein.
2. fluid in the solution bottle is under positive pressure.
3. pressure within the vein is less than atmospheric pressure.
4. pressure within the solution bottle is less than atmospheric pressure.

273. *All* of the following factors can influence the rate of an intravenous flow *except* the

1. patient's blood type.
2. viscosity of the solution.

3. patient's position in bed.

4. height of solution bottle on the standard.

274. The nurse notes that the skin near the needle of a patient receiving intravenous therapy is whitish in color and the patient states he has pain in the area. The nurse should examine the patient further for additional evidence of

1. phlebitis.

2. infiltration.

3. air embolism.

4. allergic reaction.

275. The physician orders that a patient receive 3000 ml. of solution in each 24-hour period intravenously. If there is a drop factor of 15 drops per ml., at approximately how many drops per minute should the patient receive the solution?

1. 22 drops.

2. 32 drops.

3. 42 drops.

4. 52 drops.

Mr. Anthony Dorn, a 65-year-old rancher, was admitted to the hospital with a diagnosis of chronic obstructive pulmonary disease (COPD). The patient complained of shortness of breath, lack of appetite, and feeling very discouraged about his condition. His ankles were edematous. His wife stated that he had been unusually irritable. Approximately 10 years ago, the patient was diagnosed as having emphysema. He has been living in a warm climate and taking continuous oxygen therapy for about 5 years. His orders include the following:

Oxygen therapy with nasal prongs at 1½ liters per minute.
Keep IV open with 5% dextrose in distilled water.
Theophylline ethylenediamine (aminophylline) — 250 mg. IV q 6 h.
Amitriptyline hydrochloride (Elavil)—25 mg. PO. h.s.
IPPB (intermittent positive pressure breathing) with ½ cc. isoetharine hydrochloride (Bronkosol) q.i.d.
Blood pH and arterial blood gas analysis qd X 3.

Items 276 through 305 relate to this situation.

276. Mr. Dorn was admitted to a room numbered 13. He states that he does not want to remain in the room because the number would bring him bad luck. Personnel in the admitting office say a change could be made if the nurse feels it wise to do so. Which one of the following statements offers the *best* guide for

the nurse in this situation?

1. Move the patient; fears the patient has, even when unfounded, can impede recovery.
2. Move the patient; superstitions have a good chance of coming true for those who believe in them.
3. Do not move the patient; having the patient use the room will help him overcome an unwarranted fear.
4. Do not move the patient; the patient may become unmanageable and demanding when he knows he can have his own way.

277. Which one of the following statements *best* describes why Mr. Dorn's oxygen therapy is maintained at a relatively low level?

1. When oxygen is administered by nasal prongs, the oxygen will be lost at the nostrils when given at a higher level.
2. The patient's long history of respiratory problems indicates that he would be unable to absorb oxygen given at a higher level.
3. The cells in the aveoli are so damaged by a long history of a respiratory problem that higher levels of oxygen and reduced levels of carbon dioxide are likely to cause the cells to burst.
4. The patient's respiratory center is so accustomed to high carbon dioxide and low oxygen blood concentrations that changing these concentrations with oxygen therapy may eliminate the patient's stimulant for breathing.

278. Which one of the following substances is likely to ignite spontaneously when it comes in contact with oxygen under pressure?

1. Oil.
2. Alcohol.
3. Talcum powder.
4. Sodium bicarbonate.

279. The *primary* reason for keeping an intravenous open for Mr. Dorn is to

1. keep the patient well hydrated.
2. administer intravenous drugs as indicated.
3. help make up for nourishment the patient is not taking because of his poor appetite.
4. stimulate the kidneys to rid the body of wastes which cannot be excreted via the patient's respiratory system.

280. Theophylline ethylenediamine was prescribed for Mr. Dorn because the drug acts as a

1. diuretic.
2. bronchodilator.
3. vasoconstrictor.
4. respiratory stimulant.

281. The reason amitriptyline hydrochloride was prescribed for Mr.
     Dorn is that the drug acts as an
     1. antibiotic.
     2. expectorant.
     3. antidepressant.
     4. appetite stimulant.
282. Of the following positions, which one is preferred for Mr. Dorn
     during IPPB therapy?
     1. Trendelenburg's position.
     2. Semi-Fowler's position.
     3. Flat in bed and lying on his back.
     4. Flat in bed and lying on either side.
283. By which route will the isoetharine hydrochloride be given?
     1. By inhalation.
     2. By oral administration.
     3. By intravenous injection.
     4. By intramuscular administration.
284. The positive pressure phase of an IPPB machine is activated
     when the patient
     1. makes an expiratory effort.
     2. makes an inspiratory effort.
     3. applies pressure around the mouthpiece by pursing his lips.
     4. holds his breath longer than 3 to 5 seconds after an expiration.

     Items 285 through 289 pertain to Mr. Dorn's blood gas and
pH levels, which were as follows:

	1st day	2nd day	3rd day
pH	7.35	7.34	7.29
Arterial oxygen tension (pO_2)	44	39	30
Arterial carbon dioxide tension (pCO_2)	83	76	89

Indicate as the correct answer the number

1 if the statement is supported by the laboratory findings.
2 if the statement is not supported by the laboratory findings.
3 if the statement is neither supported nor contradicted by the
laboratory findings.

285. The base excess has increased.
286. The patient appears to be slipping toward a state of acidemia.
287. The arterial carbon dioxide tension suggests alveolar hypoventi-
     lation.
288. Cardiac output is adequate to maintain proper oxygen levels in
     body tissues.

289. It appears as though oxygen therapy is helping to maintain an arterial oxygen tension within normal range.
290. Which one of the following nursing measures will be helpful in reducing Mr. Dorn's sticky bronchial secretions?
    1. Maintain an adequate fluid intake.
    2. See that his diet is low in salt.
    3. Be sure that his oxygen therapy is continuous.
    4. Keep the patient in a semisitting position as much as possible.
291. The physician interprets Mr. Dorn's ankle edema as a sign of possible heart involvement. Which chamber of Mr. Dorn's heart is *most likely* to hypertrophy in order to carry a larger-than-normal workload?
    1. The left atrium.
    2. The right atrium.
    3. The left ventricle.
    4. The right ventricle.
292. When prognosis and further care are being considered, nursing care of Mr. Dorn will be guided by understanding that he is likely to
    1. develop infections easily.
    2. require less oxygen as he becomes more sedentary.
    3. show permanent improvement following a course of IPPB therapy.
    4. show permanent improvement as long as his fluid and diet intake are well maintained.
293. The patient's wife, who cares for Mr. Dorn between hospitalizations, asks the nurse about her husband's feelings of depression, his irritability, and his poor appetite. The nurse illustrates understanding of the patient's behavior when she explains to the wife that his behavior is *most likely* the result of
    1. his illness.
    2. mental confusion.
    3. feelings of resentment for health personnel.
    4. premonitions that death is near at hand.
294. Mr. Dorn becomes angry one day when his dinner is delayed. Which one of the following courses of action would be *most appropriate* for the nurse to take *first* when Mr. Dorn becomes angry?
    1. Listen quietly to the patient as he expresses his anger.
    2. Overlook the patient's behavior until his anger subsides.
    3. Explain to the patient that his anger is interfering with his recovery.
    4. Tell the patient that the dietitian is available to discuss his problems with him.

295. Mr. Dorn had been taught early in the course of his disease to purse his lips while breathing. The primary purpose of pursed lip breathing is to help
1. promote oxygen intake.
2. strengthen the diaphragm.
3. strengthen intercostal musculature.
4. promote carbon dioxide elimination.
296. As an energy conservation measure, during which phase in his respiratory cycle should Mr. Dorn be taught to carry out as many activities of daily living as possible?
1. While inhaling.
2. While exhaling.
3. After exhaling but before the next inhalation.
4. After inhaling but before the next exhalation.
297. Percussion of his chest wall is prescribed for Mr. Dorn. The *primary* purpose of percussion is to help
1. stimulate deeper inhalations.
2. improve ciliary action in the bronchioles.
3. propel secretions along the respiratory tract.
4. loosen secretions in congested areas of the lungs.
298. The patient's wife says that Mr. Dorn often used postural drainage at home. What causes the greatest amount of movement of debris from the lower to the upper respiratory tract when the patient is using postural drainage?
1. Friction.
2. Force of gravity.
3. Sweeping motion of cilia.
4. Involuntary muscular contractions.
299. Mr. Dorn has been bedridden often and has had little exercise. The body normally reacts physiologically to prolonged periods of bed rest and inactivity by increasing the
1. retention of sodium.
2. excretion of calcium.
3. utilization of insulin.
4. production of red blood cells.
300. If these findings appear in Mr. Dorn's history, *all* may very well have played an important role in his having COPD *except*
1. having a mother who had asthma.
2. having often had bronchial infections.
3. having smoked approximately one pack of cigarettes a day for 24 years.
4. having 2 to 3 ounces of liquor almost daily for most of his adult life.

301. Neurons in the respiratory center receive their stimuli from ions of
    1. oxygen.
    2. hydrogen.
    3. potassium.
    4. bicarbonate.
302. The respiratory center is located in the
    1. cerebellum.
    2. hypothalamus.
    3. medulla oblongata.
    4. cerebral cortex.
303. The term *eupnea* means respirations that are characterized by a
    1. normal exchange of air.
    2. temporary cessation of breathing.
    3. change in the usual respiratory rhythm.
    4. marked increase in the depth of respirations.
304. Air that can be forcibly exhaled after an average normal expiration is called
    1. tidal air.
    2. reserve air.
    3. residual air.
    4. complemental air.
305. During respirations, the exchange of oxygen and carbon dioxide in the alveoli occurs by the process of
    1. osmosis.
    2. dialysis.
    3. diffusion.
    4. filtration.

      A community health nurse is caring for several patients with pulmonary tuberculosis.
      Items 306 through 317 relate to knowledge that will help the nurse give her patients competent care.

306. A positive Mantoux skin test indicates that the individual has
    1. developed clinical tuberculosis.
    2. developed a resistance to tubercle bacilli.
    3. had contact with tubercle bacilli.
    4. developed a passive immunity to tuberculosis.
307. Of the following treatment measures, which one has the *highest* priority for patients with tuberculosis?
    1. Having sufficient rest.
    2. Eating a nourishing diet.

3. Living where there is clean fresh air.

4. Taking medications as prescribed.

308. Which one of the following laboratory techniques is used *most widely* to identify tubercle bacilli in sputum?

1. Acid-fast staining.

2. Sensitivity testing.

3. Agglutination testing.

4. Darkfield illumination.

309. Most authorities believe that the single *most effective* way to decrease the spread of microorganisms is by

1. washing the hands frequently.

2. having separate personal care items for each person.

3. using disposable equipment to the greatest extent possible.

4. isolating persons known to be harboring disease-causing organisms.

310. Which one of the following forms of tuberculosis carries the *highest* death rate?

1. Miliary tuberculosis.

2. Pulmonary tuberculosis.

3. Intestinal tuberculosis.

4. Urogenital tuberculosis.

311. The *most common* means of transmitting the tubercle bacillus from person to person is by contaminated

1. dust particles.

2. food and water.

3. droplet nuclei.

4. linens and eating utensils.

312. The nurse should observe for symptoms of damage to the eighth cranial nerve when administering the tuberculostatic drug

1. streptomycin.

2. isoniazid (INH).

3. aminosalicylic acid (PAS).

4. ethambutol hydrochloride (Myambutol).

313. Which one of the following symptoms is associated with eighth cranial nerve damage?

1. Hearing loss.

2. Impaired vision.

3. Facial paralysis.

4. Difficulty in swallowing.

314. What is the *primary* reason for administering two or more tuberculostatic drugs at one time?

1. To potentiate the actions of the drugs.

2. To reduce undesirable side effects of the drugs.

3. To provide for administering lower dosages of the drugs.

4. To delay resistance of the causative organisms to the drugs.

315. *All* of the following nursing measures are important when a nurse cares for tuberculosis patients in their homes. Which one should have the *highest priority?*
   1. Offer patients emotional support.
   2. Teach patients about their disease.
   3. Meet needs of patients for various health services.
   4. Assess the environment for standards of sanitation.

316. When mortality and incidence rates of tuberculosis are examined, it has been found that the etiological factor which influences these rates *least* is one's
   1. age.
   2. sex.
   3. race.
   4. occupation.

317. In which one of the following geographic areas should the community health nurse expect to find the *largest* number of patients with tuberculosis?
   1. In rural dairy farming areas.
   2. In inner core residential areas of large cities.
   3. In areas where clean water standards are low.
   4. In suburban areas where air pollution from industrial centers is high.

Ms. Bessie Petri was admitted to the hospital with a diagnosis of bacterial pneumonia. She has a cough and an elevated temperature. She is experiencing chest pains and is having difficulty breathing.
Items 318 through 340 relate to this situation.

318. Ms. Petri is 79 years old. When the nurse obtained her admission history, she learned that the patient has arthritis and "moves about slowly." Ms. Petri said she is a vegetarian. She indicated that she "feels dirty when I can't take a bath every day, even in winter." Which one of the following findings adds *most* to the danger of her illness?
   1. Her age.
   2. Her arthritis.
   3. Being a vegetarian.
   4. Taking frequent baths year-round.

319. Ms. Petri's chest pain, which is more severe on inspiration, is *most probably* due to
   1. retained respiratory tract secretions.
   2. accumulated fluid in the alveolar sacs.

3. inadequate oxygenation of lung tissues.
4. friction rub between the pleural layers.

320. Ms. Petri appeared cyanotic upon admission, *most probably* because of
    1. cardiac involvement.
    2. malnutritional anemia.
    3. inadequate circulation.
    4. poor oxygenation of blood.

321. The physician orders aspirin for Ms. Petri. In addition to its being an antipyretic, aspirin is also classified as
    1. an analgesic agent.
    2. an adrenergic agent.
    3. a cholinergic agent.
    4. an antihistamine agent.

322. Which one of the following physiological processes is altered *most* when Ms. Petri develops abdominal distention from swallowing air during periods of dyspnea?
    1. Digestion.
    2. Circulation.
    3. Elimination.
    4. Respiration.

323. Which one of the following measures is *most likely* to be ordered for Ms. Petri to help liquify her respiratory secretions?
    1. Having her use postural drainage.
    2. Having her breathe humidified air.
    3. Using clapping and percussion on her chest wall.
    4. Having her use coughing and deep-breathing exercises.

324. The preferred site for obtaining Ms. Petri's temperature is the
    1. oral site.
    2. groin site.
    3. rectal site.
    4. axillary site.

325. The physician orders a medication to help relieve broncho-spasms which Ms. Petri is experiencing. Which one of the following drugs acts to accomplish that goal?
    1. Tyloxapol (Alevaire).
    2. Acetylcysteine (Mucomyst).
    3. Deoxyribonuclease (Dornavac).
    4. Isoproterenol hydrochloride (Isuprel).

326. Before ordering specific antibiotic therapy for Ms. Petri, the nurse should anticipate that the physician will evaluate the report of the patient's
    1. chest x-ray examinations.
    2. blood cultures.

3. throat cultures.

4. white blood count.

327. It is found that Ms. Petri has pneumococcal pneumonia. Which one of the following statements *best* describes the characteristic appearance of the causative organisms when viewed under a microscope?

1. They are arranged in pairs.

2. They are arranged in long chains.

3. They are arranged in grapelike clusters.

4. They are arranged in isolated singleness.

328. Which one of the following drugs is the physician *most likely* to order when it is learned that Ms. Petri is hypersensitive to penicillin?

1. Erythromycin (Erythrocin).

2. Amphotericin B (Fungizone).

3. Kanamycin sulfate (Kantrex).

4. Gentamycin sulfate (Garamycin).

329. The organism causing Ms. Petri's pneumonia is *most frequently* transmitted by airborne droplets. The organism is also commonly spread by contaminated

1. bed linens.

2. eating utensils.

3. hands of health personnel.

4. equipment used to obtain vital signs.

330. Which one of the following behaviors, if observed in Ms. Petri during the acute phase of her pneumonia, should be assessed by the nurse as a very possible sign of hypoxia?

1. Anger.

2. Apathy.

3. Anxiety.

4. Aggression.

331. Ms. Petri experiences diaphoresis while acutely ill. Which one of the following electrolytes is she *most likely* to lose in clinically significant amounts when she perspires profusely?

1. Sodium.

2. Potassium.

3. Phosphorus.

4. Bicarbonate.

332. A laboratory report indicates that Ms. Petri has a total white blood count of 8000 per cu. mm. on her third day of hospitalization. Which one of the following actions should the nurse take when she assesses this report?

1. Notify the physician promptly.

2. Omit the next dose of antibiotic.

3. Initiate reverse isolation techniques.

4. Continue with the current therapeutic regimen.

333. Which one of the following complications of pneumonia can *best* be prevented by giving Ms. Petri frequent oral hygiene?

1. Pleurisy.

2. Septicemia.

3. Atelectasis.

4. Otitis media.

334. The nurse cleans Ms. Petri's eyeglasses, the lenses of which are made of plastic. One disadvantage of plastic lenses is that, if they are not handled carefully, they are easily

1. warped.

2. chipped.

3. shattered.

4. scratched.

335. Ms. Petri's expectorations contain blood. The term used to describe blood-tinged sputum is

1. hemoptysis.

2. hematolysis.

3. hematemesis.

4. hemophthisis.

336. Ms. Petri complains of being constipated. Her physician prescribes dioctyl sodium sulfosuccinate (Colace) prn. This drug helps to overcome constipation by

1. softening the stool.

2. lubricating the stool.

3. increasing stool bulk.

4. stimulating peristalsis.

337. Because of Ms. Petri's constipation problem, the nurse observes her for fecal impaction. Which one of the following signs is the patient *most likely* to present if a fecal impaction develops?

1. Frequent small hard stools.

2. Frequent small liquid stools.

3. Inability to pass flatus or fecal matter.

4. Frequent passage of flatus without a bowel movement.

338. When a fecal impaction is present, the nurse should *first* prepare to give the patient a

1. glycerin suppository.

2. retention enema with oil.

3. cleansing enema with a soapsuds solution.

4. cleansing enema with a hypertonic solution.

339. The *most important* and *practical* way to help prevent the spread of the pneumonias in the general population is to have people

1. avoid large gatherings.
2. keep immunizations current.
3. observe habits of good health.
4. receive antibiotics for virus infections.

340. Which one of the following factors has contributed *most* to the reduction in pneumonia morbidity and mortality rates?
1. Active immunizations.
2. Specific antimicrobial therapy.
3. Increased use of chemoprophylaxis.
4. Sophisticated diagnostic techniques.

Ms. Sophia Lory, who is 68 years old, has pernicious anemia. She has been visiting her physician every other week for an injection of vitamin B12. Her husband, who is 69 years old, wishes to learn how to give Ms. Lory her injections.
Items 341 through 360 relate to this situation.

341. Which one of the following symptoms usually *first* brings the patient with pernicious anemia to seek medical attention?
1. Dark stools.
2. Sudden weight loss.
3. A tendency to bleed easily.
4. Feeling unusually fatigued.

342. Ms. Lory had a gastric analysis as part of her initial diagnostic studies. A typical laboratory finding when gastric samples from a patient with pernicious anemia are analyzed is
1. a high bile concentration.
2. a low bicarbonate concentration.
3. an absence of hydrochloric acid.
4. the presence of immature red blood cells.

343. Ms. Lory was given radioactive B12 in water for the Shilling test—a diagnostic procedure. The *primary* purpose of this test is to measure the patient's ability to
1. store vitamin B12.
2. digest vitamin B12.
3. absorb vitamin B12.
4. produce vitamin B12.

344. Diagnostic laboratory examinations included a study of Ms. Lory's red blood cells. Where do the red blood cells normally originate in the body?
1. The liver.
2. The spleen.
3. Bone marrow.
4. Lymphatic tissues.

345. Which one of the following conditions that typically accompanies the acute stage of pernicious anemia requires special nursing measures?
   1. Incontinence.
   2. A sore mouth.
   3. Impaired vision.
   4. Impaired hearing.

346. When Ms. Lory's pernicious anemia was diagnosed, vitamin B_{12} by intramuscular injection was prescribed. The unit of measure *most commonly* used for describing the dosage of vitamin B_{12} is a
   1. unit.
   2. milligram.
   3. microgram.
   4. milliliter.

347. When Ms. Lory was diagnosed, she asked how long it would take before she felt better. Once treatment is initiated, the time required to relieve the symptoms for *most* patients with pernicious anemia who are free of complications can be measured in terms of
   1. days.
   2. weeks.
   3. months.
   4. about 1 year.

348. Ms. Lory asks when she can stop taking injections of vitamin B_{12}. Which one of the following statements should guide the nurse when she responds to the patient's question?
   1. Injections will be necessary between remissions.
   2. Injections will be necessary for the rest of her life.
   3. Injections will be necessary until her dietary regimen has been successfully established.
   4. Injections will be necessary until the disease process has been successfully controlled.

349. Ms. Lory questions why she cannot take vitamin B_{12} by mouth. The nurse should explain that oral administration is *contraindicated* for her because
   1. gastric juices destroy oral preparations of vitamin B_{12}.
   2. there is a rapid excretion of oral preparations of vitamin B_{12} from the body.
   3. intestinal secretions impede the absorption of oral preparations of vitamin B_{12}.
   4. there is a tendency to develop a resistance to oral preparations of vitamin B_{12}.

350. In relation to the toxic effects of vitamin B12, the nurse should
teach Ms. Lory that
1. there is no known toxicity to the medication.
2. ringing in the ears is a common symptom of toxicity.
3. nausea and vomiting are common symptoms of toxicity.
4. skin rashes and itching are common symptoms of toxicity.
351. When the nurse plans a teaching program for the Lorys in relation to the patient's illness, their ages are taken into consideration. A common behavior characteristic of the elderly person,
when compared with a younger adult, is that the elderly person tends to
1. adjust more slowly to change.
2. show less interest in habits of hygiene.
3. be less concerned about having physical illnesses.
4. resent needing medical attention more strenuously.
352. Various sites for administering vitamin B12 are discussed with
Mr. Lory. Because his wife's musculoskeletal structure is
small, Mr. Lory prefers to inject the medication into the
buttocks. Which one of the sites identified in the drawing
below is the *best* one for injecting the medication?
1. Site A.
2. Site B.
3. Site C.
4. Site D.

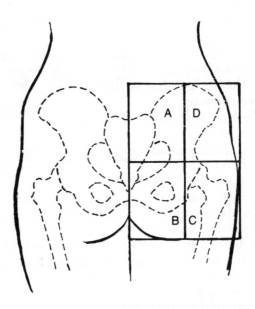

353. When the area of the buttock used for an intramuscular injection is poorly identified, the greatest danger that results is
1. damaging the iliac bone.
2. damaging the sciatic nerve.
3. injecting the medication into a vein.
4. injecting the medication into fatty tissues.

354. Which one of the following positions, all of which Ms. Lory is able to assume, will help *most* to decrease discomfort when injecting the medication?
1. Having her lie on her side with her knees sharply flexed.
2. Having her lie on her abdomen with her toes pointing inward.
3. Having her lean over the edge of a low table with her hips well flexed.
4. Having her stand in the upright position with her feet comfortably apart.

355. From which one of the following foods does the body normally obtain its best supply of vitamin B_{12}?
1. Fresh fruits.
2. Green leafy vegetables.
3. Meats and dairy products.
4. Wholewheat breads and cereals.

356. Which one of the following substances does the body fail to produce when pernicious anemia is present?
1. Pepsin.
2. Gastrin.
3. Bile salts.
4. The intrinsic factor.

357. If pernicious anemia is allowed to progress without treatment, the system of the body in which degenerative changes are *most likely* to occur is the
1. nervous system.
2. endocrine system.
3. musculoskeletal system.
4. gastrointestinal system.

358. Ms. Lory has dentures. The *chief* cause of tooth loss in adults is
1. dental caries.
2. oral infection.
3. tooth abscesses.
4. periodontal disease.

359. When cleansing Ms. Lory's dentures, which are made of plastic material, it is especially important to avoid using
1. hot water.
2. a toothbrush.
3. commercial toothpastes.

4. a vinegar soaking solution.

360. Ms. Lory comments about varicose veins she has "in this one leg. Nothing much but I know they are there." Which one of the following activities would best minimize aggravation of her varicose veins?
1. Elevating her legs several times a day.
2. Putting more weight on her uninvolved leg when standing.
3. Resting her involved leg over the other leg when sitting.
4. Using circular garters to make her stockings fit snugly.

Ms. Nancy Mott, a 34-year-old housewife, was admitted to the hospital with a diagnosis of kidney infection and chronic multiple sclerosis. Her kidney infection developed as a result of her multiple sclerosis.
Items 361 through 381 pertain to this situation.

361. Demyelinating lesions have produced bladder hypoactivity and urinary retention in Ms. Mott. In which area of her body are the lesions *most likely* located?
1. In the brain stem.
2. In the internal capsule of the brain.
3. In the motor nerve fibers in the spinal cord.
4. In the sensory nerve fibers in the spinal cord.

362. Ms. Mott has had multiple sclerosis for 5 years. Which one of the following diagnostic tests was likely to have been *most helpful* in determining her diagnosis?
1. A skull x-ray series.
2. Throat cultures.
3. An electroencephalogram.
4. Cerebrospinal fluid studies.

363. As part of her multiple sclerosis disease, which one of the following symptoms is Ms. Mott *least likely* to have experienced?
1. Double vision.
2. Sudden bursts of energy.
3. Weakness in a leg or foot.
4. Sensations of numbness and tingling in an extremity.

364. Ms. Mott has an indwelling catheter inserted into her bladder. After the catheter is removed, the nurse can help the patient to void by
1. applying heat to the patient's lower back region.
2. helping the patient to assume a sitting position.
3. running cool water over the patient's external genitalia.
4. teaching the patient to press her hands firmly over the umbilical area.

365. After Ms. Mott's catheter is removed, which one of the following signs/symptoms should suggest to the nurse that the patient is retaining urine?
1. Voiding infrequently in large quantities.
2. Having palpable distention in the suprapubic area.
3. Complaining of "cramping" sensations in her lower abdomen.
4. Drinking copious amounts of fluids with an insatiable thirst.

366. In addition to urinary problems, other common disorders of multiple sclerosis include *all* of the following complications *except*
1. ascites.
2. contractures.
3. decubitus ulcers.
4. respiratory infections.

367. Mephenesin carbamate (Tolseram) is prescribed by the physician for Ms. Mott, the *primary* purpose being to help
1. induce sleep in the patient.
2. stimulate the patient's appetite.
3. relieve muscular spasticity in the patient.
4. reduce the bacterial content in the patient's urine.

368. It is often difficult to assess the effectiveness of a particular drug in the treatment of multiple sclerosis because the patient's symptoms generally tend to
1. become worse without apparent cause.
2. persist for a time before yielding to the drug.
3. improve quickly when any new treatment is used.
4. require the use of several drug groups simultaneously.

369. Ms. Mott is troubled with slurred speech. When the nurse is communicating verbally with the patient, which one of the following nursing practices is *contraindicated?*
1. Encouraging her to speak slowly.
2. Encouraging her to speak distinctly.
3. Asking her to repeat indistinguishable words.
4. Asking her to state her needs aloud even when tired.

370. A practice the nurse should adhere to *strictly* when bathing Ms. Mott is to
1. clean the bath equipment properly after use.
2. explain the procedure of the bath briefly and clearly.
3. test the temperature of the bath water with a thermometer.
4. maintain privacy and cover the patient with a bath blanket.

371. Ms. Mott walks unsteadily and in an incoordinated manner. The term used to describe her gait is
1. ataxia.
2. vertigo.

3. paresis.

4. spasticity.

372. Ms. Mott's right hand trembles severely whenever she attempts a voluntary action. She spilled her coffee twice at lunch and could not get her dress fastened securely. Which one of the following nurses' notes offers the *best* account of these observations?

1. Has an intention tremor of the right hand.

2. Right hand tremor worsens with purposeful acts.

3. Needed assistance with dressing and eating due to severe trembling and clumsiness.

4. Slight shaking of right hand increased to severe tremor when patient tried to button her clothes or drink from a cup.

373. Because of her incoordination and weakness, Ms. Mott has become confined to a wheelchair when out of bed. Which one of the following environmental conditions is likely to be the *most* detrimental to Ms. Mott's physical well-being?

1. A wet area on the floor around the sink.

2. A drafty and cold main corridor.

3. An untidy and cluttered bedside table.

4. A bag of soiled laundry near the doorway.

374. Ms. Mott may eventually lose control of her bowels and require bowel training. In this event which one of the following measures is likely to be *least helpful?*

1. Eating a diet high in roughage.

2. Setting a regular time for elimination.

3. Raising the toilet seat for easy access by wheelchair.

4. Limiting fluid intake to 1000 ml. over a 24-hour period.

375. Patients with multiple sclerosis sometimes exhibit signs/symptoms of emotional distress which commonly fall into the general category of

1. mood disorders.

2. thought disorders.

3. psychosomatic illnesses.

4. drug dependency problems.

376. All of the following items of information concerning Ms. Mott are noteworthy. Which one should the nurse be *especially* sure to report?

1. The patient said she no longer saw spots or had pain behind the left eye.

2. The patient ate very little solid food at lunchtime but consumed most of the liquids.

3. The patient asked her visitors to leave after 20 minutes had passed because she was tired.

4. The patient asked that her "poor muscles and joints" be handled gently when being turned to her side.

377. During the rehabilitation of a patient with multiple sclerosis, occupational therapy and hobbies serve to help develop the patient's
   1. diligence and daring.
   2. muscles and motivation.
   3. intellect and imagination.
   4. productivity and personality.

378. In relation to habits of daily living at home, the nurse should encourage Ms. Mott to
   1. accept the necessity for a quiet and inactive life style.
   2. keep active while still avoiding emotional upset and fatigue.
   3. follow good health habits to change the course of the disease.
   4. practice using the mechanical aids that will be needed when future disabilities arise.

379. From which one of the following programs would Ms. Mott probably benefit *most* at home?
   1. A lengthy course of psychotherapy.
   2. A set schedule of daily activities.
   3. A day care plan for her small child.
   4. A weekly visit by another person who also has the disease.

380. Which one of the following words *best* characterizes multiple sclerosis as a disease?
   1. Fatal.
   2. Inherited.
   3. Contagious.
   4. Progressive.

381. In which one of the following types of climate does multiple sclerosis *most often* occur?
   1. In a hot, dry climate.
   2. In a hot, humid climate.
   3. In a cold, damp climate.
   4. In a mild, subtropical climate.

Ms. Harriet Cartole, age 69, has rheumatoid arthritis. She has been seeing her physician in his office for regular checkups. Items 382 and 407 relate to this situation.

382. Ms. Cartole is admitted to the hospital for surgery. She has a total knee replacement. This surgical restoration or formation of a joint is also called
   1. osteotomy.
   2. arthrodesis.
   3. arthroplasty.

4. osteosynthesis.

383. To re-educate the leg musculature after her knee surgery, Ms. Cartole is taught to do isometric exercises. The *most* important asset of isometric exercises is that they
   1. cost little in terms of both time and money.
   2. prevent joint stiffness and decrease the patient's reluctance to move.
   3. strengthen the muscles while keeping the joints stationary.
   4. involve the patient in her own care and thus improve her morale.

384. When preparing Ms. Cartole for ambulation after her joint surgery, the nurse explains the quadriceps setting exercise which is accomplished by
   1. bending the knee to form a right angle.
   2. rotating the leg slowly around in circles.
   3. pressing the back of the knee into the mattress.
   4. turning the leg inward toward the opposite thigh.

385. After Ms. Cartole was discharged from the hospital, she had her knee cast removed. On her next visit to the physician's office, she complains of stiffness in her fingers. Paraffin baths are prescribed. Before beginning the paraffin dip, which one of the following precautions should the patient be instructed to take?
   1. Shave the fingers of hair.
   2. Cover the fingers and hand with plastic wrap.
   3. Make a fist several times in rapid succession.
   4. Test the temperature of the paraffin with her elbow.

386. Which one of the following laboratory studies would be *least valuable* in confirming Ms. Cartole's diagnosis of rheumatoid arthritis?
   1. The sedimentation rate.
   2. The leukocyte count.
   3. The C-reactive protein test.
   4. The fluorescent antibody test.

387. Ms. Cartole was advised to have at least 12 hours of bed rest daily. During the rest periods, she should make sure her affected joints are kept
   1. well flexed.
   2. elevated on a pillow.
   3. supported by sandbags.
   4. as straight as possible.

388. When caring for a bedridden patient with arthritis, for which one of the following reasons should the head of the bed be kept flat?

1. To make position changes easier.
2. To decrease edema around the joints.
3. To prevent flexion deformities of the hip.
4. To increase the circulation of blood to the brain.

389. Once settled in bed, Ms. Cartole dislikes having to shift her position. To emphasize the importance of changing her position regularly and to gain her cooperation, which of the following tactics that the nurse could use would be *best*?
   1. Admonishing the patient for her negative attitude toward her therapy.
   2. Explaining to the patient why the turning and realignment are necessary.
   3. Reminding the patient that she has herself to blame if she develops complications.
   4. Pointing out signs to the patient at each office visit that indicate she is not following directions.

390. Ms. Cartole asks the nurse, "Why doesn't my doctor have me on the same drugs as my friend, Ms. Black, who also comes here for checkups? They have worked wonders for her." Which one of the following replies by the nurse would be *best*?
   1. "It would be best if you asked the doctor. He doesn't always let me in on his thinking."
   2. "Tell me more about your friend's arthritic condition. Maybe I can answer that question for you."
   3. "You shouldn't compare your condition with that of anyone else. Every patient is different and you could end up getting confused."
   4. "There are many different forms of arthritis. What may be helpful for your friend's form could be ineffective or harmful for your form."

391. Ms. Cartole takes aspirin for the relief of her arthritic pain. A symptom of toxicity the patient should be aware of when taking aspirin is
   1. dysuria.
   2. tinnitus.
   3. drowsiness.
   4. chest pain.

392. Two medications often used in the treatment of rheumatoid arthritis for their analgesic antiinflammatory effects are phenylbutazone (Butazolidin) and indomethacin (Indocin). To keep irritation to the gastric mucosa at a minimum from these drugs, when in the day should they be administered?
   1. At bedtime.
   2. Upon arising.

3. Immediately after a meal.

4. When the stomach is empty.

393. Ms. Cartole once received a corticosteroid drug for her arthritis. Because of the many adverse effects of steroid drugs, the preferred route of administration of these hormones (for example, hydrocortisone acetate [Cortef Acetate]) for a long-term arthritic patient is by

1. intravenous infusion.

2. subcutaneous injection.

3. intramuscular injection.

4. intraarticular injection.

394. Ms. Cartole wants to protect herself from unscrupulous persons offering her treatment and asks the nurse, "How can I tell what is valid and good for me and what is not?" The nurse should be guided in her reply by the fact that genuine and reputable products are *most often* sold through

1. testimonials inserted in leading magazines.

2. advertisements in circulars received in the mail.

3. prescriptions individually prescribed by physicians.

4. newspapers carrying advertisements as a direct sales campaign.

395. Ms. Cartole fears that she will become increasingly more handicapped and unable to care for herself. While all of the following resources are available, which one is *most often* recommended as a *last* resource?

1. Residential care in a local nursing home.

2. Home visits by members of the health care team.

3. Financial assistance from a social service agency.

4. Self-help devices from a regional arthritis center.

396. The food constituent that Ms. Cartole requires in *lesser* amounts than younger adults is

1. fats.

2. proteins.

3. calories.

4. carbohydrates.

397. Early in the course of the disease, a person with rheumatoid arthritis will *commonly* show signs/symptoms of

1. pallor.

2. malaise.

3. weight gain.

4. pitting edema.

398. Which one of the parts of the joint does rheumatoid arthritis *initially* affect?

1. The bursae.

2. The synovium.
3. The cartilage.
4. The ligaments.
399. In which one of the following age/sex groups is rheumatoid arthritis generally *most prevalent* at its onset?
1. In men during middle life.
2. In men during later life.
3. In women during middle life.
4. In women during later life.
400. Ms. Cartole also has glaucoma. Which one of the following medications is commonly used for treating glaucoma?
1. Atropine sulfate.
2. Pilocarpine hydrochloride (Pilocar).
3. Homatropine hydrobromide (Homatrocel).
4. Cyclopentolate hydrochloride (Cyclogyl).
401. The effects of glaucoma on ocular tissues are due to
1. a paralysis of ciliary muscles.
2. a degeneration of aqueous humor.
3. an increase in intraocular pressure.
4. a precipitation of proteins in the retina.
402. The term that means constriction of the pupils of the eyes is
1. miosis.
2. mycosis.
3. mitosis.
4. mydriasis.
403. Ms. Cartole's friend, Ms. Black, has osteoarthritis. In which one of the following joints is osteoarthritis *least likely* to occur?
1. In the knee joints.
2. In the hip joints.
3. In the finger joints.
4. In the shoulder joints.
404. Which one of the following terms is a synonym for osteoarthritis?
1. Polyarthritis.
2. Atrophic arthritis.
3. Arthritis deformans.
4. Degenerative arthritis.
405. Which two of the following factors are *most likely* to aggravate a patient's osteoarthritis?
1. Poor posture and obesity.
2. Poor hygiene and influenza.
3. Heavy smoking and laryngitis.
4. Heavy drinking and malnutrition.
406. To lessen the effects of osteoarthritis on the body, which one of the following types of diets is often recommended?

1. A ketogenic diet.
2. An acid/ash diet.
3. A low residue diet.
4. A weight reduction diet.

407. In the United States, the only illness that causes more chronic disability and incapacitation than arthritic diseases is
1. tuberculosis.
2. heart disease.
3. diabetes mellitus.
4. malignancy.

Mr. John Ketter, who has Hodgkin's disease, was admitted to the hospital for "staging." He is scheduled to have a bone marrow biopsy and mechlorethamine hydrochloride (Mustargen) therapy. His physician orders a high protein diet for him.
Items 408 through 423 relate to this situation.

408. Mr. Ketter's illness was diagnosed early in its course by his family physician. Which one of the following symptoms *most likely* first brought Mr. Ketter to seek medical attention?
1. Difficulty with swallowing.
2. Swollen cervical lymph nodes.
3. Difficulty with breathing and excessive expectorations.
4. Discomfort and a feeling of fullness over the area of his liver.

409. Which one of the following symptoms will Mr. Ketter *very likely* present upon admission that will require special nursing care measures?
1. Sore tongue.
2. Diaphoresis.
3. Itching skin.
4. Painful joints.

410. "Staging" Mr. Ketter will provide health personnel with information useful for *all* of the following purposes *except* that of
1. prescribing the patient's therapy.
2. estimating time between remissions.
3. noting where metastasis is occurring.
4. determining the cell causing the disease.

411. The nurse can anticipate that the physician is *most likely* to obtain a bone marrow specimen from Mr. Ketter's sternum or
1. rib.
2. femur.
3. vertebra.
4. iliac crest.

412. While preparing supplies for Mr. Ketter's bone marrow biopsy, the nurse should have a drug in readiness that acts as
1. an anticoagulant.
2. a muscle relaxant.
3. a heart stimulant.
4. a local anesthetic.
413. Which one of the following routes is ordinarily used to administer mechlorethamine hydrochloride?
1. Oral route.
2. Intravenous route.
3. Subcutaneous route.
4. Intramuscular route.
414. The *most common* side effects when mechlorethamine hydrochloride is used are
1. nausea and vomiting.
2. constipation and flatulence.
3. loss of hair and skin rashes.
4. headaches and visual disturbances.
415. Which one of the following blood examinations would be *most helpful* in determining whether Mr. Ketter's diet includes adequate amounts of proteins?
1. Red cell count.
2. Bilirubin level.
3. Reticulocyte count.
4. Serum albumin level.
416. Mr. Ketter develops singultus (hiccups). Singultus is due to
1. spasms of the diaphragm.
2. irritation to the glottis.
3. excessive bronchial dilatation.
4. inadequate alveolar ventilation.
417. The *primary* danger of prolonged singultus is
1. gastric ulcer.
2. paralytic ileus.
3. esophageal rupture.
4. physical exhaustion.
418. Mr. Ketter is ordered to have radiation therapy. After he receives therapy, his skin is red and moist. Which one of the following nursing measures is generally recommended for the care of his affected skin areas?
1. Wash with water and pat-dry.
2. Expose the area to air and fan-dry.
3. Apply a mild emollient and massage-dry.
4. Cover with an antiseptic ointment and sterile gauze.
419. Mr. Ketter requires oxygen therapy when he develops pneumonitis following radiation therapy. The *primary* pur-

pose for bubbling oxygen through water before it is inhaled by the patient is to help
1. measure the rate of oxygen administration.
2. remove impurities from the oxygen before it is inhaled.
3. control the pressure under which oxygen is administered.
4. add humidity to the oxygen before the patient inhales it.

420. Mr. Ketter is discharged to his home but returns to the hospital several months later when death appears imminent. One of the *greatest emotional* problems hospitalized terminally ill patients face is
1. fear of pain.
2. fear of further therapy.
3. feelings of being isolated.
4. feelings of social inadequacy.

421. When Mr. Ketter dies, Ms. Ketter cries angrily. "Why him? Why couldn't you help him?" Authorities describe such an angry emotional outburst as typical when the bereaved relative is
1. in an early stage of grief.
2. fearful of death for herself.
3. covering up her true feelings.
4. experiencing feelings of paranoia.

422. When Ms. Ketter expresses her anger, it would be *best* for the nurse to
1. offer to call a relative or friend to be with her.
2. remain with Ms. Ketter and quietly listen to what she is saying.
3. leave Ms. Ketter alone so that she can work through her emotions in privacy.
4. explain to Ms. Ketter that medical science is not perfect but that all possible was done for her husband.

423. In terms of age, Hodgkin's disease is ordinarily considered an illness that *primarily* strikes
1. children.
2. persons in their teens.
3. young adults.
4. the elderly.

Mr. Victor Day, who is 21 years old, went to a venereal disease clinic when he noted that he had a "sore" on his penis that was not healing.
Items 424 through 439 pertain to this situation.

424. A nurse had been asked to assist in setting up guidelines for the treatment of syphilis before the clinic Mr. Day visited was opened. Which of the following sources would be the *best* one for obtaining this type of information?

1. American Medical Association.
2. United States Public Health Service.
3. The American Hospital Formulary Service.
4. National Institutes of Health, Division of Biological Standards.

425. Investigations have demonstrated that the *most difficult* problem the nurse conducting Mr. Day's initial interview can anticipate is likely to be
1. motivating him to get treatment.
2. increasing his knowledge of the disease.
3. assuring him that records are confidential.
4. obtaining a complete list of his sexual contacts.

426. If the physician orders that Mr. Day receive probenecid (Benemid) in conjunction with penicillin therapy, his *primary* reason is that probenecid helps to
1. delay detoxification of penicillin.
2. potentiate the effectiveness of penicillin.
3. maintain sensitivity of organisms to penicillin.
4. decrease the likelihood of an allergic reaction to penicillin.

427. Penicillin acts on susceptible microorganisms by
1. killing them.
2. neutralizing toxins.
3. inhibiting growth rates.
4. retarding reproductive ability.

428. Penicillin is manufactured from
1. molds.
2. yeasts.
3. human serum.
4. animal serum.

429. If Mr. Day had not had therapy and eventually experienced the four stages of syphilis, during which stage would he have *most likely* been free of symptoms?
1. The primary stage.
2. The secondary stage.
3. The latent stage.
4. The tertiary stage.

430. If Mr. Day experienced the four stages of syphilis, during which stage would he *most likely* have had a negative reaction to commonly used serological tests?
1. The primary stage.
2. The secondary stage.
3. The latent stage.
4. The tertiary stage.

431. Mr. Day's care will continue on an outpatient basis at the clinic.

Approximately how long after effective treatment is begun will Mr. Day be considered infectious?

1. 24 hours.
2. 72 hours.
3. 1 week.
4. 10 days.

432. The chancre associated with syphilis is *most commonly* described as
   1. a reddened rash.
   2. an elevated wart.
   3. an itching crusted area.
   4. a painless moist ulcer.

433. The organism responsible for syphilis is classified as a
   1. virus.
   2. fungus.
   3. rickettsia.
   4. spirochete.

434. Which one of the following categories of individuals has experienced the *greatest* rise in the incidence of syphilis during the past decade?
   1. Teenagers.
   2. Divorced persons.
   3. Young married couples.
   4. Infants (congenital syphilis).

435. Which one of the following preventive measures has been found to be *most effective* in controlling the spread of syphilis?
   1. Premarital serological screening.
   2. Ongoing sex education in the schools.
   3. Serological screening of pregnant women.
   4. Prophylactic treatment of exposed individuals.

436. If Mr. Day had contracted gonorrhea instead of syphilis, his presenting symptom would *most likely* have been
   1. impotence.
   2. scrotal pain.
   3. urinary retention.
   4. urethral discharge.

437. When females acquire gonorrhea, a common observation that adds to the difficulty of preventing its spread is that many women
   1. are unaware that they have the disease.
   2. have a milder form of the disease than most men.
   3. acquire the disease without having sexual intercourse.
   4. are more reluctant to seek medical attention than men.

438. Investigations have demonstrated that the majority of individu-

als with venereal diseases receive their treatment in
1. specialty clinics.
2. hospital emergency rooms.
3. private physicians' offices.
4. student health services on school campuses.

439. The continued rise in the incidence of venereal diseases is attributed *primarily* to the
1. lack of case reporting.
2. laxity in public concern.
3. inaccessibility of treatment centers.
4. development of organisms resistent to drugs.

Mr. Charles Handy, who is 26 years old, was admitted to the hospital with a diagnosis of infectious hepatitis. He has some moderate sunburn from overexposure to the sun while swimming.
Items 440 through 454 relate to this situation.

440. Which one of the following precautionary measures should have the *lowest* priority when the nurse admits Mr. Handy?
1. Using disposable dishes.
2. Isolating his soiled linens.
3. Assigning him to a private room.
4. Wearing gowns and gloves when giving care.

441. Which one of the following diagnostic studies should the nurse anticipate the physician will likely order for Mr. Handy to help confirm the diagnosis of infectious hepatitis?
1. Diagnex blue test.
2. Bromsulphalein test (BSP).
3. Phenolsulfonphthalein test (PSP).
4. Heterophile agglutination test.

442. The virus that caused Mr. Handy's infectious hepatitis is *most often* spread by
1. infected insects.
2. infected rodents and birds.
3. contaminated food and liquids.
4. contaminated clothing and eating utensils.

443. Once having gained entrance to Mr. Handy's body, in which one of the following anatomical structures did the organisms causing his illness multiply?
1. In the liver.
2. In the intestinal tract.
3. In the circulatory system.
4. In the central nervous system.

444. The virus causing infectious hepatitis will be excreted from Mr. Handy's body *primarily* through his
1. skin.
2. urine.
3. feces.
4. nasal discharges.

445. Which one of the following characteristics applies only to viruses?
1. They multiply only by fission.
2. They produce illness only in humans.
3. They grow only inside of living cells.
4. They are visible only through a light microscope.

446. Mr. Handy expresses concern since he fears members of his family may also acquire hepatitis. Which one of the following biological preparations is *most commonly* used for prophylactic purposes for persons exposed to infectious hepatitis?
1. A vaccine.
2. An antitoxin.
3. Gamma globulin.
4. An inactivated toxin.

447. If the physician orders an adrenocorticosteroid drug during the acute phase of Mr. Handy's illness, the *primary* purpose would be to help
1. prevent mental depression.
2. limit the extent of the infection.
3. increase the patient's resistance.
4. alleviate the severity of the symptoms.

448. Which one of the following diets are *most* physicians now prescribing for patients with hepatitis?
1. A low fat diet.
2. A low protein diet.
3. A high carbohydrate diet.
4. A normally balanced diet.

449. For which one of the following symptoms, which is typical during the convalescent period following hepatitis, should the nurse be ready to offer guidelines when she prepares Mr. Handy for discharge?
1. Fatigue.
2. Insomnia.
3. Anorexia.
4. Constipation.

450. Which of the following symptoms would *usually be present* in patients with infectious hepatitis but *generally absent* in patients with serum hepatitis?

1. Jaundice.
2. Low grade fever.
3. Malaise and general weakness.
4. Abdominal and epigastric distress.

451. Serum hepatitus if often called
1. hepatitis Type A.
2. hepatitis Type B.
3. catarrhal jaundice.
4. epidemic hepatitis.

452. Which one of the following practices *best* explains the marked increase in the number of cases and carriers of serum hepatitis in the United States today?
1. Using "pep" pills.
2. Smoking marihuana.
3. Injecting illicit drugs.
4. Increasing sexual permissiveness.

453. It is generally agreed that the safest method for sterilizing reusable equipment that has been contaminated with the hepatitis virus is to use
1. boiling water.
2. a dry heat oven.
3. chemical solutions.
4. steam under pressure.

454. In which one of the following hospital units do nurses run the *greatest* risk of acquiring hepatitis from their patients?
1. In birthing rooms.
2. In isolation units.
3. In emergency rooms.
4. In hemodialysis units.

Mr. James Corning, a 34-year-old business executive, was admitted to the hospital with a diagnosis of duodenal ulcer. He has smoked approximately two packs of cigarettes a day for 15 years and has been taking household soda bicarbonate for "indigestion and heartburn" for about a year. The physician's admission orders included the following:

Gastric analysis.
Upper gastrointestinal tract x-rays (GI series).
Propantheline bromide (Pro-Banthine) 15 mg. with meals and H.S.
Aluminum hydroxide (Amphojel) 8 ml. q 2 h while awake.
Allow patient to sip milk as desired.

Items 455 through 482 relate to this situation.

455. The physician indicates that Mr. Corning demonstrated signs of bleeding from his ulcer before admission. Shortly after admission, Mr. Corning vomits. Unless Mr. Corning is hemorrhaging and vomiting bright, red blood, it would be *typical* that his vomitus contains
   1. duodenal fecal matter.
   2. undigested particles of food.
   3. chyme streaked with black syrupy material.
   4. materials having a coffee-ground appearance.
456. Which one of the following statements concerning food and fluid intake prior to gastric analysis is *most accurate*?
   1. There is no special preparation of food and fluid intake prior to gastric analysis.
   2. Fluids and food are withheld for 6 to 8 hours prior to gastric analysis.
   3. Fluids and food, except for water, are withheld for 6 to 8 hours prior to gastric analysis.
   4. The evening meal the night before gastric analysis is withheld; the patient may have clear liquids for breakfast prior to the examination.
457. If the physician had ordered a tubeless gastric analysis for Mr. Corning, the patient would have ingested a dye after which the nurse should expect to collect a specimen of
   1. stool.
   2. blood.
   3. urine.
   4. gastric content.
458. Roentgenography of the upper gastrointestinal tract is carried out after and while the patient receives
   1. a resin dye, given orally.
   2. barium sulfate, given orally.
   3. magnesium citrate, given orally.
   4. a radiopaque dye, given intravenously.
459. The nurse should anticipate that following a GI series, measures are *usually* used to guard against
   1. diarrhea.
   2. heartburn.
   3. fecal impaction.
   4. nausea and vomiting.
460. Propantheline bromide is an anticholinergic agent that acts to help
   1. suppress secretions of gastric glands.
   2. neutralize hydrochloric acid in the stomach.
   3. shorten the time required for digestion in the stomach.
   4. improve the mixing of foods and normal gastric secretions.

461. Of the following side effects, the two *most commonly* associated with drugs classified as anticholinergics are
1. drowsiness and headaches.
2. photophobia and blurred vision.
3. bleeding and prolonged clotting times.
4. urinary suppression and calculi formation.
462. Although none of the following fluids is necessarily contraindicated for Mr. Corning, it is generally recommended that aluminum hydroxide gel be mixed with or followed by sips of
1. milk.
2. water.
3. a bland fruit juice.
4. a carbonated beverage.
463. A problem frequently associated with the use of aluminum hydroxide gel is
1. anorexia.
2. pylorospasms.
3. constipation.
4. frequent belching.
464. Mr. Corning requests that a container of milk be left at his bedside. The nurse uses measures to keep the milk cold *primarily* because the coldness helps to
1. improve the milk's antacid action.
2. depress acid secretions in the stomach.
3. constrict vessels in the stomach mucosa.
4. inhibit the growth of bacteria in the milk.
465. Ms. Corning wishes to bring Mr. Corning a midafternoon snack from home the day after his admission. Which one of the following foods would be best and still allow Mr. Corning to adhere to a suitable diet?
1. Pizza pie.
2. Baked custard.
3. Fruit turnover.
4. Fresh fruit salad with cream.
466. The heartburn for which Mr. Corning had been taking soda bicarbonate *usually* occurs as a result of
1. overeating.
2. food allergies.
3. reverse peristalsis.
4. dilatation of the pyloric valve.
467. When soda bicarbonate is used indiscriminately, the patient may be in danger of developing
1. renal calculi.
2. fluid retention.

3. metabolic alkalosis.

4. iron deficiency anemia.

468. If the nurse notes the following items on Mr. Corning's dinner tray, which one should she remove before serving the patient?

1. Salt.

2. Sugar.

3. Cream.

4. Pepper.

469. If Mr. Corning's ulcer perforates, which one of the following signs/symptoms is the patient *most likely* to demonstrate?

1. Bloody vomitus.

2. Relief from pain.

3. A boardlike abdomen.

4. A sudden increase in blood pressure.

470. Which one of the following statements *best* describes current opinion concerning diet during convalescence for the patient with peptic ulcers?

1. The type of diet appears to be less important than the time at which the patient eats.

2. A regulated diet remains the most effective medical treatment for peptic ulcers.

3. Dietary restrictions appear to be most helpful among elderly persons but are rarely helpful among young and middle-aged adults.

4. Eliminating specific foods from the diet is no longer recommended, as long as the diet contains an abundant amount of milk and cream.

471. Which one of the following beverages should Mr. Corning be instructed to avoid after his discharge?

1. Carbonated beverages.

2. Low calorie soft drinks.

3. Drinks containing alcohol.

4. Drinks that are artificially sweetened.

472. Although Mr. Corning appears calm, the nurse assesses that he is experiencing anxiety. *All* of the following signs/symptoms serve as a good basis for concluding that an otherwise calm person is nevertheless suffering from anxiety *except*

1. flushed skin.

2. rapid heart rate.

3. dry lips and mouth.

4. increased blood pressure.

473. Mr. Corning cannot avoid stressful situations in his occupation which he realizes does not help his ulcer to heal. Which one of the following statements describes the *best* guide for help-

ing to develop a healthful attitude toward stress?

1. Eliminating fear will overcome stress.
2. Perseverance will usually overcome the effects of stress.
3. The body returns to normal functioning rapidly after experiencing stress.
4. The method of coping with stress is more important than its common causes.

474. The physician recommends that Mr. Corning try to stop smoking because of the effects of nicotine which increases the body's secretions of
1. thyroxin.
2. epinephrine.
3. pancreatic juices.
4. gastrointestinal mucus.

475. In addition to the difficulty of breaking a firm habit, Mr. Corning is likely to find that suddenly giving up cigarettes is a difficult undertaking because
1. smoking helps digestion.
2. smoking relieves tensions.
3. tar in tobacco gives it a pleasant taste.
4. nicotine in tobacco is an addictive substance.

476. The nature of discomfort that *typically* brings patients like Mr. Corning to seek medical attention is pain that
1. is relieved by rest.
2. is relieved by eating.
3. increases with physical activity.
4. increases with excretory efforts.

477. Research on the etiology of duodenal ulcers has demonstrated a familial tendency which is commonly associated with
1. blood grouping.
2. genetic mutations.
3. enzyme deficiencies.
4. hormonal activities.

478. A diet consisting primarily of milk and cream eventually leads to health problems because the two foods will affect the blood by increasing the
1. amylase level.
2. uric acid content.
3. cholesterol level.
4. prothombin content.

479. Which one of the following secretions causes foods rich in fat content to be digested more slowly than foods rich in carbohydrate and protein content?
1. Ptyalin.

2. Gastrin.

3. Pepsinogen.

4. Enterogastrone.

480. Which one of the following substances is normally absorbed in the stomach?

1. Alcohol.

2. Peptones.

3. Glycerol.

4. Amino acids.

481. Absorption of food in the small intestines occurs *primarily* through structures known as

1. rugae.

2. villi.

3. taeniae.

4. papillae.

482. Which one of the following substances is absorbed in largest amounts in the colon?

1. Water.

2. Glucose.

3. Fatty acids.

4. Amino acids.

Mr. Joseph Smith has been ordered to receive hypothermia. A cooling blanket will be used.
Items 483 through 491 relate to this situation.

483. Which one of the following signs is *most likely* to be present if Mr. Smith's temperature rises to 40° C. (104° F.)?

1. The patient can be expected to have cyanosed skin.

2. The patient can be expected to have a drop in blood pressure.

3. The patient can be expected to have a faster than average pulse rate.

4. The patient can be expected to have a slower than average respiratory rate.

484. By which method is *most* heat removed from this patient's body while he is receiving hypothermia?

1. Radiation.

2. Convection.

3. Conduction.

4. Evaporation.

485. A drug is to be administered while the patient is receiving hypothermia. If the following routes are available and it is safe to administer the drug by any of them, the nurse should be prepared to give the drug

1. intravenously.
2. subcutaneously.
3. intramuscularly.
4. by rectal instillation.

486. The nurse caring for Mr. Smith should understand that the primary danger when body temperatures drop below approximately 32° C. (90° F.) is a complication involving the
1. liver.
2. lungs.
3. heart.
4. kidneys.

487. The four statements below describe observations made on Mr. Smith. Which finding should indicate to the nurse that the downward drift of the patient's temperature after the cooling device is removed is likely to be more than the average amount?
1. The patient weighs 238 pounds.
2. The patient is a 32-year-old black male.
3. The patient was unconscious before hypothermia was started.
4. The patient suffered a head injury in an automobile accident.

488. The preferred method of rewarming Mr. Smith is to
1. sponge the patient with warm water.
2. allow the patient to rewarm naturally at room temperature.
3. apply a warming device, as a warming blanket, to the surface of the body.
4. apply heating pads to areas where large vessels are superficial, as in the groins and axillae.

489. Consider the relationship between statements A and B.
Statement A: Heat loss from the body is increased when evaporation of moisture from the body can occur readily.
Statement B: After having a chill, Mr. Smith had a body temperature of 40° C. (104° F.). A humidifier was placed in Mr. Smith's room.
1. Statement A is true and explains why statement B describes correct nursing action.
2. Statement A is true and explains why statement B describes incorrect nursing action.
3. Statement A is true but does not explain why statement B is either correct or incorrect nursing action.
4. Statement A is false and has no relationship to statement B.

490. Consider the relationship between statements A and B.
Statement A: Water tends to shift from intravascular to intracellular and interstitial spaces during periods of immobility, thereby increasing the viscosity of the blood.

Statement B: Patients who are receiving hypothermia therapy should have their positions changed and passive range-of-motion exercises carried out frequently in order to help prevent the formation of emboli.
1. Statement A is true and explains why statement B describes correct nursing action.
2. Statement A is true and explains why statement B describes incorrect nursing action.
3. Statement A is true but does not explain why statement B is either correct or incorrect nursing action.
4. Statement A is false and has no relationship to statement B.

491. The body's heat regulating center is located in the
1. cerebrum.
2. cerebellum.
3. hypothalamus.
4. spinal cord.

Ms. Lorraine Myerby has had migraine headaches for approximately 10 years. She started biofeedback training and is learning to use appropriate monitoring of her physiological activities in an effort to control the headaches.
Items 492 through 496 relate to this situation.

492. The purpose of biofeedback is to enable Ms. Myerby to exert control over physiological processes by
1. shocking her when an undesirable response is elicited.
2. regulating her body processes by electrical control.
3. monitoring her body processes for the therapist to interpret.
4. translating signals of her body processes into observable forms.

493. The pain associated with migraine headaches is believed to be due to
1. a temporary increase in intracranial pressure.
2. dilatation of the dural arteries of the scalp.
3. irritation and inflammation of the openings to the sinuses.
4. sustained contraction of the muscles around the scalp and face.

494. Which one of the following medications was *most likely* prescribed for Ms. Myerby in the past to abort and control an attack of migraine?
1. Dipyridamole (Persantine).
2. Ergotamine tartrate (Gynergen).
3. Papaverine hydrochloride (Pavabid).
4. Isoproterenol hydrochloride (Isuprel).

495. What will Ms. Myerby be taught to observe on her monitors as a

sign that biofeedback is having its desired effect?
1. Decreasing musculature tension.
2. Increasing temperature of the hands.
3. Decreasing heart rate and blood pressure.
4. Increasing frequency and amplitude of the brain's alpha waves.

496. One of the *most important* prerequisites of Ms. Myerby's biofeedback training is that she must
1. have no physiological deficits.
2. have exhausted all other means of treatment.
3. be passive and relaxed at the therapist's direction.
4. take an active and responsible part in the training.

A nurse working in a junior college is preparing a class on the physiology of menstruation. She anticipates that questions concerning menopause may also arise.

Items 497 through 512 pertain to information the nurse reviewed for the class.

497. Which one of the following bodily changes occurs *first* in the prepubertal girl as evidence that sexual maturity is beginning?
1. Development of the breasts.
2. Growth spurt in height and weight.
3. Growth of axillary and pubic hair.
4. Increase in the size of external genitalia.

498. Which one of the following factors exerts the *least* amount of influence on the age at which the beginning of menstrual functioning occurs?
1. Climate.
2. Heredity.
3. Nutrition.
4. Physical activity.

499. Which one of the following hormones is contained in follicular fluid prior to ovulation?
1. Estrogen.
2. Progesterone.
3. Luteinizing hormone.
4. Follicle-stimulating hormone.

500. The release of gonadotropic hormone by the pituitary gland is controlled by the
1. medulla.
2. cerebrum.
3. cerebellum.
4. hypothalamus.

501. When the ovum is not fertilized, menstruation is precipitated *primarily* because of a cessation in the secretion of hormones from the
1. endometrium.
2. corpus luteum.
3. pituitary gland.
4. graafian follicle.

502. The *primary* function of cervical secretions which become watery at the time of ovulation is to help
1. cleanse the cervical canal.
2. facilitate the passage of sperm.
3. neutralize the normal acidity of vaginal secretions.
4. prepare the uterus for implantation of a fertilized ovum.

503. Which one of the following hormones is *especially* important in preparing the endometrium for implantation of the fertilized ovum?
1. Oxytocin.
2. Progesterone.
3. Luteinizing hormone.
4. Follicle-stimulating hormone.

504. The time in the month when a woman is *most likely* to be fertile is *best* determined by a study of her
1. sex desires.
2. blood pressure.
3. menstrual history.
4. body temperatures.

505. The pelvic discomfort experienced by some women during ovulation is called
1. climacteric.
2. metrorrhagia.
3. dysmenorrhea.
4. mittleschmerz.

506. For which one of the following females is the wearing of tampons *contraindicated*?
1. Jane, age 14, having her third menstrual period.
2. Ms. Jones, age 21, who is 3 days postpartum.
3. Ms. Rose, age 39, who has irregular periods.
4. Ms. Becker, age 45, who has a cystocele.

507. Since the question of activities that are contraindicated during menstruation can be anticipated, the nurse should be prepared with a response guided by knowledge that *most* authorities are of the opinion that
1. dental work should be avoided.
2. sexual intercourse should be avoided.

3. any activity involving active sports should be avoided until a gynecological evaluation has been done.

4. no usual activities of daily living are contraindicated.

508. When compared with women who have not given birth, menstrual cramps are less frequent in women who have had children because the

1. endometrium has been replaced.

2. cervix remains slightly opened.

3. doubts about femininity have been removed.

4. preoccupation with menstruation is less intense.

509. The changes noted by a woman at menopause are caused *primarily* by a lack of the hormone

1. estrogen.

2. progesterone.

3. luteinizing hormone.

4. chorionic gonadotropin.

510. The nurse should explain that a change in the body that is *least* often observed following menopause is

1. an increase in emotional instability.

2. an increase in the dryness of the skin.

3. a change in the distribution of adipose tissues.

4. a loss of a normal interest in sexual activities.

511. "Hot flashes" that many women experience during and after menopause are caused *primarily* by

1. hereditary factors.

2. vasomotor instability.

3. pituitary disturbances.

4. psychological responses.

512. If a woman feels that her usefulness in life has ended when she reaches menopause, it is generally helpful to assure her that

1. most women feel the same way.

2. worrying about it intensifies the problem.

3. feelings of discouragement and self-pity are normal signs.

4. finding new interests has helped many women overcome the feeling.

A group of nurses studied together in preparation for writing the state board licensing examinations.

Items 513 through 557 relate to material they reviewed in relation to trends influencing nursing, legal and ethical considerations in nursing, nursing organizations, education for nursing, and the like.

513. Historians generally agree that Florence Nightingale's *greatest*

contribution to nursing was in her efforts to promote
1. licensure for nurses.
2. research programs for nursing.
3. educational programs for nursing.
4. professional organizations for nurses.
514. The Social Security Act has provisions for *all* of the following
types of service *except*
1. life insurance.
2. disability insurance.
3. funds for the needy blind.
4. grants-in-aid for welfare for children.
515. Public Law 93-360, which amended the National Labor Relations Act (Taft-Hartley Act) in 1974, influenced nursing by
1. including nonprofit hospitals and their employees under its
jurisdiction.
2. disallowing a nursing supervisor from being a member of the
American Nurses' Association.
3. excluding nurses with a rank of head nurse, team leader, and
staff nurse from its jurisdiction.
4. stating that professional nursing organizations can no longer
maintain economic security programs.
516. Being responsible and answerable for services the nurse provides is a common definition of
1. advocacy.
2. endorsement.
3. accountability.
4. professionalism.
517. Which one of the following statements describes a trend which
has become apparent in hospital populations in the United
States within the last decade?
1. Hospital populations remain hospitalized longer than those of
previous decades.
2. Hospital populations tend to be more acutely ill than those of
previous decades.
3. Hospital populations are voicing opposition concerning nursing taking over responsibilities previously carried out by
physicians.
4. Hospital populations reflect the post World War II baby boom
with more young patients (under 30) than older patients (over
50).
518. The *primary* purpose of investigations described in the publication *An Abstract For Action* was to promote better health for
Americans by improving
1. relationships among health workers.

2. nursing care and nursing education.

3. the distribution of health practitioners.

4. hospital and clinic facilities for patient care.

519. A consistent trend in preservice education for nursing within the last decade or so has been

1. lengthening the amount of clinical practice required of students.

2. placing education for nursing in institutions of higher learning.

3. developing a greater variety of basic educational programs for nursing.

4. providing increasingly large numbers of students with scholarship aid.

520. Which one of the following nursing organizations allows non-nurse members?

1. Academy of Nursing.

2. National League for Nursing.

3. American Nurses' Association.

4. American Association of Industrial Nurses.

521. Which one of the following organizations has the *most active* national program for recruiting minority groups into nursing careers?

1. National League for Nursing.

2. American Nurses' Association.

3. National Student Nurses' Association.

4. American Association of Colleges of Nursing.

522. Which one of the following factors has helped nurse mobility *most* in this country?

1. Having individual state nursing boards.

2. Having national licensing examinations.

3. Having professional employment agencies for nurses.

4. Having national accreditation for schools of nursing.

523. Continuing education is generally considered important for nurses *primarily* so that they may

1. obtain college credit.

2. keep current in their practice.

3. gain recognition as health professionals.

4. return to work after a period of retirement.

524. Which one of the following magazines publishes a list of nursing programs that have been accredited by the National League for Nursing?

1. *Nursing Update.*

2. *Nursing Outlook.*

3. *American Journal of Nursing.*

4. *Journal of Nursing Education.*
525. The national honorary society for nurses in the United States is
1. Alpha Phi Omega.
2. Alpha Tau Delta.
3. Phi Delta Kappa.
4. Sigma Theta Tau.
526. The official organ of the National Student Nurses' Association is
1. *Image.*
2. *Imprint.*
3. *Nursing Care.*
4. *Nursing Review.*
527 Of the following educational concepts, the American Nurses' Association has taken a stand *against*
1. external degree study programs.
2. continuing education on a voluntary basis.
3. degree-granting status for service agencies.
4. interdisciplinary programs for doctoral degrees.
528. At the present time, one of the greatest problems concerning transplanting organs and tissues from a dead body to a living person relates to the definition of
1. death.
2. cryonics.
3. euthanasia.
4. thanatology.
529. Upon graduation, a student nurse plans to move to another state where she wishes to become licensed and work. Of the following sources, in which one will she find the title and address of the board of nursing in the state to which she plans to move?
1. *Nursing Forum.*
2. *Nursing Outlook.*
3. *Nursing Research.*
4. *American Journal of Nursing.*
530. A physician's office nurse who also served as his cashier was found guilty of taking small amounts of money regularly from the office cash box. According to the law, she has committed a wrong called
1. robbery.
2. larceny.
3. burglary.
4. embezzlement.
531. A concept clearly implied in the 1973 Code for Nurses of the International Council of Nurses that had not been present in previous codes is that nurses should
1. be accountable for their practice.

2. work toward meeting criteria of a profession.

3. include health promotion in their services to humanity.

4. assume leadership for health care in developing countries.

532. When the New York State Nurses' Association proposed legislation that would require a baccalaureate degree for nurse licensure, the proposal included a provision to exempt persons already licensed from complying. An exemption of this sort is called

1. a waiver.

2. a precedent.

3. an endorsement.

4. a private law.

533. The *primary* purpose of having a body of common law is that it helps to prevent

1. one person from being tried under both criminal and civil law.

2. one person from being tried for the same crime more than once.

3. persons being brought to trial without benefit of legal counsel.

4. persons in similar circumstances being judged by different sets of rules.

534. A mandatory nurse practice act is one that requires a nurse to be

1. employed under the general supervision of a licensed physician.

2. currently licensed in the state where she wishes to practice nursing.

3. graduated from a school accredited by a national nursing organization.

4. enrolled at least yearly in courses approved by the state to meet requirements for continuing education.

535. Laws in this country derive from *all* of the following sources *except*

1. the legislatures.

2. the judiciary system.

3. administrative regulations.

4. preambles to the federal and state constitutions.

536. A common criticism of nurse licensure laws in this country is that they fail to provide for

1. revocation of licenses.

2. reciprocity between states.

3. proof of continued competence.

4. licensure of nurses educated in foreign countries.

537. A nurse told several friends and co-workers that a patient, who was a physician, was unsafe for medical practice because he was paralyzed from the waist down and acted "slightly silly."

The nurse's action can constitute the offense known as
1. libel.
2. fraud.
3. slander.
4. malpractice.

538. A patient was not allowed to leave a hospital upon discharge until his bill was paid. The hospital's action can constitute the offense known as
1. assault.
2. battery.
3. false imprisonment.
4. invasion of privacy.

539. A nurse who refuses to give or imply endorsement for promoting health-related commercial products is observing
1. the patient's bill of rights.
2. the code of ethics for nurses.
3. her state's nurse practice act.
4. her state's consumer fraud act.

540. A law derived from a court decision is called
1. a common law.
2. a statutory law.
3. a constitutional law.
4. an administrative law.

541. A nurse has been sued for negligence following the administration of an intramuscular injection. Which one of the following persons would *most likely* be asked to serve as a witness to describe standards of care?
1. An experienced nursing supervisor.
2. A lawyer who had successfully defended another nurse sued for negligence.
3. A judge who is considered to be an expert in the field of professional negligence.
4. Another patient who had received an injection by the same nurse but without complications.

542. For which one of the following actions could an experienced nurse be held liable and possibly sued for gross negligence?
1. Giving cardiac and pulmonary resuscitation for only 2 hours on a child found in a swimming pool even though the child did not show signs of responding to therapy.
2. Keeping a tourniquet in place continuously on an extremity when bleeding was present during the 2-hour trip required to reach the nearest hospital.
3. Refusing to allow a person to sit up while being moved following an accident when he said he had no feelings in his legs but

had feelings in his arms.

    4. Slapping a man in a restaurant on his upper back so vigorously while trying to remove food from his throat that he complained of muscular aches and pains in his back following the incident.

543. The United States is represented in the International Council of Nurses by the
1. American Red Cross.
2. National League for Nursing.
3. American Nurses' Association.
4. American Association of Colleges of Nursing.

544. A nurse was of the opinion that to carry out a certain order written by a physician could constitute unethical behavior. Which one of the following courses of action would be *best* for the nurse to take in this situation?
1. Carry out the order; then discuss it with the physician.
2. Carry out the order; then discuss it with her supervisor.
3. Do not carry out the order; report the situation to the physician.
4. Do not carry out the order; report the situation to the supervisor.

545. A current trend in legislation is that laws pertaining to nursing are increasingly moving toward
1. indicating qualifications for nurses in individual practices.
2. including physicians on official boards for certifying nursing specialists.
3. removing restrictions that would hamper the preparation of nurses for expanded roles.
4. giving employing agencies more responsibility for licensing nurses educated in foreign countries.

546. *All* of the following types of patients must be reported to the proper official agency *except*
1. a suicide victim.
2. a battered child.
3. a patient with a gunshot wound.
4. an unmarried pregnant woman who requests an abortion.

547. *All* of the following drugs are regulated by federal law *except*
1. codeine sulfate.
3. reserpine (Serpasil).
3. meperidine hydrochloride (Demerol).
4. methadone hydrochloride (Dolophine).

548. How many states in all must ratify the bill calling for equality of rights (ERA) before it can become an amendment to the federal constitution?
1. 14.

2. 26.
3. 38.
4. 50.
549. The federal act that has provided money for hospital construction
is the
1. Hill-Burton Act.
2. Social Security Act.
3. Health Amendments Act.
4. Health Maintenance Organization Act.
550. Which one of the following nursing organizations makes professional liability insurance available for its members?
1. National League for Nursing.
2. American Nurses' Association.
3. National Black Nurses' Association.
4. American Association of Industrial Nurses.
551. The official organ of the American Nurses' Association is
1. *Nursing Forum.*
2. *Nursing Outlook.*
3. *Nursing Research.*
4. *American Journal of Nursing.*
552. The honorary chairman of the American National Red Cross is
the president of the
1. United States.
2. United Nations.
3. American Medical Association.
4. American Nurses' Association.
553. The so-called ladder concept in education for nursing is based on
the philosophy that a nurse should be able to
1. be placed in an educational program on the basis of results
obtained in a challenge examination.
2. study basic knowledge in nursing through a universally accepted 21 problem-centered approach.
3. enroll in basic courses that are appropriate for students regardless of their occupational choice in the health field.
4. move from one level of education for nursing to the next higher
level without repeating previous educational experiences.
554. Which one of the following organizations requires evidence of an
outstanding contribution to nursing as one criterion for membership?
1. Academy of Nursing.
2. American Nurses' Foundation.
3. Congress for Nursing Practice.
4. N-Cap (Nurses' Coalition for Action in Politics).
555. Which one of the following proposals has been under attack by

professional nursing organizations because they consider the proposal contrary to the best interests of the patient?
1. Having nurses rather than physicians monitor nurses practicing in an expanded role.
2. Having institutions rather than states issue licenses to the nurses they employ.
3. Having nurses considered as professionals under the national labor relations act.
4. Setting standards for graduate as well as for basic educational programs for nurses.

556. A woman says her father became blind from glaucoma and she wishes to see a "specialist" to learn if she too is developing the disease. It would be *best* for the nurse to recommend that this woman be examined by an
1. optician.
2. ocularist.
3. optometrist.
4. ophthalmologist.

557. A chiropodist is a person who specializes in the care of the
1. ears.
2. skin.
3. feet.
4. spine.

Items 558 through 609 are miscellaneous items.

558. The body's normal buffering system, which maintains an acid-base balance, is geared toward either taking up or releasing the ion
1. sodium.
2. oxygen.
3. hydrogen.
4. potassium.

559. To obtain accurate daily weights of a patient, it would be *least* important to
1. use the same scales for every weighing.
2. weigh the patient at the same time each day.
3. have the same person weigh the patient each day.
4. have the patient wear approximately the same amount of clothing for each weighing.

560. While the following factors may all influence the course of ulcerative colitis, the one that tends to aggravate the disease *most* is
1. allergies.

2. bacterial infections.
3. dietary indiscretions.
4. emotional disturbances.

561. The *most life-threatening* complication of ulcerative colitis is
   1. intussusception.
   2. electrolyte disturbances.
   3. obstruction of the bowel.
   4. perforation of the bowel.

562. If a patient is bleeding from a stomach ulcer, the nurse can expect the color of his stools to be
   1. grey.
   2. black.
   3. dark red.
   4. light brown.

563. A serologic test is done on a patient's blood to determine an antigen-antibody reaction and an agglutination reaction occurs. An agglutin is a substance that causes bacteria to
   1. decrease in number.
   2. increase in number.
   3. scatter about at random.
   4. stick together in clumps.

564. Which one of the following blood disorders responds *best* to diet therapy?
   1. Agranulocytosis.
   2. Aplastic anemia.
   3. Sickle cell anemia.
   4. Iron deficiency anemia.

565. An alert adult is to be taught how to give himself insulin. Most authorities agree that it is *best* when the goals of learning are
   1. left unstated because discussing them usually becomes a distraction during the learning process.
   2. left unstated because discussing them has been found to be unimportant when the patient is an alert adult.
   3. determined cooperatively by the nurse and patient so that the patient feels he is participating.
   4. determined cooperatively by the nurse and patient's physician so that the nurse knows what the physician wishes taught.

566. A patient has shown all of the following types of behavior while learning how to give himself insulin. The behavior which *most accurately* indicates that he has learned the procedure is when the patient
   1. demonstrates that he can carry out the procedure correctly.
   2. demonstrates a sincere interest and readiness for what is being taught.

3. correctly explains how to prepare the insulin and syringe and how to inject himself.
4. satisfactorily answers oral and written questions the nurse poses about the procedure.

567. The nurse can anticipate that *all* of the following measures are commonly ordered for patients with acute pulmonary edema *except*
1. performing a pericardiocentesis.
2. rotating tourniquets on the extremities.
3. maintaining the patient in Fowler's position.
4. administering morphine sulfate subcutaneously.

568. The *most common* purpose for performing a liver biopsy is to help evaluate the liver's
1. size.
2. tissue.
3. blood supply.
4. detoxification abilities.

569. The *primary* reason for having a patient lie on his right side with a pillow under his lower rib cage after a liver biopsy is to help
1. immobilize the diaphragm.
2. facilitate full chest expansion.
3. minimize the danger of infection.
4. reduce the likelihood of bleeding.

570. A patient is scheduled to have an abdominal paracentesis. The nurse should check the patient's preparation for the procedure by seeing to it that he has
1. had a cleansing enema.
2. had an abdominal x-ray examination.
3. not had fluids for 3 hours.
4. emptied his urinary bladder.

571. One of the *most effective* methods for preventing rheumatic fever is to obtain prompt care whenever persons experience symptoms of
1. cystitis.
2. sinusitis.
3. nephritis.
4. pharyngitis.

572. If a patient with angina pectoris has a choice, it is *best* for him to avoid weather that is
1. dry.
2. warm.
3. cold.
4. humid.

573. A patient who is subject to angina attacks wishes to visit a friend

who lives in a second-floor walk-up apartment. As a prophylactic measure, it would be *best* for the patient to
1. visit the friend as early in the day as possible.
2. take prescribed nitroglycerin before walking the stairs.
3. rest for approximately an hour before walking the stairs.
4. plan to rest immediately after arriving at the friend's apartment.

574. The term, essential hypertension, refers to an elevated blood pressure, the cause of which is
1. unknown.
2. repeated infections.
3. endocrine disturbances.
4. congenital malformations.

575. Which one of the following physical phenomena accounts for the relief of symptoms of fainting (syncope) when the head is lowered?
1. Torque.
2. Gravity.
3. Capillary action.
4. Centrifugal force.

576. When a disease is classified as being idiopathic, the cause is considered to be
1. unknown.
2. hereditary.
3. an allergy.
4. an endocrine deficiency.

577. The system in the body that causes an increase in the activity of the sweat glands is the
1. endocrine system.
2. hemolytopoietic system.
3. sympathetic nervous system.
4. parasympathetic nervous system.

578. During which season of the year do persons with acne vulgaris generally experience noticeable improvement?
1. Fall.
2. Winter.
3. Spring.
4. Summer.

579. The name of the type of skin lesion which causes moisture and weeping of the skin's surface is a
1. macule.
2. papule.
3. pustule.
4. vesicle.

580. It is generally agreed that skin warts are caused by a
  1. virus.
  2. fungus.
  3. protozoa.
  4. bacillus.
581. The louse that causes pediculosis pubis is *most often* spread by
  1. excreta.
  2. sexual contact.
  3. clothing and linens.
  4. bathing and showering facilities.
582. The *most predominant* symptom in affected body areas when a person has scabies is
  1. pain.
  2. itching.
  3. swelling.
  4. numbness.
583. A characteristic of the organisms that cause Vincent's gingivitis (trench mouth) is that they
  1. succumb readily to heat.
  2. survive without free oxygen.
  3. live within protective cysts.
  4. are resistant to most antibiotics.
584. A nurse caring for a patient with tic douloureux (trigeminal neuralgia) should be prepared to care for a patient whose *most common* symptom in the affected area is
  1. pain.
  2. swelling.
  3. numbness.
  4. paralysis.
585. The instrument required for examining a patient by auscultation is a
  1. speculum.
  2. tonometer.
  3. stethoscope.
  4. mercury manometer.
586. Which one of the following abbreviations mean "before meals"?
  1. a.a
  2. a.c.
  3. p.c.
  4. q.s.
587. A patient hospitalized for diabetes mellitus made this comment: "I forgot to save a urine specimen, but why bother? I know I am all right and don't even know why I am here." In which stage of illness can the nurse judge this patient is *most likely* to

be?

1. Late stage.
2. Early stage.
3. State of dependency.

588. A patient with a diagnosis of osteoporosis should be taught to be *particularly* careful to avoid accidents involved with
   1. cuts.
   2. burns.
   3. falls.
   4. abrasions.

589. Addison's disease is characterized by an increase in the body's excretion of the electrolyte
   1. sodium.
   2. calcium.
   3. chloride.
   4. potassium.

590. Most authorities are of the opinion that the *best* way to decide whether respiratory failure is present is to
   1. determine levels of blood gases.
   2. determine levels of serum electrolytes.
   3. compare respiratory rates with severity of dyspnea.
   4. compare amounts of cyanosis with respiratory rates.

591. Of the measures listed below, the *first* one to carry out when managing an acute respiratory emergency is to
   1. start oxygen therapy.
   2. provide an open airway.
   3. give mouth-to-mouth resuscitation.
   4. start giving sodium bicarbonate intravenously.

592. The body's chemoreceptors for respirations influence breathing because these receptors are particularly sensitive to blood levels of
   1. oxygen.
   2. uric acid.
   3. bicarbonates.
   4. carbon dioxide.

593. *All* of the following drugs are used to relax and dilate bronchial musculature *except*
   1. potassium iodide.
   2. isoproterenol (Isuprel).
   3. methoxyphenamine (Orthoxine).
   4. theophylline ethylenediamine (aminophylline).

594. The *primary* purpose of using the "sigh" mechanism for a patient on a volume respirator is to help
   1. clear the upper respiratory tract of debris.

2. inflate areas of the lung that are hypoventilating.

3. increase the turbulance of the air as it enters the lungs.

4. decrease the monotony of the respirator's rhythm and depth.

595. Which one of the following pieces of equipment should the nurse have in readiness when she is assisting with the insertion of an endotracheal tube?
1. An S tube.
2. A bronchoscope.
3. A laryngoscope.
4. A flashlight and tongue blade.

596. A patient has splashed acid in his eye while cleaning his swimming pool. Of the following courses of action, which one should the nurse suggest that the patient do *first*?
1. Place any mild ointment or white petrolatum in his eye.
2. Irrigate his eye repeatedly with generous amounts of tap water.
3. Place an eye patch over his eye and go to the nearest hospital emergency room.
4. Instill at least 3 or 4 drops of any commercial brand of eyedrops into his eye.

597. Which one of the following agents is often recommended to be stocked in a first aid kit because, in an emergency, it can be used to produce vomiting quickly and effectively?
1. Acetic acid.
2. Tannic acid.
3. Ipecac syrup.
4. Potassium permanganate.

598. If a patient in shock is breathing satisfactorily, the nurse should next direct her efforts toward assisting with
1. restoring blood volume
2. supporting kidney functioning.
3. providing psychological support.
4. replacing lost serum electrolytes.

599. A patient has a sucking stab wound in the chest wall. Of the following courses of action, the nurse should *first*
1. start to administer oxygen.
2. prepare to do a tracheostomy.
3. apply a pressure bandage over the wound.
4. prepare to intubate the respiratory tract.

600. Statement A below is a correct statement. What is the relationship between statements A and B?
Statement A: The peritoneum is a semipermeable membrane.
Statement B: Peritoneal dialysis is *ineffective* for helping to restore the body's electrolyte balance.

1. Statement B is true; statement A explains or confirms statement B.
2. Statement B is true; statement A neither helps explain nor confirm statement B.
3. Statement B is false; statement A contradicts or indicates the falsity of statement B.
4. Statement B is false; statement A neither contradicts nor indicates the falsity of statement B.

601. Steam under pressure is especially effective for sterilization purposes because the pressure acts to
1. penetrate the items being sterilized.
2. increase the temperature of the steam.
3. penetrate cell walls of microorganisms.
4. retain a constant temperature in the autoclave.

602. Which of the following types of cells are *most sensitive* to radiation therapy?
1. Bone cells.
2. Muscle cells.
3. Connective tissue cells.
4. Gastrointestinal epithelial cells.

603. Most authorities agree that the *best* way to get rid of unused portions of medications is to
1. burn them in an incinerator.
2. return them to the pharmacy from which they were purchased.
3. place them in the toilet and flush them into the sewage system.
4. wrap them in several thicknesses of heavy plastic and place them in the garbage.

604. It has been observed that people who continue working after age 65 tend to live longer than those who retire. Which one of the following statements *best* expresses the opinion most authorities take regarding this observation?
1. Most authorities take the position that there is as yet no good explanation for the observation.
2. More health care is available to workers than to nonworkers after age 65.
3. The majority of people who are in good health at age 65 continue to work and those in failing health tend to retire.
4. Working people tend to be motivated people and are inclined to practice more healthful living habits than nonworkers.

605. Preoccupation with one's own culture and judging other cultures as inferior to one's own is called
1. holism.
2. relativism.
3. acculturation.

4. ethnocentrism.

606. *All* of the following acts use nonverbal communication *except*
   1. crying.
   2. painting a picture.
   3. listening to a speech.
   4. grasping the hand in greeting.

607. According to sociological research, which one of the following statements is *most accurate* in relation to marriage/divorce in the United States?
   1. Couples in high income brackets have higher divorce rates than couples in low income brackets.
   2. Couples who are quarrelsome are no more likely to divorce than couples who appear to be congenial.
   3. Teenage marriages are less likely to end in divorce than those contracted between persons in their 20's and 30's.
   4. Couples having children during the first year of marriage are less likely to divorce than couples having children later in marriage.

608. As a cause of death in the United States, malignant diseases rank
   1. first.
   2. second.
   3. third.
   4. fourth.

609. In contrast to statistics gathered early in this century, statistics today demonstrate that cardiovascular diseases are a major cause of death in the United States, *primarily* because
   1. there has been an increase in amounts of tension in daily living.
   2. the number of elderly persons in the population has been on the increase.
   3. genetic factors related to these diseases have not been controlled effectively.
   4. public education in relation to methods of controlling these diseases has been largely ineffective.

answer sheet for medical nursing

Read each question in the examination carefully and select which one of the options is the *best* or *correct* answer. If the answer you would prefer is not given, select the one which seems *most appropriate*.

Locate on the answer sheet the number of the item you are answering. With a pencil, blacken the circle corresponding to the answer you have selected. Be sure you are recording your answer in the proper space.

	1 2 3 4		1 2 3 4		1 2 3 4		1 2 3 4
1	○○○○	18	○○○○	35	○○○○	52	○○○○
2	○○○○	19	○○○○	36	○○○○	53	○○○○
3	○○○○	20	○○○○	37	○○○○	54	○○○○
4	○○○○	21	○○○○	38	○○○○	55	○○○○
5	○○○○	22	○○○○	39	○○○○	56	○○○○
6	○○○○	23	○○○○	40	○○○○	57	○○○○
7	○○○○	24	○○○○	41	○○○○	58	○○○○
8	○○○○	25	○○○○	42	○○○○	59	○○○○
9	○○○○	26	○○○○	43	○○○○	60	○○○○
10	○○○○	27	○○○○	44	○○○○	61	○○○○
11	○○○○	28	○○○○	45	○○○○	62	○○○○
12	○○○○	29	○○○○	46	○○○○	63	○○○○
13	○○○○	30	○○○○	47	○○○○	64	○○○○
14	○○○○	31	○○○○	48	○○○○	65	○○○○
15	○○○○	32	○○○○	49	○○○○	66	○○○○
16	○○○○	33	○○○○	50	○○○○	67	○○○○
17	○○○○	34	○○○○	51	○○○○	68	○○○○

	1 2 3 4		1 2 3 4		1 2 3 4		1 2 3 4
69	○○○○	91	○○○○	113	○○○○	135	○○○○
70	○○○○	92	○○○○	114	○○○○	136	○○○○
71	○○○○	93	○○○○	115	○○○○	137	○○○○
72	○○○○	94	○○○○	116	○○○○	138	○○○○
73	○○○○	95	○○○○	117	○○○○	139	○○○○
74	○○○○	96	○○○○	118	○○○○	140	○○○○
75	○○○○	97	○○○○	119	○○○○	141	○○○○
76	○○○○	98	○○○○	120	○○○○	142	○○○○
77	○○○○	99	○○○○	121	○○○○	143	○○○○
78	○○○○	100	○○○○	122	○○○○	144	○○○○
79	○○○○	101	○○○○	123	○○○○	145	○○○○
80	○○○○	102	○○○○	124	○○○○	146	○○○○
81	○○○○	103	○○○○	125	○○○○	147	○○○○
82	○○○○	104	○○○○	126	○○○○	148	○○○○
83	○○○○	105	○○○○	127	○○○○	149	○○○○
84	○○○○	106	○○○○	128	○○○○	150	○○○○
85	○○○○	107	○○○○	129	○○○○	151	○○○○
86	○○○○	108	○○○○	130	○○○○	152	○○○○
87	○○○○	109	○○○○	131	○○○○	153	○○○○
88	○○○○	110	○○○○	132	○○○○	154	○○○○
89	○○○○	111	○○○○	133	○○○○	155	○○○○
90	○○○○	112	○○○○	134	○○○○	156	○○○○

	1 2 3 4		1 2 3 4		1 2 3 4		1 2 3 4
157	○○○○	179	○○○○	201	○○○○	223	○○○○
158	○○○○	180	○○○○	202	○○○○	224	○○○○
159	○○○○	181	○○○○	203	○○○○	225	○○○○
160	○○○○	182	○○○○	204	○○○○	226	○○○○
161	○○○○	183	○○○○	205	○○○○	227	○○○○
162	○○○○	184	○○○○	206	○○○○	228	○○○○
163	○○○○	185	○○○○	207	○○○○	229	○○○○
164	○○○○	186	○○○○	208	○○○○	230	○○○○
165	○○○○	187	○○○○	209	○○○○	231	○○○○
166	○○○○	188	○○○○	210	○○○○	232	○○○○
167	○○○○	189	○○○○	211	○○○○	233	○○○○
168	○○○○	190	○○○○	212	○○○○	234	○○○○
169	○○○○	191	○○○○	213	○○○○	235	○○○○
170	○○○○	192	○○○○	214	○○○○	236	○○○○
171	○○○○	193	○○○○	215	○○○○	237	○○○○
172	○○○○	194	○○○○	216	○○○○	238	○○○○
173	○○○○	195	○○○○	217	○○○○	239	○○○○
174	○○○○	196	○○○○	218	○○○○	240	○○○○
175	○○○○	197	○○○○	219	○○○○	241	○○○○
176	○○○○	198	○○○○	220	○○○○	242	○○○○
177	○○○○	199	○○○○	221	○○○○	243	○○○○
178	○○○○	200	○○○○	222	○○○○	244	○○○○

	1 2 3 4		1 2 3 4		1 2 3 4		1 2 3 4
245	○○○○	267	○○○○	289	○○○○	311	○○○○
246	○○○○	268	○○○○	290	○○○○	312	○○○○
247	○○○○	269	○○○○	291	○○○○	313	○○○○
248	○○○○	270	○○○○	292	○○○○	314	○○○○
249	○○○○	271	○○○○	293	○○○○	315	○○○○
250	○○○○	272	○○○○	294	○○○○	316	○○○○
251	○○○○	273	○○○○	295	○○○○	317	○○○○
252	○○○○	274	○○○○	296	○○○○	318	○○○○
253	○○○○	275	○○○○	297	○○○○	319	○○○○
254	○○○○	276	○○○○	298	○○○○	320	○○○○
255	○○○○	277	○○○○	299	○○○○	321	○○○○
256	○○○○	278	○○○○	300	○○○○	322	○○○○
257	○○○○	279	○○○○	301	○○○○	323	○○○○
258	○○○○	280	○○○○	302	○○○○	324	○○○○
259	○○○○	281	○○○○	303	○○○○	325	○○○○
260	○○○○	282	○○○○	304	○○○○	326	○○○○
261	○○○○	283	○○○○	305	○○○○	327	○○○○
262	○○○○	284	○○○○	306	○○○○	328	○○○○
263	○○○○	285	○○○○	307	○○○○	329	○○○○
264	○○○○	286	○○○○	308	○○○○	330	○○○○
265	○○○○	287	○○○○	309	○○○○	331	○○○○
266	○○○○	288	○○○○	310	○○○○	332	○○○○

	1 2 3 4		1 2 3 4		1 2 3 4		1 2 3 4
333	○○○○	355	○○○○	377	○○○○	399	○○○○
334	○○○○	356	○○○○	378	○○○○	400	○○○○
335	○○○○	357	○○○○	379	○○○○	401	○○○○
336	○○○○	358	○○○○	480	○○○○	402	○○○○
337	○○○○	359	○○○○	381	○○○○	403	○○○○
338	○○○○	360	○○○○	382	○○○○	404	○○○○
339	○○○○	361	○○○○	383	○○○○	405	○○○○
340	○○○○	362	○○○○	384	○○○○	406	○○○○
341	○○○○	363	○○○○	385	○○○○	407	○○○○
342	○○○○	364	○○○○	386	○○○○	408	○○○○
343	○○○○	365	○○○○	387	○○○○	409	○○○○
344	○○○○	366	○○○○	388	○○○○	410	○○○○
345	○○○○	367	○○○○	389	○○○○	411	○○○○
346	○○○○	368	○○○○	390	○○○○	412	○○○○
347	○○○○	369	○○○○	391	○○○○	413	○○○○
348	○○○○	370	○○○○	392	○○○○	414	○○○○
349	○○○○	371	○○○○	393	○○○○	415	○○○○
350	○○○○	372	○○○○	394	○○○○	416	○○○○
351	○○○○	373	○○○○	395	○○○○	417	○○○○
352	○○○○	374	○○○○	396	○○○○	418	○○○○
353	○○○○	375	○○○○	397	○○○○	419	○○○○
354	○○○○	376	○○○○	398	○○○○	420	○○○○

	1 2 3 4		1 2 3 4		1 2 3 4		1 2 3 4
421	○○○○	443	○○○○	465	○○○○	487	○○○○
422	○○○○	444	○○○○	466	○○○○	488	○○○○
423	○○○○	445	○○○○	467	○○○○	489	○○○○
424	○○○○	446	○○○○	468	○○○○	490	○○○○
425	○○○○	447	○○○○	469	○○○○	491	○○○○
426	○○○○	448	○○○○	470	○○○○	492	○○○○
427	○○○○	449	○○○○	471	○○○○	493	○○○○
428	○○○○	450	○○○○	472	○○○○	494	○○○○
429	○○○○	451	○○○○	473	○○○○	495	○○○○
430	○○○○	452	○○○○	474	○○○○	496	○○○○
431	○○○○	453	○○○○	475	○○○○	497	○○○○
432	○○○○	454	○○○○	476	○○○○	498	○○○○
433	○○○○	455	○○○○	477	○○○○	499	○○○○
434	○○○○	456	○○○○	478	○○○○	500	○○○○
435	○○○○	457	○○○○	479	○○○○	501	○○○○
436	○○○○	458	○○○○	480	○○○○	502	○○○○
437	○○○○	459	○○○○	481	○○○○	503	○○○○
438	○○○○	460	○○○○	482	○○○○	504	○○○○
439	○○○○	461	○○○○	483	○○○○	505	○○○○
440	○○○○	462	○○○○	484	○○○○	506	○○○○
441	○○○○	463	○○○○	485	○○○○	507	○○○○
442	○○○○	464	○○○○	486	○○○○	508	○○○○

	1 2 3 4		1 2 3 4		1 2 3 4		1 2 3 4
509	○○○○	531	○○○○	553	○○○○	575	○○○○
510	○○○○	532	○○○○	554	○○○○	576	○○○○
511	○○○○	533	○○○○	555	○○○○	577	○○○○
512	○○○○	534	○○○○	556	○○○○	578	○○○○
513	○○○○	535	○○○○	557	○○○○	579	○○○○
514	○○○○	536	○○○○	558	○○○○	580	○○○○
515	○○○○	537	○○○○	559	○○○○	581	○○○○
516	○○○○	538	○○○○	560	○○○○	582	○○○○
517	○○○○	539	○○○○	561	○○○○	583	○○○○
518	○○○○	540	○○○○	562	○○○○	584	○○○○
519	○○○○	541	○○○○	563	○○○○	585	○○○○
520	○○○○	542	○○○○	564	○○○○	586	○○○○
521	○○○○	543	○○○○	565	○○○○	587	○○○○
522	○○○○	544	○○○○	566	○○○○	588	○○○○
523	○○○○	545	○○○○	567	○○○○	589	○○○○
524	○○○○	546	○○○○	568	○○○○	590	○○○○
525	○○○○	547	○○○○	569	○○○○	591	○○○○
526	○○○○	548	○○○○	570	○○○○	592	○○○○
527	○○○○	549	○○○○	571	○○○○	593	○○○○
528	○○○○	550	○○○○	572	○○○○	594	○○○○
529	○○○○	551	○○○○	573	○○○○	595	○○○○
530	○○○○	552	○○○○	574	○○○○	596	○○○○

	1 2 3 4		1 2 3 4		1 2 3 4		1 2 3 4
597	○○○○	600	○○○○	603	○○○○	606	○○○○
598	○○○○	601	○○○○	604	○○○○	607	○○○○
599	○○○○	602	○○○○	605	○○○○	608	○○○○

	1 2 3 4
609	○○○○

answer sheet for medical nursing

Read each question in the examination carefully and select which one of the options is the *best* or *correct* answer. If the answer you would prefer is not given, select the one which seems *most appropriate*.

Locate on the answer sheet the number of the item you are answering. With a pencil, blacken the circle corresponding to the answer you have selected. Be sure you are recording your answer in the proper space.

	1 2 3 4		1 2 3 4		1 2 3 4		1 2 3 4
1	○○○○	18	○○○○	35	○○○○	52	○○○○
2	○○○○	19	○○○○	36	○○○○	53	○○○○
3	○○○○	20	○○○○	37	○○○○	54	○○○○
4	○○○○	21	○○○○	38	○○○○	55	○○○○
5	○○○○	22	○○○○	39	○○○○	56	○○○○
6	○○○○	23	○○○○	40	○○○○	57	○○○○
7	○○○○	24	○○○○	41	○○○○	58	○○○○
8	○○○○	25	○○○○	42	○○○○	59	○○○○
9	○○○○	26	○○○○	43	○○○○	60	○○○○
10	○○○○	27	○○○○	44	○○○○	61	○○○○
11	○○○○	28	○○○○	45	○○○○	62	○○○○
12	○○○○	29	○○○○	46	○○○○	63	○○○○
13	○○○○	30	○○○○	47	○○○○	64	○○○○
14	○○○○	31	○○○○	48	○○○○	65	○○○○
15	○○○○	32	○○○○	49	○○○○	66	○○○○
16	○○○○	33	○○○○	50	○○○○	67	○○○○
17	○○○○	34	○○○○	51	○○○○	68	○○○○

	1 2 3 4		1 2 3 4		1 2 3 4		1 2 3 4
69	○○○○	91	○○○○	113	○○○○	135	○○○○
70	○○○○	92	○○○○	114	○○○○	136	○○○○
71	○○○○	93	○○○○	115	○○○○	137	○○○○
72	○○○○	94	○○○○	116	○○○○	138	○○○○
73	○○○○	95	○○○○	117	○○○○	139	○○○○
74	○○○○	96	○○○○	118	○○○○	140	○○○○
75	○○○○	97	○○○○	119	○○○○	141	○○○○
76	○○○○	98	○○○○	120	○○○○	142	○○○○
77	○○○○	99	○○○○	121	○○○○	143	○○○○
78	○○○○	100	○○○○	122	○○○○	144	○○○○
79	○○○○	101	○○○○	123	○○○○	145	○○○○
80	○○○○	102	○○○○	124	○○○○	146	○○○○
81	○○○○	103	○○○○	125	○○○○	147	○○○○
82	○○○○	104	○○○○	126	○○○○	148	○○○○
83	○○○○	105	○○○○	127	○○○○	149	○○○○
84	○○○○	106	○○○○	128	○○○○	150	○○○○
85	○○○○	107	○○○○	129	○○○○	151	○○○○
86	○○○○	108	○○○○	130	○○○○	152	○○○○
87	○○○○	109	○○○○	131	○○○○	153	○○○○
88	○○○○	110	○○○○	132	○○○○	154	○○○○
89	○○○○	111	○○○○	133	○○○○	155	○○○○
90	○○○○	112	○○○○	134	○○○○	156	○○○○

	1 2 3 4		1 2 3 4		1 2 3 4		1 2 3 4
157	○○○○	179	○○○○	201	○○○○	223	○○○○
158	○○○○	180	○○○○	202	○○○○	224	○○○○
159	○○○○	181	○○○○	203	○○○○	225	○○○○
160	○○○○	182	○○○○	204	○○○○	226	○○○○
161	○○○○	183	○○○○	205	○○○○	227	○○○○
162	○○○○	184	○○○○	206	○○○○	228	○○○○
163	○○○○	185	○○○○	207	○○○○	229	○○○○
164	○○○○	186	○○○○	208	○○○○	230	○○○○
165	○○○○	187	○○○○	209	○○○○	231	○○○○
166	○○○○	188	○○○○	210	○○○○	232	○○○○
167	○○○○	189	○○○○	211	○○○○	233	○○○○
168	○○○○	190	○○○○	212	○○○○	234	○○○○
169	○○○○	191	○○○○	213	○○○○	235	○○○○
170	○○○○	192	○○○○	214	○○○○	236	○○○○
171	○○○○	193	○○○○	215	○○○○	237	○○○○
172	○○○○	194	○○○○	216	○○○○	238	○○○○
173	○○○○	195	○○○○	217	○○○○	239	○○○○
174	○○○○	196	○○○○	218	○○○○	240	○○○○
175	○○○○	197	○○○○	219	○○○○	241	○○○○
176	○○○○	198	○○○○	220	○○○○	242	○○○○
177	○○○○	199	○○○○	221	○○○○	243	○○○○
178	○○○○	200	○○○○	222	○○○○	244	○○○○

	1 2 3 4		1 2 3 4		1 2 3 4		1 2 3 4
245	○○○○	267	○○○○	289	○○○○	311	○○○○
246	○○○○	268	○○○○	290	○○○○	312	○○○○
247	○○○○	269	○○○○	291	○○○○	313	○○○○
248	○○○○	270	○○○○	292	○○○○	314	○○○○
249	○○○○	271	○○○○	293	○○○○	315	○○○○
250	○○○○	272	○○○○	294	○○○○	316	○○○○
251	○○○○	273	○○○○	295	○○○○	317	○○○○
252	○○○○	274	○○○○	296	○○○○	318	○○○○
253	○○○○	275	○○○○	297	○○○○	319	○○○○
254	○○○○	276	○○○○	298	○○○○	320	○○○○
255	○○○○	277	○○○○	299	○○○○	321	○○○○
256	○○○○	278	○○○○	300	○○○○	322	○○○○
257	○○○○	279	○○○○	301	○○○○	323	○○○○
258	○○○○	280	○○○○	302	○○○○	324	○○○○
259	○○○○	281	○○○○	303	○○○○	325	○○○○
260	○○○○	282	○○○○	304	○○○○	326	○○○○
261	○○○○	283	○○○○	305	○○○○	327	○○○○
262	○○○○	284	○○○○	306	○○○○	328	○○○○
263	○○○○	285	○○○○	307	○○○○	329	○○○○
264	○○○○	286	○○○○	308	○○○○	330	○○○○
265	○○○○	287	○○○○	309	○○○○	331	○○○○
266	○○○○	288	○○○○	310	○○○○	332	○○○○

	1 2 3 4		1 2 3 4		1 2 3 4		1 2 3 4
333	○○○○	355	○○○○	377	○○○○	399	○○○○
334	○○○○	356	○○○○	378	○○○○	400	○○○○
335	○○○○	357	○○○○	379	○○○○	401	○○○○
336	○○○○	358	○○○○	480	○○○○	402	○○○○
337	○○○○	359	○○○○	381	○○○○	403	○○○○
338	○○○○	360	○○○○	382	○○○○	404	○○○○
339	○○○○	361	○○○○	383	○○○○	405	○○○○
340	○○○○	362	○○○○	384	○○○○	406	○○○○
341	○○○○	363	○○○○	385	○○○○	407	○○○○
342	○○○○	364	○○○○	386	○○○○	408	○○○○
343	○○○○	365	○○○○	387	○○○○	409	○○○○
344	○○○○	366	○○○○	388	○○○○	410	○○○○
345	○○○○	367	○○○○	389	○○○○	411	○○○○
346	○○○○	368	○○○○	390	○○○○	412	○○○○
347	○○○○	369	○○○○	391	○○○○	413	○○○○
348	○○○○	370	○○○○	392	○○○○	414	○○○○
349	○○○○	371	○○○○	393	○○○○	415	○○○○
350	○○○○	372	○○○○	394	○○○○	416	○○○○
351	○○○○	373	○○○○	395	○○○○	417	○○○○
352	○○○○	374	○○○○	396	○○○○	418	○○○○
353	○○○○	375	○○○○	397	○○○○	419	○○○○
354	○○○○	376	○○○○	398	○○○○	420	○○○○

	1 2 3 4		1 2 3 4		1 2 3 4		1 2 3 4
421	○○○○	443	○○○○	465	○○○○	487	○○○○
422	○○○○	444	○○○○	466	○○○○	488	○○○○
423	○○○○	445	○○○○	467	○○○○	489	○○○○
424	○○○○	446	○○○○	468	○○○○	490	○○○○
425	○○○○	447	○○○○	469	○○○○	491	○○○○
426	○○○○	448	○○○○	470	○○○○	492	○○○○
427	○○○○	449	○○○○	471	○○○○	493	○○○○
428	○○○○	450	○○○○	472	○○○○	494	○○○○
429	○○○○	451	○○○○	473	○○○○	495	○○○○
430	○○○○	452	○○○○	474	○○○○	496	○○○○
431	○○○○	453	○○○○	475	○○○○	497	○○○○
432	○○○○	454	○○○○	476	○○○○	498	○○○○
433	○○○○	455	○○○○	477	○○○○	499	○○○○
434	○○○○	456	○○○○	478	○○○○	500	○○○○
435	○○○○	457	○○○○	479	○○○○	501	○○○○
436	○○○○	458	○○○○	480	○○○○	502	○○○○
437	○○○○	459	○○○○	481	○○○○	503	○○○○
438	○○○○	460	○○○○	482	○○○○	504	○○○○
439	○○○○	461	○○○○	483	○○○○	505	○○○○
440	○○○○	462	○○○○	484	○○○○	506	○○○○
441	○○○○	463	○○○○	485	○○○○	507	○○○○
442	○○○○	464	○○○○	486	○○○○	508	○○○○

	1 2 3 4		1 2 3 4		1 2 3 4		1 2 3 4
509	○○○○	531	○○○○	553	○○○○	575	○○○○
510	○○○○	532	○○○○	554	○○○○	576	○○○○
511	○○○○	533	○○○○	555	○○○○	577	○○○○
512	○○○○	534	○○○○	556	○○○○	578	○○○○
513	○○○○	535	○○○○	557	○○○○	579	○○○○
514	○○○○	536	○○○○	558	○○○○	580	○○○○
515	○○○○	537	○○○○	559	○○○○	581	○○○○
516	○○○○	538	○○○○	560	○○○○	582	○○○○
517	○○○○	539	○○○○	561	○○○○	583	○○○○
518	○○○○	540	○○○○	562	○○○○	584	○○○○
519	○○○○	541	○○○○	563	○○○○	585	○○○○
520	○○○○	542	○○○○	564	○○○○	586	○○○○
521	○○○○	543	○○○○	565	○○○○	587	○○○○
522	○○○○	544	○○○○	566	○○○○	588	○○○○
523	○○○○	545	○○○○	567	○○○○	589	○○○○
524	○○○○	546	○○○○	568	○○○○	590	○○○○
525	○○○○	547	○○○○	569	○○○○	591	○○○○
526	○○○○	548	○○○○	570	○○○○	592	○○○○
527	○○○○	549	○○○○	571	○○○○	593	○○○○
528	○○○○	550	○○○○	572	○○○○	594	○○○○
529	○○○○	551	○○○○	573	○○○○	595	○○○○
530	○○○○	552	○○○○	574	○○○○	596	○○○○

	1 2 3 4		1 2 3 4		1 2 3 4		1 2 3 4
597	○○○○	600	○○○○	603	○○○○	606	○○○○
598	○○○○	601	○○○○	604	○○○○	607	○○○○
599	○○○○	602	○○○○	605	○○○○	608	○○○○

	1 2 3 4
609	○○○○

medical nursing examination

correct answers and rationales

1. 2. The various parts of a heartbeat on the electrocardiogram are
2. 4. uniformly identified by letters. The area beginning with the
3. 4. P wave and ending with the QRS complex is called the PR
        interval. The area beginning where the QRS complex termi-
        nates and the T wave begins is the ST segment.
4. 1. Electrocardiogram paper is uniformly calibrated so that a
        small square represents 0.04 second. A large square repre-
        sents 0.20 second.
5. 3. Complete emptying of the atria promotes efficient heart func-
        tioning. The slight delay of electrical impulse at the AV node
        allows this to occur.
6. 4. The heartbeat normally begins in cardiac muscle cells. The
        autonomic nervous system provides nervous innervation.
7. 2. Cardiac muscle cells that have the most rapid inherent rhythm
        are found in the SA node. This knot of modified myocardium
        is called the pacemaker because the heartbeat normally be-
        gins in this area of the heart.
8. 1. Each deflection on an electrocardiogram represents an elec-
9. 1. trical phenomenon in heart muscle. The P wave represents
        atrial depolarization; the QRS segment represents ventricular
        depolarization; and the T wave represents ventricular re-
        polarization.
10. 2. Atrial repolarization is slow and of low amplitude and, hence,
        is not ordinarily visible on an electrocardiogram.

11. 3. Each QRS complex represents a heartbeat. Refer to item 4. There is 0.60 second between each QRS complex: $60 \div 0.6 = 100$ beats per minute.

12. 3. The heart rate of the patient is below 60 per minute. A slow heart rate is called sinus bradycardia.

13. 4. An abnormally large Q wave is characteristic of a patient who had a myocardial infarction some time ago.

14. 4. The electrical stimulus of an artificial pacemaker appears as a small line on the electrocardiogram, immediately preceding the QRS complex.

15. 3. In contrast to a fixed rate pacemaker, a demand pacemaker functions only when the heart requires electrical stimulation.

16. 2. It is recommended to allow the frightened patient opportunity to express his fears rather than suggesting that there is no need for concern or handing him a manual to read. Listening to the patient's fears offers the nurse an opportunity for selecting appropriate nursing intervention measures that may be possible to help alleviate fears.

17. 3. The microwave range *may* interfere with proper pacemaker functioning. Microwaves are of a particular frequency and wave length of electromagnetic energy. They may be picked up by the pacemaker and cause heart stimulation. Some of the newest microwave ranges on the market are advertised as safe for patients with pacemakers.

18. 1. The P wave, which represents atrial contraction, is distorted when atrial contractions are distorted. PAC's and PAT's describe improper atrial functioning.

19. 1. Impulses begin in the atria but outside the SA node when PAC's and PAT's are present.

20. 3. Ventricular tachycardia results when contractions occur from an ectopic focus below the AV node in the ventricles. Hence, the atria and the ventricles contract independently of each other.

21. 4. PVC's originate below the AV node in the heart in the myocardium of the ventricles.

22. 4. The commonly accepted definition of sinus tachycardia is a cardiac rate of over 100 beats per minute.

23. 3. Cardioversion is a timed electrical shock. It is synchronized so that the electrical output does not hit a T wave. Electrical defibrillation requires no timing and synchronization since there are no T waves in ventricular fibrillation.

24. 1. If the operator touches the patient or the bed, the operator may act as a ground for the current and receive a shock.

25. 4. For best results, the center of one paddle is applied just to the right of the upper sternum in the second interspace; the rim of

the second paddle is placed just below the left nipple.

26. 3. Distortions on the electrocardiogram occur, as illustrated here, when the patient moves about in bed.

27. 4. The U wave follows the T wave on the electrocardiogram. It *may* be present in healthy persons. However, its presence is commonly seen when there is a deficiency of potassium in the blood, and the nurse should be prepared to carry out orders that will help to correct hypokalemia.

28. 3. Elasticized stockings are commonly used to decrease the threat of emboli formation because they help prevent venous stasis in the legs, thus decreasing the threat of emboli. Allowing commode privileges provides minimum exercise and, therefore, will be relatively ineffective to help prevent emboli formation. Digoxin acts to influence the heartbeat and heart rate.

29. 1. Digitalis acts to slow the conduction of electrical impulses in the heart. It is useful for the treatment of congestive heart failure and of various arrhythmias.

30. 1. Atropine sulfate has a blocking effect upon cholinergic nerve pathways and, hence, blocks vagal responses. Side effects of atropine sulfate include heart palpitations and tachycardia, owing to loss of vagal control.

31. 3. Metaraminol bitartrate constricts arterioles and increases the strength of the heartbeat. These actions result in an increase in blood pressure.

32. 3. Lidocaine hydrochloride acts as an anesthetic. Because it helps decrease heart muscle irritability, it is especially useful in controlling cardiac arrhythmias.

33. 3. The most common practice is to notify the physician when the heart rate of a patient taking digitalis falls below 60 beats per minute. Toxicity may be present when the heartbeat becomes excessively slow; the drug may need to be discontinued.

34. 2. Of the electrolytes given, only calcium has been found to be involved in the release of the contractile substances of actin and myosin.

35. 3. Nervous innervation via the autonomic nervous system performs the task of allowing the heart to change its rate or rhythm to meet the body's physiological demands.

36. 4. The innermost surface of the heart is called the endocardium. The fibrous pericardium is the outer layer; the serous pericardium under the fibrous pericardium consists of two layers, one of which is called the epicardium. The middle layer of the heart is called the myocardium.

37. 2. The heart chamber normally receiving blood from body tis-

sues is the right atrium. The blood normally proceeds in this order: right atrium to right ventricle; right ventricle to lungs; lungs to left atrium; left atrium to left ventricle.

38. 2. The valve located between the right ventricle and the right atrium is the tricuspid valve. The bicuspid valve is between the left atrium and the left ventricle. The pulmonary semilunar valve prevents blood from entering the right ventricle from the pulmonary artery. The aortic semilunar valve prevents blood from entering the left ventricle from the aorta.

39. 2. Cardiogenic shock, which often occurs when the circulation is inadequate for body tissues, is characterized by a low blood pressure. A rapid pulse rate is also usually present.

40. 1. It is generally agreed that estrogen helps to protect the female from atherosclerotic changes. Factors described in options 2, 3, and 4 have not been found significant.

EDWARD BROWN

41. 4. Humidity added to oxygen during oxygen therapy does not decrease fire hazards; oxygen, even though humidity has been added, supports combustion. Humidity is added to oxygen in order to help prevent drying of respiratory membranes when oxygen therapy is prescribed.

42. 4. The technique of rotating tourniquets helps to remove blood from the central circulation by temporarily pooling blood in the extremities.

43. 3. Authorities recommend that no one extremity should have a decreased blood flow for longer than 45 minutes in order to help avoid tissue damage in the extremity. Shorter periods are less effective and unnecessary for safety purposes.

44. 3. One extremity is free of a tourniquet while three extremities have tourniquets applied to help prevent risks of tissue damage and emboli formation.

45. 4. The amount of inflation should be slightly above diastolic pressure. Venous flow should be occluded; however, arterial flow should not be completely impeded.

46. 3. Releasing the tourniquets one at a time helps prevent central circulatory overload.

47. 3. The sitting position decreases venous return to the heart, thus helping to lower the right ventricle output and lung congestion. Also, the sitting position allows for maximum space for lung expansion.

48. 2. The characteristic sound when lungs are congested with fluid is a bubbling sound when auscultation is used.

49. 2. Morphine sulfate is given to help alleviate anxiety that is

ordinarily present when patients are suffering with acute pulmonary edema and associated respiratory distress. It is an ineffective drug for affecting nausea, blood pressure, and bronchial secretions.

50. 1. Meralluride sodium acts to help promote the excretion of sodium which if reabsorbed into the blood in the kidneys tends to cause fluid retention. Not all diuretics promote sodium excretion.

51. 2. Digoxin is a glycoside which, in this instance, was used to help strengthen the patient's heartbeat. Digitalis preparations do not decrease the electrical conductivity of the myocardium; rather, they decrease the heart rate by blocking vagal stimulation.

52. 2. Anorexia is a common symptom of digitalis toxicity. So also are nausea and vomiting. The three symptoms given in options 1, 3, and 4 are not associated with digitalis toxicity.

53. 2. A slow pulse rate is indicative of digitalis toxicity. The other three symptoms are not ordinarily associated with digitalis toxicity. See also item 33.

54. 2. A characteristic of a low potassium level is that it sensitizes the heart to digitalis intoxification.

55. 2. A characteristic of chlorthalidone is that it is long-lasting, up to 72 hours after administration. This is probably due to slow absorption from the gastrointestinal tract. Meralluride sodium is fast-acting and, thus, often used when prompt diuresis is desired.

56. 1. A study of daily weights will help decide whether a patient is excreting excess fluid. The other three measures are poor methods for determining the effects of diuretic therapy.

57. 4. When diuretics are given early in the day, the patient's more frequent need to void will not disturb his nighttime rest.

58. 1. Edematous areas are subject to the development of decubitus ulcers since there is interference with the proper blood supply to the skin and underlying tissues. The cause of decubitus ulcers is poor circulation to tissues.

59. 1. The American Heart Association has recommended no more than 0.5 Gm. of salt be used in the daily diet of a patient whose sodium intake is strictly limited.

60. 1. Of the four foods given, only apples are salt free.

61. 3. Bananas are the best source of potassium. The other three foods are low in or free of potassium.

62. 3. Catsup contains salt and is, therefore, contraindicated for this patient. The other three seasonings are salt free.

63. 4. Shortness of breath is a characteristic symptom of congestive

heart failure. It is due to inadequate pulmonary circulation which causes engorgement of the pulmonary vessels and pulmonary edema, thus interfering with adequate lung functioning.

64. 2. Left-sided heart failure most commonly begins in the left ventricle, that chamber of the heart primarily responsible for generating enough pressure to pump blood to all parts of the body.

65. 4. Right-sided heart failure causes an increase in pressure in the right atrium, thus producing pressure in the vena cava. This phenomenon will cause an increase in the central venous pressure.

66. 1. Echocardiography, which is noninvasive, uses sound vibrations which are sent to the heart through the chest wall. The other three measures require needle perforation of the skin and, hence, require sterile technique.

67. 4. Research findings indicate that the most common reason for patients' not taking medications as prescribed is failure to understand directions. The other three reasons, it is reported, were of less significance.

MYRA CONE

68. 4. A myocardial infarction interferes or blocks blood circulation to heart muscle. This causes poor myocardial oxygenation, producing the pain that is characteristically associated when myocardial infarction occurs.

69. 1. The patient suffering from pain characteristically becomes very anxious. Anxiety tends to increase the body's secretions of epinephrine, resulting in an increase in blood pressure.

70. 2. The pain associated with a myocardial infarction is characteristically severe and, therefore, the nurse should first administer the drug prescribed primarily for the relief of pain. In this case, the drug is meperidine hydrochloride.

71. 4. The patient who has had a myocardial infarction may develop complications, such as cardiac arrhythmias, which require prompt intervention measures. Having an intravenous open allows various agents to be administrated intravenously as quickly as necessary.

72. 1. Salt (sodium chloride) is restricted in order to help prevent edema. Sodium retention delays fluid excretion.

73. 2. Furosemide is a diuretic and is often used when pulmonary rales are present. The rales occur when fluid accumulates in lung tissues. The drug is ineffectual for the control of the other three signs/symptoms.

74. 4. When the heart muscle is damaged, the cells release enzymes. The characteristic laboratory finding when the patient has had an acute myocardial infarction is an elevation of serum enzymes. They are reported to be above normal in option 4; the normal range for SGOT is between approximately 8 and 40; the normal range in the female for CPK is between approximately 0 and 14.

75. 4. Levarterenol bitartrate is the drug of choice since it acts to increase blood pressure by constricting peripheral blood vessels. Among the most characteristic signs of cardiogenic shock is a low blood pressure.

76. 3. A serious arrhythmia most often observed in patients who have experienced an acute myocardial infarction is ventricular fibrillations. The other three arrhythmias are not ordinarily associated with a myocardial infarction.

77. 2. A deviation in readings on a scale when a liquid is in a cylinder is due to spaces between the liquid and the cylinder where a miniscus forms. The deviation is called parallax.

78. 3. When reporting the blood pressure, it is common practice to use three numbers when recording the point when muffled sound was first heard (86) and the point when the last distinct sound was heard (76). The number 130, given in this stem, represents systolic pressure.

79. 2. Diastole is that period when the heart's ventricles are relaxed and filling with blood from the atria. Diastolic blood pressure describes the minimum pressure exerted on the walls of the arteries, which occurs when the heart is relaxed between beats.

80. 2. Exercise helps prevent stasis of blood. Stasis predisposes to thrombophlebitis and blood clot formation. Leg exercises *may* help prepare the patient for ambulation and *may* help divert the patient's attention, but these are not reasons of prime importance.

81. 2. The three wrong options state questions which allow the patient the opportunity of answering "yes" or "no," a response that gives the nurse very little information. To plan appropriate intervention, option 2 encourages the patient to express herself more fully and helps the nurse learn more about the patient's feelings.

82. 3. The motion described results in straightening of the shoulder. Motion that increases or straightens an angle between two adjoining parts is called extension. Adduction is motion that moves a part toward the body's midline; abduction is motion that moves a part away from the body's midline; pronation is

used to describe the forearm when the palm of the hand faces downward, or the body when one is lying on the abdomen.

83. 2. See item 82 above.

84. 4. For this patient, physical effort should be limited. Reaching for articles on the night stand is contraindicated. Since this patient is not in pain or shock, the other three activities are not ordinarily contraindicated.

85. 1. It is generally recommended to use nursing measures, such as those described in options 2, 3, and 4, to promote sleep before resorting to the use of sedatives. However, when nursing measures fail, the nurse may judge that a sedative is necessary in order to promote rest and sleep. The indiscriminate use of sedatives is indefensible.

86. 1. There appears to be no rigid formula concerning what is normal in relation to periodicity and duration of sleep. The important thing is that each person follow a pattern of rest that maintains well-being.

87. 4. Research findings have demonstrated that the depth of unconsciousness during deep sleep is greatest for the sense of smell. The depth is least for pain and hearing.

88. 1. When persons have been wakened during REM sleep, they almost all report that they were dreaming. During certain stages of sleep, when REM is absent, persons are in deep sleep; blood pressure is low and oxygen needs are low.

89. 2. Many drugs have been shown to decrease the amount of dreaming during sleep. An example of a drug that does not appear to suppress dreams is chloral hydrate.

90. 3. A person who customarily uses a hypnotic has had dream suppression. When the hypnotic is omitted, REM sleep increases in order for the body to make up for loss of dreaming. This increase in dreaming is often associated with nightmares.

91. 1. Of the signs given, research has demonstrated that the most common symptom when persons are deprived of dreaming is anxiety.

92. 4. This patient, who has had an acute myocardial infarction and is in a coronary care unit, is not ready to be moved to the patio. However, the other three activities are appropriate for helping to prevent sensory deprivation and do not require physical effort. Television programs of a violent nature are usually contraindicated.

93. 3. Of the guides described, the amount of dyspnea the patient experiences offers the best one in relation to activity.

94. 4. As collateral vessels develop, normal blood supply returns to

the heart muscle. Rehabilitation is planned in a manner to allow time for the body to develop collateral vessels in the heart to replace those occluded by the infarction.

95. 1. The nicotine inhaled during smoking stimulates the secretion of epinephrine in the body, and, hence, predisposes the smoker to atherosclerosis.

96. 3. A basic principle of behavior modification is that behavior that is learned and continued is behavior that has been rewarded. No other technique of reinforcement has been found to be as effective as reward.

97. 1. The coronary arteries arise from the aorta; they encircle the heart.

98. 4. There are approximately 2.2 pounds per 1 kilogram;
$3.2 \times 2.2 = $ approximately 7 pounds.

99. 1. Among environmental factors, diet appears to be linked to coronary heart disease most significantly, according to research.

100. 1. When atherosclerosis is present, it has been found that affected arteries show calcified plaques in the intima; there is a tendency for thrombus formation in the presence of these plaques.

101. 2. A certain amount of stress and anxiety appears helpful for the development of normal adaptive behavior. For example, the stress of an examination encourages the student to do extra study, concern about an abnormal symptom helps the person seek out medical attention.

RALPH BERNARD

102. 1. This position allows for best maintenance of the patient's airway by promoting drainage of secretions from the mouth. Adequate ventilation is desirable but an environment that has extra ventilation is not as important as keeping an airway open. Placing the patient's head lower than his body is contraindicated since this position increases intracranial pressure which may promote bleeding in this patient.

103. 3. Incontinence may occur later but the other three symptoms are typical of impending stroke.

104. 1. Hemiplegia is defined as a paralysis of one side of the body. When both legs are paralyzed, the condition is called paraplegia; paralysis of all four extremities is called quadriplegia.

105. 3. Receptive aphasia is defined as a difficulty in understanding the spoken word.

106. 4. An aphasic person is not necessarily deaf or hard of hearing and, hence, speaking more loudly than normal is of little value.

107. 1. The patient may not respond to normal stimuli but may well be able to hear what is being said. Therefore, conversing away from the bedside offers the best action in this situation. Options 2 and 4 avoid the problem at hand.

108. 3. The involved leg of a patient who has hemiplegia characteristically falls into external rotation. Unless the leg is properly supported, as described in the stem, the patient may develop a deformity of the hip.

109. 1. Placing the affected arm into a sleeve first, adjusting the sleeve with the unaffected arm, and then placing the unaffected arm in the other sleeve make it easier to help dress the patient. When undressing the patient, it is usually easier to remove the unaffected arm from the sleeve first.

110. 1. Although decubitus ulcers may develop on the head, the other three areas of the body are more often affected when proper preventive measures are not taken.

111. 3. When blood flow is impeded, the normal pink color of the skin disappears. Therefore, the earliest sign of a decubitus ulcer, which is caused by impaired circulation to the skin and underlying tissues, is that the area appears blanched.

112. 3. Options 1, 2, and 4 are inaccurate statements. Joint motion exercises are an important part of care during the rehabilitation of a patient who has had a stroke. Unless the physician orders to the contrary, the nurse ordinarily starts passive range-of-motion exercises.

113. 3. Bishydroxycoumarin is an anticoagulant. The drug is ordinarily discontinued at the first sign of bleeding. Therefore, if the patient develops epistaxis, the nurse should record and report the condition promptly.

114. 3. For the unconscious patient, it is ordinarily recommended that body temperature be taken rectally. However, the thermometer may stimulate the vagus nerve which is distributed in the abdominal organs as well as in the thorax and neck. This stimulation tends to increase intracranial pressure and increase hemorrhaging. Axillary temperatures would be recommended for this patient while he is unconscious.

115. 3. Fear stimulates the body to produce epinephrine which, in turn, increases the work of the heart. This may add to cerebral hemorrhaging.

116. 2. The patient's airway should be open and free of secretions before beginning oxygen therapy. These goals are best accomplished by keeping the chin up and clearing secretions from the mouth.

117. 4. The stroke patient may have damage to nerves that control the

blinking reflex in the eye. This usually results in the eyelid remaining open which causes drying and irritation to the cornea.

118. 4. The application of pressure often stimulates swallowing. Options 1, 2, and 3 describe methods that are ineffective to stimulate swallowing; placing food on the back of the tongue is likely to produce choking.

119. 4. The most positive method of offering emotional support to this patient is by displaying encouragement and patience. Sympathy, charitableness, and firm discipline have been found to have little supportive value.

120. 4. After the patient's condition improves, being with other patients offers a favorable environment. Options 1, 2, and 3 may be desirable but are of less significance than option 4.

121. 3. When emotional expression is uncontrollable because of organic damage, the behavior is usually most easily interrupted by sharply diverting the patient's attention.

122. 2. To increase the visual field, the partially blind person should be taught to turn his head from side to side. Neglecting to do so may result in accidents, especially when ambulating. Options 1, 3, and 4 are of little value when helping a patient increase his visual field.

123. 1. Wearing an eyepatch is unimportant. Options 2, 3, and 4 increase the patient's ability to ambulate safely. The sling helps prevent subluxation on the affected side.

124. 2. A brain-damaged patient often has good memory for old information but a poor memory for new information. Therefore, practicing in a familiar setting requires less ability to generalize new information.

125. 2. Statistics have shown that hemiplegia most frequently accompanies cerebral thrombosis.

126. 2. An elevated temperature and slow pulse and respiratory rates are most indicative of central nervous system damage and increasing intracranial pressure.

127. 2. Infection in the parotid glands is likely to occur when oral hygiene for an unconscious patient is neglected. The parotid glands have a duct that opens into the vestibule of the mouth.

128. 1. Restricting fluids is an unsatisfactory way to help overcome incontinence and may do the patient harm. Options 2, 3, and 4 are advised.

129. 4. Keeping the environment as simple as possible is less frustrating for a patient with perceptual and visual defects.

130. 3. For the patient with right brain damage, verbal cues are more often effective than visual cues. The opposite is true for the

patient with left brain damage. The location of the damage in the brain tissues determines the specific symptoms the patient will demonstrate.

CARL JONES

131. 4. Options 1, 2, and 3 describe recommended procedure. When the operator flexes the elbows, cardiac compression is likely to be inadequate.
132. 2. The liver, because of its location near the xiphoid process, is the organ most easily damaged when the pressure is exerted over the xiphoid process during resuscitation.
133. 3. Authorities recommend that cardiac compression be carried out 60 times per minute during resuscitation. It is important to have adequate blood flow through the brain; a slower rate may not make this possible and a faster rate does not seem indicated.
134. 2. Authorities recommend that 12 complete respiratory cycles be administered per minute during resuscitation. This rate promotes proper oxygenation of the blood.
135. 2. It has been determined that the patient being resuscitated by mouth-to-mouth resuscitation receives air containing approximately 16 percent oxygen. Normal air contains approximately 20 percent oxygen.
136. 3. The carotid artery is recommended because it is nearest the operator, it is ordinarily easily accessible, and it will usually have a pulse when smaller and less central arteries may be pulseless.
137. 1. When the airway is not clear, it is impossible to inflate the lungs.
138. 3. The reaction of the pupils is the best indication of whether oxygenated blood is reaching the patient's brain. If the pupils remain widely dilated and do not respond, serious brain damage is likely to have occurred.
139. 4. Epinephrine is administered during resuscitation primarily for its ability to improve cardiac activity. Epinephrine has great affinity for adrenergic receptors in cardiac tissue and acts to strengthen and speed the heart rate, as well as increase impulse conduction from atria to ventricles. Epinephrine will constrict arterioles but this is not the primary reason for administering it during resuscitation.
140. 1. The intravenous route is used most frequently for the rapid administration of drugs and solutions in emergency situations.
141. 3. Sodium bicarbonate is very nearly always necessary to combat

metabolic acidosis. The other three drugs *may* be indicated but usually only for selected patients.

142. 3. Option 3 offers a truthful and positive response. Options 1, 2, and 4 are comments less likely to help the anxious patient.
143. 3. The pulse pressure is obtained by subtracting the diastolic pressure from the systolic pressure: $160 - 80 = 80$.
144. 1. Communicating by touch, as for example, holding the patient's hand firmly, is often an effective way to offer the patient emotional support. Options 2, 3, and 4 offer little if any emotional support to the patient in distress.
145. 1. A precordial thump is not recommended for young children. Options 2, 3, and 4 do not describe patients for whom a precordial thump is contraindicated.
146. 1. When cardiac rest is *observed*, the first course of action is to administer a precordial thump. This procedure often is enough to start the heart beating again. Measures described in options 2, 3, and 4 can follow.

MARIA CASELLI

147. 1. Phenformin functions by potentiating the action of insulin; that is, it is insulin-supporting or -inforcing. It does not stimulate the production of insulin, as do oral hypoglycemic agents of the sulfonylureas group.
148. 3. Activities described in options 1, 2, and 4 predispose to poor circulation in the feet. Wearing low-heeled shoes does not. The diabetic patient is prone to serious foot problems when circulation is impeded.
149. 1. To minimize injury to the feet, a patient with diabetes mellitus should avoid going barefoot. Options 2, 3, and 4 are not ordinarily contraindicated.
150. 2. Options 1, 3, and 4 describe satisfactory ways to care for toenails. Cutting the corners of the nails is likely to damage tissues and predispose to ingrown toenails, and can result in serious foot problems, especially for the diabetic patient.
151. 4. Of those agents given, vegetable oil is the preferred one for massaging the feet. The other agents will tend to dry the skin, making abrasions more likely.
152. 2. The diabetic patient should be advised to consult her physician when corns occur. Removing corns for this patient is serious business! There is danger of traumatizing foot tissues.
153. 4. Statistics demonstrate that diabetes mellitus is frequently associated with atherosclerosis.
154. 2. It *may* be necessary to consult a physician, but it is essential

that his patient be taught that a skin break, no matter how small, is worthy of concern.

155. 3. There are 4 calories in each Gm. of carbohydrate and protein and 9 calories in each Gm. of fat:

$190 \times 4 = 760$
$90 \times 9 = 810$
$100 \times 4 = 400$

Total   1970, or approximately 2000

156. 4. It has been determined that one small apple is most nearly equivalent to one-half cup of orange juice.*

157. 1. It has been determined that one slice of bread is most nearly equivalent to one-third cup of corn.*

158. 4. It has been determined that one slice of crisply fried bacon is equivalent to one fat exchange.*

159. 1. It has been determined that 1 ounce of lean meat is equivalent to one egg.*

160. 3. Of the foods given in these 4 options, green and yellow vegetables offer the best supply of vitamin A. Cereals and breads and lean meats are good sources of vitamin B. Citrus fruits are good sources of vitamin C.

161. 2. Statement B is true but not for the reason given in statement A. Since pasta products have been an important part of this patient's diet, she should be taught how to include them in her dietary regimen. To exclude them in her diet may cause the patient to rebel against her diet and/or fail to follow a satisfactory diet.

162. 4. Exercise promotes metabolism and the utilization of carbohydrates, thereby reducing the body's insulin requirements. Exercise is also a healthful diversional activity, is a helpful way to aid weight control, and promotes circulation.

163. 4. Patients described in options 1, 2, and 3 are most likely to require insulin injections. Maturity-onset diabetes is very often effectively controlled with oral antidiabetic drugs.

164. 3. There has been a marked rise in deaths among diabetics due to renal complications. Damage to organs other than the kidneys and cardiovascular system are less life-threatening.

165. 3. Options 1, 2, and 4 describe common eye problems of persons with diabetes. Astigmatism has not been associated with the disease.

*The American Dietetic Association, the American Diabetes Association, and the U.S. Public Health Service have developed four-exchange lists to help the diabetic select a balanced and varied diet. Foods are arranged in exchange lists with foods in each exchange list having about the same caloric and sugar content.

166. 4. The tissues in the body that consume the highest rate of oxygen are in the retina of the eye.
167. 4. Carbohydrates are stored in the body as glycogen. It is formed from glucose into which it is again convertible.
168. 1. When fat is poorly oxidized, ketone bodies begin to accumulate in the bloodstream.
169. 3. Statistics have demonstrated that, of the ethnic groups given here, Eskimos have the lowest incidence of diabetes mellitus. Jews have a particularly high incidence of diabetes, as do American Indians.
170. 1. It is in the kidney tubules that glucose is reabsorbed.
171. 4. Insulin functions in the body to stimulate the proper metabolism of carbohydrates. It plays no role in functions described in options 1, 2, and 3.
172. 3. Adverse reactions have been reported when antiinflammatory agents, such as aspirin, are taken with the sulfonylureas because the combination tends to increase the hypoglycemic effects of these agents.
173. 3. Diabetes insipidus is a disorder characterized by a deficiency of vasopressin, a hormone secreted by the posterior lobe of the pituitary gland.
174. 2. The most characteristic symptoms of diabetes insipidus is a large output of urine with the resulting symptom of thirst.

UROLOGIC PATIENTS

175. 2. Padding the stirrups increases comfort by decreasing pressure on the nerves and blood vessels at the back of the knees. Options 1, 3, and 4 are likely to add to discomfort.
176. 3. Since the discomfort is generally minimal during a cystoscopy, the most commonly used anesthesia is a surface anesthesia which acts to penetrate free nerve endings below the mucosal surface.
177. 4. Using steam under pressure is the safest and most frequently recommended method of sterilization.
178. 4. In the option 4 figure, the nurse is likely to contaminate her gloved hand by grasping that part of the second glove she will pull over the hand and wrist. Better technique would be to slip the fingers of the gloved hand under the cuffed part of the glove and push the glove over the hand without touching any part of the glove that will be in contact with skin.
179. 3. The nurse should avoid plugging the eye of the catheter with lubricant in order to allow for the free flow of urine. Options 1 and 4 are not contraindicated procedures. The lubricant

should be sterile and, therefore, some of it on the gloves will not contaminate the nurse's hand.

180. 1. The bladder will be empty when the urine near the exit of the bladder is also removed. The bladder may not be empty if option 2 behavior is used. Options 3 and 4 are contraindicated because of the danger of introducing organisms into the bladder.

181. 2. While continuing to hold the labia apart, voiding in a forcible manner helps to collect urine which has not "dribbled" about the meatus and external genitalia. Sterile containers are used for the specimen.

182. 4. The urethral meatus should be cleansed *before* obtaining the specimen in order to minimize organisms normally found at the meatus from entering the specimen.

183. 1. The pH of normal urine varies between approximately 4.8 and 8.0. Options 2, 3, and 4 describe findings that are not typical of normal.

184. 1. When collecting a 24-hour urine specimen, the recommended and most accurate procedure is to begin the 24-hour period with an empty bladder and end the collecting period with an empty bladder 24 hours later. *All* urine is saved during the 24-hour collecting period.

185. 3. The most effective exercise for strengthening muscles at and around the urinary meatus is to alternately contract and relax the perineal muscles. This exercise is accomplished when the patient moves muscles as though she wished to alternately stop and start a urinary flow.

186. 1. The most likely cause of discomfort would be that the balloon was inflated in the urethra, causing stretching of the tissues. Options 2, 3, and 4 describe situations that are very unlikely to cause discomfort.

187. 1. An effective way to learn whether a patient is passing renal calculi is to strain his urine. Practices described in options 2, 3, and 4 will not assist effectively in making the diagnosis.

188. 1. Many constituents in the glomerular filtrate are reabsorbed into the bloodstream in the renal tubules. The PSP test examines the ability of the tubules to eliminate (that is, refuse to reabsorb) the injected dye.

189. 2. The most frequently used route for administering dye used in the PSP test is the intravenous route, although the intramuscular route is not contraindicated and is used occasionally.

190. 2. To help avoid diluting the contrast media used for an intravenous pyelogram, preparation of the patient ordinarily includes limiting the fluid intake.

191. 3. Although a variety of conditions may result in cystitis, authorities hold that the most common cause is an ascending infection from the urethra.

192. 4. It is possible that the patient, whose work requires her to be on her feet all day, has orthostatic albuminuria. This is a circulatory phenomenon rather than a disease condition. The patient should be asked to collect a specimen immediately upon arising in the morning in order to help confirm whether or not disease exists.

193. 4. The stresses of hemodialysis therapy, chronic illness, limited life expectancy, and the like, tend to cause patients to suffer depression and feelings of worthlessness. A rather high percentage of patients using hemodialysis demonstrate suicidal tendencies.

194. 1. A study of the patient's weight is most commonly used to estimate how much fluid a patient loses during hemodialysis.

195. 3. Protamine sulfate is presently the drug of choice to counteract the effects of heparin for a patient receiving hemodialysis. The agent is a specific chemical antagonist of heparin.

196. 2. An amendment to the Social Security Act made patients who need hemodialysis eligible for financial assistance.

197. 4. Tea, cocoa, and coffee contain caffeine which acts as a diuretic. Root beer does not contain caffeine.

198. 4. The stretch receptors found in the urinary bladder wall normally arouse the urge to void.

199. 3. Peristaltic waves along the ureters are primarily responsible for moving urine along the ureters.

200. 3. The renal tubules function to reabsorb substances from glomerular filtrate. See item 188 also.

201. 1. The reabsorption of water is accomplished by osmosis. Other substances are reabsorbed by complicated mechanisms that use diffusion and active transport.

202. 2. The antidiuretic hormone (ADH) is *released* from the pituitary gland. The hormone is *produced* in the hypothalamus.

203. 2. Emotional stress causes the body to secrete epinephrine which causes an elevation in the blood sugar level. When the level of blood sugar surpasses the renal threshold concentration, glycosuria can be expected to occur.

204. 2. All of the constituents listed are found in normal urine except albumin. Its presence suggests kidney pathology. See also item 192.

205. 1. *Escherichia coli* have been found to be responsible for approximately 85 percent of urinary tract infections.

206. 4. Circulatory disturbances which cause changes in the renal

blood vessels are responsible for most chronic kidney diseases.

207. 4. The safest method for destroying spores is using steam under pressure. Spores are particularly resistant and are best destroyed by the high temperatures generated in autoclaves.

STEVE OLDEN

208. 3. Oliguria is defined as the subnormal production of urine, less than approximately 20 ml. of urine per hour. Anuria refers to the total suppression of urine. Dysuria is painful urination. Enuresis refers to involuntary urination that occurs during sleep.

209. 1. Acute glomerulonephritis is most often a complication of streptococcal infections.

210. 4. Half-strength hydrogen peroxide is most often recommended for cleansing the mouth and lips of crusted mucus.

211. 2. For the patient whose intake is restricted, it is usually best to serve the patient ice chips. They help moisten the mouth and lips while keeping the fluid intake low. Salty and sweet liquids tend to add to thirst.

212. 2. Nocturnal emissions have been found to be common in about 85 percent of all men. They may occur at any age but usually begin during the teen years. A relatively common misconception is that "wet dreams" are a sign of a sexual disorder. They do not assure the presence of sperm and are not a sign of disease.

213. 2. The person who handles and solves his problems of daily living with relative ease usually has an attitude of self-confidence. Degree of intelligence, relationship with parents, and membership in a particular socioeconomic class in themselves do not appear as essential as attitudes in relation to self-confidence.

214. 3. Proteins and highly spiced foods are ordinarily restricted when acute glomerulonephritis is present. Carbohydrates as described in options 1, 2, and 4 are generally offered liberally.

215. 2. Generally, teenagers enjoy activities with their peers in preference to socializing with younger persons and parents.

216. 2. Teenagers are prone to be moody, concerned with personal appearance, and interested in members of the opposite sex. They are less likely to be submissive.

217. 1. The rate of growth varies among individuals. Options 2, 3, and 4 are false statements in relation to human growth.

218. 1. Few authorities would deny that options 2, 3, and 4 describe

experiences that influence one's personality. The issue of heredity and its effects on personality continues to be more controversial.

LOIS JANTER

219. 4. Increased protein breakdown accounts for the patient's elevated BUN.
220. 4. Protein breakdown which is characteristic of acute renal failure results in the release of cellular potassium and potassium intoxication. Hence, sodium polystyrene sulfonate is given because of its ability to cause the body to excrete potassium through the gastrointestinal tract when the agent exchanges sodium ions for potassium ions.
221. 1. Potassium intoxication predisposes to serious cardiac arrhythmias and cardiac arrest.
222. 4. Protein intake is limited during acute renal failure. The body's caloric needs are met by high carbohydrate feedings.
223. 1. Low protein was prescribed to help minimize protein breakdown.
224. 4. Bananas should be avoided for this patient because they are high in potassium content. Since potassium intoxication may be a threat, potassium intake should be restricted.
225. 2. Although the nurse should check all of the care given here, special precautions should be used to be sure that the patient's intake and output are being recorded accurately since fluid retention often presents a problem for the patient with renal failure.
226. 2. Of the procedures listed, it is most important before dialysis can be started to be sure that the patient has signed a permit form.
227. 3. The peritoneum functions as a semipermeable membrane during dialysis. The dialyzing solution must be hypertonic in order to prevent absorption of water from the solution by the body.
228. 2. Turning the patient from side to side and/or elevating the head of the bed facilitates drainage. The other procedures given here will not promote drainage.
229. 3. Heat causes dilatation of peritoneal vessels and thereby increases urea clearance. Warmed solution also adds to the patient's comfort.
230. 4. Option 4 describes the least helpful report. It is indefinite and describes only one facet of the patient's care.
231. 4. The kidneys have remarkable ability to recover from serious

insult. In view of prompt and effective treatment, the patient's prognosis should be very good.

232. 4. The behavior described here is normal in both men and women as they seek to meet needs for self-esteem and self-respect.

233. 1. Meeting a personal need for status and prestige means paying attention to the person and treating him as a person different from all others. For the patient to feel included and important involves the nurse relating to the patient in a way so that the patient feels as though the nurse is interested in her.

237. 2. Most authorities hold the opinion that organisms are most often spread in health agencies by health practitioners whose hands are not clean. Practices described in options 1, 3, and 4 help to spread organisms but not to the same extent as unclean hands of health personnel.

235. 3. Acute renal failure is defined as a sudden and almost complete loss of kidney function. In this patient's case, kidney function failed because renal circulation was impaired by hemorrhage.

WATER AND ELECTROLYTE BALANCE AND IMBALANCE

236. 3. The level of HCO_3 in arterial and venous blood is approximately the same, between 22 and 26 mEq. per L.

237. 2. pO_2 in venous blood is approximately 35 to 40 mm. Hg. It is approximately 80 to 100 mm. Hg. in arterial blood.

238. 1. pCO_2 in venous blood is approximately 41 to 51 mm. Hg. It is approximately 35 to 45 mm. Hg. in arterial blood.

239. 1. Sodium is the most prevalent extracellular electrolyte. It comprises more than 90 percent of the total cations at its normal concentration of approximately 142 mEq. per L.

240. 3. Normally, the total number of cations is equal to the total number of anions. The total number of cations and anions is approximately 308 mEq. per L., or total cations of 154 mEq. per L. and total anions of 154 mEq. per L.

241. 3. The same holds true for intracellular fluid as for extracellular fluid. See item 240.

242. 2. Potassium is the principal cation of cellular fluid with a normal concentration of approximately 150 mEq. per L. Its plasma concentration is about 5 mEq. per L.

243. 4. Energy and a carrier are necessary to remove ions from cytoplasm through cell membranes. The process is called active transport.

244. 2. Water is formed during the metabolism of food (enogenous water). Relatively little or no fluid is taken into the body by processes described in options 1, 3, and 4.

245. 1. An average well adult eating a balanced diet and exercising moderately loses the following approximate amounts of water daily from the body:

Lungs	350 ml.
Gastrointestinal tract	150 ml.
Skin	500 ml.
Kidneys	1800 ml.

246. 4. Potassium is vitally important for proper neuromuscular changes. It plays no significant role on factors described in options 1, 2, and 3.

247. 1. Sodium excess is most commonly manifested by edema. A predictable outcome follows this rule: The water goes where the salt is.

248. 2. A low calcium plasma concentration increases the excitability of the nervous system until at a critical level, the nerve fibers discharge spontaneously causing skeletal muscles to develop spasms called tetany.

249. 4. Vitamin D is essential for proper calcium absorption.

250. 1. Sodium concentrations in the body influence aldosterone secretions.

251. 3. Potassium is excreted via the body's sweat, urine, and feces. However, the final and greatest responsibility for potassium balance in the body rests with the kidneys.

252. 2. Most diuretics interfere with reabsorption of substances in the kidney tubules. One imbalance resulting from the indiscriminate use of diuretics is hypokalemia when potassium is not being absorbed sufficiently well in the tubules.

253. 4. To compensate when respiratory acidosis is present, the kidneys excrete more acid and less bicarbonate.

254. 2. The equation depicts reversible actions. Options 1, 3, and 4 are false statements.

255. 4. Ridding the body of carbon dioxide is an important function of the lungs. Hence, an important relationship exists between amount of ventilation and the pCO_2 of arterial blood. Values described in options, 1, 2, and 3 are less valuable to determine adequacy of ventilation.

256. 4. The normal relationship is 20:1, at which point the pH is also normal.

257. 2. There are two characteristic conditions associated with abnormalities in HCO_3^- or the base excess: low levels of HCO_3^- and low B.E. are present in metabolic acidosis and high levels of HCO_3^- are present in metabolic alkalosis.

258. 2. When glucose is being excreted via the kidneys in large amounts, the obligatory loss of water and salt may be excessive, resulting in a sodium deficit.

259. 2. The statement is not supported by laboratory findings. A pCO_2 of 40 mm. Hg. falls within the normal range of 35 to 45 mm. Hg.

260. 1. Normal HCO_3^- is between 22 and 26 mEq. per L. Normal B.E. is between -2 and $+2$. The patient's HCO_3^- and B.E. are below normal.

261. 3. The patient who has insufficient ventilation (hypoventilation) will have a high pCO_2. This patient's pCO_2 is within normal range (see item 259). In addition, it is generally considered unwise to base therapy on the findings of one laboratory report.

262. 3. Data for comparison purposes are necessary to make the judgment.

263. 1. The major abnormality when metabolic acidosis is present is a low HCO_3^- which this patient has. See item 257.

264. 1. Normal values for pO_2 and pCO_2 are approximately as follows:

	Alveolar Air	Venous Blood	Arterial Blood
	Measured in mm. Hg.		
pO_2	104	40	100
pCO_2	40	45	40

The patient's laboratory findings fall within normal.

265. 2. When carbon dioxide diffuses into interstitial fluids, most of it diffuses into red blood cells. Some of it then is carried in the bloodstream. This is illustrated in the circle which shows Hgb : CO_2.

266. 1. The equation given near the venous end of the vessel illustrates this phenomenon. The complete equation is usually illustrated as follows:

$$CO_2 + H_2O \rightleftarrows H_2CO_3 \rightleftarrows H^+ + HCO_3^-$$

267. 3. This judgment cannot be made on the basis of information given although all parameters appear within normal.

268. 1. A damaged vein high on the arm makes entry into veins lower on the arm difficult. If a vein low on the arm is damaged, the veins high in the arm are still available.

269. 3. The gauge of a needle describes its diameter. The length of a needle is described in inches. The circumference of the hub and the length of the bevel are not described in terms of size.

270. 1. When cleansing the skin prior to injection, it is recommended that cleansing start at the site of injection and continue outward around it in order to avoid carrying organisms toward the injection site.
271. 2. The thumb helps stabilize the vein. Options 1, 3, and 4 describe factors that are not influenced by the procedure of stabilizing the vein.
272. 1. Options 2, 3, and 4 are inaccurate concerning pressure in the intravenous bottle and in the vein. Gravity normally carries fluids into the vein during intravenous therapy. An exception would be when a pump is used to instill substances into the vein.
273. 1. The patient's blood type does not influence the rate of flow. Factors described in options 2, 3, and 4 can influence it.
274. 2. The stem of this item describes typical findings when infiltration occurs. Phlebitis is characterized by pain, swelling, and redness over the affected vein. There are many different symptoms of allergic reactions, two common ones related to the skin being itching and the appearance of a rash. An air embolism ordinarily is symptom-free, unless the embolism is so large as to threaten life.
275. 2. The number of drops the patient should receive each minute is determined as follows:

$$\frac{3000}{24} = 125 \text{ ml. to be given every hour}$$

$$\frac{125 \text{ ml.} \times 15 \text{ (drop factor)}}{60 \text{ (minutes)}} = \frac{1875}{60} = \text{approximately 32 drops per minute}$$

ANTHONY DORN

276. 1. It has been demonstrated that fear, even when unfounded, can stand in the way of recovery. In this instance, it would be best to eliminate the reason for the patient's fear. Options 3 and 4 do not describe care that has the best interests of the patient in mind. Option 2 has not been proven true, except by chance.
277. 4. Option 4 accurately describes the reason for oxygen therapy being administered at a low level. Options 1, 2, and 3 are inaccurate statements.
278. 1. The friction of oxygen molecules may cause oil to flare up of its own accord.
279. 2. The intravenous is kept open for this patient primarily in order to avoid repeated injections of veins for the administration of prescribed drugs. Also, keeping an intravenous open pro-

vides easy access, should an emergency situation arise that requires intravenous injections of various agents.

280. 2. Theophylline ethylenediamine was prescribed because of the patient's shortness of breath. The prescribed drug acts as a bronchodilator which helps provide maximum passageways for the exchange of air.

281. 3. Amitriptyline hydrochloride acts as an antidepressant.

282. 2. The diaphragm has maximum room for functioning when the patient is in the semi-Fowler's position, since the abdominal organs tend to shift lower and toward the pelvis.

283. 1. Isoetharine hydrochloride is nebulized during IPPB therapy. The drug is then inhaled by the patient.

284. 2. The IPPB machine is constructed so that an inspiratory effort will activate it.

285. 3. The base excess is neither contradicted nor supported since it has not been reported in this example.

286. 1. The patient's pH is falling; acidosis is ordinarily considered to be present when the pH is below 7.35.

287. 1. Alveolar hypoventilation is ordinarily considered to be present when the pCO_2 in arterial blood is above approximately 50 mm. Hg.

288. 3. There is no sound way to judge cardiac output on the basis of these reports. The statement given here cannot be considered supported nor contradicted by laboratory findings.

289. 2. The patient's arterial pO_2 is below normal and falling still farther below normal. Normal pO_2 in arterial blood is between approximately 80 and 100 mm. Hg.

290. 1. Maintaining an adequate fluid intake helps liquify bronchial secretions. Measures described in options 2, 3, and 4 will not influence the nature of secretions.

291. 4. Due to lung pathology (congestion), the right ventricle is carrying a larger-than-normal workload to force blood to the lungs. Hence, the right ventricle is likely to hypertrophy.

292. 1. This patient is very subject to infections, especially along respiratory passages. Permanent improvement and less oxygen requirements are unrealistic.

293. 1. The patient's behavior is characteristic of persons with COPD. The types of behavior described in options 2, 3, and 4 are unlikely explanations.

294. 1. Allowing the patient to express his anger while quietly listening usually helps the patient overcome his feelings of frustration and anxiety. The nurse can then look toward nursing intervention measures so that the cause of the anger may possibly be corrected.

295. 4. Pursed lip breathing increases pressure within the alveoli and makes it easier for the patient to empty the air in the lungs, thereby promoting carbon dioxide elimination.

296. 2. Inhalation normally requires more energy than exhalation. Therefore, in order to use energy when the body is demanding least during respirations, it is helpful to carry out activities during exhalations.

297. 4. Percussion helps loosen mucus mechanically. Deeper inhalations *may* sometimes result but this is not the primary purpose of percussion. Percussion in itself does not improve ciliary action nor propel secretions along respiratory passages.

298. 2. Postural drainage helps move secretions to larger airways through the force of gravity. It is best used after percussion, when secretions have been loosened.

299. 2. Laboratory studies have shown that prolonged periods of inactivity cause the body to excrete larger-than-normal amounts of calcium.

300. 4. Predisposing factors to COPD are characteristically those described in the first three options. Liquor intake is not associated with the disease.

301. 2. It is the hydrogen ion that influences respirations through respiratory center stimulation.

302. 3. The respiratory center is located in the medulla oblongata.

303. 1. Eupnea is defined as normal respirations, or the normal exchange of air.

304. 2. Tidal air is the amount of air exchanged in each normal respiration. Inspiratory reserve air is the volume of air, in excess of the tidal, that can be inhaled by the deepest possible inspiration. Expiratory air is the volume of air, in excess of tidal, that can be exhaled by the deepest possible expiration. Residual air is air remaining in the lungs following maximum exhalation.

305. 3. Oxygen and carbon dioxide diffuse through alveolar tissues.

CARE OF PATIENTS WITH PULMONARY TUBERCULOSIS

306. 3. A positive Mantoux test indicates only that the person has had contact with tubercle bacilli.

307. 4. Although the four treatment measures may all be important, taking medications as prescribed has the highest priority. The modern treatment of tuberculosis with drug therapy has been so successful in arresting and curing tuberculosis that most patients no longer need sanitarium care or surgery.

308. 1. The most commonly used technique to identify tubercle bacilli is acid-fast staining.

309. 1. Authoritative opinion is that unclean hands spread most organisms. All of the techniques described here will help control the spread of organisms but most important, washing the
hands is essential.

310. 1. According to statistics, miliary tuberculosis carries the highest
death rate.

311. 3. Tubercle bacilli may be spread in various ways, the most
common one being by droplet nuclei.

312. 1. The most common side effect of streptomycin is vertigo as a
result of damage to a part of the eighth cranial nerve.

313. 1. Of the symptoms given, deafness is the one associated with
eighth cranial nerve damage. See item 312 above also.

314. 4. It has been found that using a combination of tuberculostatic
drugs slows the rate at which organisms develop resistance to
drugs.

315. 2. While all measures given may play a part in the nursing care of
patients with tuberculosis, being sure the patient is well-
educated about his disease has highest priority.

316. 2. Males and females appear to be about equally susceptible to
tuberculosis. Age, race, and occupation are important
etiological factors.

317. 2. Statistics demonstrate that, of the four geographic areas described, the nurse can expect to find most cases of tuberculosis
in inner core residential areas of large cities, where health and
sanitation standards tend to be low.

BESSIE PETRI

318. 1. Of factors given, this patient's age (79) adds most danger to the
patient's illness. Older patients handle infections, especially
respiratory infections, less well than do younger persons.

319. 4. Friction rub is the most likely cause of the patient's pain and is
frequently present when a patient has pneumonia. The other
options do not describe situations that are likely to cause pain.

320. 4. Due to infection and congestion in her lungs, the patient's
blood is being poorly oxygenated which causes cyanosis.

321. 1. Aspirin is an analgesic since it helps control pain.

322. 4. Abdominal distention minimizes the area in the body in which
normal respiratory functioning occurs, thus adding to the patient's difficulty with breathing.

323. 2. Humidified air helps liquify respiratory secretions. The
measures described in options 1, 3, and 4 may be used for
respiratory hygiene but will not influence the nature of secretions, as humidified air will.

324. 3. Because the patient is having difficulties with breathing and is

coughing, the preferred site to obtain her temperature is the rectum. The groin or axillary sites are usually used only when the oral and rectal sites are contraindicated.

325. 4. Isoproterenol hydrochloride acts to relieve bronchospasms. Acetylcysteine and tyloxapol are mucolytic agents. Deoxyribonuclease helps liquify secretions by its action on cell enzymes.

326. 2. The physician will wish to know what organism is causing the patient's illness in order to prescribe the antibiotic that has been found to be most effective to destroy it.

327. 1. Pneumococci are of the species Diplococcus pneumoniae. These cocci are usually arranged in pairs, although short chains are sometimes observed.

328. 1. Of the agents given, the physician is most likely to prescribe erythromycin since it is an antibiotic with a spectrum similar to penicillin.

329. 3. The organism can be spread in a variety of ways, but of those given, the hands of health personnel are considered most guilty.

330. 3. When hypoxia is present, patients characteristically show evidence of anxiety, and less frequently, signs of the emotions described in options 1, 2, and 4.

331. 1. The electrolyte lost in largest amounts through perspiration is sodium. This accounts for the salty taste of perspiration.

332. 4. Normal total white blood count is between 5,000 and 10,000 per cu. mm. of blood in adults. Since this patient's count is within normal range, there is no need to take action other than to continue with her current regimen.

333. 4. Because of the danger of organisms entering the patient's eustachian tubes, oral hygiene is especially important.

334. 4. Plastic lenses are easily scratched. Chipping, shattering, or warping them is uncommon.

335. 1. Hymoptysis is defined as sputum containing blood. Hematolysis refers to the destruction of red blood cells. Hematemesis is defined as vomitus containing blood. Hemophthisis is a type of anemia.

336. 1. Dioctyl sodium sulfosuccinate is a stool softener and does not function in ways described in options 2, 3, and 4.

337. 2. The patient with a fecal impaction very often passes frequent liquid stools. The watery fecal material seeps around the hardened stool impaction in the rectum.

338. 2. To help soften and lubricate the stool, an oil retention enema is usually used first when a fecal impaction is present.

339. 3. Observing habits of good health serves the body well as a

defense against respiratory infections. Options 1, 2, and 4 describe practices that are impractical or ill-advised.

340. 2. Drugs that control infections have done most to reduce pneumonia morbidity and mortality rates.

SOPHIA LORY

341. 4. The patient with pernicious anemia characteristically seeks medical attention because of fatigue. Symptoms described in options 1, 2, and 3 are uncommon. Energy is poor because of the drop in the red blood count; the body is being poorly oxygenated.

342. 3. Patients with pernicious anemia demonstrate a lack of hydrochloric acid in gastric secretions.

343. 3. Pernicious anemia is caused by the body's inability to absorb vitamin B_{12}. This is caused by a lack of the intrinsic factor in the gastric juices. The Shilling test helps diagnose pernicious anemia by determining the patient's ability to absorb vitamin B_{12}.

344. 3. The red blood cells normally originate in red bone marrow.

345. 2. Patients with pernicious anemia almost always complain of a sore mouth.

346. 3. Vitamin B_{12} is measured in micrograms. One microgram is a millionth of a Gram.

347. 1. Dramatically quick recoveries have been observed in patients, even those very ill with pernicious anemia, after only a few days of therapy. However, permanently damaged tissues will not recover.

348. 2. Vitamin B_{12} therapy must continue for life in order to prevent recurrence of symptoms since the intrinsic factor does not return to gastric secretions, even with therapy.

349. 4. Many patients have been observed to become resistant to vitamin B_{12} when the agent is taken orally. Options 1, 2, and 3 are false statements.

350. 1. Vitamin B_{12} is remarkably free of toxicity.

351. 1. The elderly patient tends to adjust more slowly as a rule than younger persons. Options 2, 3, and 4 have not been found to be related to age.

352. 4. Site D is the preferred site, primarily in order to avoid possible damage to the sciatic nerve and in order to reach substantial muscle tissues.

353. 2. The sciatic nerve is most often damaged when the buttock is injected without due care.

354. 2. The position described in option 2 promotes the greatest

amount of relaxation of muscles which, in turn, tends to help decrease discomfort.

355. 3. Of the foods given, the best sources of vitamin B12 are meats and dairy products. Many fresh fruits are good sources of vitamin C. Green leafy vegetables are good sources of vitamin A, vitamin B2, and vitamin B (folic acid). Whole wheat breads and cereals are good sources of vitamin B1, vitamin B2, vitamin B3, vitamin B6, and vitamin E.

356. 4. The body fails to produce the intrinsic factor which is secreted in the gastric mucosa and is essential for vitamin B12 absorption.

357. 1. Patients who do not have therapy will eventually have damaged neurons. The damage becomes irreversible.

358. 4. The most common cause of loss of teeth in adults is periodontal disease which is a progressive disease of the gums and other supporting structures of the teeth.

359. 1. Hot water may cause the dentures to warp. Options 2, 3, and 4 are measures that are not necessarily contraindicated.

360. 1. To promote good circulation and help prevent venous stasis, it is recommended that this patient elevate her legs several times a day. Options 2, 3, and 4 would be contraindicated.

NANCY MOTT

361. 3. Studies reveal that these lesions occur in the motor nerve fibers in the spinal cord.

362. 4. Many diagnostic tests could be used but of those given, the most helpful would be studies of cerebrospinal fluid.

363. 2. Symptoms described in options 1, 3, and 4 are likely to occur. The patient is least likely to note bursts of energy.

364. 2. It would be best to help the patient assume a sitting position when she attempts to void. Measures described in options 1, 3, and 4 are ineffective to encourage voiding.

365. 2. Distention of the bladder, which makes it palpable in the suprapubic area, is a sign of distention. Signs/symptoms described in options 1, 3, and 4 are unrelated to retention.

366. 1. Typical problems the patient with multiple sclerosis encounters are described in options 2, 3, and 4. Ascites is not associated with multiple sclerosis.

367. 3. Mephenesin carbamate is a centrally acting skeletal muscle relaxant and, hence, tends to relieve reflex spasms that patients with multiple sclerosis often experience.

368. 3. Studies have noted that generally, a patient with multiple sclerosis shows a period of improvement when new treatments are instigated. The reason is not clear.

369. 4. Practices described in options 1, 2, and 3 tend to improve the ability of the patient with multiple sclerosis to communicate. Option 4 is an unsatisfactory practice and may aggravate the problem.

370. 3. It is especially important to test the temperature of bath water with a thermometer because a patient with multiple sclerosis can be burned easily due to sensory changes.

371. 1. Ataxia is defined as an inability to coordinate walking movements. Vertigo refers to dizziness. Paresis refers to a type of paralysis. Spasticity refers to the state of muscular contraction.

372. 4. The most useful account describes specific behavior demonstrated by the patient and indicates the circumstances that produced it.

373. 2. Being cold and in drafty areas tend to aggravate the symptoms of multiple sclerosis. Practices described in options 1, 3, and 4 may be undesirable but not necessary detrimental.

374. 4. Limiting fluid intake is more likely to aggravate rather than help in a program of bowel training. Measures described in options 1, 2, and 3 are helpful.

375. 1. Of the disorders given, it can be expected that a patient with multiple sclerosis is most likely to demonstrate mood disorders.

376. 1. The change in vision and discomfort in the patient's eye is noteworthy. Activities described in options 2, 3, and 4 are of less significance unless they become regular behavior.

377. 2. There may be desirable results of rehabilitation in options 1, 3, and 4 but for the patient with multiple sclerosis, care is directed toward muscle rehabilitation and helping the patient remain motivated. The disease is chronic and, hence, goals should be those with the most benefit over a long period of time.

378. 2. The most positive approach is to help a patient with multiple sclerosis to keep active while still avoiding emotional upset and fatigue. A quiet and inactive life style is not necessarily indicated and good health habits will not be likely to alter the course of the disease although they may avoid complications. Option 4 describes activity that may be helpful to a certain extent but also may discourage the patient.

379. 2. The patient with multiple sclerosis usually does best and is least frustrated at home when a schedule of daily activities is observed. Options 1, 3, and 4 describe activity which may be unnecessary (1 and 3) or not as helpful (4).

380. 4. Multiple sclerosis is a progressive disease. Death is most

often caused by intercurrent infections. The disease has not been demonstrated to be contagious nor is it considered to be an inherited disease although it appears more often among relatives.

381. 3. The rate of occurrence is higher in northern climates. The reason is unknown.

HARRIET CARTOLE

382. 3. Arthroplasty is defined as plastic surgery on a joint. An osteotomy refers to cutting upon a bone. Surgical fixation of a joint is called arthrodesis. Osteosynthesis is unrelated to surgical procedures.

383. 3. An exercise program is recommended to strengthen muscles following arthroplasty. Isometric exercises (muscle setting) strengthen muscles but keep the joint stationary during the healing process. Options 1 and 4 may be true but do not explain the most important purpose for exercising. Isometric exercises will not help prevent joint stiffness since the joint remains stationary.

384. 3. The quadriceps setting exercises strengthen the quadriceps femoris, muscles in the leg that are important for proper walking. They can be exercised in bed by pushing the back of the knee into the mattress.

385. 1. Paraffin is applied directly to the skin. The fingers can be shaven in order to prevent discomfort when the cooled paraffin is removed. The temperature should be tested with a thermometer before applying the paraffin. Exercising the fingers and hand is recommended after the dip has been completed.

386. 4. The studies described in options 1, 2, and 3 are often used to help diagnose rheumatoid arthritis. A fluorescent antibody test is not.

387. 4. Keeping the joints in good alignment helps prevent contracture deformities. The measures described in options 1, 2, and 3 are likely to lead to deformities.

388. 3. If the hips are flexed, the patient is likely to develop contracture deformities. Reasons given in options 1, 2, and 4 do not apply in this situation.

389. 2. When a patient understands why an activity is ordered, he is more likely to carry it out. Admonitions and threats are unsatisfactory.

390. 4. Option 4 gives the patient information. Scolding, implying criticism of the physician, and forcing attention on another patient are poor ways to help this patient.

391. 2. Tinnitus is a very common symptom of aspirin toxicity. The other three symptoms are not associated with aspirin toxicity.

392. 3. Drugs that cause gastric irritation are best taken after a meal when stomach contents help minimize the local irritation.

393. 4. The preferred route is the one which results in the least systemic absorption, that is, the intraarticular route.

394. 3. Using prescriptions from the patient's physician is the best way to avoid misuse of drugs. Using testimonials and advertisements is a poor way to select drug therapy.

395. 1. It is generally best policy to keep a patient independent and in his home environment for as long as it is feasible. Therefore, residing in a nursing home is usually used as a last resort.

396. 3. With increasing age and decreasing activity, most elderly patients require fewer calories than younger persons. Fats, proteins, and carbohydrates are a necessary part of diet throughout life.

397. 2. Of the signs/symptoms given, most patients will complain of general malaise. The other signs/symptoms given here are not commonly associated with rheumatoid arthritis.

398. 2. The synovium is ordinarily involved at first. However, the disease commonly progresses to other parts of the joint.

399. 3. Rheumatoid arthritis affects women chiefly and characteristically begins during middle life. The reason is not understood.

400. 2. Pilocarpine hydrochloride is most commonly used because it acts to constrict the pupil and to cause the iris to draw away from the cornea. This promotes drainage of aqueous humor. The other three drugs given here act to cause dilatation of the pupils.

401. 3. The increase in the pressure within the eye decreases circulation to ocular tissues which will eventually lead to blindness. Options 1, 2, and 4 are not related to the pathology of glaucoma.

402. 1. Miosis is defined as pupillary constriction. Mydriasis refers to pupillary dilatation. Mycosis is a fungi or bacterial disease. Mitosis refers to cell reproduction.

403. 4. Joints described in options 1, 2, and 3 are common sites of osteoarthritis. The shoulder joints are least likely to be involved.

404. 4. A synonym for osteoarthritis is degenerative arthritis.

405. 1. A variety of factors may aggravate arthritis but of those given, poor posture and obesity are most likely to aggravate the disease because of their effects on diseased joints.

406. 4. Excess weight aggravates osteoarthritis and contributes to de-

formities. Hence a weight reduction diet is most often prescribed. See also item 405. Diets described in options 1, 2, and 3 are not indicated.

407. 2. According to statistics, only heart diseases cause more disability than arthritic diseases.

JOHN KETTER

408. 2. A characteristic and early symptom of Hodgkin's disease is the presence of swollen lymph nodes.

409. 3. The nurse should be prepared with measures that will relieve the discomforts of itching skin. This symptom is often a very distressing part of Hodgkin's disease.

410. 4. "Staging" is done to determine the extent and activity of the disease. The nature of the cell causing the disease is studied microscopically.

411. 4. The iliac crest and the sternum are the most common sites for obtaining bone marrow specimens, although other bones *may* be used.

412. 4. To decrease discomfort, a local anesthesia is usually used. Types of agents described in options 1, 2, and 3 are not ordinarily necessary unless other complications exist.

413. 2. Mechlorethamine hydrochloride is too irritating to tissue to be administered by other than the intravenous route.

414. 1. The most common side effects of mechlorethamine hydrochloride are nausea, vomiting, and anorexia. Headaches *may* occur but visual disturbances are not associated with toxicity of this agent.

415. 4. Proteins are broken down into amino acids during digestion. Amino acids are absorbed in the small intestine. Albumin is built from amino acids. Hence, serum albumin levels help determine protein intake sufficiency.

416. 1. Singultus is due to spasms of the diaphragm. The factors given in options 2, 3, and 4 have not been observed to be related to singultus.

417. 4. Singultus interferes with proper rest and, therefore, the danger of prolonged singultus is physical exhaustion. Complications given in options 1, 2, and 3 have not been reported.

418. 1. The procedure of washing the area with water and patting it dry is most often recommended. It is least irritating and most comfortable. Other types of care are not recommended.

419. 4. Oxygen is humidified in order to prevent drying and irritation of respiratory membranes. Bubbling oxygen through water plays no role in accomplishing purposes described in options 1, 2, and 3.

420. 3. Terminally ill patients most often report feelings of isolation, since they tend to be ignored, are often left out of conversations concerning the future, and sense attitudes of discomfort that many persons feel in their presence.
421. 1. The stages of grief are fairly predictable. Anger is an early sign of grief. The characteristic expression of anger is "Why him?"
422. 2. During anger, it is best to allow the person time to express anger and to listen quietly while the angry behavior relieves a charged emotional situation. Option 1 turns a nursing responsibility over to someone else. Option 3 offers the person no help. Explanations, as described in option 4, are of little value when given in an emotional situation.
423. 3. Statistics reveal that young adults are most often struck with Hodgkin's disease.

VICTOR DAY

424. 2. The United States Public Health Service has defined guidelines for setting up venereal disease clinics.
425. 4. Many patients with a venereal disease are most reluctant to reveal their sexual contacts. Problems given in options 1, 2, and 3 are usually relatively easy to handle when present.
426. 2. Probenecid acts to potentiate the effectiveness of penicillin. Reasons described in options 1, 3, and 4 are unrealistic for this drug.
427. 1. Penicillin is noted primarily for its ability to kill selected organisms.
428. 1. Molds provide the source of penicillin.
429. 3. There are typical symptoms for each stage of syphilis except for the latent stage when the patient is most likely to be symptom-free. The latent stage generally occurs several years after the primary stage and may last as long as 50 years.
430. 1. Serological tests are most likely to be negative during the primary stage. It is the most infectious stage and is characterized by the appearance of a chancre and swollen lymph nodes.
431. 1. It has been observed that the patient becomes noninfectious in approximately 24 hours after initiating effective treatment.
432. 4. The chancre is characteristically a painless, moist ulcer, and its serous discharge is very infectious. It is most often seen on the male genital organs; it is seldom seen in the female.
433. 4. The organism causing syphilis is the Treponema pallidum. It is classified as a spirochete because of its corkscrew appearance.

434. 1. Statistics reveal that the incidence of venereal diseases among teenagers is rising more rapidly than it is among persons of other ages. Many factors have been stated to influence this trend, one being a change in morals and increasing sexual activity among the young. See also item 439.

435. 4. Treating the exposed individual promptly has done more to control the spread of syphilis than practices described in options 1, 2, and 3. This is the reason why it is important to obtain a complete list of sexual contacts who may then be encouraged to have treatment.

436. 4. Gonorrhea in the male is characterized by a mucopurulent urethral discharge. Gonorrhea is the most common reportable communicable disease in this country today.

437. 1. Unfortunately, many females are unaware that they have gonorrhea because they are free of symptoms or experience only the mildest symptoms. These women compose a large pool of unsuspecting carriers of the disease.

438. 3. Although treatment is offered in many different settings, most persons visit a private physician.

439. 2. Of the factors mentioned, laxity of public concern appears to contribute most to the rise in the incidence of venereal diseases. Reports indicate that some organisms have become resistant to drugs (gonorrhea) but evidence of public concern appears lacking.

CHARLES HANDY

440. 3. According to the United States Public Health Service guidelines, enteric precautions are recommended for patients with infectious hepatitis but a private room for an adult patient is not necessary.

441. 2. Infectious hepatitis is a disease primarily of the liver. Of the tests given, the BSP test is used to help diagnose hepatitis. A dye is given and the liver's ability to excrete the dye is studied. Dye excretion is abnormal in the presence of liver disease.

442. 3. Infectious hepatitis may be spread in several ways, but the most common one is by contaminated water and food.

443. 1. The organism causing infectious hepatitis travels to the liver where it grows and multiplies.

444. 3. The organism causing infectious hepatitis leaves the body primarily through the feces. The respiratory route has not been ruled out but is not considered to be the most common route of transmission.

445. 3. Of the characteristics given, the one typical of viruses is their inability to grow outside of living cells.

446. 3. Gamma globulin is used for prophylactic purposes for persons exposed to infectious hepatitis. There are no vaccines, antitoxins, or inactivated toxins available.

447. 4. It has been found that adrenocorticosteroid therapy helps alleviate the symptoms of infectious hepatitis but the therapy is not considered effective for conditions described in options 1, 2, and 3.

448. 4. Although various diets have been tried in the past, most authorities are now of the opinion that a normally balanced diet is best for persons with infectious hepatitis.

449. 1. Of those given, fatigue is the most common symptom of infectious hepatitis during the convalescing period.

450. 2. A low-grade fever is atypical of serum hepatitis.

451. 2. Serum hepatitis is also called hepatitis Type B. It is also often called long incubation hepatitis because of its long incubation period when compared with infectious hepatitis. Infectious hepatitis is also called hepatitis Type A or short incubation period hepatitis.

452. 3. Serum hepatitis is most often spread by blood and plasma and by contaminated instruments used to puncture the skin. Persons injecting illicit drugs have a high rate of serum hepatitis because they use contaminated needles and spread the disease among themselves.

453. 4. The safest method is to use steam under pressure when sterilizing equipment contaminated with the hepatitis virus.

454. 4. Health personnel working in hemodialysis units have been noted to have a higher-than-average rate of hepatitis which they acquire from contaminated blood and equipment.

JAMES CORNING

455. 4. Fresh blood that is partially digested in the stomach and then vomited has a coffee-ground appearance. Particles of undigested food may be present but they would not be evidence of bleeding.

456. 2. Usual preparation for gastric analysis includes avoiding all fluids and food for 6 to 8 hours in order to obtain a specimen that is free of fluid and foods.

457. 3. Tubeless gastric analysis includes ingesting a dye which, if acid is present in the stomach, is excreted in the urine.

458. 2. Barium sulfate is given orally prior to roentgenography of the upper gastrointestinal tract. The substance is radiopaque and is not digested so that it illustrates the outlines of the tract on the x-ray film.

459. 3. The barium sulfate used for x-ray study is likely to produce

fecal impactions since it dries into a chalky, hard substance.

460. 1. Anticholinergic drugs act to reduce the rate of secretion by the gastric glands, as well as by the salivary, bronchial, and sweat glands. These drugs act by preventing postganglionic parasympathetic nerves from exerting full control over, among other things, exocrine gland cells.

461. 2. Anticholinergic drugs act to dilate the pupils and paralyze eye accommodations. Common side effects include photophobia and blurred vision.

462. 2. It is generally recommended that aluminum hydroxide gel be offered with water.

463. 3. Aluminum hydroxide gel tends to cause constipation.

464. 4. The temperature of the milk has no significant effects on factors described in options 1, 2, and 3 but a low temperature will inhibit the growth of bacteria.

465. 2. Baked custard is preferred because it is bland and relatively easy to digest.

466. 3. Reverse peristalsis causes acid stomach content to reach the distal end of the esophagus. The burning sensation this causes is commonly called heartburn.

467. 3. Sodium bicarbonate taken in excess may result in metabolic alkalosis. Ingestion of bicarbonate is unrelated to problems described in options 1, 2, and 4.

468. 4. Pepper should be removed because of its possible irritating effects on gastrointestinal mucosa.

469. 3. The body reacts to perforation by "immobilizing" the area as much as possible. This results in a boardlike rigidity of the abdomen and the abdomen is ordinarily extremely tender. The blood pressure will fall.

470. 1. The type of diet has been found to be of less significance than once was thought. However, frequent meals/snacks are recommended in order to help protect the mucosa from the irritating effects of gastric acidity.

471. 3. Alcohol is ordinarily poorly tolerated by the patient with peptic ulcers because of its irritating effects on the mucosa.

472. 1. Options 2, 3, and 4 are typical signs/symptoms of anxiety. So also is blanched skin which results from vasoconstriction, because during anxiety, the body increases its secretions of epinephrine. This hormone is a vasoconstrictor.

473. 4. Behaviors described in options 1, 2, and 3 are not necessarily possible (1) or true (2 and 3). The method of coping with stress is of most importance.

474. 2. One of nicotine's influences on the body is to increase the secretion of epinephrine.

475. 4. Nicotine is an addictive substance. Options 1, 2, and 3 describe commonly held opinions about smoking but they are largely untrue.

476. 2. The pain of a duodenal ulcer is ordinarily relieved by eating. The food helps neutralize excess acids and offers protection to the mucosa.

477. 1. Research has demonstrated that persons in blood group O are 35 percent more susceptible to ulcers than persons in other blood groups.

478. 3. Whole milk and cream contain significant amounts of cholesterol. High blood levels of cholesterol are believed to predispose to various cardiovascular disorders.

479. 4. Fat stimulates the secretion of enterogastrone which inhibits the secretion of gastric juices and muscular contractions in the stomach.

480. 1. Of the substances given, only alcohol is absorbed in the stomach.

481. 2. Villi provide the absorptive surface in the small intestines. Rugae are ridges formed in the stomach when empty Taeniae refer to musculature in the large intestine. Papillae are structures found in the tongue and in the skin.

482. 1. Large quantities of water are absorbed in the large intestine. There is no significant absorption of food in the large intestine.

JOSEPH SMITH

483. 3. Pyrexia causes an elevation in body metabolism and the respiratory and pulse rates will increase, usually proportionately with the body temperature.

484. 3. Heat is removed by conduction; the blanket removes heat by its contact with the patient's body, because the heat is transmitted directly from the body to the blanket. Radiation involves the transfer of heat through the form of waves. Convection requires a current of air; heat is absorbed by the air and transferred elsewhere. Heat is also lost from the body when a liquid (perspiration) changes to vapor.

485. 1. The absorption of drugs will be slow when hypothermia is present due to a decrease in body activities. Hence, it is better to administer drugs during hypothermia intravenously.

486. 3. Myocardial irritability may occur during hypothermia, most probably due to potassium movement in the body.

487. 1. It has been observed that obese persons have a greater-than-average degree of downward drift in temperature after the cooling device is removed.

488. 2. Although various methods may be used to rewarm the patient following hypothermia, the preferred method is to allow the patient to rewarm naturally.

489. 2. Evaporation of moisture from the body is enhanced when humidity of environmental air is low and it is retarded when humidity of environmental air is high.

490. 1. Statement A is true. The shifting of water, as described, produces hemoconcentration. Therefore, nursing measures, such as position changes and range-of-motion exercises, help prevent emboli formation.

491. 3. The heat-regulating center is located in the hypothalamus.

LORRAINE MYERBY

492. 4. The purpose of biofeedback is to translate body processes into observable signs. Statements in options 1, 2, and 3 are false in relation to biofeedback.

493. 2. Dilatation of dural arteries on the scalp is generally believed to be responsible for the pain associated with migraine headaches.

494. 2. Ergotamine tartrate acts to constrict dilated arterioles and is, therefore, the drug of choice to abort and control attacks of migraine. See item 493 above.

495. 2. It has been observed that migraine headaches are relieved by a regulation of blood flow from the head to the hands. This transfer of blood to the hands increases the temperature of the hands.

496. 4. Patients are trained to carry out biofeedback procedures themselves. Hence, this requires the patient to take an active and responsible part in the program.

PHYSIOLOGY OF MENSTRUATION AND MENOPAUSE

497. 3. Of the changes given, the first to appear when sexual maturity begins is the growth of axillary and pubic hair.

498. 4. Climate, heredity, and nutrition may influence the age at which menstruation occurs. Physical activity does not.

499. 1. Estrogen is the hormone contained in the graafian follicle. Progesterone is produced by the corpus luteum. The other two hormones are released by the anterior lobe of the pituitary gland.

500. 4. The hypothalamus controls the release of gonadotropin hormone. See also item 499 above.

501. 2. The corpus luteum secretes both estrogen and progesterone. Unless the ova is fertilized, the corpus luteum is short-lived

and as a result, the endometrium degenerates and menstruation begins.

502. 2. The watery cervical secretions function primarily to facilitate the passage of sperm.

503. 2. Progesterone, which supplements the action of estrogen, helps prepare the endometrium for implantation. Progesterone is so named because the word means *for gestation.*

504. 4. Of the factors given, the most important indication that ovulation has occurred is a rise in body temperature.

505. 4. The term mittleschmerz (middle pain) is used to describe discomfort during ovulation.

506. 2. Wearing of tampons is not recommended during the postpartal period.

507. 4. It is generally agreed that no usual activities are necessarily contraindicated during menstruation in healthy females.

508. 2. Following childbirth, the cervix tends to be slightly open, which is believed to be the reason why menstrual cramps become less frequent in women who have had children. Menstrual flow is enhanced when the cervix is slightly open.

509. 1. It is a decrease in estrogen that is responsible for changes noted by most women at menopause.

510. 4. Loss of normal interest in sexual activity is least often observed in women at menopause. Many women report just the opposite phenomenon, one reason often given being that pregnancy is no longer a threat.

511. 2. "Hot flashes" are the result of vasomotor instability—they are not myths. Estrogen is often prescribed for relieving them. See also item 509.

512. 4. Finding new interests tends to improve self-esteem and has most often helped women who feel usefulness has ended. Suggestions offered in options 1, 2, and 3 are generally of little value and offer no positive guidance.

TRENDS, LEGAL AND ETHICAL CONSIDERATIONS,
ORGANIZATIONS, AND THE LIKE

513. 3. Florence Nightingale is most often remembered for her efforts to establish educational programs for nursing. She was largely responsible for the development of a school at St. Thomas's Hospital in London although she never directly administered it.

514. 1. The Social Security Act includes provisions for disability insurance, funds for the needy blind, and grants-in-aid for children, among others. It has no provision for life insurance.

515. 1. Public Law 93-360 includes nonprofit hospitals and their em-

ployees. Options 2, 3, and 4 are inaccuracies in relation to this law.

516. 3. Accountability is defined as being responsible and answerable for one's acts. Advocacy, a commonly recognized responsibility of nursing, refers to acts performed for another person, as the patient. An endorsement sanctions or upholds an act. Professionalism is a broad term and is often used to refer to all aspects of a particular occupation.

517. 2. With improved diagnostic techniques and therapy, hospital populations tend to be more acutely ill. Although chronic illness and an increasingly elderly population are part of today's life, they have not produced effects described in option 1. There has been no evidence that option 3 is true. Young persons tend to have conditions requiring hospitalization less frequently than older persons.

518. 2. The study reported in *An Abstract For Action* focused on supply and demands for nurses, nursing roles, nursing functions, nursing education, and nursing careers. Factors given in options 1, 3, and 4 have been researched in other studies.

519. 2. The most obvious and consistent trend in preservice education for nursing within the last couple of decades has been to move these programs into institutions of learning (colleges and universities) and from service agencies (hospitals).

520. 2. Only the National League for Nursing allows non-nurse members. Organizations in options 1, 3, and 4 require members to be nurses.

521. 3. Although all of the organizations listed have interests in minority groups in nursing, the National Student Nurses' Association has taken the most active role to recruit them and began by launching the National Recruitment Project in 1965.

522. 2. Although factors given in options 1, 3, and 4 exist, it was having one licensing examination used by all states that helped make nurse mobility less cumbersome than it had been.

523. 2. With an ever-increasing concern to keep up-to-date on knowledge influencing the practice of nursing, continuing education for nurses has increased markedly. Factors given in options 1, 3, and 4 may be influenced by continuing education but they are not primary purposes of such programs.

524. 2. *Nursing Outlook*, the official periodical of the National League for Nursing, publishes lists of accredited programs.

525. 4. The honorary society for nurses is Sigma Theta Tau. Alpha Tau Delta membership is open to nurses joining its chapters in schools having baccalaureate or higher degree programs.

526. 2. The National Student Nurses' Association official organ is

Imprint. Image is a Sigma Theta Tau organ. *Nursing Care* is a National Federation of Licensed Practical Nurses' publication.

527. 3. The American Nurses' Association supports educational concepts expressed in options 1, 2, and 4 but has taken a strong stand against having service agencies, such as hospitals, grant degrees for graduates of educational programs for nurses.

528. 1. Because of being able to sustain life by using biomedical equipment, controversy has arisen concerning the definition of death which has created legal problems in relationship to procuring tissues and organs. Cryonics refers to the freezing of dead bodies. Euthanasia is defined as painless or mercy killing. Thanatology is the study of death.

529. 4. Information concerning addresses of boards of nursing is published in the *American Journal of Nursing* in Directory issues. These issues also contain information concerning organizations of interest to nurses.

530. 4. The act described is called embezzlement. Taking property entrusted to his care distinguishes embezzlement from robbery (taking by violence), larceny (simple thievery), or burglary (breaking and entering to commit a crime).

531. 1. The 1973 Code for Nurses of the International Council of Nurses includes accountability. Concepts described in options 2, 3, and 4 were previously and still are included in the Code.

532. 1. The exemption described is called a waiver because the proposed law would refrain from applying (waive) to persons previously licensed.

533. 4. Common law helps protect persons being judged by different sets of rules. Actions described in options 1, 2, and 3 are unrelated to the purpose of common law.

534. 2. A mandatory nurse practice act commands (mandates) that a nurse must be licensed to practice. A permissive nurse practice act offers methods for obtaining a license but does not mandate that licensure is required to practice. Some states are now beginning to require that continuing education is necessary to maintain one's license to practice.

535. 4. Laws do not derive from preambles of constitutions. Laws derive from legislatures (statutory law), the judiciary system (common law), and administrative regulations (administrative law).

536. 3. Although some states are presently making changes, the common criticism of present licensure laws is that they do not provide for proof of continued competence. Present laws provide for factors in options 1, 2, and 4.

537. 3. The comments described can constitute slander. Had the person written these comments, the nurse could be guilty of libel. Fraud is willful misrepresentation that causes harm to another. Malpractice is an act of negligence.

538. 3. The hospital's action can constitute false imprisonment. Assault is a threat or attempt to make bodily contact without consent. Battery is an assault that is carried out. Invasion of privacy violates the right of a person to be let alone.

539. 2. Endorsements for promoting health-related products is not supported by the Code of Ethics. The act of endorsing is not forbidden by law or by the patient's bill of rights.

540. 1. See item 535.

541. 1. To determine negligence, a standard of care is described in order to decide what should, or should not, have been done under similar circumstances. Juries and judges turn to expert witnesses who are capable of describing standards of care. Of the persons given, only the experienced nurse is qualified to describe standards of nursing care.

542. 2. There is no evidence of negligence in statements made in options 1, 3, and 4. However, an experienced nurse could be considered negligent by leaving a tourniquet in place on an extremity for 2 hours. Her action may cause loss of the limb due to inadequate circulation for a prolonged period of time.

543. 3. According to membership rules of the International Council of Nurses, only the American Nurses' Association can represent the United States in the International Council of Nurses.

544. 4. It would be best not to carry out the order. The nurse should consult the nurse under whose supervision she is employed.

545. 3. To meet the increasing demands for health care better, nurses are functioning increasingly in roles that include considerably more responsibility than previously recognized roles. A current legislative trend is to change laws that are so restrictive that assuming expanded roles in nursing places the nurse in legal jeopardy. Options 1, 2, and 4 do not describe current trends.

546. 4. Since the act of having an abortion is legal, a woman requesting one is not in violation of a law and, hence, if she has the abortion, her act is not reportable. The other patients are reportable by law.

547. 2. The Comprehensive Drug Abuse Prevention and Control Act regulates the use of opium, cocaine, and their derivatives. Reserpine is a rauwolfia alkaloid and not under the regulation of federal law although it cannot be sold without a physician's prescription.

548. 3. According to the federal constitution, three-fourths of the 50

states (38) are required to ratify a bill before it may become an amendment to the constitution.

549. 1. Of those given, only the Hill-Burton Act has provided money for hospital construction.

550. 2. Of the organizations given, only the American Nurses' Association makes professional liability insurance available to its members.

551. 4. The *American Journal of Nursing* is the official organ of the American Nurses' Association. *Nursing Forum* and *Nursing Research* are not official organs of organizations. *Nursing Outlook* is the official organ of the National League for Nursing.

552. 1. Since 1913, the honorary chairman of the American Red Cross has been the president of the United States. The ARC was chartered by an Act of Congress in 1905.

553. 4. The "ladder concept" holds that a student should be able to move from one level of education to the next higher level without repetition of previous educational experiences. Options 1 and 3 describe concepts that guide educational administrators in some schools; some curricula use a 21 problem-centered approach in courses of study for nursing; however, these are not examples of the ladder concept.

554. 1. Only the Academy of Nursing requires evidence of an outstanding contribution to nursing for membership.

555. 2. There is nothing generally considered contrary to the best interests of the patient described in options 1, 3, and 4. See item 527 for further discussion.

556. 4. The ophthalmologist is a physician licensed to diagnose and treat disease; a synonym is oculist. The optician is responsible for making optical glasses. The ocularist makes artificial eyes. An optometrist refracts eyes and makes glasses.

557. 3. A chiropodist specializes in the care of feet.

MISCELLANEOUS ITEMS

558. 3. The acid-base balance of the body is controlled primarily by the hydrogen ion. It can combine with other elements quickly to increase or decrease acidity or alkalinity. The concentration of hydrogen (H^+) and hydroxyl (OH^-) ions determine the degree of acidity/alkalinity of body fluids, that is, their pH.

559. 3. Different persons are capable of weighing a patient accurately. Accuracy is often influenced by factors described in options 1, 2, and 4.

560. 4. The importance of emotional factors in the course of ulcerative

colitis is etiologically well established. Emotional disturbances tend to influence gastrointestinal secretions, motility,
and/or absorption ability.

561. 4. Although perforation with peritonitis does not occur frequently, it is the most common cause of death in fatal cases.

562. 2. The digested blood in the stool causes it to be black in color.
The odor of the stool also becomes particularly offensive.

563. 4. The term, agglutination, refers to a clumping together and the
substance causing it is called an agglutin. An agglutin does
not influence events described in options 1, 2, and 3.

564. 4. The conditions described in options 1, 2, and 3 do not respond
favorably to diet therapy. Simple iron deficiency anemia,
which is caused by inadequate absorption or excessive loss of
iron, does.

565. 3. The patient who is participating tends to be motivated to learn
and is meeting a need for self-esteem and feelings of importance. The learner directs learning toward goals he sees as
satisfactory for him. Hence, goals should be developed with
the learner for best results.

566. 1. Learning is said to have occurred when there is evidence of a
change in behavior. Option 1 offers the best method for
determining whether a behavioral skill (giving himself an
injection) has been learned.

567. 1. A pericardiocentesis is not commonly indicated in this situation. See also items 42, 47, and 49.

568. 2. A liver biopsy is done to evaluate tissue. A biopsy will not
furnish information in relation to the liver's size, blood supply,
or detoxification abilities.

569. 4. Placing a patient on his right side with a pillow under his
lower rib cage helps reduce the likelihood of bleeding by
causing pressure on the liver.

570. 4. It is essential to perform a paracentesis only after it has been
determined that the urinary bladder is empty in order to avoid
the risk of puncturing the full bladder.

571. 4. It has been stated that if every person with streptococcic
pharyngitis had prompt and adequate treatment with an effective antibiotic, rheumatic fever would practically cease to
exist.

572. 3. It has been observed that cold weather tends to aggravate
angina pectoris. Dry, warm, or humid weather has not been
noted to influence the condition.

573. 2. It is generally recommended that a person subject to angina
attacks use the prophylactic measure of taking his prescribed
nitroglycerin prior to activity that is likely to produce an attack.

Suggestions offered in options 1, 3, and 4 have not been demonstrated to be effective prophylactic measures.

574. 1. The cause of essential, or primary, hypertension has not been identified. Essential hypertension accounts for approximately 90 percent of cases of hypertensive cardiovascular diseases.

575. 2. Gravity accounts for relief of symptoms of fainting. Blood circulation to the brain is enhanced when the head is lowered, thereby overcoming the symptoms of fainting.

576. 1. The word idiopathic is used to describe a disease, the cause of which is unknown.

577. 3. The sympathetic (thoracolumbar) division of the autonomic nervous system carries impulses that increase the activity of sweat glands.

578. 4. Most patients with acne vulgaris notice improvement during the summer months, possibly because of the drying effects of the sun and warmth on the skin.

579. 4. A vesicle contains fluid and causes moisture and weeping. A macule is a small dry skin lesion of a color different from its surroundings; it is not raised. A papule is a solid elevated lesion. A pustule contains pus and tends to drain but is not characterized by watery moisture and weeping.

580. 1. The organism believed responsible for warts is a virus.

581. 2. Pediculosis pubis may be spread in several ways, one of which could be contaminated clothing and linen. However, it is most often spread by sexual contact.

582. 2. The predominate symptom of scabies, which is caused by a mite that burrows under the skin, is itching, usually most pronounced during the night.

583. 2. Trench mouth is caused by Borrelia vincentii and Fusobacterium fusiforme organisms in a symbiotic relationship. Both organisms are anaerobic, that is, they survive without free oxygen.

584. 1. Trigeminal neuralgia which involves the fifth cranial nerve is characterized by excrutiating pain in the skin in the affected area. Pain is easily brought on by simple noxious agents, such as a draft of cold air.

585. 3. The stethoscope is used for auscultation. A speculum is used to examine a body cavity, such as the vagina. A tonometer is used to measure intraocular pressure. The mercury manometer is used for obtaining blood pressure.

586. 2. a.c. means before meals; a.a. means of each; p.c. means after meals; and q.s. means quantity sufficient.

587. 2. The patient is most likely to be in an early stage of illness which is characterized by behavior that expresses denial or

disbelief in being ill. Later stages of illness are characterized by acceptance and interest in care.

588. 3. Osteoporosis, which means a decrease in the density of bone,
is a metabolic bone disorder. Falls are particularly dangerous
because of the ease with which affected bones fracture.

589. 1. Addison's disease is characterized by a deficiency of aldosterone which is a hormone that normally regulates sodium
and potassium levels. In Addison's disease, sodium is excreted in excessive amounts; potassium is retained.

590. 1. Determining levels of blood gases is the most accurate method
for determining whether the patient is well ventilated. Other
methods, such as those described in options 3 and 4, give only
rough estimates.

591. 2. Unless the airway is open for the entry of air/oxygen, other
measures, such as described in options 1, 3, and 4, will not be
of value.

592. 1. Chemoreceptors in the carotid bodies in the neck and aortic
arch monitor blood oxygen levels. These chemoreceptors are
not as powerful for respiratory stimulus as are carbon dioxide
and hydrogen-ion concentrations in the blood.

593. 1. Of those given, only potassium iodide does not relax and dilate
bronchioles. Potassium iodide is an expectorant.

594. 2. The "sigh" mechanism produces a deep breath which helps to
inflate areas of the lung that are hypoventilating during ordinary breathing. It does not clear respiratory passages nor
increase air turbulence. It may decrease monotony but that is
not its primary purpose.

595. 3. A laryngoscope is required for endotracheal intubation. The
instrument allows the operator to view the larynx and vocal
cords and provides a passageway for inserting the tube.

596. 2. The best initial action when the eye has been splashed with an
acid is to dilute it as quickly as possible with water. Other
types of care, such as described in other options, *may* be used
later.

597. 3. Ipecac syrup is an effective emetic and is commonly used
when vomiting is indicated. The other agents have entirely
different uses.

598. 1. Factors described in options 2, 3, and 4 are important when
caring for a patient in shock but can be safely delayed until
measures are started to restore blood volume.

599. 3. The first course of action is to take steps to help stop air from
entering the chest cavity which will cause the lungs to collapse. Other measures *may* be necessary but do not have the
same priority as closing the wound.

600. 3. Because the peritoneum is a semipermeable membrane,

peritoneal dialysis is effective for helping to restore electrolyte balance.

601. 2. The pressure increases the temperature of the steam. The pressure has no relationship with penetrating items, with penetrating cell walls, nor with retaining a constant temperature.

602. 4. It has been observed that gastrointestinal epithelial cells are more sensitive to radiation therapy than are connective tissue, muscle, or bone cells.

603. 3. Poison control experts recommend flushing unused drugs into the toilet. Other methods allow persons to acquire the drugs. Burning is not effective for many drugs, such as liquids, and because of pollution control measures, many places do not allow burning of a nature that would destroy drugs.

604. 4. People who continue to work after usual ages for retirement are motivated and, hence, tend to take better care of themselves. The majority of people in good health still do not continue to work after usual retirement age and health care is generally equally available to all elderly persons, especially with Medicare and Medicaid programs that are in wide use.

605. 4. Ethnocentrism is defined as preoccupation with one's own culture. Holism is a concept based on the assumption that a whole has many parts, each related to others. Acculturation is the process of mixing cultures by contact with others. Relativism refers to a philosophical doctrine in relation to knowledge and truth.

606. 3. Verbal communication includes listening to a speech. Communications described in options 1, 2, and 4 do not involve words and, hence, they are examples of nonverbal communication.

607. 2. Couples who are quarrelsome are no more likely to divorce than couples who appear congenial. Options 1, 3, and 4 are statements that oppose research findings.

608. 2. Malignant diseases rank second; diseases of the heart rank first; cerebrovascular accidents rank third; and accidents rank fourth.

609. 2. While there may be some elements of truth in options 1, 3, and 4, cardiovascular diseases are diseases of the elderly and on the increase as the number of elderly in the population continues to grow.

surgical nursing

An industrial nurse set up an educational program for women employees. Classes that deal with health care of the breasts are included in the program.

Items 1 through 13 pertain to information included in these classes.

1. One of the *most important* reasons for teaching women how to examine their breasts correctly is that
    1. most women still do not care to have a male physician palpate the breasts for tumors.
    2. most breast tumors are discovered by women themselves during their normal activities of daily living.
    3. most women are less reluctant to have treatment when they find a breast tumor than if someone else finds it.
    4. self-examination of the breasts has been shown to be a more accurate method for detecting tumors than examinations by someone else.
2. At what time in the menstrual cycle is it *best* to examine the breasts?
    1. During the week ovulation occurs.
    2. During the week menstruation occurs.
    3. During the first week after menstruation.
    4. During the week immediately before menstruation.
3. Which of the following positions is the one of choice for the woman whose breasts are being examined by another person?
    1. A sitting position.
    2. A standing position.
    3. Flat on her back with a pillow under her head.
    4. Flat on her back with a pillow under the shoulder on the side being examined.
4. Ms. Victor asks the nurse what the firm ridge is that she feels un-

der the lower part of her breasts. The nurse should base her response to Ms. Victor's question on knowledge that this ridge is

1. tumorous tissue which requires further investigation.
2. connective tissue which is a normal part of the lower breast.
3. muscular tissue which normally develops with exercise and work.
4. glandular tissue which normally enlarges prior to menstruation.

5. Ms. Colson, who is 18 years old, says she noticed that her brassiere fits more snugly at certain times of the month. She asks the nurse if this is a sign of breast disease. The nurse should base her reply on knowledge that

1. benign cysts tend to cause the breasts to vary in size.
2. it is normal for the breasts to increase in size prior to menstruation.
3. a change in breast size is sufficiently uncommon at Ms. Colson's age to warrant further investigation.
4. at Ms. Colson's age, differences in the size of her breasts are related to her normal growth and development.

6. Ms. Winost asks the nurse why a friend of hers had her ovaries removed after having a radical mastectomy. The nurse should be guided in her response by knowledge that an oophrectomy helps to prevent metastasis of malignant growths by eliminating the body's source of the hormone

1. estrogen.
2. prolactin.
3. progesterone.
4. testosterone.

7. Which one of the following characteristics is *most typical* of malignant cells?

1. They are encapsulated.
2. They usually grow rapidly.
3. They rarely recur after removal.
4. They closely resemble the tissues whence they arise.

8. One woman in the class exclaims, "Men are lucky! They don't have to worry about breast tumors." Which one of the following possible responses to the comment is *most accurate?*

1. "You are correct; tumors do not attack the male breast."
2. "Men can have breast cancers just as women, but they occur relatively infrequently."
3. "The types of cancers that attack the male breast do not spread as do those in women."
4. "You are partly correct; tumors attack the male breast, but they are benign rather than cancerous."

9. From the sketch below, select the quadrant of the breast in which most malignant tumors occur.
   1. Quadrant A.
   2. Quadrant B.
   3. Quadrant C.
   4. Quadrant D.

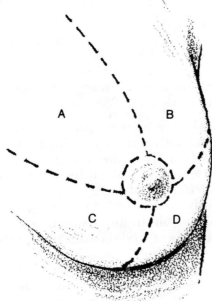

10. The incidence of carcinoma of the breast is *lowest* among women who
    1. have nursed their babies.
    2. have had no children.
    3. have not been married.
    4. are in a high socioeconomic class.
11. Of the following ethnic groups, the *lowest* incidence of carcinoma of the breast has been found among women who are
    1. Black.
    2. Jewish.
    3. Japanese.
    4. Scandinavian.
12. The nurse explains to the group that Paget's disease is a malignancy in the breast's
    1. muscle fascia.
    2. adipose tissue.
    3. connective tissue.
    4. lactiferous ducts.
13. Chronic cystic mastitis is discussed. The nurse explains that a

symptom of chronic cystic mastitis that is rarely a symptom of a malignancy (except in late stages) is

1. an elevated temperature.
2. asymmetry of the breasts.
3. a feeling of discomfort in the affected breast.
4. retraction of the nipple in the affected breast.

Ms. Ruth Maitt told the industrial nurse that she felt a lump in her right breast, which the nurse confirmed. After the physician examined Ms. Maitt, she was admitted to the hospital. A biopsy was done, the growth proved to be malignant, and a right radical mastectomy was performed.

Items 14 through 28 pertain to this situation.

14. Ms. Maitt asked numerous questions after she was admitted to the hospital and appeared anxious. Which one of the following statements offers the *best* guide for the nurse when she answered questions raised by an apprehensive preoperative patient such as Ms. Maitt?

1. It is usually best to tell the patient as much as she wants to know and is able to understand.
2. It is usually best to delay discussing the patient's questions with her until she is convalescing.
3. It is usually best to delay discussing the patient's questions with her until her apprehension subsides.
4. It is usually best to explain to the patient that she should discuss her questions first with the physician.

15. Ms. Maitt was ordered to have atropine sulfate preoperatively. The *primary* reason for giving this drug preoperatively is that it helps to

1. promote general muscular relaxation.
2. decrease the pulse and respiratory rates.
3. inhibit secretions in the mouth and respiratory tract.
4. facilitate maintaining blood pressure within normal range.

16. Which one of the following assessments should be made *first* by the recovery room nurse upon receiving Ms. Maitt from the operating room?

1. Taking and recording the patient's vital signs.
2. Observing that drainage tubes are open and functioning.
3. Noting that the patient's airway is free of obstructions.
4. Checking the patient's dressings for drainage and bleeding.

17. When Ms. Maitt returns from the operating room, her right arm is free of the dressings that cover her chest wall. Which one of the following positions is the one of choice for her right arm?

1. Across her chest wall.
2. At her side at the same level as her body.

3. On pillows: hand lower than her elbow and elbow lower than her shoulder.

4. On pillows: hand higher than her elbow and elbow higher than her shoulder.

18. A drainage tube is left in Ms. Maitt's operative area and is attached to a suctioning apparatus. The *primary* purpose of this procedure is to help

1. decrease intrathoracic pressure and facilitate breathing.
2. increase collateral lymphatic flow toward the operative area.
3. remove accumulations of serum and blood in the operative area.
4. prevent the formation of adhesions between the skin and chest wall in the operative area.

19. On the third postoperative day, the drainage tube is removed and the dressings changed. Ms. Maitt appears shocked when she sees the operative area and exclaims, "I look horrible! Will it ever look better?" Which one of the following responses would be *best* for the nurse to make?

1. "Don't worry. You know the tumor is gone and the area will heal soon."
2. "You are shocked by the sudden change with this operation, aren't you?"
3. "Would you like to meet Ms. Paul? She looks just great and she had a mastectomy too."
4. "After it heals and you are wearing your normal clothing, you will never know you had an operation."

20. Of the exercises illustrated in the sketches below and on page 168, which one would be *least effective* in promoting good range of joint motion for Ms. Maitt's right shoulder joint?

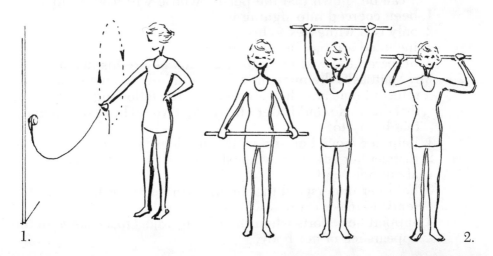

1.

2.

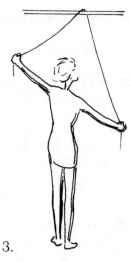

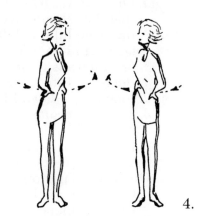

3.

4.

21. Ms. Maitt tells the nurse that her three children, ages 9, 15, and 17, are annoying her. Which one of the following questions would be the *most appropriate* for the nurse to ask?
1. "Are you saying that your children bother you?"
2. "Can't you stop whatever your children are doing that annoys you?"
3. "Can your husband help by doing something about your children's behavior?"
4. "Let's try to get to the bottom of this. Why are your children annoying you?"

22. Mr. Maitt comments to the nurse one day after visiting his wife that, in view of this scare with illness, he feels it is time the family prepares a will. A will would *not* be considered valid if it can be shown that the person whose will it was had
1. been coerced into signing it.
2. only two witnesses to his signature.
3. included a minor as a beneficiary.
4. prepared the will more than 2 years before his death.

23. Mr. Maitt asks the nurse how he could help his wife when she returns home after her surgery. Of the following suggestions that the nurse could offer Mr. Maitt, it would be *best* to suggest that he try to
1. help her move her arm while she does her exercises.
2. distract her attention when she seems unnecessarily anxious about her condition.
3. help her understand that being worried about her condition tends to make matters worse.
4. support her efforts when she tries to adjust to a change in the appearance of her body.

24. Radiation therapy is ordered for Ms. Maitt following her discharge from the hospital. Regarding the care of her skin at the site of the therapy, Ms. Maitt should be taught to avoid *all* of the following practices *except*
   1. using talcum powder.
   2. applying an ointment.
   3. washing the area with water.
   4. exposing the area to sunlight.
25. Normal local tissue response to radiation *most often* appears as
   1. atrophy of the skin.
   2. scattered pustule formation.
   3. redness of the surface tissues.
   4. sloughing of two layers of the skin.
26. Which one of the following activities of daily living is *contraindicated* for Ms. Maitt after discharge?
   1. Taking a daily tub bath.
   2. Taking a late evening swim.
   3. Working in her rose garden.
   4. Caring for her tropical fish.
27. What advantage does using a silicone prosthesis following a radical mastectomy have over using ordinary sponge or cotton padding?
   1. A silicone prosthesis is permanent.
   2. A silicone prosthesis is less expensive.
   3. A silicone prosthesis adheres to the chest wall.
   4. A silicone prosthesis is fitted to the individual.
28. The *primary* purpose of the American Cancer Society's Reach For Recovery program is to
   1. help rehabilitate patients who have had radical mastectomies.
   2. raise funds to support early breast cancer detection programs.
   3. provide free dressings for patients who have had radical mastectomies.
   4. collect statistics for research from patients who have had radical mastectomies.

   Ms. Carol Shaw, who is 45 years old, has had intermittent vaginal bleeding for several months. She calls her physician's office for an appointment and is scheduled to have a pelvic examination, including a Papanicolaou (Pap) test.
   Items 29 through 56 pertain to this situation.

29. The nurse speaks to Ms. Shaw when she schedules the appointment. In relation to douching, the nurse should instruct Ms. Shaw to
   1. avoid douching for about a week before the appointment.
   2. avoid douching for about 24 hours before the appointment.

3. douche the morning of the appointment with warm tap water only.

4. douche the night before the appointment with a solution of 1 quart of water and 1 tablespoon of white vinegar.

30. Which one of the following responses would be *best* for the nurse to make when Ms. Shaw says she is "nervous" about the pelvic examination the physician is about to perform?

1. "Can you tell me more about the nervousness you feel concerning the examination you are to have?"

2. "Are you fearful of having a disease that may not be related to the bleeding you have been having?"

3. "If you are nervous about your doctor, you need not feel concern. He is a specialist in women's diseases."

4. "Feeling concern about one's sex life is common when women have gynecological illnesses. But your problem is not related to sexual relations."

31. The *primary* purpose for performing a Papanicolaou test is to help determine whether Ms. Shaw has

1. cancer of the cervix.

2. fibroids of the uterus.

3. pelvic inflammatory disease.

4. infection of the Bartholin's glands.

32. Which one of the following positions is *most often* preferred for the patient who is to have a vaginal examination?

1. Sims's position.

2. Lithotomy position.

3. Genupectoral position.

4. Dorsal recumbent position.

33. Ms. Shaw's physician recommends that an abdominal hysterectomy be performed, and the patient is admitted to the hospital. Which one of the following statements offers the nurse the *best* guide when she responds to fears Ms. Shaw expresses concerning surgery?

1. The nurse should assure the patient of her physician's competency.

2. The nurse should allow the patient opportunities to express her fears.

3. The nurse should teach the patient how fears stand in the way of recovery.

4. The nurse should change the subject of conversation to pleasantries when fear appears to be present.

34. Ms. Shaw observes Judaism and refuses to eat since the hospital does not serve kosher food. It is against hospital policy to allow family members to bring food to patients. In this situa-

tion, it would be *best* for the nurse to

1. teach the patient that it is important for her to eat what she is served.
2. discuss the problem and possible courses of action with the dietitian.
3. tell the patient's family to bring food for the patient because of the special circumstances.
4. explain to the patient that if she does not eat, it will be necessary for her physician to order intravenous therapy.

35. The darkened areas in the drawings below indicate possible areas to shave a patient preoperatively. Which drawing *most accurately* depicts the area to be shaved prior to an abdominal hysterectomy?

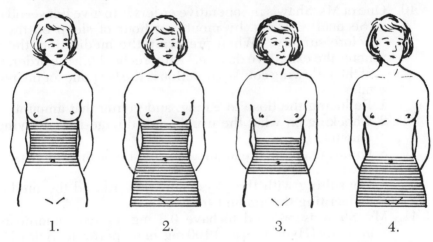

1.   2.   3.   4.

36. For legal reasons, *all* of the following information should appear on the operative permit before Ms. Shaw's surgery *except* the
1. surgeon's signature.
2. patient's signature.
3. name of the surgical procedure.
4. date of signing the operative permit.
37. Ms. Shaw's nursing care plan includes teaching her how to deep breathe and cough in preparation for her postoperative period. Which one of the following techniques should Ms. Shaw be taught to use while she coughs?
1. Support her abdomen with a pillow or her hands.
2. Support her rib cage with a binder or her hands.
3. Lie on her abdomen with her arms at her side.
4. Lie flat in bed with her hands behind her head.
38. Which one of the following *early* signs/symptoms is the patient

most likely to experience if she is hyperventilating while she practices deep breathing?

1. Dyspnea.
2. Dizziness.
3. A rapid pulse rate.
4. A drop in blood pressure.

39. Ms. Shaw had been taking prednisone (Deltasone) daily for several years. Which one of the following complications is *most likely* to occur if this drug is discontinued abruptly?
   1. Adrenal crisis.
   2. Paralytic ileus.
   3. Pulmonary emboli.
   4. Thrombophlebitis.

40. One of Ms. Shaw's preoperative orders is to give her secobarbital (Seconal) 300 mg. by mouth, at hour of sleep on the night before surgery. When preparing the medication, the nurse notes the excessive dosage. After rechecking the order, which of the following courses of action is the *best* one for the nurse to take?
   1. Reducing the dose to 20 mg. and giving that amount.
   2. Checking on what the usual adult dosage is and giving that amount.
   3. Omitting giving the medication and recording the reason why it was not given.
   4. Consulting with the physician who ordered the medication concerning the amount to give.

41. Ms. Shaw is ordered to have 0.3 mg. of scopolamine hydrobromide (Hyoscine) and 100 mg. of meperidine hydrochloride (Demerol) intramuscularly 1 hour prior to surgery. The stocked ampules indicate that there are 0.4 mg. of scopolamine hydrobromide in each ml. and 50 mg. of meperidine hydrochloride in each ml. If the two medications are placed in one syringe in the amounts prescribed for the patient, how many ml. should there be in the syringe?
   1. 1.30 ml.
   2. 2.30 ml.
   3. 2.75 ml.
   4. 3.10 ml.

42. Ms. Shaw has still not voided 10 hours after surgery. Which one of the following measures is *least likely* to help her void?
   1. Offering her a cool bedpan.
   2. Running water in a nearby sink.
   3. Having her use a bedside commode.
   4. Pouring warm water over her perineal area.

43. Ms. Shaw has to be catheterized. The arrows in the drawings below indicate the direction in which each cotton ball could be moved when cleansing the area at the meatus before catheterizing the patient. Which drawing depicts the *best* method?

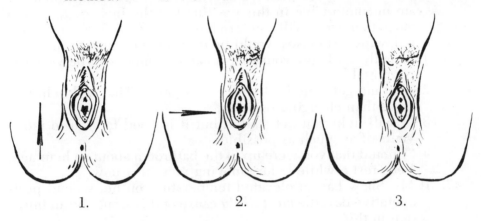

1.   2.   3.

44. In the drawing below, which letter indicates the urethral meatus in a female patient?
   1. A.
   2. B.
   3. C.
   4. D.

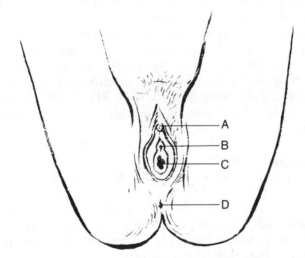

45. About 8 hours after catheterization, Ms. Shaw has the urge to void frequently but voids only a few ml. of urine each time. This symptom is *most commonly* associated with

1. bladder damage.
2. a kidney infection.
3. an inadequate fluid intake.
4. retention of urine with overflow.

46. On the second postoperative day, Ms. Shaw says to the nurse, "I am uncomfortable in this position but the incision hurts too much to move. Will you turn me, please?" Which one of the following responses would be *best* for the nurse to make?
   1. "Gladly! I know your incisional area must still be very uncomfortable."
   2. "Let me get a medication for your pain. That will help you more than changing position."
   3. "I will help you get started but it is good for you to move yourself as much as possible."
   4. "I noted that you were up to the bathroom about an hour ago. Let's rest a while before moving more just now."

47. If Ms. Shaw has an elevated temperature on her second postoperative day, the *most likely* cause of this would be an infection in the
   1. wound.
   2. urinary bladder.
   3. respiratory tract.
   4. veins of the legs (phlebitis).

48. The vaginal drainage on the perineal pad for the first few days after a hysterectomy *normally* consists of
   1. minimal amounts of serous drainage.
   2. minimal amounts of mucoid drainage.
   3. moderate amounts of bright bloody drainage.
   4. moderate amounts of serosanguineous drainage.

49. Which one of the following procedures is *best* to use when removing a dressing that sticks to Ms. Shaw's incisional area?
   1. Pulling off the dressings quickly and then applying slight pressure over the area.
   2. Lifting up an easily moved portion of the dressing and then removing it slowly.
   3. Moistening the dressing with sterile normal saline and then removing the dressing.
   4. Removing part of the dressing and then removing the remainder gradually over a period of an hour or two.

50. The *primary* reason for applying fluffed dressings to a draining wound is that fluffed dressings
   1. incorporate air that helps keep the dressing dry.
   2. are more comfortable than flatly packed dressings.
   3. allow drainage to be lifted from its source by capillary action.

4. permit drainage to leave its source readily by the force of gravity.

51. Ms. Shaw complains of gas pains postoperatively. If none of the following nursing measures is contraindicated, it would be *best* for the nurse to
   1. have the patient walk about.
   2. apply a snugly fitting abdominal binder.
   3. offer the patient a hot beverage, such as tea.
   4. provide extra warmth with an additional blanket.

52. *All* of the following measures have been found to be beneficial in helping to reduce the incidence of postoperative thrombophlebitis *except*
   1. ambulating the patient.
   2. massaging the patient's legs.
   3. having the patient use elasticized stockings.
   4. having the patient move her legs about in bed.

53. If Ms. Shaw's abdominal wound opens and tissues are exposed, the nurse should take immediate steps to
   1. replace the tissues carefully while wearing sterile gloves.
   2. apply a snugly fitting sterile abdominal binder over the wound.
   3. approximate the wound edges by applying strips of adhesive over the wound.
   4. cover the exposed tissues with sterile dressings moistened with sterile normal saline.

54. Approximately how many days postoperatively is abdominal wound dehiscence *most likely* to occur?
   1. 1 to 3 days.
   2. 4 to 5 days.
   3. 6 to 8 days.
   4. 9 to 11 days.

55. The physician removed Ms. Shaw's ovaries, tubes, and uterus and plans hormonal replacement therapy for the patient. Which one of the following hormones can the nurse anticipate the physician will prescribe for Ms. Shaw?
   1. Thyroxin.
   2. Estrogen.
   3. Prolactin.
   4. Progesterone.

56. Which one of the following statements should the nurse use to guide her response when Ms. Shaw asks about having sexual relations again in her life?
   1. Usual sexual responses will be reduced.
   2. Sexual intercourse should be avoided as much as possible.

3. Following convalescence, some sexual counseling usually is necessary.
4. After the postoperative checkup, normal sexual activity can usually be resumed.

Seventy-year-old Steven Johnson was brought to the hospital by his daughter. He has an indirect inguinal hernia on his right side and a herniorrhaphy is scheduled.
Items 57 through 98 pertain to this situation.

57. Which one of the following positions that Mr. Johnson might take would permit the *best* assessment of his inguinal hernia?
1. The sitting position.
2. The standing position.
3. The left side-lying position.
4. The right side-lying position.

58. While admitting Mr. Johnson, the nurse notes that he is wearing a hearing aid. Which one of the following courses of action would be *best* for the nurse to take in relation to the hearing aid?
1. Send it home with his daughter for safe-keeping.
2. Label it and place it in a locked cupboard for safe-keeping.
3. Encourage the patient to wear it as he ordinarily does at home.
4. Instruct the patient to keep it in the drawer of his bedside stand.

59. Mr. Johnson tells the nurse that he fears he will die during surgery. Which one of the following actions would be *most appropriate* for the nurse to take in this situation?
1. Sit down at the patient's bedside and express an interest in knowing more about his feelings and fears.
2. Explain to the patient that his fears are unnecessary and try to instill confidence by carrying on with routine tasks.
3. Assure the patient that a written message will be left on his chart so that the physician can discuss the patient's fears with him.
4. Tell the patient that fears before surgery are normal and that he will receive medication to help him rest and forget his fears.

60. If the physician wishes to have Mr. Johnson's bowel cleansed preoperatively, the nurse can anticipate that he will *most likely* order that, on the evening before surgery, Mr. Johnson be given a
1. laxative.
2. suppository.
3. cleansing enema.

4. colonic irrigation.
61. Which adjustment in the average adult dosage of preoperative medications should the nurse expect for Mr. Johnson?
    1. A larger than average dosage; elderly patients tend to have a decreased ability to absorb drugs.
    2. A larger than average dosage; elderly patients tend to have a decreased ability to maintain adequate blood levels of most drugs.
    3. A smaller than average dosage; elderly patients tend to have an increased sensitivity to most drugs.
    4. A smaller than average dosage; elderly patients tend to have increased susceptibility to allergic reactions to most drugs.
62. The *primary* goal of the preoperative skin preparation is to
    1. render the operative area free of organisms.
    2. decrease the number of organisms on the skin.
    3. improve the field of vision for the physician.
    4. enhance the skin's natural defenses against organisms.
63. The physician orders atropine sulfate to be given to Mr. Johnson preoperatively. The nurse should explain to the patient that the medication will *most probably* cause him to experience
    1. thirst.
    2. hunger.
    3. sleepiness.
    4. incontinence.
64. If one of the following procedures is to be carried out after Mr. Johnson receives a narcotic drug preoperatively, it would be *best* for the nurse to select to delay
    1. having him void.
    2. caring for his dentures.
    3. giving him a sponge bath.
    4. having him sign the operative permit.
65. The hospital's preoperative checklist is *least likely* to include the
    1. patient's early morning vital signs.
    2. time and amount of the patient's last voiding.
    3. fact that the patient had a physical examination.
    4. signature of the patient on the checklist form.
66. After Mr. Johnson is transported to the operating room, a short delay in starting his surgery becomes necessary. Which one of the following courses of action would be *most appropriate* for the nurse to take in this situation?
    1. Place him in a quiet room so that he can relax.
    2. Stay with him so that his questions can be answered.
    3. Take him back to his room where he can wait comfortably with his family.

4. Place him where the staff can observe him at frequent intervals.

67. Mr. Johnson receives spinal anesthesia. The position of choice for this procedure is to have the patient lie on his
   1. side with his legs well flexed.
   2. side with his legs well extended.
   3. abdomen with his arms at his side.
   4. abdomen with his arms folded under his head.

68. The recovery room nurse wishes to have Mr. Johnson cough but he has difficulty understanding her because he is without his hearing aid. Which one of the following actions would be *best* for the nurse to take?
   1. Sending for his daughter to come speak to him.
   2. Tapping his shoulder and speaking loudly into his good ear.
   3. Standing where the patient can observe her face and speaking clearly to him.
   4. Asking the nurse who learned to know him preoperatively to come to the recovery room to speak to him.

69. If the anesthetic rises too high in the spinal canal, the nurse should be prepared to
   1. elevate the foot of the bed.
   2. apply heat to the extremities.
   3. begin external cardiac massage.
   4. administer artificial respirations.

70. What is the body's first physiological response when shock from fluid loss occurs?
   1. Vasoconstriction which increases blood volume in the vascular system.
   2. Vasoconstriction which decreases the loss of plasma into interstitial spaces.
   3. Vasodilatation which improves blood flow to the capillary beds.
   4. Vasodilatation which improves oxygen and carbon dioxide exchange in tissue cells.

71. Of the following conditions, which one is the *most common* cause of postoperative shock?
   1. Adrenal failure.
   2. Excessive bleeding.
   3. A transfusion reaction.
   4. An untoward drug reaction.

72. Which one of the following signs/symptoms should the nurse describe in the patient's record to document Mr. Johnson's recovery from the spinal anesthesia?
   1. The color of his extremities.

2. The tingling sensation in his toes.

3. His pushing the airway out of place.

4. His orientation to time and place.

73. The physician orders that Mr. Johnson be catheterized if he has not voided 12 hours postoperatively. When he has not, Mr. Johnson asks that he be given another hour or two to try to void. The nurse's action should be guided by knowledge that, in Mr. Johnson's case,

1. a wait of an hour or two carries no risk.

2. a distended bladder will cause undue pressure on the patient's operative area.

3. the patient's motivation to void will help, making catheterization unnecessary.

4. if the patient's bladder cannot be palpated, there is insufficient urine present to necessitate catheterizing him.

74. When Mr. Johnson develops hiccups, of the following courses of action, it would be *best* for the nurse to

1. change his position in bed.

2. give him several whiffs of 100 percent oxygen.

3. have him take several sips of hot tea or coffee.

4. apply pressure with a finger on his closed eyelids.

75. On the second postoperative day, Mr. Johnson complains that his shoulders are too stiff to move. Which one of the following activities of daily living should Mr. Johnson be encouraged to carry out in order to help prevent loss of shoulder motion?

1. Feeding himself.

2. Combing his hair.

3. Shaving himself.

4. Cleaning his dentures.

76. Mr. Johnson's scrotum is swollen and painful 2 days postoperatively. A nursing measure that promotes comfort for many patients experiencing this condition is

1. applying a snug binder low on the patient's abdomen.

2. having the patient wear a truss to support the inguinal area.

3. elevating the scrotum and placing ice bags to the area intermittently.

4. having the patient lie on his side and placing a pillow between his legs.

77. The purpose of having Mr. Johnson wear a scrotal support postoperatively is to help

1. prevent prostatitis.

2. decrease local discomfort.

3. retain ejaculatory ability.

4. increase abdominal support.

78. Which one of the following types of drugs can the nurse anticipate the physician will *most likely* order for Mr. Johnson to
help prevent epididymitis?
   1. A hormone.
   2. A narcotic.
   3. An antibiotic.
   4. A urinary disinfectant.
79. Which one of the following nursing measures will be *most helpful* in preventing Mr. Johnson's developing postoperative
atelectasis?
   1. Having him cough every 1 to 2 hours.
   2. Having him wear elasticized stockings.
   3. Placing him in a semisitting position while he eats.
   4. Helping him to take at least 1200 ml. of oral fluids daily.
80. When Mr. Johnson's physician reads the nurses' notes on the
third postoperative day concerning the condition of the operative site, he says the patient might possibly be developing a
wound infection because the nurses recorded that there was
   1. progressive drying of the sutures.
   2. mild tenderness in the inguinal area.
   3. generalized itching in the operative area.
   4. a small amount of drainage on the dressing.
81. The hospital's admitting office scheduled four patients for admission, one of whom will be sharing Mr. Johnson's room.
Until it can be determined whether Mr. Johnson has a wound
infection, it would be *best* to have him share his room with a
patient whose diagnosis is
   1. pneumonia; causative organism is to be determined.
   2. gastric ulcers; his medical regimen is to be evaluated in view
   of bleeding.
   3. inguinal hernia; a herniorrhaphy is scheduled for his second
   day of hospitalization.
   4. gallbladder disease; a cholecystectomy is scheduled for his
   third day of hospitalization.
82. Mr. Johnson develops an incisional abscess. A debridement is
done and a small drain is left in the wound. The *primary*
reason for using a drain is to
   1. allow air to circulate in the wound.
   2. decrease the pain in the surrounding tissues.
   3. permit the escape of blood and lymph from the wound.
   4. use it for irrigating the entire length and depth of the wound.
83. The physician orders that Mr. Johnson receive 1 Gm. of
cephalothin sodium (Keflin) in 50 ml. of 5% dextrose in water
every 6 hours. The drip factor of equipment the nurse uses is
10 drops per ml. At what rate should the antibiotic solution be

given in order that Mr. Johnson will receive the entire amount in 30 minutes?
1. 10 to 11 drops per minute.
2. 16 to 17 drops per minute.
3. 23 to 24 drops per minute.
4. 29 to 30 drops per minute.

84. Mr. Johnson expresses concern about his wound infection. In addition to allowing the patient to express his concern, the nurse touches him gently on his arm. Which one of the following statements *most accurately* describes this use of touch in nursing practice?
1. It is very often misinterpreted as an aggressive act.
2. It decreases the effectiveness of most verbal communication.
3. It is interpreted largely on the basis of one's cultural background.
4. It is used so infrequently with success that it is usually considered insignificant in the nurse-patient relationship.

85. In contrast to younger patients, elderly patients have a higher incidence of postoperative infections *primarily* because older persons
1. have atrophy of lymph nodes.
2. tend to react unfavorably to stress.
3. have reduced cardiovascular circulation.
4. tend to observe careless habits of health.

86. After giving Mr. Johnson a bath, the nurse lowers his bed but keeps the bottle containing his intravenous fluid at the same height on the intravenous pole. What effect will this have on the rate of his intravenous flow?
1. The rate will increase.
2. The rate will decrease.
3. The rate will remain unchanged.
4. The solution will stop flowing.

87. Obesity contributes to the incidence of wound infections because a characteristic of adipose tissue is that it has a relatively
1. poor blood supply.
2. poor lymph supply.
3. high water content.
4. high cellular osmolality.

88. Which one of the following blood values is indicative of an infection?
1. A low calcium level.
2. A low hemoglobin level.
3. An elevated red cell count.
4. An elevated white cell count.

89. A "clean catch" urine specimen is ordered to be obtained from

Mr. Johnson. If the nurse uses the following steps while carrying out the procedure, which one will be in *error?*

1. Donning sterile goves to wear during the procedure.
2. Retracting the foreskin to cleanse the glans penis with soap and water.
3. Having the patient void directly into a clean container.
4. Returning the foreskin to its reduced position.

90. Which portion of the urinary stream *best* reflects the consistency of the bladder urine?
    1. The first portion.
    2. A midstream portion.
    3. The last portion.
    4. Equal samples from the three above portions.

91. Mr. Johnson's urine has a specific gravity of 1.012, a finding which is *most accurately* assessed as being
    1. below normal.
    2. above normal.
    3. within normal range.

92. If Mr. Johnson's urinalysis report includes the following findings, which one should the nurse assess as being *abnormal?*
    1. pH—5.2.
    2. Casts—rare.
    3. White blood cells—2.
    4. Qualitative protein—small amount.

93. The laboratory examination *most often* used to assess the quality of kidney functioning is one that determines the level of blood
    1. glucose.
    2. serum calcium.
    3. urea nitrogen.
    4. protein-bound iodine.

94. The *most common* predisposing factor for a postoperative bladder infection is
    1. limited ambulation.
    2. urinary incontinence.
    3. inadequate fluid intake.
    4. bladder catheterization.

95. Mr. Johnson is concerned about his bowels. Nursing techniques that will help to promote intestinal elimination include *all* of the following measures *except* seeing that Mr. Johnson
    1. has a generous fluid intake.
    2. is ambulating as often as prescribed.
    3. avoids drinking coffee or cola soft drinks.
    4. uses his bedside commode or bathroom instead of a bedpan.

96. If none of the following snacks is contraindicated for Mr. Johnson, which one offers him the best source of protein?
   1. Pretzels.
   2. Corn puffs.
   3. Potato chips.
   4. Peanut butter crackers.
97. Mr. Johnson's daughter tells the nurse that she is concerned about her father's disinterest in food. The nurse should explain that the nutritional requirement that decreases with age is
   1. protein.
   2. calcium.
   3. vitamins.
   4. calories.
98. Which one of the following agencies would provide skilled nursing care to assess Mr. Johnson's progress at home?
   1. A visiting nurse service.
   2. An extended care facility.
   3. The State Nurses' Association.
   4. The American Heart Association.

   Ms. Madeleine Crawford, who is 45 years old, was admitted to the hospital with a diagnosis of renal calculi (kidney stones). Her history includes having had renal calculi in the past. She complained of pain upon admission. The physician's orders include the following:

Schedule for an intravenous pyelogram and for a KUB x-ray examination.
Observe for passage of kidney stones.

   Items 99 through 123 pertain to this situation.

99. When preparing the kidneys, ureters, and bladder (KUB) for x-ray study, the nurse should anticipate that
   1. an enema will be ordered to be given prior to the x-ray examination.
   2. fluids and food will be withheld the morning of the examination.
   3. a tranquilizer will be ordered to be given prior to the examination.
   4. there is ordinarily no special preparation required for the x-ray examination.
100. The intravenous pyelogram indicates that Ms. Crawford has a 2-cm. stone in her left kidney pelvis. Hydronephrosis is also

present. If hydronephrosis goes unchecked, nephritis is likely to develop due to

1. low acidity of the urine.
2. stagnation of urine in the renal pelvis.
3. impaired circulation to the renal pelvis.
4. poor filtration of blood in the nephrons.

101. Which one of the following nursing measures would be *least effective* as a means of finding renal calculi after a patient has voided?
    1. Straining the urine through gauze.
    2. Examining the urine for acetone level.
    3. Inspecting the bedpan for calculi after emptying it.
    4. Breaking up blood clots that may appear in the urine.

102. Intravenous fluids are ordered for Ms. Crawford. When the nurse starts the patient's intravenous therapy, she applies a tourniquet and selects the site for introducing the needle. When should the tourniquet be removed?
    1. When the skin has been cleansed.
    2. As soon as the needle is in the vein.
    3. As soon as the needle is in position under the skin.
    4. When the needle has been secured in place with tape strips.

103. If all of the following areas on Ms. Crawford contain veins that appear easy to enter, which area should the nurse *avoid?*
    1. An area on the back of the hand.
    2. An area on the inner aspect of the elbow.
    3. An area on the inner aspect of the forearm.
    4. An area on the outer aspect of the forearm.

104. Ms. Crawford develops signs of circulatory overload when the intravenous solution is allowed to enter her vein too rapidly. When this occurs, it will be *best* for the nurse to position Ms. Crawford in bed so that she is
    1. lying on her back.
    2. lying on her right side.
    3. in a semisitting position.
    4. in a position with her head lower than her trunk.

105. Ms. Crawford's earlier renal calculi were found to have a high phosphorus content. Which one of the following pharmaceutical preparations is often prescribed to help the body eliminate excess phosphorus through the gastrointestinal tract in order to help prevent renal calculi?
    1. Calcium carbonate (Titralac).
    2. Aluminum hydroxide (Amphojel).
    3. Sodium bicarbonate (baking soda).
    4. Magnesium hydroxide (Milk of Magnesia).

106. Ms. Crawford experiences an episode of renal colic. The nature of the pain associated with renal colic can *best* be described as
    1. dull.
    2. diffuse.
    3. gnawing.
    4. excruciating.
107. Pain resulting from having renal calculi is *most often* referred from the region of the affected kidney to the
    1. other kidney.
    2. coccyx and buttocks.
    3. genitalia and bladder.
    4. umbilicus and epigastric area.
108. Ms. Crawford has nephritis which destroys nephrons in her left kidney. Where in the kidney are the nephrons located?
    1. In the hilus.
    2. In the pelvis.
    3. In the medulla and cortex.
    4. In the capsule and calyces.
109. Ms. Crawford is scheduled to have a left nephrectomy. During the surgical procedure, care will be taken to avoid damaging the adrenal gland. Where is the adrenal gland located?
    1. In the kidney's medulla.
    2. On the top of the kidney.
    3. Next to the ureter where it leaves the kidney.
    4. On the side of the kidney opposite the exit from the kidney pelvis.
110. If adrenal failure occurs, which of the following signs/symptoms is *very common?*
    1. Low blood pressure.
    2. Slow bounding pulse.
    3. Warm skin temperature.
    4. Projectile vomiting without nausea.
111. Postoperatively, Ms. Crawford is ordered to have a daily urine specimen sent to the laboratory. She has continuous bladder drainage with an indwelling catheter, and urine is collected in a bag with a spigot at the bottom for emptying the bag. Which one of the following procedures is *most often* recommended for obtaining a urine specimen with this type of continuous bladder drainage?
    1. Opening the spigot on the collecting bag and allowing urine to empty into the specimen container.
    2. Disconnecting the drainage tube from the collecting bag and allowing urine to flow from the tubing into the specimen container.

3. Disconnecting the drainage tube from the indwelling catheter and allowing urine to flow from the catheter into the specimen container.
4. Removing urine from the drainage tube with a sterile needle and syringe and placing urine from the syringe into the specimen container.

112. How should the drainage tube that is attached to Ms. Crawford's indwelling catheter be fixed in place so that tension on the bladder will be prevented?
1. By taping it to her gown.
2. By taping it to her thigh.
3. By taping it to her lower abdomen.
4. By taping it to her bottom bed linen.

113. Ms. Crawford develops paralytic ileus postoperatively at which time the physician writes the orders given below. Which order should the nurse question before carrying it out?
1. Begin continuous gastric suction.
2. Encourage patient to take carbonated beverages.
3. Neostigmine methyl sulfate (Prostigmin) 0.5 mg. IM stat.
4. Continue intravenous therapy—1000 ml. of 5% dextrose in water every 8 hours.

114. Which one of the following assessments *best* indicates that Ms. Crawford's peristaltic activity is returning to normal after having experienced paralytic ileus?
1. The patient is passing flatus.
2. The patient is complaining of thirst.
3. Bowel sounds are absent when auscultation is used.
4. Peristalsis can be felt when the abdomen is palpated.

115. When observing for signs of hemorrhage from the patient's operative site, the nurse should be certain to check Ms. Crawford's
1. top dressing.
2. bladder drainage.
3. bottom bed linen.

116. If Ms. Crawford develops thrombophlebitis postoperatively, the complication which typical therapy attempts to help prevent is
1. pulmonary emboli.
2. ateriole collapse.
3. cerebrovascular accident.
4. contracture deformities of the leg.

117. Which one of the following agents should the nurse anticipate will most likely be ordered to decrease the likelihood of clotting when a diagnosis of thrombophlebitis is made?
1. Vitamin K.

2. Vitamin B$_{12}$.

3. Folic acid (Folvite).

4. Heparin sodium (Panheprin).

118. Ms. Crawford is ordered to receive warfarin sodium (Coumadin). This drug is classified as an

1. anticoagulant agent.

2. antiarrhythmic agent.

3. anticholinergic agent.

4. antiinflammatory agent.

119. After Ms. Crawford's continuous bladder drainage is discontinued, the physician orders a "clean catch" urine specimen for routine urinalysis. The *minimum* number of milliliters of urine the nurse should collect from the patient for this examination is approximately

1. 25 to 50 ml.

2. 75 to 100 ml.

3. 150 to 200 ml.

4. 250 to 300 ml.

120. If all of the following findings appear in Ms. Crawford's nursing history, which finding is *least likely* to have predisposed her to having renal calculi?

1. Having had several urinary infections.

2. Having less than the recommended amount of milk intake in her diet.

3. Have had a prolonged period of bed rest following an accident the previous year.

4. Having lived in the southwestern part of the United States for most of her life.

121. Which one of the following four patients for whom a nurse is caring is *most* prone to develop renal calculi?

1. A patient with gout.

2. A patient with a gastric ulcer.

3. A patient with Addison's disease.

4. A patient who is a heroin addict.

122. If normal urine is allowed to stand at room temperature for several hours, which one of the following changes will occur?

1. Its color will fade.

2. It will become alkaline.

3. It will develop a strong odor.

4. Its specific gravity will decrease.

123. For which one of the following kidney diseases does heredity appear to be an etiological factor?

1. Nephrosis.

2. Pyelonephritis.

3. Glomerulonephritis.
4. Polycystic disease.

A public health nurse calls on 63-year-old Ms. Elizabeth
Walker who reported having dark urine. She has a history of
recurrent bladder infections.

Items 124 through 140 pertain to this situation.

124. Ms. Walker's daughter indicates to the public health nurse that
she believes her mother imagines her illnesses and is perfectly
well. She says, "For example, the clinic findings show that
mother does not have diabetes but she insists she does."
The nurse should base her response to the daughter's comments on knowledge that
1. psychosomatic illnesses usually occur because of the patient's
conscious desire.
2. emotional support is usually sufficient to treat most
psychosomatic illnesses.
3. physical problems rarely occur as a result of psychological
stresses of daily living.
4. serious physical illnesses have been observed to originate
from psychological problems.

125. Ms. Walker is scheduled to have a cystogram at the hospital on an
outpatient basis. One purpose for performing a cystogram is
to study ureterovesical valve reflux, which means an examination to determine the amount of urine that
1. enters the ureters from the bladder.
2. leaves each kidney from the ureters.
3. remains in the bladder after a normal voiding.
4. escapes from the internal opening of the urethra.

126. When preparing a patient scheduled to have a cystogram, it is
generally recommended that the patient's fluid intake be
1. encouraged.
2. restricted.
3. as desired.

127. After the cystogram, Ms. Walker calls from home to say she has
lower abdominal pain. Of the following nursing measures,
which one is recommended to relieve Ms. Walker's discomfort?
1. Massaging her abdomen.
2. Having her sit in a tub of warm water.
3. Applying an ice bag to her abdomen.
4. Having her void while in the standing position.

128. Ms. Walker is admitted to the hospital when laboratory studies
indicate that she has a malignant tumor of the bladder. Kid-

ney needle biopsy is ordered. Prior to the biopsy, an x-ray examination (plain film) of her kidneys is done, *primarily* in order to

1. determine the size of each kidney.
2. locate the position of each kidney.
3. locate the position of the ureters.
4. determine whether there are kidney stones present.

129. Following kidney needle biopsy, for which one of the following complications should the nurse be especially alert?

1. Hemorrhage.
2. Pulmonary edema.
3. Acute renal failure.
4. Rupture of the kidney.

130. The physician recommends that Ms. Walker have surgery for urinary diversion, using an ileal conduit. Which one of the following techniques will help *most* to protect Ms. Walker from hemorrhage during the surgical procedure?

1. Removing blood clots from the operative site.
2. Flushing the operative area with normal saline.
3. Clamping bleeding vessels in the operative site.
4. Using pressure on bleeding areas in the operative site.

131. Postoperatively, it will be normal for Ms. Walker to excrete (through the ileal conduit) urine that contains

1. pus.
2. feces.
3. blood.
4. mucus.

132. The physician told Ms. Walker that she will have a tube placed in her stomach. The nurse should explain to her that the purpose for having the stomach tube postoperatively is that it will help to

1. prevent aspiration of stomach contents.
2. provide a means for feeding her by gastric gavage.
3. prevent the accumulation of gas in her intestinal tract.
4. allow rest for her stomach until convalescence is underway.

133. Ms. Walker becomes disoriented postoperatively. Which one of the following nursing measures is *most likely* to help Ms. Walker to become oriented?

1. Helping her understand where she is.
2. Calling her by familiar family titles, such as "Granny."
3. Limiting her personal possessions in her unit that remind her of home.
4. Providing her with privacy, such as using pull curtains near her bed.

134. The nurse teaches Ms. Walker to empty her urine collecting device whenever it contains approximately 100 ml. of urine, the *primary* reason being that emptying it before it becomes too full will help prevent
1. rupturing the ileal conduit.
2. suppressing the production of urine.
3. forcing urine from the device back into the kidneys.
4. having the device become so heavy that it will not adhere to her skin.

135. To prevent urine leakage when she changes her collecting device, Ms. Walker should be taught to
1. insert a gauze wick into the stoma.
2. close the opening temporarily with a cellophane seal.
3. suction the conduit for a few minutes before changing the device.
4. withhold oral fluids for several hours before changing the device.

136. Ms. Walker is taught how to clean and deodorize her collecting device. For cleansing purposes, it is *most often* recommended that the device be washed in a solution of water and
1. baking soda.
2. hydrogen peroxide.
3. soap or detergent.
4. alcohol or witch hazel.

137. If the following solutions are available at home, which one will be *best* for deodorizing Ms. Walker's collecting device after it is clean?
1. Salt solution.
2. Ammonia solution.
3. Vinegar solution.
4. Bleaching solution.

138. Maintaining urine acidity will help decrease Ms. Walker's chances of developing a urinary tract infection. Which one of the following juices is *most often* recommended to help maintain urine acidity?
1. Apple juice.
2. Carrot juice.
3. Pineapple juice.
4. Cranberry juice.

139. Ms. Walker wears her collecting device at the site of her stoma on her abdomen. Which one of the following preparations is *most often* recommended for protecting the skin around the stoma from irritation?
1. Baking soda.

2. Cornstarch.
3. Karaya powder.
4. Antibiotic ointment.

140. Another method for collecting urine following an ileal conduit is to drain the urine into a bag fastened to the patient's thigh. This is often used when the patient
1. tends to drink fewer fluids than the average person.
2. has a life style that is more sedentary than active.
3. has considerable adipose tissue in the abdominal region.
4. complains that the stoma appliance is uncomfortable.

Ms. Gloria Dunn was admitted to the hospital with acute right upper quadrant pain which radiates to her back. Her admitting diagnosis was cholecystitis and possible cholelithiasis.
Items 141 through 171 pertain to this situation.

141. The physician orders nitroglycerin (Glyceryl trinitrate) and meperidine hydrochloride (Demerol) for the control of Ms. Dunn's pain. The rationale for using nitroglycerin is that it acts to help
1. relax smooth muscles.
2. reduce nausea and vomiting.
3. enhance the action of meperidine hydrochloride.
4. decrease the secretion of gastric hydrochloric acid.

142. An intravenous infusion is ordered for Ms. Dunn. During the venipuncture procedure, a tourniquet is applied to Ms. Dunn's arm in order to
1. distend the veins.
2. immobilize the arm.
3. stabilize the veins.
4. occlude arterial circulation.

143. If a gallstone were to become lodged in Ms. Dunn's common bile duct, the color of her stools would *most likely* be
1. gray.
2. green.
3. black.
4. yellow.

144. If there is an obstruction in the common bile duct, in addition to a change from normal in the color of the stool, Ms. Dunn is also *most likely* to have signs of
1. circulatory overload.
2. respiratory distress.
3. urinary tract infection.
4. prolonged bleeding time.

145. On Ms. Dunn's second day of hospitalization, the physician orders a low fat diet for her. Which of the following foods would be *most appropriate* for Ms. Dunn's lunch?
    1. Cheese omelet and chocolate pudding.
    2. Ham salad sandwich and baked custard.
    3. Egg salad sandwich and fresh fruit cup.
    4. Roast beef sandwich and tapioca pudding.
146. As preparation for a cholecystogram, Ms. Dunn is ordered to have iopanoic acid (Telepaque) after her evening meal. Prior to administering the iopanoic acid, it is important for the nurse to ask Ms. Dunn if she is allergic to
    1. eggs.
    2. seafoods.
    3. organ meats.
    4. food colorings.
147. At bedtime on the evening before her cholecystogram, Ms. Dunn asks the nurse for a glass of milk. Since milk is contraindicated when a patient is being prepared for a cholecystogram, the nurse should suggest that, as a substitute, Ms. Dunn drink a glass of
    1. water.
    2. lemonade.
    3. orange juice.
    4. tomato juice.
148. Ms. Dunn's x-ray films reveal the presence of gallstones and she is prepared for a cholecystectomy and choledochotomy. The nurse should interpret the term choledochotomy to mean
    1. drainage of the gallbladder.
    2. opening of the common bile duct.
    3. removal of stones from the common bile duct.
    4. insertion of a drainage tube into the cystic duct.
149. The physician orders that Ms. Dunn receive no food or fluids after midnight before having surgery. Oral foods and fluids are generally withheld before surgery for patients who will receive general anesthesia *primarily* to help prevent
    1. constipation during the immediate postoperative period.
    2. vomiting and possible aspiration of vomitus during surgery.
    3. pressure on the diaphragm with poor lung expansion during surgery.
    4. gas pains and distention during the immediate postoperative period.
150. The nurse chooses to give Ms. Dunn her preoperative intramuscular medication in the ventrogluteal site. The muscle into which the nurse will inject the medication is the
    1. gluteus medius muscle.

2. rectus femoris muscle.

3. gluteus maximus muscle.

4. vastus lateralis muscle.

151. Ms. Dunn returns from surgery with a T tube sutured into the common bile duct. Which one of the following statements explains the *primary* purpose of the T tube?
    1. It helps in the removal of wound drainage.
    2. It prevents bile from entering the duodenum.
    3. It prevents the bile from entering the peritoneum.
    4. It provides a mechanism for irrigating the biliary tract.

152. To maintain accurate intake and output records, the amount of T tube drainage is measured and then recorded by
    1. adding it to the patient's urinary output.
    2. charting it separately on the output record.
    3. adding it to the amount of nasogastric drainage.
    4. subtracting it from the total intake for the day.

153. A scultetus (many-tailed) binder is used when Ms. Dunn ambulates. Which one of the following techniques should the nurse use for the correct application of the binder?
    1. Wrapping it from bottom to top.
    2. Wrapping it from top to bottom.
    3. Beginning in the middle and wrapping it in either direction.

154. Ms. Dunn uses blow bottles postoperatively, *primarily* because they help to
    1. stimulate circulation.
    2. prepare for ambulation.
    3. strengthen abdominal muscles.
    4. increase respiratory effectiveness.

155. The nurse observes that Ms. Dunn's intravenous solution is infusing very slowly and there is swelling and hardness at the needle site. Which of the following courses of action should the nurse take?
    1. Apply a warm dressing to the site and continue the infusion very slowly.
    2. Discontinue the infusion and assemble equipment for another venipuncture.
    3. Stop the flow temporarily and resume the flow when the swelling and hardness decrease.
    4. Disconnect the infusion tubing from the needle and irrigate the needle with normal saline.

156. Ms. Dunn states that she is nauseated on her first postoperative day. Of the following medications, the one *most commonly* used to relieve the postoperative discomforts of nausea and vomiting is
    1. diazepam (Valium).

2. meprobamate (Miltown).

3. chlordiazepoxide (Librium).

4. prochlorperazine (Compazine).

157. On the third postoperative day, the physician assesses that Ms. Dunn has developed paralytic ileus. Which of the following signs did the nurse *most probably* report to aid the physician with his diagnosis?

1. Passage of flatus.

2. Absence of bowel sounds.

3. Vomiting of fecal material.

4. Uncontrolled singultus (hiccups).

158. The physician orders that Ms. Dunn have continuous nasogastric suction. In which of the following positions should Ms. Dunn be placed for passage of the nasogastric tube?

1. Sitting with the neck hyperextended.

2. Lying on her left side with a pillow under the head.

3. Low Fowler's position with a rolled towel under the shoulders.

4. Lying on her right side with the head of the bed elevated approximately 15°.

159. Which one of the following techniques is *least acceptable* for assessing whether the nasogastric tube is in the stomach?

1. Applying suction to the tube and observing for the return of gastric contents.

2. Irrigating the tube with normal saline and observing for the return of solution.

3. Inverting the free end of the tube in a glass of water and observing for air bubbles.

4. Instilling air into the tube and auscultating over the epigastric area for air sounds.

160. The physician orders neostigmine methyl sulfate (Prostigmin) for Ms. Dunn. This drug is classified as

1. a beta blocking agent.

2. an alpha blocking agent.

3. an anticholinergic agent.

4. an anticholinesterase agent.

161. Neostigmine methyl sulfate facilitates transmission of impulses across the myoneural junction by

1. competing with catecholamines.

2. inhibiting adrenergic stimulation.

3. blocking the effects of muscarine.

4. prolonging the activity of acetylcholine.

162. Nasogastric replacement therapy is used for Ms. Dunn, the *primary* purpose being to help

1. maintain acid-base balance.
2. facilitate osmotic diuresis.
3. equalize the intake and output record.
4. maintain water and electrolyte balance.
163. How should solution that is *not* returned when the nasogastric
   tube is irrigated be recorded on the patient's intake and output
   record?
   1. It should be recorded separately.
   2. It should be added to the patient's intake.
   3. It should be added to the patient's output.
   4. It should be subtracted from the patient's intake.
164. Which one of the following nursing measures is *most often*
   recommended for a patient with a nasogastric tube in place to
   help reduce throat discomfort?
   1. Having the patient use anesthetic lozenges as indicated.
   2. Having the patient take frequent small sips of warm water.
   3. Irrigating the tube with warm solution at frequent intervals.
   4. Having the patient rinse her mouth with an antiseptic solu-
      tion.
165. Which one of the following characteristics do the Miller-Abbott,
   Cantor, and Harris tubes have in common?
   1. There are two channels for drainage of gastrointestinal con-
      tents.
   2. There is a lumen for the constant intake of air from the atmos-
      phere.
   3. There is a mechanism to help move the tubes into the intesti-
      nal tract.
   4. There is a self-inflating balloon to hold the tubes securely in
      the intestinal tract.
166. The nurse planned dietary teaching for Ms. Dunn prior to her
   discharge. Ms. Dunn will ordinarily feel *most* comfortable
   when she restricts her intake of
   1. fats.
   2. proteins.
   3. minerals.
   4. carbohydrates.
167. Of the following health problems, which one predisposes *most*
   to the development of gallbladder disease?
   1. Obesity.
   2. Alcoholism.
   3. Hypertension.
   4. Chronic constipation.
168. The gallbladder and biliary tract normally are responsible for *all*
   of the following functions *except*

1. storing bile.
2. secreting bile.
3. transporting bile.
4. concentrating bile.

169. Which of the following bile components is responsible for the effective digestion of fat in the small intestines?
   1. Lecithin.
   2. Bilirubin.
   3. Bile salts.
   4. Cholesterol.

170. The structure that controls the passage of bile and pancreatic enzymes into the duodenum is the
   1. common bile duct.
   2. ampulla of Vater.
   3. pyloric sphincter.
   4. sphincter of Oddi.

171. Which one of the following physiological processes occurs when the intestinal mucosa secretes cholecystokinin?
   1. Peristalsis is inhibited.
   2. The sphincter of Oddi relaxes.
   3. The gallbladder contracts and empties.
   4. Food passes from the stomach to the duodenum.

Mr. Robert Shelly, who is 57 years old, was admitted to the hospital for cardiac surgery.   He has mitral stenosis.
Items 172 through 208 relate to this situation.

172. Mr. Shelly's apical-radial pulse rate is obtained regularly, the *primary* reason being to determine the pulse
   1. rhythm.
   2. deficit.
   3. pressure.
   4. strength.

173. Which one of the following nursing measures has the *most potential* for decreasing the patient's anxieties preoperatively?
   1. Allowing the patient time to express his fears.
   2. Taking the patient on a tour of the operating room suite.
   3. Explaining the nature of the surgery the patient will have.
   4. Encouraging the patient's family to visit as much as hospital policy allows.

174. When planning a teaching program for Mr. Shelly, which one of the following steps should the nurse take *first?*
   1. Defining the medical terms the nurse will use.
   2. Telling the patient the goal the nurse has in mind.

3. Determining the patient's knowledge on the subject.

4. Explaining the nurse's qualifications for teaching him.

175. Preoperatively, the nurse teaches Mr. Shelly about various devices that will be used during and after his heart surgery. Which one of the following devices is *least likely* to be used for Mr. Shelly?

1. An arterial line.

2. An indwelling catheter.

3. Alternating tourniquets.

4. Electrocardiogram monitor.

176. Mr. Shelly will have an endotracheal tube in place when he leaves the operating room. The nurse should prepare the patient by explaining to him that the tube will

1. require that he lie quietly on his back.

2. make it impossible for him to speak while the tube is in place.

3. be removed within 2 or 3 hours after he awakens following surgery.

4. require that he have a small neckline incision in order to insert the tube.

177. Mr. Shelly asks why he will have a tube in his chest. The nurse's response should be based on knowledge that the tube will assist in accomplishing *all* of the following goals *except*

1. preventing hemorrhage.

2. preventing clotting in the wound area.

3. indicating blood loss for replacement.

4. identifying the type of wound drainage.

178. During visiting hours one afternoon, Mr. Shelly's wife and children discuss new responsibilities each will have at home during Mr. Shelly's illness and convalescence. Mr. Shelly does not join in the conversation as he normally would have. His quietness is *most probably* due to

1. anxieties about possible death.

2. concern about his sudden role change.

3. an inability to comprehend his illness.

4. confidence in his family's ability to adjust.

179. If a drug Mr. Shelly has been taking is discontinued a day or two before he is to have heart surgery, the nurse should question the discontinuation order if the drug is classified as

1. a sedative.

2. a diuretic.

3. a cardiotonic.

4. an antihypertensive.

180. Mr. Shelly is placed on a hypothermia pad prior to surgery. The patient should be cooled slowly when hypothermia is

used to help prevent shivering which causes an undesirable increase in the
1. metabolic activity of brain cells.
2. level of glucose in the bloodstream.
3. secretion of the hormone epinephrine.
4. level of carbon dioxide in the bloodstream.

181. Which one of the following sketches illustrates where the incision line is *most often* located when open heart surgery is performed?

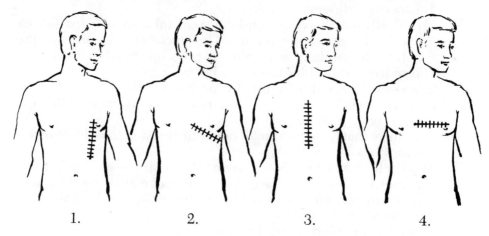

1.   2.   3.   4.

182. Which one of the following types of devices is very commonly used to replace a diseased mitral valve?
1. Ball-in-cage valve.
2. Metal flap closure.
3. Rubber cover implant.
4. Silicone gate structure.

183. During surgery, Mr. Shelly receives heparin sodium (Panheprin) while he is on the cardiopulmonary bypass machine. For which one of the following complications should the nurse be *especially* alert when a patient is receiving this drug?
1. Hemorrhage.
2. Cardiac arrest.
3. Thrombophlebitis.
4. Pulmonary embolus.

184. From which of the following structures does blood leave Mr. Shelly's body when he is placed on the cardiopulmonary bypass machine?
1. Aorta.
2. Left ventricle.
3. Pulmonary artery and vein.

4. Superior and inferior vena cavae.

185. When Mr. Shelly is removed from the cardiopulmonary machine, what agent will *most likely* be ordered for him to neutralize the effects of the heparin sodium?
1. Vitamin A.
2. Vitamin C.
3. Protamine sulfate.
4. Warfarin sodium (Coumadin).

186. Postoperatively, nursing efforts will include helping Mr. Shelly avoid activities that result in Valsalva's maneuver (bearing down against a closed glottis). Which one of the following nursing orders should appear on his care plan to help prevent the Valsalva's maneuver?
1. Have the patient take fewer but deeper breaths.
2. Have the patient clench his teeth while moving in bed.
3. Have the patient take oral fluids through a drinking tube.
4. Have the patient avoid holding his breath during activity.

187. Mr. Shelly develops premature ventricular contractions (PVCs). Which one of the following patterns traced by an electrocardiograph illustrates this type of arrhythmia?

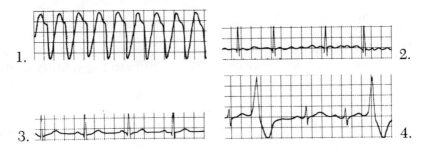

188. The physician orders lidocaine hydrochloride (Xylocaine), 1000 mg. in 500 ml. of 5% dextrose in water intravenously at the rate of 3 mg. of lidocaine hydrochloride per minute when Mr. Shelly develops multiple PVCs. If the equipment used for administering the drug and solution indicates that 60 microdrops are equal to 1 ml., how many microdrops would provide 3 mg. of lidocaine hydrochloride each minute?
1. 12 microdrops.
2. 24 microdrops.
3. 60 microdrops.
4. 90 microdrops.

189. After some excitation, which one of the following symptoms is *typical* of a toxic reaction to lidocaine hydrochloride?

1. Dyspnea.
2. Drowsiness.
3. Ringing in the ears.
4. Numbness in the extremities.

190. The nurse assesses peripheral circulation by checking Mr. Shelly's dorsalis pedis pulse. At which location on the diagram below can the dorsalis pedis pulse be assessed *best?*

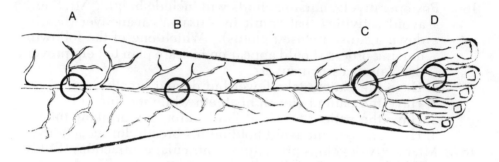

1. Site A.
2. Site B.
3. Site C.
4. Site D.

191. If the pedal pulses are not palpable, what assessment should the nurse perform *next* in order to estimate the quality of peripheral circulation?
1. Check the patient's pulses at the femoral arteries.
2. Check the patient's feet for their color and warmth.
3. Check the patient's lower back (sacral area) for color and edema.
4. Check the patient's pedal pulses after he coughs and deep breathes several times.

192. Mr. Shelly is ordered to have his central venous pressure (CVP) monitored. The purpose for determining Mr. Shelly's central venous pressure is to help in assessing the
1. circulatory volume in his arteries.
2. blood pressure in the left ventricle.
3. heart's ability to receive and pump blood.
4. oxygen and carbon dioxide pressure in the blood.

193. Mr. Shelly's chest tube accidently slips out when he is turning onto his side. Of the following possible actions, which one should the nurse take *first?*
1. Disconnecting the suction machine.

2. Applying a dressing to the chest wall.

3. Placing a closed hand over the chest opening.

4. Clamping the chest tube at its connection to the suction machine.

194. When the nurse uses auscultation on Mr. Shelly's chest wall, she hears rales which should indicate to her that the patient has *very likely* developed

1. endocarditis.

2. an asthmatic attack.

3. pleural friction rub.

4. pulmonary congestion.

195. For which one of the following complications should the nurse observe if Mr. Shelly's prothrombin time is longer than normal?

1. Emboli.

2. Hemorrhage.

3. Renal shutdown.

4. Respiratory failure.

196. What vitamin is necessary in order for the liver to produce prothrombin?

1. Vitamin A.

2. Vitamin B$_{12}$.

3. Vitamin D.

4. Vitamin K.

197. Mr. Shelly is ordered to have elastic bandages applied to his lower legs. Which one of the following statements describes proper technique when applying elastic bandages to the lower legs?

1. The bandages should cover the toes of the feet.

2. The bandages should expose bony prominences at the ankles.

3. The bandages should be started just below the knees with a circular turn.

4. The bandages should be applied so that tension on each turn is approximately equal.

198. Of the following practices of asepsis that the nurse should observe when changing Mr. Shelly's dressings, which one is usually credited as being the *most effective* in helping to prevent a wound infection?

1. Washing her hands before beginning the procedure.

2. Using prepackaged sterile dressings to cover the incision.

3. Cleansing the incisional area with an antiseptic solution.

4. Placing the soiled dressings in a water-proof bag before disposing of them.

199. Mr. Shelly asks the nurse to "break" or gatch his bed in a manner that would support his knees in a flexed position. The nurse should explain that the position he requested is *contraindicated primarily* in order to avoid
1. placing the feet in a dropped position.
2. causing the knees to ankylose ("freeze").
3. causing stagnation of blood in his lower extremities.
4. placing pressure on nerves in the area under his knees.

200. Mr. Shelly often speaks of his memberships and responsibilities in the Optimist and The Lions' Clubs. According to Erik Erikson's theory on human development, this type of activity reflects Mr. Shelly's concern with
1. intimacy versus isolation.
2. ego integrity versus despair.
3. identity versus role confusion.
4. generativity versus stagnation.

201. Patients like Mr. Shelly who become accustomed to care in specialized hospital units, such as a cardiac care unit, often experience uneasiness and fear when they are transferred to a general care unit. Which one of the following nursing measures is likely to help these patients *most* while they are adjusting to less intensive care?
1. Checking them at frequent intervals.
2. Emphasizing their progress toward recovery.
3. Orienting them especially carefully to their new environment.
4. Placing them in a room with a patient who also has been in a specialized unit.

202. Mr. Shelly delayed having surgery longer than his physician had wished. Which one of the following statements has the *least* amount of scientific support as a reason why some people neglect obtaining proper health care?
1. Fear of having a disease often leads to ignoring its symptoms.
2. An attitude often influences behavior more strongly than a fact.
3. Neglecting to have health care often appears to be an inherited trait.
4. Lack of knowledge of a disease often results in neglecting to seek proper care.

203. While the nurse is preparing Mr. Shelly for discharge, she teaches him how to use his body effectively when carrying out activities of daily living. Which one of the following sketches illustrates poor body mechanics?

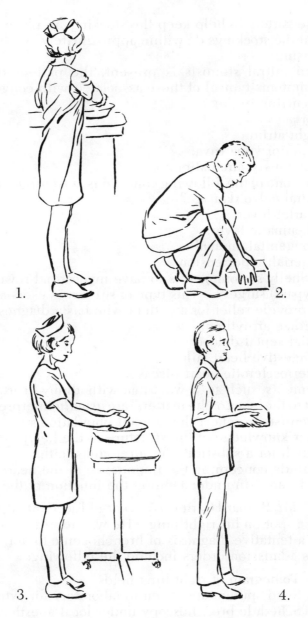

1.

2.

3.

4.

204. Mr. Shelly is to wear elasticized stockings after discharge. He should be taught to
1. discard them when they become soiled.
2. inspect his legs daily while bathing.

3. use garters to help keep the stockings in place.
4. put the stockings on within approximately one-half hour after arising.

205. When mitral stenosis is present, the patient demonstrates symptoms typical of those associated with congestion that is occurring in the
   1. aorta.
   2. right atrium.
   3. superior vena cava.
   4. pulmonary circulation.

206. Which one of the following conditions *most often* predisposes to mitral valve damage?
   1. Scarlet fever.
   2. Rheumatic fever.
   3. Congenital anomalies.
   4. Arterial hypertension.

207. Mr. Shelly's roommate is to have myocardial revascularization (bypass) surgery. This type of surgery is used *most common* to provide relief for a patient who has a diagnosis of
   1. cardiac arrhythmia.
   2. atrial septal defect.
   3. congestive heart failure.
   4. arteriosclerotic heart disease.

208. Statements, such as "I want that with all my heart," and "Let's get to the heart of the matter," are *usually* interpreted by social scientists to reflect the general population's
   1. poor knowledge of the structure of the heart.
   2. search for a substitute for a religious faith.
   3. attitude concerning the importance of the heart.
   4. disinterest in understanding the function of the heart.

Mr. Bernard Carter, a 55-year-old accountant, was found to have a spot on his right lung. He was admitted to the hospital with a tentative diagnosis of bronchogenic tumor. The physician's admission orders include the following:

Tomogram of right lung fields.
Send sputum specimen to laboratory for cytology.
Schedule bronchoscopy under local anesthesia.
Schedule pulmonary function tests.

Items 209 through 258 pertain to this situation.

209. Tomography is a radiographic examination of the chest that provides for visualization of
   1. pulmonary motion.

2. the bronchiole tree.

3. sections of the lung from various planes.

4. the thickness of membranes surrounding alveoli sacs.

210. Cytologic examination of Mr. Carter's sputum is done in order to determine the presence of

1. mucous casts.

2. blood cells.

3. malignant cells.

4. pathogenic bacteria.

211. If Mr. Carter is given oral fluids before the local anesthetic has worn off following the bronchoscopy, he is very likely to

1. choke.

2. cough.

3. vomit.

4. sneeze.

212. The *primary* purpose for conducting a variety of pulmonary function tests on Mr. Carter prior to surgery is to

1. evaluate the extent of the spread of the lung cancer.

2. estimate the amount of anesthesia needed for the surgery.

3. determine the amount of lung tissue that will need to be removed.

4. calculate whether the contemplated surgery will leave enough functioning lung tissue.

213. The term tidal air means the volume of air that

1. remains in the lungs after a forced expiration.

2. is exhaled after the deepest possible inhalation.

3. is inhaled after the greatest possible expiration.

4. is inhaled and exhaled with one normal respiration.

214. Mr. Carter is ordered to receive intermittent positive pressure breathing (IPPB) therapy. The *primary* purpose for using preoperative IPPB therapy for Mr. Carter is to

1. dilate his bronchioles.

2. aerate dead air spaces in his lungs.

3. reduce the carbon dioxide in his blood.

4. clear his airway to the greatest extent possible.

215. Mr. Carter complains of feeling dizzy and lightheaded during his first IPPB treatment. The *most probable* cause for Mr. Carter's symptoms is that he is

1. breathing too rapidly.

2. receiving air that is too humid.

3. using poorly functioning equipment.

4. receiving an insufficient amount of oxygen.

216. Mr. Carter has high voltage radiation therapy preoperatively, the *primary* purpose of this therapy being to

1. alleviate his symptoms.
2. decrease the size of the tumor.
3. minimize the risk of metastasis.
4. depress the formation of red blood cells.

217. Mr. Carter is scheduled for chest surgery. He has a preoperative order for atropine sulfate, gr. 1/6 (10 mg.), subcutaneously. The nurse questions the order because it is
   1. a larger than normal dose.
   2. a smaller than normal dose.
   3. unusual to give atropine sulfate subcutaneously.
   4. unusual to give atropine sulfate before chest surgery.

218. Mr. Carter's surgical report states that he had an exploratory thoracotomy with a right lower lobectomy. Which of the following muscles was transsected by the thoracotomy incision?
   1. Teres major.
   2. Scalenus medius.
   3. Latissimus dorsi.
   4. Quadratus lumborum.

219. Mr. Carter is ordered to have oxygen by nasal cannula at 3 liters per minute. Approximately what percentage of oxygen is Mr. Carter receiving via the cannula?
   1. 5 percent.
   2. 12 percent.
   3. 32 percent.
   4. 50 percent.

220. Which one of the following assessment procedures should the nurse use to determine when Mr. Carter needs tracheal suctioning postoperatively?
   1. Auscultation of breath sounds.
   2. Inspection of chest movements.
   3. Percussion of the lung borders.
   4. Palpation of diaphragm movements.

221. The *chief* purpose of performing tracheal suctioning on Mr. Carter is to
   1. excite the cough reflex.
   2. remove pharyngeal secretions.
   3. re-expand collapsed lung tissues.
   4. break up obstructing mucous plugs.

222. Which of the following measures will help prevent hypoxia due to suctioning?
   1. Positioning the patient properly.
   2. Using a catheter of appropriate size.
   3. Oxygenating the patient before suctioning.
   4. Checking for patency of the suctioning equipment.

223. Mr. Carter is ordered to have central venous pressure readings

every hour. During the first and second postoperative hours, his central venous pressure readings ranged between 3 and 4 cm. of water pressure. The nurse should interpret these readings as reflecting

1. loss of fluids.
2. normal pressure.
3. overload of fluids.
4. a nonfunctioning pressure gauge.

224. In addition to monitoring his pressure, the nurse should anticipate that the patient's central venous pressure catheter is also often used for *all* of the following purposes *except*

1. infusing fluids.
2. administering medications.
3. administering a blood transfusion.
4. drawing blood for laboratory purposes.

225. Mr. Carter is ordered to receive morphine sulfate for the control of pain. An undesirable effect of the indiscriminate use of morphine sulfate is that it acts to

1. decrease mental awareness.
2. increase the blood pressure.
3. depress the respiratory center.
4. inhibit the secretion of mucus.

226. If the following nursing measures are planned for Mr. Carter, it would be *best* to medicate him for pain prior to carrying out

1. coughing routines.
2. deep-breathing exercises.
3. range-of-motion exercises.
4. repositioning of the patient.

227. To close the glottis before starting a cough, the nurse should teach Mr. Carter to

1. swallow immediately before starting to cough.
2. exert pressure with his hand on his voice box.
3. bear down by contracting his abdominal muscles.
4. hold his breath for a few seconds and then cough.

228. A blood transfusion, to be administered at 60 ml. of blood per hour, is ordered for Mr. Carter. The equipment has a drop factor of 15 drops per ml. How many drops per minute should the patient receive?

1. 10 drops.
2. 15 drops.
3. 20 drops.
4. 25 drops.

229. Since Mr. Carter is receiving 60 ml. of blood per hour, approximately how long will it take for him to receive one unit of whole blood?

1. 2 hours.
2. 4 hours.
3. 6 hours.
4. 8 hours.

230. It is generally contraindicated to administer blood intravenously to Mr. Carter at a rate faster than 60 ml. per hour because more rapid infusion predisposes to
1. pulmonary edema.
2. emboli formation.
3. hemolysis of red blood cells.
4. allergic reactions to the blood.

231. Mr. Carter has an anterior (upper) and a posterior (lower) chest catheter. Each is attached with tubing to a single-bottle closed chest drainage system. Four hours after surgery, the measuring tape on the side of Mr. Carter's posterior chest drainage bottle reads 350 ml. At the time the system was initiated, 100 ml. of sterile water were put into the bottle. How much chest drainage did Mr. Carter have in 4 hours?
1. 150 ml.
2. 250 ml.
3. 350 ml.
4. 450 ml.

232. The nurse should anticipate that the return from the catheter in the anterior (upper) chest wall should normally consist mainly of
1. air.
2. blood.
3. mucus.
4. serosanguineous fluid.

233. Which one of the following diagrams illustrates the correct setup for a one-bottle closed chest drainage system?

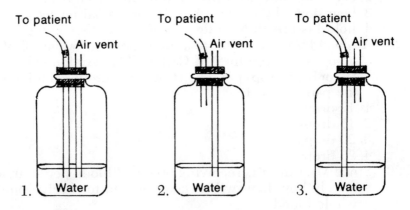

234. Which one of the following aspects of a closed chest drainage system prevents backward, or return, flow of air and fluid into the pleural space?
1. Water seal.
2. Force of gravity.
3. Mechanical suction.
4. Atmospheric pressure.

235. "Milking," or "stripping," the chest tubes is done *primarily* to
1. prevent kinking of the drainage tube.
2. maintain the patency of the drainage tube.
3. re-establish negative intrapleural pressure.
4. avoid backflow of fluid into the pleural space.

236. On his second postoperative day, Mr. Carter's oral temperature is noted to be 100.4° F. On the Celsuis scale, his temperature was equivalent to
1. 37.6° C.
2. 38.0° C.
3. 38.4° C.
4. 38.8° C.

237. At approximately what time in a 24-hour period is the body temperature for most people the *lowest?*
1. Noon.
2. Midnight.
3. Early in the morning.
4. Early in the evening.

238. Which one of the following statements explains *best* how a glass mercury thermometer functions to determine body temperature?
1. Mercury expands when it is heated.
2. Glass contracts when it is in contact with heat.
3. The specific gravity of mercury decreases when warmed.
4. The thermal coefficient is greater for mercury than it is for glass.

239. Mr. Carter states that he is worried about whether his wife will be able to visit him. Worry differs from anxiety in that worry can usually be
1. traced to unfound fears and doubts.
2. identified and expressed as a concern.
3. put out of mind easily with willpower.
4. suppressed effectively with tranquilizers and sedatives.

240. Which one of the following statements describes a correct assessment when the nurse observes intermittent bubbling in Mr. Carter's drainage bottle?
1. The system is functioning in a normal manner.

2. The water level has dropped too low in the drainage bottle.
3. One of the catheters has slipped out of the patient's chest.
4. The tube connecting the drainage bottle with the patient's chest catheter has developed a leak.

241. For the closed drainage system to function effectively, at what level, in relation to the patient's chest, should the bottle(s) be placed?
1. At the level of the chest.
2. Below the level of the chest.
3. Above the level of the chest.

242. Which one of the following items should be kept readily available while Mr. Carter has chest tubes in place?
1. An airway.
2. A tracheostomy tray.
3. A rubber-capped hemostat.
4. An additional drainage bottle.

243. On the third postoperative day, the physician removes Mr. Carter's posterior chest tube. Which one of the following items is ordinarily placed directly over the wound when the chest tube is removed?
1. A Montgomery strap.
2. A butterfly bandage.
3. A petrolatum gauze dressing.
4. A fine mesh gauze dressing.

244. What is the *most probable* cause when, on Mr. Carter's fifth postoperative day, the fluctuation of the water level in the long glass tube(s) in the chest drainage bottle stops?
1. The tubing is kinked.
2. The lung has re-expanded.
3. There is a leakage of air in the seal.
4. The tubing is blocked with mucous plugs.

245. When the nurse reports that the fluid fluctuation has stopped in Mr. Carter's chest drainage system, she should anticipate that the physician will instruct her to
1. milk the tubing.
2. order a chest x-ray examination.
3. remove the chest tube.
4. double clamp the tubing.

Another type of chest drainage that could have been used for Mr. Carter, uses mechanical suction. The diagram on page 211 and items 246 through 248 pertain to a 3-bottle suction setup for closed chest drainage.

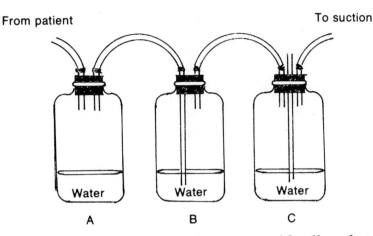

From patient

To suction

Water | Water | Water

A   B   C

246. Which one of the bottles in the diagram would collect drainage from the pleural space?
   1. Bottle A.
   2. Bottle B.
   3. Bottle C.
247. Which one of the bottles in the diagram is the pressure regulator bottle?
   1. Bottle A.
   2. Bottle B.
   3. Bottle C.
248. If it becomes necessary to turn off the motor that provides suction in the diagrammed setup, an air vent must be provided in the system. Which one of the following methods is generally recommended for opening the system to the atmosphere?
   1. Disconnecting the patient's chest tube from the setup at bottle A.
   2. Raising the long tube in bottle B above water level.
   3. Removing the cap which seals Bottle C.
   4. Disconnecting the tube leading to the suction motor from the setup.
249. Which one of the following positions in bed is generally *contraindicated* for the patient following chest surgery?
   1. Side-lying position.
   2. Lying on the abdomen.
   3. Semisitting position.
   4. Trendelenburg's position.
250. Which of the following rehabilitative measures should the nurse instruct Mr. Carter to perform to prevent the development of "frozen shoulder" after his chest surgery?
   1. Turning from side to side.

2. Lifting and lowering his head.

3. Raising his right arm over his head.

4. Flexing and extending his right elbow.

251. At the time of discharge, Mr. Carter asks the nurse for the name of an organization where he could volunteer to help teach others about lung cancer. Of the following organizations, which one would be *best* for the nurse to recommend?

1. The American Red Cross.

2. The American Cancer Society.

3. The State Health Department.

4. The American Medical Association.

252. Mr. Carter has a history of cigarette smoking. One of the respiratory tract's functions, that of cleaning its passages of debris, is damaged by cigarette smoking, through smoking's effects on the tract's

1. cilia.

2. alveoli.

3. the pleura.

4. mucous secretions.

253. A common *early* symptom of bronchogenic cancer is

1. a hacking cough.

2. general malaise.

3. dull chest pain.

4. difficulty with breathing.

254. The examination used *most often* for screening for bronchogenic cancer is a

1. chest x-ray.

2. lung scanning.

3. sputum examination.

4. test of pulmonary function.

255. It is recommended that persons who are habitual cigarette smokers have screening examinations for bronchogenic cancer every

1. 6 weeks.

2. 3 months.

3. 6 months.

4. 12 months.

256. Which one of the following statements *best* describes a current trend in cigarette smoking in the United States today?

1. Fewer teenagers are beginning to smoke each year than was true a decade ago.

2. The number of women who start smoking annually has been increasing in recent years.

3. The daily average number of cigarettes each smoker uses has

been decreasing in recent years.

4. There has been a slow but steady decline in the last decade in the total number of cigarette smokers in the general population.

257. When a lung tumor is called a secondary tumor, it means that a characteristic of the primary (original) tumor cells is that the primary cells
1. were malignant and are now benign.
2. were benign and have become malignant.
3. have spread to the lungs from another organ.
4. responded to therapy while the secondary growth is resistant to containment.

258. Which of the following types of cells line the bronchioles?
1. Simple squamous epithelium.
2. Ciliated columnar epithelium.
3. Stratified squamous epithelium.
4. Cuboidal glandular epithelium.

Mr. Glenn Hopkin, who is 46 years old, was admitted to the hospital with a diagnosis of bleeding gastric ulcers. He has a history of "stomach trouble" and bleeding. Surgical intervention is planned.

Items 259 through 281 pertain to this situation.

259. Mr. Hopkin had been taking an antacid containing magnesium salts. If he experienced adverse side effects from the antacid, he would *most likely* complain of
1. diarrhea.
2. flatulence.
3. bloody stools.
4. abdominal cramping.

260. If Mr. Hopkin had been taking an antacid containing aluminum compounds and experienced adverse side effects, he would *most likely* have complained of
1. faintness.
2. headaches.
3. constipation.
4. respiratory congestion.

261. While interviewing Mr. Hopkin, the nurse learns that he had been taking the types of pharmaceutical preparations listed below. From an etiological viewpoint, which type may well have contributed to his having gastric ulcers?
1. Diuretics.
2. Cathartics.

3. Salicylates.

4. Antihistamines.

262. Because of Mr. Hopkin's history, the nurse should be particularly alert for evidence of perforation, the *most common first* sign/symptom being

1. projectile vomiting.

2. sharp abdominal pain.

3. marked abdominal distention.

4. sudden decrease in blood pressure.

263. Mr. Hopkin is scheduled to have a subtotal gastrectomy with a jejunotomy. This surgical procedure allows the stomach contents to bypass the

1. ileum.

2. duodenum.

3. cardiac sphincter.

4. fundus of the stomach.

264. Preoperatively Mr. Hopkin demonstrates symptoms of anxiety. Which part of the nervous system normally carries innervation to produce symptoms of anxiety?

1. The brain.

2. The spinal cord.

3. The somatic division of the nervous system.

4. The autonomic division of the nervous system.

265. When Mr. Hopkin returns from surgery, he is ordered to have continuous gastric suction. During the first 12 to 24 hours postoperatively, the nurse can expect that the normal color of his stomach contents will be

1. brown.

2. green.

3. yellow.

4. cloudy white.

266. If gastric suction is used indiscriminately, Mr. Hopkin will *most probably* develop

1. renal failure.

2. paralytic ileus.

3. abdominal distention.

4. electrolyte imbalances.

267. The nurse wishes to position Mr. Hopkin in bed postoperatively in a manner that will minimize tension on his abdominal incision and allow his cardiovascular and respiratory systems to function well. To accomplish these goals, which of the following positions would be the *best* one for Mr. Hopkin?

1. Lying on his abdomen.

2. Lying flat on his back.

3. Lying in a low semisitting position.

4. Lying on either side with his knees flexed.

268. Mr. Hopkin is ordered to have inhalations of carbon dioxide postoperatively, the *primary* reason being to help

1. promote gastric drainage.

2. prevent metabolic alkalosis.

3. stimulate deep respirations.

4. improve the strength of his heartbeat.

269. For the first 3 or 4 days postoperatively, the nurse can anticipate that Mr. Hopkin's needs for nourishment will be met by giving him

1. clear liquids by mouth.

2. liquid nourishment through his gastric tube.

3. essential electrolytes and glucose introduced with intravenous therapy.

4. essential proteins and electrolytes introduced with parenteral hyperalimentation therapy.

270. Nursing orders include irrigating Mr. Hopkin's gastric tube at regular intervals. Of the following fluids that could be used for irrigating purposes, the one of choice is

1. normal saline.

2. distilled water.

3. mild antiseptic solution.

4. soda bicarbonate solution.

271. The amount of drainage observed on Mr. Hopkin's dressing was recorded by a different nurse at four different times. Which one of the following entries on Mr. Hopkin's record describes observations in the *most useful* manner?

1. "There is a moderate amount of drainage on the dressing."

2. "The amount of drainage has doubled since the last observation."

3. "The amount of drainage that has stained his dressing is the size of a quarter."

4. "There is no increase in amount of drainage since dressing change yesterday."

272. Mr. Hopkin complains of a sore throat while the gastric tube is in place. The discomfort caused by the tube is *most probably* due to

1. dehydration.

2. an infection.

3. a chemical irritation.

4. a mechanical irritation.

273. Mr. Hopkin's electrolyte blood findings include a potassium level of 3.8 mEq. per L. Which one of the following interpre-

tations of this finding is *most accurate?*
   1. The electrolyte level is above normal range.
   2. The electrolyte level is below normal range.
   3. The electroylte level is within normal range.
274. Which one of the following changes in his stomach should Mr. Hopkin be taught to expect as time goes on postoperatively?
   1. It will likely shrink in size.
   2. It will likely accommodate larger meals.
   3. It will likely tolerate spicy foods poorly.
   4. It will likely develop a sphincter at the site of anastomosis.
275. At the time Mr. Hopkin is ready for discharge, he notices that he is belching small amounts of emesis after eating. He asks the nurse why this is happening. The nurse should explain that the *most probable* cause is that he is
   1. eating too rapidly.
   2. taking too much food with each meal.
   3. being too active immediately after eating.
   4. swallowing large amounts of air while eating.
276. About 2 weeks after discharge from the hospital, Mr. Hopkin develops the "dumping syndrome," a condition believed due to rapid emptying of stomach contents. Which one of the following symptoms strongly suggests that the patient is suffering from the "dumping syndrome"?
   1. Nausea.
   2. Diarrhea.
   3. Faintness.
   4. Abdominal cramping.
277. To help prevent the "dumping syndrome," Mr. Hopkin should be taught to avoid foods that are especially high in
   1. roughage.
   2. fat content.
   3. protein content.
   4. carbohydrate content.
278. The intrinsic factor, a component of gastric juice, is often in low supply when a large portion of the stomach has been removed. Unless remedial steps are taken, the patient is likely to develop signs/symptoms very typical of
   1. hypoglycemia.
   2. pernicious anemia.
   3. diabetes mellitus.
   4. ulcerative colitis.
279. The production of gastric juices is stimulated by secretions of
   1. pepsin.

2. gastrin.

3. enterogastrone.

4. gastric lipase.

280. Which one of the following substances converts pepsinogen to pepsin?
1. Ptylin.
2. Secretin.
3. Cholecystokinin.
4. Hydrochloric acid.

281. The incidence of peptic ulcers (gastric and duodenal) is highest among persons who are
1. over 50 years of age.
2. under emotional stress.
3. of the Oriental race.
4. in the higher socioeconomic groups.

Sixty-one-year-old Mr. Carl Short was admitted to the hospital with complaints of recent weight loss, diarrhea, and bloody stools. The physician's orders include the following:

Low residue diet.
Schedule for sigmoidoscopy.
Schedule for a barium enema.
Send stool specimen to laboratory for blood for 3 successive days.

Items 282 through 323 pertain to this situation.

282. Which of the following breakfast cereals would Mr. Short be allowed while on a low residue diet?
1. Puffed Wheat.
2. Rice Krispies.
3. Shredded Wheat.
4. Grapenuts Flakes.

283. Which one of the following measures is *most commonly* carried out prior to a sigmoidoscopy?
1. Giving the patient an enema 1 hour before the examination.
2. Having the patient fast 8 to 10 hours prior to the examination.
3. Giving a liquid diet to the patient the evening before the examination.
4. Giving the patient a colonic irrigation the evening prior to the examination.

284. The evening before the barium enema, Mr. Short is ordered to have 60 ml. of castor oil. Castor oil facilitates evacuation of the bowel *primarily* by

1. softening the feces.
2. lubricating the feces.
3. increasing the volume of intestinal contents.
4. irritating the nerve endings in the intestinal mucosa.

285. After administering barium, orally or rectally, the nurse can anticipate that the physician will *most likely* write an order for
   1. an emetic.
   2. an antacid.
   3. a digestant.
   4. a cathartic.

286. Which one of the following situations *most often* leads to false positive results when the stool is examined for blood?
   1. Having eaten foods containing iron.
   2. Having high bilirubin level in the blood serum.
   3. Having meat residue in the gastrointestinal tract.
   4. Having failed to add a preservative to the specimen.

287. Following diagnostic examinations, Mr. Short is scheduled for an abdominoperineal resection and colostomy. Bowel preparation by chemical means prior to the patient's surgery is done *primarily* in order to help reduce
   1. electrolyte disturbances.
   2. bacterial content in the colon.
   3. peristaltic action in the colon.
   4. inflammation caused by the tumor.

288. Mr. Short is ordered to receive succinylsulfathiazole (Sulfasuxidine), the rationale for using this particular drug being that it
   1. diffuses quickly into body fluids.
   2. produces undesirable side effects infrequently.
   3. is poorly absorbed from the gastrointestinal tract.
   4. is excreted rapidly before toxic accumulations occur.

289. If a choice is possible, the preferred site in the colon to create a permanent colostomy is in the
   1. hepatic flexure.
   2. splenic flexure.
   3. lower portion of the descending colon.
   4. middle portion of the transverse colon.

290. Which site in the sketch on page 219 represents the splenic flexure in the large intestine?
   1. Site A.
   2. Site B.
   3. Site C.
   4. Site D.

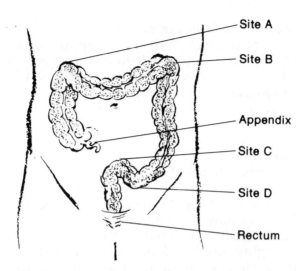

Site A

Site B

Appendix

Site C

Site D

Rectum

291. On the second postoperative day, Mr. Short is ordered to receive a unit of whole blood. When using a tandem setup for administering the blood, the intravenous solution of choice with which to start the therapy is
1. distilled water.
2. 0.9% saline solution.
3. 10% dextrose in normal saline.
4. 5% dextrose in distilled water.

292. Which of the following actions should the nurse take *first* when Mr. Short complains of a headache and tingling sensations in his fingers shortly after the blood transfusion is started?
1. Notify the physician.
2. Check for infiltration.
3. Slow the rate of the infusion.
4. Stop the infusion of the blood.

293. Which one of the following activities would be *contraindicated* for Mr. Short during his postoperative period?
1. Using diaphragmatic breathing.
2. Coughing against a closed glottis.
3. Wearing elastic bandages on both legs.
4. Resting his knees over a blanket roll.

294. Which one of the following observations should lead the nurse to anticipate that the physician will *most likely* order removal of Mr. Short's nasogastric tube, which was inserted at the time of surgery?
1. Absence of bowel sounds.
2. Passage of mucus from the rectum.

3. Passage of gas from the colostomy.

4. Absence of stomach drainage for approximately 24 hours.

295. After removing the nasogastric tube, the physician orders a clear liquid diet for Mr. Short. Which one of the following foods is *inappropriate* for Mr. Short's diet?

1. Beef broth.

2. Apple juice.

3. Tea and sugar.

4. Vanilla ice cream.

296. If Mr. Short has demonstrated readiness for the following nursing interventions, which one is likely to be the *most effective* in preparing him for the sight of his colostomy?

1. Telling him how normal body functions will continue.

2. Using illustrative material during teaching sessions.

3. Encouraging him to ask questions about his colostomy.

4. Asking a member of the local ostomy club to visit him.

297. A colostomy irrigation is ordered for Mr. Short on his fifth postoperative day. The *primary* purpose of this irrigation is to

1. cleanse the colon.

2. regulate the bowel.

3. dilate the sphincter.

4. stimulate peristalsis.

298. If Mr. Short complains of abdominal cramping after receiving approximately 150 ml. of solution during a colostomy irrigation, the nurse should temporarily

1. stop the flow of solution.

2. remove the irrigating tube.

3. have the patient sit up in bed.

4. insert the tube further into the colon.

299. If the nurse uses the following measures of intervention while changing Mr. Short's soiled colostomy bag, which one would be *least likely* to convey her acceptance of his altered body image?

1. Discussing subjects of interest with the patient.

2. Putting on gloves before starting the procedure.

3. Encouraging the patient to assist to the extent that he wishes.

4. Explaining that the patient will be taught the procedure when he is ready.

300. A clue that the patient is ready to participate in his care would be if, while the nurse is changing Mr. Short's colostomy bag and dressing, he

1. asks what time his physician would call that day.

2. asks about the supplies used during the dressing change.

3. talks about something he read in the morning newspaper.

4. complains about the way the night nurse changed the dressing.

301. Of the following preparations, which one would be *best* to apply around Mr. Short's surgical site to help prevent skin irritation due to drainage from his colostomy?
    1. Zinc oxide.
    2. Petrolatum.
    3. Cornstarch.
    4. Antiseptic cream.

302. Which of the following measures would *most effectively* promote healing of Mr. Short's perineal wound after the drain has been removed?
    1. Taking sitz baths.
    2. Taking daily showers.
    3. Applying warm moist dressings to the area.
    4. Applying a protected heating pad to the area.

303. When planning dietary instructions for Mr. Short, the nurse should develop her teaching plan based on knowledge that
    1. foods containing roughage should be eliminated from the diet of a person with a colostomy.
    2. each person with a colostomy must experiment to determine what balance of foods is best for him.
    3. gas-forming foods taken in moderate amounts are generally well tolerated by the person with a colostomy.
    4. a constipating diet will produce a formed stool that can be passed with more regularity through a colostomy.

304. Which one of the following long-term objectives would be *unrealistic* if Mr. Short had had an ileostomy rather than a colostomy?
    1. Managing his own care.
    2. Returning to normal nutrition.
    3. Resuming normal sexual activity.
    4. Controlling evacuation of the bowel.

305. Six months after his surgery, Mr. Short is readmitted to the hospital for cancer chemotherapy. Mr. Short is ordered to receive the antimetabolite fluorouracil (5 FU) when it is found that his cancer has spread to the liver. Antimetabolites function to control cancer by
    1. decreasing the blood supply to malignant cells.
    2. interfering with the nutrition of malignant cells.
    3. producing an acid that is toxic to malignant cells.
    4. destroying the capsules surrounding malignant cells.

306. At 4 P.M. on the third day after chemotherapy is started, the nurse notes that Mr. Short's temperature is 101° F. (38.3° C.).

Which one of the following actions should the nurse take *first?*

1. Notify the patient's physician.
2. Give the patient a cool-water sponge bath.
3. Obtain a urine specimen for culturing.
4. Omit the dose of fluorouracil due at this time.

307. Mr. Short is placed on reverse (protective) isolation. Which one of the following statements *best* describes the primary purpose of reverse isolation?
    1. It helps prevent the spread of organisms to the patient from sources outside his environment.
    2. It helps prevent the spread of organisms from the patient to health personnel, visitors, and other patients.
    3. It helps prevent the spread of organisms by using special techniques to destroy discharges from the patient's body.
    4. It helps prevent the spread of organisms by using special techniques to handle the patient's bed and personal linens.

308. Of the following body tissues, drugs commonly used to treat malignant tumors are *most often* also toxic to
    1. muscle cells.
    2. hair follicles.
    3. the lungs' alveoli.
    4. the kidneys' capsules of Bowman.

309. A disadvantage in the use of antineoplastic drugs is that they
    1. fail to distinguish between tumor and normal cells.
    2. tend to cause focal infections in tumor and normal cells.
    3. tend to accumulate with resulting dangerously high drug blood levels.
    4. occupy normal defenses that would normally help control the growth of tumor cells.

310. The *most common* toxic reaction observed among patients receiving cytotoxic drugs for malignant diseases is
    1. nausea.
    2. joint pains.
    3. renal failure.
    4. bone marrow depression.

311. It is determined that Mr. Short is suffering with thrombocytopenia, which means that his blood values reveal a
    1. low platelet count.
    2. high red cell count.
    3. low lymphocyte count.
    4. high eosinophil count.

312. Mr. Short responds to cancer chemotherapy very poorly and his physical condition deteriorates rapidly. During which stage

of dying will Mr. Short *most appreciate* having the nurse recognize his need for privacy?
1. The stage of anger.
2. The stage of bargaining.
3. The stage of depression.
4. The stage of acceptance.

313. Which one of the following observations indicates central nervous system deterioration when death is imminent?
1. The patient complains of severe pain while being turned.
2. The patient constantly drools saliva from a drooping chin.
3. The patient presents a blank stare through half closed eyelids.
4. The patient's body temperature is elevated while the extremities are moist and cool.

314. After seeing Mr. Short, a family member asks the nurse, "How much longer will it be?" Which one of the following responses would be *most appropriate* for the nurse to make?
1. "It is very difficult to say. He has such a strong will."
2. "I really couldn't say. What did the doctor tell the family?"
3. "We cannot say definitely. The matter is no longer in our hands."
4. "It is only a matter of a few minutes now. He is deteriorating very rapidly."

315. As death approaches, it is believed that the *last* body sense to fall into unconsciousness is the sense of
1. smell.
2. touch.
3. sight.
4. hearing.

316. Mr. Short expires and his family is leaving the room. Which of the following actions should the nurse take to demonstrate recognition of the family's needs at this time?
1. Take the family to a private area where they can be alone for a while.
2. Extend her sympathy and ask them if there is anything she can do for them.
3. Ask the family to wait a few minutes while the patient's personal belongings are gathered.
4. Ask the family if they wish the nurse to call their clergyman and a mortician of their choice.

317. Which one of the following behaviors demonstrates *best* that a family member is in the stage of grief when he is developing an awareness of a loss through death?
1. Crying about the death.
2. Talking repeatedly of fond memories.

3. Appearing to manage and organize everything.

4. Directing anger and aggression at everything.

318. Which of the following statements *best* explains the common observation that, in many instances, the terminally ill patient is avoided by health personnel?
1. The family members that are present are able to provide essential care.
2. Staff members have failed to understand their own feelings on death and dying.
3. The dying patient requires a minimal amount of physical care to be comfortable.
4. It is best to avoid interrupting the patient frequently in order to protect his right to die in dignity.

319. From which anatomical portion of the lower gastrointestinal tract do *most* malignancies arise?
1. From the sigmoid and rectum.
2. From the cecum and ascending colon.
3. From the splenic flexure and descending colon.
4. From the hepatic flexure and transverse colon.

320. A diagnostic measure that provides the *most* conclusive information concerning whether a tumor exists in the colon is an examination of the
1. abdomen by palpating for masses.
2. stools for the presence of blood.
3. blood for the level of hemoglobin.
4. lower gastrointestinal tract with a contrast media.

321. Bacteria in the large intestine act to
1. synthesize vitamin K.
2. break down cellulose.
3. reduce the fluid content of chyme.
4. neutralize acidity of waste products.

322. The cephalic stage of digestion which begins with the sight, smell, and taste of food, aids digestion by stimulating
1. peristaltic waves.
2. the secretion of gastric juices.
3. the production of enterogastrone.
4. muscular contractions in the stomach.

323. The act of defecation is normally stimulated *primarily* by
1. toxins produced by intestinal bacteria.
2. relaxation of the external anal sphincter.
3. distention of the rectum with fecal matter.
4. phenol normally found in the end products of digestion.

Ms. Hilda Towe, a 32-year-old homemaker and mother of

two children, visited her physician because of "nervousness and irritability." The physician orders the following examinations for the patient:

Basal metabolism rate (BMR).
Protein-bound iodine test (PBI).
Radioactive iodine test (^{131}I uptake).

Items 324 through 355 pertain to this situation.

324. In preparing Ms. Towe for her basal metabolism rate examination, it would be inappropriate for the nurse to tell the patient that she will
   1. receive a medication before the examination.
   2. fast for approximately 10 hours prior to the examination.
   3. have the examination early in the morning before breakfast.
   4. breathe into a machine for several minutes during the examination.

325. Of the following basal metabolism rate values, the nurse can anticipate that the one typical of a patient with hyperthyroidism is
   1. +15 percent and above.
   2. −15 percent and below.
   3. −15 percent to +15 percent.

326. The PBI and ^{131}I uptake tests will be falsely elevated if Ms. Towe was or had recently been taking medications containing
   1. iodine.
   2. cortisone.
   3. salicylates.
   4. sulfonamides.

327. Ms. Towe is given radioactive iodine by mouth in the laboratory at 11 A.M. and scheduled to return for an appointment at 11 A.M. the next morning. The nurse should instruct Ms. Towe to prepare for the next morning's appointment by
   1. fasting for 10 hours before her morning appointment.
   2. anticipating that a minimum of three blood samples will be taken.
   3. saving her urine for the 24-hour period and bringing it with her for examination.
   4. limiting her fluid intake to 800 ml. during the 24-hour period and avoiding coffee and tea.

328. Which of the following assessment techniques would be of *least value* when the nurse examines Ms. Towe's thyroid gland?
   1. Palpation.
   2. Percussion.

3. Inspection.

4. Auscultation.

329. After the laboratory tests are completed, the physician makes a diagnosis of hyperthyroidism with exophthalmus. Which of the following symptoms, related to the eyes, characterizes exophthalmus?

1. Floating eyeballs.

2. Protrusion of the eyeballs.

3. Inability to see in the dark.

4. Halos around colored objects.

330. Which one of the following measures is *most helpful* in preventing drying of the eyeballs while Ms. Towe is sleeping?

1. Massaging the eyes before retiring.

2. Instilling artificial tears before retiring.

3. Covering both eyes with moistened gauze pads.

4. Taping the eyelids shut with nonirritating tape.

331. In addition to Ms. Towe's presenting complaints of nervousness and irritability, she would *most likely* also demonstrate

1. fine hand tremors.

2. a decreased appetite.

3. thinning of her hair.

4. a subnormal temperature.

332. Which symptom related to Ms. Towe's menstrual periods is also *very likely* to be present?

1. Amenorrhea.

2. Menorrhagia.

3. Dysmenorrhea.

4. Polymenorrhea.

333. Which one of the following types of reactions should the nurse anticipate when she assesses Ms. Towe's deep tendon reflex of the Achilles tendon?

1. Decreased response.

2. Prolonged response.

3. Exaggerated response.

4. Absent jerking reflex.

334. The physician orders propylthiouracil (Propacil) for Ms. Towe. Which of the following symptoms should the nurse teach Ms. Towe to report *immediately* if they occur?

1. A sore throat and general malaise.

2. Painful and excessive menstruation.

3. Constipation and abdominal distention.

4. Increased urinary output and itching skin.

335. Mr. Towe tells the nurse that his wife has become very irritable, especially with the children at mealtime since they are

"picky" eaters. The nurse illustrates understanding of the patient's behavior when she explains to Mr. Towe that it is
1. usually the result of temporary mental confusion.
2. commonly observed in patients with hyperthyroidism.
3. fairly typical when a patient thinks her illness may be terminal.
4. frequently associated with an impending drop in the patient's serum thyroxin level.

336. Ms. Towe is admitted to the hospital and scheduled for a subtotal thyroidectomy. If the following hospital rooms are available, which one would be *best* for the nurse to select for Ms. Towe?
1. A private room located in an area where the patient has privacy and quietness.
2. A semiprivate room which the patient can share with another patient who has a sinus infection.
3. A private room next to the nurses' station so that the patient can be checked frequently with convenience.
4. A semiprivate room which is presently empty but has one bed which is used only for emergency admissions.

337. The physician orders saturated solution of potassium iodide for Ms. Towe, the *primary* reason being that the drug helps to
1. reduce the size of the thyroid gland.
2. decrease the progression of exophthalmus.
3. decrease the body's ability to store thyroxin.
4. increase the body's ability to absorb thyroxin.

338. Which one of the following measures is *most often* recommended to prepare a saturated solution of potassium iodide for administration?
1. Pouring it over ice chips.
2. Mixing it with an antacid.
3. Diluting it with water, milk, or fruit juice.
4. Disguising it with a puréed fruit or vegetable.

339. The nurse prepares Ms. Towe's saturated solution of potassium iodide by placing the prescribed number of drops in a medicine glass. An emergency arises and 45 minutes later when the nurse plans to give Ms. Towe the medication, she finds everything as she left it in the locked cupboard except that the medicine glass is empty. A good explanation for what has occurred is that
1. the medication has most likely evaporated.
2. someone apparently discarded the medication.
3. another nurse undoubtedly has administered the medication.
4. the nurse most probably did not pour the medication as she thought she had.

340. A high caloric diet is prescribed for Ms. Towe. She receives 300 Grams of carbohydrates, 150 Grams of protein, and 150 Grams of fat daily. How many calories will her daily diet be providing?
  1. 1950 calories.
  2. 2200 calories.
  3. 3150 calories.
  4. 4650 calories.

341. A friend who visits Ms. Towe expresses concern to the nurse by saying, "She seems worse and is unable to sit still and concentrate, even for a minute." Which one of the following responses would be *best* for the nurse to make to the patient's friend?
  1. "Thank you for telling me. I shall check on Ms. Towe immediately."
  2. "Ms. Towe had a bad night but she will be better, we are sure, after some rest."
  3. "Unfortunately, I cannot discuss Ms. Towe's condition with you since you are not a family member."
  4. "Ms. Towe's behavior is part of her illness, but she is receiving medication that will help her."

342. Meperidine hydrochloride (Demerol) and diazepam (Valium) are ordered to be given to Ms. Towe preoperatively. When preparing these drugs for intramuscular injection, the nurse should draw up
  1. each medication in a separate syringe and give two injections.
  2. the diazepam first and then add the meperidine hydrochloride to the same syringe.
  3. the merperidine hydrochloride first and then add the diazepam to the same syringe.
  4. both medications in one syringe; it makes no difference which medication is drawn up first.

343. Ms. Towe is of average height and weighs 115 pounds. When the following needles are available, which one should be the nurse's *first* choice for administering Ms. Towe's preoperative medications?
  1. 19 gauge by 1½ inches.
  2. 20 gauge by 1 inch.
  3. 22 gauge by 1½ inches.
  4. 26 gauge by 1 inch.

344. As soon as Ms. Towe responds after surgery, the nurse asks the patient to state her name and repeats this request every 30 minutes. The nurse carries out this activity *primarily* in order to assess for evidence of

1. hemorrhage.
2. consciousness.
3. damage to the laryngeal nerve.
4. obstruction in the upper airway.

345. Ms. Towe is ordered to receive morphine sulfate for the control of pain. Which one of the following assessments should be made before administering the drug to Ms. Towe?
1. Pupil size.
2. Pulse deficit.
3. Respiratory rate.
4. Radial pulse rate.

346. Two hours after Ms. Towe is returned to her room, she complains of pain in the operative area, her breathing becomes noisy, and she is showing signs of cyanosis. If orders by the physician are available to carry out the following courses of action, which one should the nurse take *first?*
1. Begin oxygen therapy.
2. Administer morphine sulfate.
3. Suction the mouth and trachea.
4. Begin steam inhalations in the patient's room.

347. Which one of the following techniques *best* enables the nurse to assess Ms. Towe's wound for hemorrhaging?
1. Gently slipping her hand behind the patient's neck and checking for blood on the back of the neck and bed linens.
2. Carefully loosening the dressings at both ends and having the patient turn her head to one side while observing for blood on the dressings.
3. Carrying out a routine change of dressings every 2 hours for at least 12 hours and then every 4 hours for the next 2 to 3 days.
4. Checking the patient's blood pressure and pulse and respiratory rates every hour for the first 24 hours and then every 2 hours for the next 24 hours.

348. Certain items should be placed in Ms. Towe's room in order to treat complications, should they develop postoperatively. Of the following items, which one is *least likely* to be necessary?
1. Cutdown equipment.
2. Suctioning equipment.
3. Tracheostomy equipment.
4. Equipment for administering oxygen.

349. If Ms. Towe presents the following signs/symptoms postoperatively, which should suggest to the nurse that the patient may be developing tetany?
1. Backache and joint pain.
2. Tingling sensation in the fingers.

3. Hoarseness and weakness of the voice.

4. Retraction of neck muscles with inspirations.

350. Which one of the following medications should the nurse anticipate the physician will order if Ms. Towe has tetany?

1. Sodium phosphate.

2. Calcium gluconate.

3. Phospholine iodide.

4. Sodium bicarbonate.

351. To minimize tension on the suture line, which one of the following techniques should the nurse teach Ms. Towe when she moves herself to the sitting position?

1. Pressing the chin against the chest while moving to the sitting position.

2. Supporting the head by placing both hands behind the head while moving to the sitting position.

3. Rolling to the side first and then moving to the sitting position while holding the head perfectly still.

4. Grasping flexed knees with both arms while in the back-lying position and then rocking forward to the sitting position.

352. Ms. Towe expresses concern about the appearance of her suture line after the skin clips are removed. Which one of the following measures has proven helpful in minimizing scarring?

1. Applying cold cream or petrolatum over the suture line each day.

2. Alternately tensing and relaxing the neck muscles several times a day.

3. Wiping the suture line every day with cotton balls moistened with hydrogen peroxide or alcohol.

4. Keeping a sterile dressing over the wound for at least 2 to 3 days after the suture line is completely healed.

353. Prior to Ms. Towe's discharge, the nurse teaches the patient to call her physician if she begins developing hypothyroidism. Typical symptoms of hypothyroidism include

1. increased appetite and weight loss.

2. joint pain and frequency of urination.

3. consistent weight gain and increasing fatigue.

4. muscle twitching and difficulty with swallowing.

354. The *most common* cause of death when hyperthyroidism progresses without abatement is

1. liver failure.

2. kidney failure.

3. cardiac failure.

4. respiratory failure.

355. The thyroid gland receives its stimulus from the "target" or

"master" gland, which is the
1. pancreas.
2. pituitary gland.
3. suprarenal gland.
4. parathyroid gland.

Mr. Peter Hoyt, who is 80 years old, is brought to the emergency room of the local hospital by his son. He complains of great discomfort because he has been unable to void for approximately 12 hours. Two days previously when Mr. Hoyt was in the emergency room with the same symptoms, the physician diagnosed Mr. Hoyt as having an enlarged prostate gland. At that time, he refused to be admitted to the hospital.
Items 356 through 385 pertain to this situation.

356. The method of choice for assessing a patient for a distended bladder is that the nurse check for a
   1. rounded swelling above the pubis.
   2. discharge from the urethral meatus.
   3. dullness in the lower left quadrant.
   4. rebound tenderness below the symphysis.
357. Mr. Hoyt is prepared for digital examination of the prostate gland. Although various positions can be used, the position of choice for this examination is to have the patient.
   1. lie on his back on the examining table with his legs separated and his knees bent.
   2. lie on his left side on the examining table with his right knee flexed and drawn up toward his chest.
   3. stand while leaning over the edge of an examining table with his body bent at approximately a right angle to his hips.
   4. rest on his knees and upper chest and elbows on the examining table with his body bent at approximately a right angle to his hips.
358. While taking Mr. Hoyt's history, the nurse can anticipate that the patient will *most likely* report having experienced *all* of the following symptoms *except*
   1. voiding at more frequent intervals.
   2. difficulty starting the flow of urine.
   3. excessive voiding during nighttime hours.
   4. having a urinary stream of greater force than usual.
359. Mr. Hoyt is to be catheterized. The *primary* reason for lubricating the catheter *well* before inserting it is that this technique helps to reduce
   1. spasms at the orifice of the bladder.

2. friction along the urethra when the catheter is being inserted.
3. the number of organisms gaining entrance to the bladder.
4. formation of encrustations that may occur at the end of the catheter.

360. Mr. Hoyt's bladder is emptied gradually. The *best* rationale for the nurse's action is that emptying an overdistended bladder completely at one time tends to cause
1. renal collapse and failure.
2. abdominal cramping and pain.
3. hypotension and possible shock.
4. weakening and atrophy of bladder musculature.

361. If Mr. Hoyt has had a long history of urinary retention, it is possible that he may have hydronephrosis. Which one of the following mechanisms would *most likely* account for this?
1. Abnormally high retention of blood urea and nitrogen.
2. Atrophy of the muscle fibers along the walls of the ureters.
3. Gradual backing up of stagnant urine into the pelvis of the kidneys.
4. Insufficient arterial blood pressure that results in poor kidney circulation.

362. Mr. Hoyt is prepared for admission to the hospital after his bladder is emptied in the emergency room. Which one of the following reports that the emergency room nurse could make would be *most helpful* to the nurse responsible for admitting Mr. Hoyt?
1. "A urine specimen was obtained and sent to the laboratory for analysis."
2. "Mr. Hoyt was catheterized for 1100 ml. of urine. The urine appeared cloudy and a specimen was sent to the laboratory."
3. "Mr. Hoyt is a very cooperative patient. He is comfortable now that his bladder has been emptied. He had no ill effects from catheterization."
4. "Mr. Hoyt was in the emergency room for 3 hours because of bladder distention. He is fine now but is being admitted as a possible candidate for surgery."

363. An intravenous pyelogram (IVP) examination is ordered for Mr. Hoyt. This examination will produce visualization of *all* of the following anatomical structures *except* the
1. ureters.
2. kidneys.
3. bladder.
4. urethra.

364. Mr. Hoyt's blood urea nitrogen (BUN) level is reported to be 32 mg. per 100 ml. The nurse correctly assesses this finding when she concludes that Mr. Hoyt *most probably* has

1. acute renal failure.
2. normally functioning kidneys.
3. a minimal amount of kidney damage.
4. a disturbance in his acid-base balance.

365. Mr. Hoyt is examined for residual urine. Residual urine is *best* described as urine that
1. remains in the bladder after voiding.
2. stagnates in the pelvis of the kidneys.
3. contains a sediment when a specimen is centrifuged.
4. escapes involuntarily from the bladder between voidings.

366. The physician orders that Mr. Hoyt have an indwelling catheter inserted. After inserting the catheter, the nurse tapes it to the patient's thigh, as illustrated below.

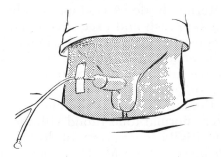

The *primary* reason for taping the catheter in this particular manner is to help in
1. eliminating pressure at the penoscrotal angle.
2. preventing the catheter from kinking in the urethra.
3. preventing the catheter from being pulled accidently.
4. allowing the patient to turn without kinking the catheter.

367. Of the following actions which the nurse could take when giving catheter care, which one should have *highest* priority?
1. Changing the catheter if it is not draining.
2. Cleansing the area around the urethral meatus.
3. Irrigating the catheter with several ounces of normal saline.
4. Changing the location where the catheter is taped to the patient's leg.

368. The report on a culture of Mr. Hoyt's urine indicates that there are numerous white and red blood cells present and a moderate amount of bacterial growth. The nurse interprets these findings accurately when she deduces that Mr. Hoyt *most probably* has a
1. urethral stricture.
2. chronic renal failure.
3. urinary tract infection.
4. malignancy of the prostate gland.

369. A urinary sensitivity test is ordered for Mr. Hoyt. The *primary* purpose for doing this test is to help the physician to
1. detect drugs to which the patient may be allergic.
2. detect the amount of tissue to remove from the patient's prostate gland.
3. identify the microorganisms found in the culture of the patient's urine.
4. select drugs to which microorganisms found in the patient's urine are susceptible.

370. Chloral hydrate is ordered for Mr. Hoyt for sleeplessness. If Mr. Hoyt has untoward side effects to the drug, the signs he is *most likely* to demonstrate include
1. being confused and disoriented.
2. being alternately depressed and euphoric.
3. having a skin rash and excessive perspiration.
4. having constricted pupils and edema of the eyelids.

371. The *most common* preoperative problem of patients over 65 years of age has been observed to be
1. presence of various diseases.
2. dehydration and malnourishment.
3. lower than normal total blood volume.
4. hypersensitivity to a variety of drugs.

372. The physician schedules Mr. Hoyt for a transurethral resection of the prostate gland and a bilateral vasectomy. Spinal anesthesia is to be used. Mr. Hoyt is ordered to receive meperidine hydrochloride (Demerol) 30 mg. intramuscularly preoperatively. The nurse notes that there are 50 mg. of meperidine hydrochloride per ml. in the prepackaged syringe. How many minims should the nurse *discard* to have the correct dosage for Mr. Hoyt?
1. 6 minims.
2. 9 minims.
3. 12 minims.
4. 15 minims.

When Mr. Hoyt returns to his room after surgery, he has a 3-way catheter in place and is ordered to have continuous bladder irrigations for 24 hours. Items 373 and 374 pertain to the catheter sketched below.

373. To which lumen of the catheter should the nurse attach the irrigation apparatus to begin the inflow of solution for continuous irrigation?
1. Lumen A.
2. Lumen B.
3. Lumen C.

374. To which lumen should the nurse attach the drainage tube for the outflow of urine and irrigation solution?
   1. Lumen A.
   2. Lumen B.
   3. Lumen C.
375. In which one of the following instances, if it occurred approximately 3 hours postoperatively, should the nurse increase the rate of the solution entering Mr. Hoyt's continuous irrigating system?
   1. When the return is continuous but slow.
   2. When the return appears cloudy and dark yellow.
   3. When the drainage has become brighter red in color.
   4. When there is no return of urine and irrigating solution.
376. A nursing assistant reports to the nurse, "I think Mr. Hoyt is confused. He keeps telling me he has to void but that isn't possible because he has a catheter in place." Which one of the following possible responses to the nursing assistant's comment is *most appropriate* for the nurse to make?
   1. "His catheter is probably plugged. I'll irrigate it in a few minutes."
   2. "This is a common complaint following prostate surgery. The urge to void is being imagined."
   3. "The urge to void is usually created by the catheter and he may be having some bladder spasms."
   4. "I think he may be somewhat confused and possibly may be having some internal bleeding."
377. Which one of the following symptoms can normally be expected temporarily when Mr. Hoyt's indwelling catheter is removed postoperatively?
   1. Urinary retention.
   2. Dribbling incontinence.
   3. Loss of urine while straining.
   4. Suppression of urinary output.
378. Mr. Hoyt is to receive bethanechol chloride (Urecholine) postoperatively, as necessary. The nurse should give the patient the drug when he demonstrates signs of
   1. painful voidings.
   2. urinary retention.
   3. frequency of urination.
   4. urinary tract infection.
379. Mr. Hoyt is readied for ambulation postoperatively. Which one of the following bed exercises has been found to be especially helpful in preparing a patient for early ambulation?
   1. Alternately flexing and extending the knees.
   2. Alternately abducting and adducting the legs.

3. Alternately tensing and relaxing the Achilles tendons.
4. Alternately flexing and relaxing the quadriceps femoris muscles.

380. Mr. Hoyt's son asks the nurse why the physician performed a vasectomy on his father. The nurse's response should be guided by knowledge that a vasectomy was done to
1. reduce the risk of epididymitis.
2. eliminate hormone stimulus to the prostate gland.
3. decrease the possibility of traumatic urethritis.
4. help prevent the recurrence of prostatic enlargement.

381. In many instances, older gentlemen with prostatic hypertrophy do not seek medical attention until urinary obstruction is almost complete. Investigations have found that the *primary* reason for their delay in seeking attention is that they
1. tend to feel too self-conscious to seek help when reproductive organs are involved.
2. expect that it is normal to have to live with some urinary problems as they grow older.
3. are fearful that sexual indiscriminations in earlier life may be the cause of their problem.
4. have little discomfort in relation to the amount of pathology as responses to pain stimuli fade with age.

382. Of the four approaches used for prostatic tissue removal, which one *most frequently* requires that the patient will need surgery for tissue removal again?
1. Perineal.
2. Retropubic.
3. Suprapubic.
4. Transurethral.

383. Which one of the following functions does the prostate gland serve?
1. It stores underdeveloped sperm prior to ejaculation.
2. It regulates the acidity/alkalinity environment for proper sperm development.
3. It produces a secretion that aids in the nourishment and passage of the sperm.
4. It secretes a hormone that stimulates the production and maturation of the sperm.

384. Of the following complications, for which one should the nurse be particularly alert when a patient has had spinal anesthesia?
1. Hypotension.
2. Convulsions.
3. Cardiac arrest.
4. Renal shutdown.

385. Of the following complications, the *most common* one following
a prostatectomy is
1. renal failure.
2. septic infection.
3. respiratory failure.
4. circulatory collapse.

Ms. Florence Hill, who is 73 years old, was admitted to the
hospital after suffering a fall in her home. She complains of pain
in her right hip and is unable to move her right leg.
Items 386 through 416 pertain to this situation.

386. The physician orders hydromorphone hydrochloride (Dilaudid)
2 mg. subcutaneously immediately and every 4 hours as necessary for the relief of Ms. Hill's pain. Hydromorphone hydrochloride is administered in relatively small doses *primarily* because the drug
1. is irritating to subcutaneous tissues.
2. tends to be excreted extremely slowly.
3. is more potent than many other analgesics.
4. is less likely to cause dependency when administered in small
doses.

387. Which of the following factors is of *most importance* when
selecting the length of the needle the nurse should use when
giving Ms. Hill a subcutaneous injection in her arm?
1. The diameter of the needle.
2. The size of the patient's arm.
3. The dosage to be administered to the patient.
4. The viscosity of the solution to be injected.

388. Two hours after Ms. Hill receives an injection of hydromorphone
hydrochloride, she complains of pain. Which of the following
actions would be *best* for the nurse to take at this time?
1. Call the physician for guidance.
2. Give the patient a back massage.
3. Offer the patient a hot cup of tea.
4. Offer to sit with the patient for a short time.

389. Following a hip fracture, which Ms. Hill has, the *most common*
observation is that the leg on the affected side will be
1. rotated internally.
2. held in a flexed position.
3. moved away from the body's midline.
4. shorter than the leg on the unaffected side.

390. Which one of the following phenomena is produced when broken bone fragments are rubbed against each other?

1. Crepitation.
2. Ossification.
3. Proliferation.
4. Consolidation.
391. Which of the following pieces of equipment can be used *most effectively* to help prevent external rotation of Ms. Hill's right leg?
1. Sandbags.
2. A high footboard.
3. A rubber air ring.
4. A metal frame cradle.
392. X-ray studies of Ms. Hill's right hip reveal an intertrochanteric fracture. Which site on the diagram below *best* identifies the intertrochanteric area of the femur?
1. Site A.
2. Site B.
3. Site C.
4. Site D.

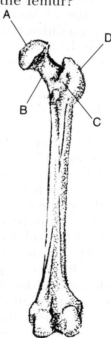

The femur

393. Ms. Hill has a history of diabetes mellitus and has been taking tolbutamide (Orinase) 500 mg. twice a day. Tolbutamide acts to lower the blood sugar level by
1. stimulating the pancreas to secrete more insulin.
2. reducing the number of circulating ketone bodies.
3. increasing peripheral cell utilization of glucose.

4. decreasing the rate of conversion of glycogen to glucose.

394. What metabolic defect produces diabetic acidosis?
   1. Rapid breakdown of fat.
   2. Depletion of stored minerals.
   3. Increased production of insulin.
   4. Inadequate destruction of proteins.

395. Ms. Hill's fracture is corrected by surgical internal fixation with the insertion of a pin. This procedure is the treatment of choice for most older persons because, in contrast to other surgical procedures, internal fixation with a pin
   1. is a simpler procedure.
   2. promotes more rapid healing.
   3. carries less danger of infection.
   4. makes earlier mobilization possible.

396. Ms. Hill has a drainage tube in her surgical wound. A portable suction device is attached to the tube. The *primary* purpose for using this apparatus is to help
   1. detect a wound infection.
   2. eliminate the need for wound irrigations.
   3. prevent fluid from accumulating in the wound.
   4. provide a mechanism for instilling antibiotics into the wound.

397. The physician orders an intravenous infusion for Ms. Hill with 10 Units of insulin added. Which of the following types of insulin should the nurse anticipate has been ordered to be given in the intravenous solution?
   1. Insulin zinc suspension (Lente).
   2. Crystalline zinc insulin (Regular).
   3. Isophane insulin suspension (Neutral-Protamine-Hagedorn).
   4. Protamine zinc insulin suspension (Protamine Zinc Iletin).

398. Prior to turning Ms. Hill onto her left side, two nurses first plan to slide her as far as possible to the right side of the bed. The nurses can increase their own stability before moving Ms. Hill by
   1. bending at the waist.
   2. widening their base of support.
   3. leaning against the edge of the bed.
   4. moving the patient in a rocking manner.

399. Which one of the following measures would help to prevent flexion contracture of Ms. Hill's hip?
   1. Having an overbed trapeze for Ms. Hill's use.
   2. Using bedboards under Ms. Hill's mattress.
   3. Using an alternating pressure mattress on Ms. Hill's bed.
   4. Having Ms. Hill's feet rest against a footboard.

400. In which one of the following positions would it be *best* to place

Ms. Hill when giving her an enema with a hypertonic solution?
1. Knee-chest position.
2. Left lateral position.
3. Right lateral position.

401. Whenever Ms. Hill is lying on her side, a pillow is placed between her legs to help prevent
1. flexion of the knees.
2. abduction of the thighs.
3. adduction of the hip joint.
4. hyperextension of the knees.

402. Which one of the following signs/symptoms is of *least importance* when the nurse assesses Ms. Hill for postoperative peripheral nerve damage?
1. Pain.
2. Pallor.
3. Porosis.
4. Pulselessness.

403. Which one of the following chairs would be *best* to use for Ms. Hill when she sits up for the first time postoperatively?
1. A desk-type swivel chair.
2. A padded upholstered chair.
3. A recliner chair with attached foot rest.
4. A high-backed straight chair with arm rests.

404. Which of the following leg positions should be discouraged while Ms. Hill sits in the chair?
1. Crossing the legs.
2. Elevating the legs.
3. Flexing the ankles.
4. Extending the knees.

405. When changing Ms. Hill's surgical wound dressings, it is *least important* for the nurse to wear
1. a gown.
2. a mask.
3. sterile gloves.

406. For many elderly persons, crutch-walking is an *impractical* goal *primarily* because of their decreased
1. visual acuity.
2. reaction time.
3. motor coordination.
4. level of comprehension.

407. If Ms. Hill is going to learn crutch-walking, which of the following activities should she be encouraged to perform to strengthen her hand muscles in preparation for using crutches?

1. Brushing her hair.
2. Squeezing a rubber ball.
3. Alternately flexing and extending her wrists.
4. Pushing her hands into the mattress while raising herself in bed.

408. Which one of the following medications, all of which Ms. Hill is receiving postoperatively, predisposes to constipation?
1. Tolbutamide.
2. Ascorbic acid.
3. Nicotinic acid.
4. Codeine sulfate.

409. Ms. Hill had been taking psyllium hydrophilic mucilloid (Metamucil) for occasional constipation. This agent stimulates peristalsis by
1. moistening the fecal material.
2. lubricating the fecal material.
3. irritating the nerve endings in the mucosa.
4. increasing bulk within the intestinal tract.

410. The *greatest* hazard when insufficient water is taken with bulk-producing laxatives containing fibers, seeds, and granules is that the drug may
1. ulcerate the duodenum.
2. dehydrate the patient.
3. obstruct the esophagus.
4. cause an allergic reaction.

411. Which foods should the nurse encourage Ms. Hill to include in her diet to help overcome constipation?
1. Lean meats.
2. Bran cereals.
3. Dairy products.
4. Carbonated beverages.

412. The progress of bone healing is *best* determined by
1. follow-up x-ray studies.
2. healing of the surgical wound.
3. the absence of pain during weight-bearing.
4. the ability to put the hip through full range of motion.

413. Ms. Hill has the items listed below and two pets in her home. Which ones present the *greatest* hazard to her when she is using her crutches?
1. The pets.
2. Scatter rugs.
3. Snack tables.
4. Rocking chairs.

414. Which one of the following tests provides information about skeletal metabolic activity?

1. Synovial fluid analysis.
2. Radioactive isotope skeletal surveys.
3. Blood sedimentation rate and red cell count.
4. Serum and urine calcium and phosphorus levels.

415. Which one of the following terms is used to indicate infection in the bone?
   1. Osteolysis.
   2. Osteomalacia.
   3. Osteoporosis.
   4. Osteomyelitis.

416. Which of the following anatomical structures attaches muscles to bones?
   1. Fascia.
   2. Tendons.
   3. Ligaments.
   4. Cartilage.

Ms. Beverly Sloan was hospitalized because of a herniated intervertebral disc. Surgical intervention was planned. The physician's orders include the following:

Position of comfort.
Schedule for myelography.

Items 417 through 437 pertain to this situation.

417. Which one of the following symptoms is Ms. Sloan *least likely* to complain of as a result of the pressure on her spinal cord caused by the herniated disc?
   1. Loss of urinary control.
   2. Impaired skin sensations.
   3. Poor muscle coordination.
   4. Weakness in her extremities.

418. Since hyperextension of her spine causes discomfort for Ms. Sloan, which one of the following positions in bed is likely to be the *most comfortable* for her?
   1. Lying flat in bed.
   2. Lying on either side.
   3. Lying on her abdomen.
   4. Lying on her back with the head of the bed elevated.

419. Ms. Sloan asks about the myelogram. The nurse explains that Ms. Sloan's spinal cord will be x-rayed after it has been injected with
   1. air.
   2. sterile water.

3. radioactive oil.
4. a radiopaque dye.
420. When Ms. Sloan is scheduled to have a laminectomy, Ms. Sloan asks what the physician will do to her back. The nurse's response should be based on knowledge that the physician will remove the herniated disc and
1. the nerve roots affected by the cord compression.
2. a portion of the involved vertebrae's posterior arches.
3. a major portion of the vertebrae in the affected area.
4. the spinous processes of the vertebrae in the affected area.
421. Ms. Sloan asks what the physician meant when he said she would have a spinal fusion. A spinal fusion immobilizes part of the spine by using a
1. metal pin.
2. bone graft.
3. skeletal clamp.
4. chemical cement.
422. Immediately postoperatively, vomitus accumulates in Ms. Sloan's mouth. After turning Ms. Sloan's head to the side, which of the following measures should the nurse take next?
1. Insert an oral airway.
2. Lower the head of the bed.
3. Apply a sharp blow to the chest.
4. Place Ms. Sloan's head on a small pillow.
423. Many drugs that help to prevent nausea and vomiting have undesirable side effects, one of which is
1. diarrhea.
2. headache.
3. constipation.
4. low blood pressure.
424. Ms. Sloan is ordered not to be turned postoperatively. When she complains of pain, the nurse chooses the deltoid muscle for injecting the analgesic ordered for her. Which area in the diagram below illustrates the *best* site for injecting a drug into the deltoid muscle?
1. Site A.
2. Site B.
3. Site C.
4. Site D.

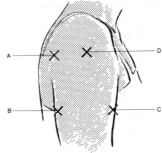

425. When Ms. Sloan demonstrates signs of shock from blood loss postoperatively, the physician orders a plasma extender. Which one of the following preparations serves the same function as plasma when used intravenously?
   1. Normal saline.
   2. Human serum albumin.
   3. Packed red blood cells.
   4. Balanced electrolyte solution.
426. In which one of the following positions should the bed be placed for a patient who is in a state of shock and for whom the position is not contraindicated for any reason?

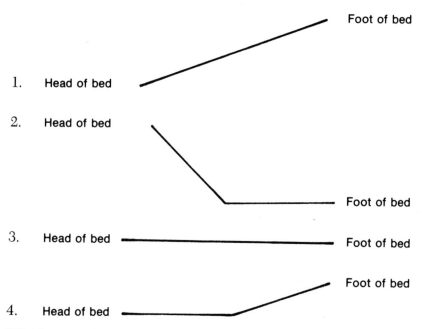

427. Which one of the following urinary signs is *most likely* to occur when glomerular filtration is impaired as a result of shock?
   1. Increased urinary output.
   2. Increased urine pH level.
   3. Decreased urinary output.
   4. Decreased urine pH level.
428. When Ms. Sloan's arterial blood gases are studied, findings demonstrate that she is experiencing metabolic acidosis. Which one of the following adaptive mechanisms helps the body initially to rid itself of carbon dioxide when metabolic acidosis is present?
   1. The heart rate slows.

2. The body temperature rises.
3. The urinary output increases.
4. The respiratory rate increases.

429. As soon as Ms. Sloan's shock is under control, which one of the following orders regarding the administration of intravenous therapy should the nurse anticipate?
1. The intravenous therapy will be discontinued.
2. The rate of administering the solution will be increased.
3. The rate of administering the solution will be decreased.
4. The rate of administering the solution will be the same as when shock was present.

430. Ms. Sloan complains of pain due to abdominal distention on her second postoperative day. If none of the following measures is contraindicated for the patient, which one is *most likely* to give her relief?
1. Massaging her abdomen.
2. Inserting a rectal tube.
3. Having her eat some cooked fruit.
4. Having her drink a carbonated beverage.

431. When Ms. Sloan complains of abdominal distention, the nurse notes that the patient's prescribed medications include those listed below. Which one would be *best* to use to help relieve Ms. Sloan's abdominal discomfort?
1. Codeine sulfate.
2. Diazepam (Valium).
3. Psyllium hydrophilic mucilloid (Metamucil).
4. Neostigmine bromide (Prostigmin).

432. Ms. Sloan needs to be moved from her bed to a stretcher and a 3-carrier lift is used. Her bed is elevated to the same height as the stretcher. Which one of the following actions should the carriers take *next*?
1. Place the patient on the edge of her bed.
2. Place the patient in the middle of her bed.
3. Place the patient so that her body is at right angles to the length of the bed with her legs off the bed resting on one carrier's arms.
4. Place the patient so that her body is at right angles to the length of the bed with her trunk off the bed resting on two carriers' arms.

433. When Ms. Sloan first walks with the nurse and the nurse's arm is under hers in an arm-in-arm manner, the patient begins to feel faint. After stopping the walking, what would be *best* for the nurse to do next until help arrives?
1. Have the patient close her eyes for a few minutes.

2. Slowly maneuver the patient to a sitting position on the floor.
3. Separate the nurse's feet to form a wide base of support and have the patient rest on the nurse's hip.
4. Have the patient separate her feet to form a wide base of support and have her bend at the waist to place her head near her knees.

434. Ms. Sloan is allowed to sit in a chair. In which one of the following positions should she be instructed to place her feet?
1. Flat on the floor.
2. On a low footstool.
3. In any position of comfort while keeping the legs uncrossed.
4. On a high footstool so that her feet are approximately at the same level as the chair seat.

435. The physician orders that Ms. Sloan wear a back brace. Which one of the following positions should Ms. Sloan assume to start applying the brace?
1. The standing position.
2. Lying on her side in bed.
3. Lying on her abdomen in bed.
4. The sitting position in a straight chair.

436. To protect Ms. Sloan's skin under the brace, it would be *best* for the nurse to
1. place padding as necessary for a snug fit.
2. have the patient wear a thin cotton shirt under the brace.
3. lubricate the areas where the patient's brace will contact skin surfaces.
4. apply powder to the areas where the patient's brace will contact skin surfaces.

437. While preparing Ms. Sloan for discharge, which one of the following activities is suitable during the period immediately following discharge?
1. Squatting.
2. Climbing stairs.
3. Bending at the waist.
4. Driving an automobile.

Twenty-year-old Mr. John Marlen was brought to the emergency room of a hospital about 20 minutes after being in a motorcycle accident. He has multiple abrasions on his body, has a head injury, and is unconscious upon arrival. Signs of increasing intracranial pressure are present. An adult friend and his fiancée accompanied Mr. Marlen.

Items 438 through 478 pertain to this situation.

438. Which one of the following methods is *best*, from a legal point of

view, for obtaining permission to treat Mr. Marlen when he arrives in the emergency room in an unconscious state?

1. Having his fiancée sign the consent form.
2. Having three physicians agree on treatment the patient requires.
3. Receiving a verbal consent by telephone from a responsible relative.
4. Obtaining written consent from the adult friend who accompanied the patient to the emergency room.

439. When Mr. Marlen arrives in the emergency room, which one of the following considerations in his care should have *highest* priority?

1. Establishing an airway.
2. Replacing blood losses.
3. Stopping bleeding from open wounds.
4. Determining whether he has a fractured neck.

440. Which one of the following biological products will provide Mr. Marlen with passive immunity for tetanus?

1. Tetanus toxoid.
2. Tetanus antigen.
3. Tetanus vaccine.
4. Tetanus antitoxin.

441. The nurse should withhold the injection for tetanus immunity if it is learned that Mr. Marlen has a history of an allergic reaction to

1. eggs.
2. bee sting.
3. penicillin.
4. horse serum.

442. The pathological condition which tetanus immunity helps to prevent is

1. tetany.
2. lockjaw.
3. meningitis.
4. gas gangrene.

443. Mr. Marlen's initial blood pressure was 124/80 mm. Hg. As his condition worsens, Mr. Marlen's pulse pressure increases. Which one of the following blood pressure readings illustrates a pulse pressure greater than the patient's initial measurement?

1. 102/60 mm. Hg.
2. 110/90 mm. Hg.
3. 140/100 mm. Hg.
4. 160/100 mm. Hg.

444. In which area in the diagram below is the respiratory center located?
   1. Area A.
   2. Area B.
   3. Area C.
   4. Area D.

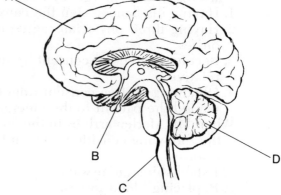

445. Which one of the following signs is *least* typical of terminal increasing intracranial pressure?
   1. Slow pulse rate.
   2. Periods of apnea.
   3. Elevated blood pressure.
   4. Subnormal body temperature.

446. Through which one of the following structures does the brain herniate if intracranial pressure is allowed to progress without relief?
   1. Frontal sinus.
   2. Mastoid process.
   3. Foramen magnum.
   4. Occipital suture.

447. In which of the sites illustrated in the diagram below had bleeding occurred when Mr. Marlen developed an extradural hematoma?
   1. Site A.
   2. Site B.
   3. Site C.
   4. Site D.

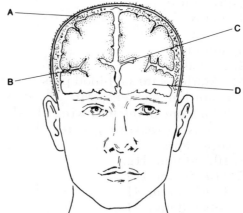

448. Which one of the following assessments of the eyes is *least helpful* when determining increasing intracranial pressure?
   1. The visual acuity.
   2. The size of the pupils.
   3. The pupils' reaction to light.
   4. The reaction of the corneas to touch.
449. Which one of the following cranial nerves controls pupil accommodation?
   1. Optic.
   2. Acoustic.
   3. Olfactory.
   4. Oculomotor.
450. The nurse obtains a specimen when she observes clear fluid draining from Mr. Marlen's nose. An examination of the fluid that will assist the physician in determining whether the fluid is mucus or cerebrospinal fluid is one that tests for the
   1. pH level.
   2. specific gravity.
   3. presence of glucose.
   4. presence of microorganisms.
451. Mr. Marlen is taken to the operating room for surgery to relieve intracranial pressure. Which one of the following nursing actions would be *least helpful* in supporting the family and friends while the patient is in the operating room?
   1. Suggesting that they wait at home where they can relax in comfort.
   2. Telling them where the patient will be cared for when surgery is completed.
   3. Explaining that they will be notified when the patient's surgery is completed.
   4. Preparing them for equipment that will be used during the patient's postoperative period.
452. The physician orders that Mr. Marlen receive mannitol (Osmitrol) intravenously during surgery to help decrease intracranial pressure. Which one of the following nursing observations will help the physician *most* to conclude that the desired effect of the drug is being obtained?
   1. Urinary output is increasing.
   2. The pulse rate is decreasing.
   3. The blood pressure is decreasing.
   4. Muscular relaxation is increasing.
453. Which one of the following comments that the nurse could make would help Mr. Marlen *most* to become oriented following surgery when he regains consciousness?

1. "I am your nurse and will take care of you."
2. "Can you tell me your name and where you live?"
3. "Can you move your hands and feet a few inches from side to side?"
4. "You are in a hospital where you had an operation after your accident."

454. When Mr. Marlen is fully conscious, it would be *best* to examine his motor strength by having him
1. feed himself with a spoon.
2. squeeze the nurse's hands.
3. demonstrate his ability to move his legs.
4. signal as soon as pressure applied to the soles of his feet becomes discernible.

455. Mr. Marlen becomes very restless and attempts to pull out his intravenous needle when he is regaining consciousness. As a protective measure to prevent injury without increasing intracranial pressure and until a medication becomes effective to control the restlessness, it would be *best* for the nurse to
1. wrap Mr. Marlen's hands in washcloths.
2. place Mr. Marlen in a jacket restraint.
3. apply a wristlet restraint to each of Mr. Marlen's arms.
4. hold Mr. Marlen's hands firmly in place at his sides.

456. Which one of the following normal body activities is *least likely* to cause a temporary increase in intracranial pressure?
1. Sneezing.
2. Coughing.
3. Vomiting.
4. Swallowing.

457. A tracheostomy is done on Mr. Marlen and he is placed on a mechanical ventilator. A cuffed tracheostomy tube is used, the *primary* reason being that, in contrast to an uncuffed tube, the cuffed tube
1. is more difficult to dislodge.
2. is easier to clean and suction.
3. prevents air from escaping around it.
4. makes it possible for the patient to speak.

458. Mr. Marlen dislodges his tracheostomy tube when he coughs. If all of the equipment listed below is available to the nurse, her *first* course of action should be to
1. maintain the opening into the trachea with the hemostat.
2. intubate the patient orally with the endotracheal tube.
3. place the tracheostomy tube's obturator into the tracheal opening.

4. start continuous suctioning with a catheter inserted through the patient's mouth.

459. While suctioning Mr. Marlen's tracheostomy tube, it is important that the nurse use intermittent suction *primarily* in order to help prevent
   1. stimulating the patient's cough reflex.
   2. dislocating the position of the patient's tracheostomy tube.
   3. depriving the patient of a sufficient supply of oxygen.
   4. clogging the suctioning catheter with the patient's exudate.

460. Most authorities recommend that the longest period of time that the nurse should maintain continuous suction when cleansing the respiratory passages of a patient with a tracheostomy is
   1. 3 to 5 seconds.
   2. 10 to 15 seconds.
   3. 20 to 25 seconds.
   4. 28 to 30 seconds.

461. Even though Mr. Marlen has no cardiovascular problems, cardiac arrest could occur if suctioning his tracheostomy tube is prolonged, due to
   1. oxygen overload.
   2. alveoli collapse.
   3. very viscid secretions.
   4. vagus nerve stimulation.

462. In relation to aseptic technique and the catheter used to suction Mr. Marlen's tracheostomy tube, it is recommended that
   1. a clean catheter be used with each suctioning and then discarded or disinfected for reuse.
   2. a sterile catheter be used with each suctioning and then discarded or sterilized for reuse.
   3. a sterile catheter be used for all suctioning during an 8-hour shift and then discarded or sterilized for reuse.
   4. a sterile catheter be used for all suctioning during a 24-hour period and then discarded or sterilized for reuse.

463. To prevent tracheal trauma, it is important that the pressure in the cuff of Mr. Marlen's tracheostomy tube be
   1. maintained continuously.
   2. increased while suctioning the tube.
   3. released at regular intervals for a few minutes.
   4. decreased while giving the patient fluids through a gastric tube.

464. Which one of the following signs indicates *most accurately* that respiratory airway suctioning has been effective?
   1. Observing that the patient's respirations are not labored.

2. Hearing a hollow sound when the patient's chest is percussed.
3. Observing that the patient is not raising mucus while coughing.
4. Hearing clear breath sounds during auscultation of the patient's chest.

465. If the following orders appear on Mr. Marlen's nursing care plan, which one would be *inappropriate?*
1. Don sterile gloves for suctioning procedure.
2. Change the tracheostomy tube every other day.
3. Administer oxygen prior to suctioning procedure.
4. Cleanse the wound with half strength hydrogen peroxide.

466. The oxygen supplied through Mr. Marlen's mechanical ventilator should be humidified to help
1. decrease the viscosity of respiratory secretions.
2. promote normal secretions in respiratory passages.
3. prevent the destruction of surfactant in the alveoli.
4. prevent the oxygen concentration from becoming too high.

467. What action should the nurse take *first* when condensation due to humidity collects in the mechanical ventilator's tubing?
1. Decrease the amount of humidity.
2. Measure the amount and mark it on the tubing.
3. Record the amount and report it to the physician.
4. Empty the fluid from the tubing and reconnect the system.

468. While Mr. Marlen is using the mechanical ventilator, certain of his blood laboratory findings are as follows:

> Arterial oxygen tension (pO_2)—88
> Arterial carbon dioxide tension (pCO_2)—30
> pH—7.47
> Bicarbonate level—22
> Base excess—0
> Oxygen saturation—97%

These findings indicate that the type of acid-base abnormality the patient is experiencing is
1. metabolic acidosis.
2. metabolic alkalosis.
3. respiratory acidosis.
4. respiratory alkalosis.

469. The normal range for the pH of arterial blood is between
1. 7.15 and 7.25.
2. 7.25 and 7.35.
3. 7.35 and 7.45.
4. 7.45 and 7.55.

470. The degree of acidity or alkalinity of the blood (its pH) involves

the relationship between the two ions,
1. calcium and chloride.
2. hydroxyl and hydrogen.
3. magnesium and sulfate.
4. sodium and bicarbonate.

471. If the following nursing orders appear on Mr. Marlen's care plan, which one would be *most helpful* in determining whether Mr. Marlen may be developing diabetes insipidus?
1. Obtain vital signs every 2 hours.
2. Measure specific gravity of urine hourly.
3. Determine arterial blood gases every other day.
4. Send urine specimen to laboratory every morning for glucose determination.

472. Mr. Marlen is placed on an alternating air pressure mattress, the *primary* purpose being to help
1. keep his body in good alignment.
2. stimulate occasional muscle contractions.
3. relieve continuous pressure on body parts.
4. improve circulation of air on pressure prone body parts.

473. Many nurses are finding that an effective way to prevent footdrop is to
1. reposition the patient every 2 to 3 hours.
2. have the patient wear ankle-high tennis shoes.
3. massage the patient's feet and ankles regularly.
4. support the patient's bed linen over a cradle placed on the bed.

474. To prevent external rotation of Mr. Marlen's hips while he is lying on his back, it would be *best* to place
1. firm pillows under the length of his legs.
2. sandbags alongside his legs from knees to ankles.
3. trochanter rolls alongside his legs from ilium to midthigh.
4. a footboard that supports his feet in the normal anatomical position.

475. Mr. Marlen is placed in a right side-lying position, as described below. Which aspect of the positioning will cause *improper* body alignment?
1. His head is placed on a small pillow.
2. His right leg is extended without pillow support.
3. His left arm rests on the mattress with the elbow flexed.
4. His left leg is supported on a pillow with the knee flexed.

476. Mr. Marlen's skin care includes frequent massage over areas prone to develop decubitus ulcers. The *primary* reason for massage is to help
1. relax tense muscles.
2. improve blood circulation.

3. allow the skin to stay dry.

4. reduce the number of organisms on the skin.

477. Which of the following bony prominences has the *least potential* for developing a decubitus ulcer?
   1. The knees.
   2. The heels.
   3. The coccyx.
   4. The back of the head.

478. During Mr. Marlen's recovery period, the nurse notes at 4 P.M. that Mr. Marlen seems disinterested in his visitors and is more lethargic than usual. If the following notations appear on the patient's record, which one indicates the *most probable* cause for his lethargy?
   1. 12:30 P.M. - Refused lunch; drank glass of milk only.
   2. 3:00 P.M. - Placed in side-lying position after being in semisitting position for 3 hours.
   3. 3:00 P.M. - Meperidine hydrochloride (Demerol) 100 mg. given IM for pain in area of bruises on back.
   4. 3:30 P.M. - Intake 800 ml. and output 300 ml. since 8:00 A.M.

   Mr. Sidney Clate is a 76-year-old man admitted to the hospital for cataract extraction.
   Items 479 through 499 pertain to this situation.

479. If the nursing care plan for Mr. Clate takes the following items into account preoperatively, which one will be of *prime* importance for this patient following his surgery?
   1. Obtaining his health history.
   2. Assessing his visual acuity.
   3. Orienting him to his physical surroundings.
   4. Explaining the purpose of eyedrops he will be receiving.

480. As a result of having a cataract, the visual symptoms Mr. Clate is *most likely* to comment about are
   1. halos and rainbows around lights.
   2. pain and irritation that is worse at night.
   3. eye strain and headache when doing close work.
   4. blurred vision and hazy appearance of objects.

481. Mr. Clate asks the nurse, "What causes cataracts in older persons?" Which one of the following statements offers the nurse the *best* guide in answering the patient's question?
   1. Cataracts usually result from chronic systemic diseases.
   2. The cause of cataracts in the elderly is not clearly understood.
   3. Cataracts usually result from prolonged use of toxic substances, such as alcohol and tobacco.

4. The cause of cataracts is believed to be due to eye injuries sustained early in the patient's life.

482. One of Mr. Clate's preoperative orders is written as follows: Phenylephrine hydrochloride (Neo-Synephrine) 10% and cyclopentolate hydrochloride (Cyclogyl) 1%: 1 drop of each, O.D., every 5 minutes for 3 times. According to this information, the preoperative medications are to be placed into
   1. both eyes.
   2. the left eye.
   3. the right eye.

483. Phenylephrine hydrochloride acts in the eye to produce
   1. dilatation of the pupil and dilatation of blood vessels.
   2. dilatation of the pupil and constriction of blood vessels.
   3. constriction of the pupil and constriction of blood vessels.
   4. constriction of the pupil and dilatation of the blood vessels.

484. Of the following reasons, which one serves as a rationale for using cyclopentolate hydrochloride preoperatively?
   1. It paralyzes the ciliary muscles.
   2. It increases intraocular pressure.
   3. It reduces pathogenic bacterial count.
   4. It depresses the formation of aqueous humor.

485. After instilling eyedrops, the nurse should apply slight pressure against the nose at the inner angle of the closed eye in order to
   1. prevent the drug from escaping and running down the face.
   2. prevent absorption of the drug into the general systemic system.
   3. allow the sensitive cornea to become adjusted to the medication.
   4. facilitate distribution of the drug over the entire surface of the eye.

486. Mr. Clate tells the nurse that he does not like to think about being awake during the eye surgery. Of the following responses, which one is the *most appropriate* for the nurse to make?
   1. "Can you tell me more about not liking the idea of being awake?"
   2. "Have you ever had any reactions to local anesthetics in the past?"
   3. "By using a local anesthetic, you will not have nausea and vomiting after the surgery."
   4. "There is really nothing to fear about being awake. You will be given a medication that will help you relax."

487. If Mr. Clate has both eyes patched postoperatively, which of the following nursing interventions would be *most helpful* in preventing sensory deprivation?

1. Maintaining a quiet, dark environment.
2. Administering sedation as often as necessary.
3. Providing frequent verbal and physical stimulation.
4. Isolating the patient from possible sources of infection.

488. During the evening on the day of surgery, the patient states he is "sick to my stomach." The *best* action for the nurse to take at this time is to
1. have the patient take a few deep breaths until the nausea subsides.
2. explain to the patient that this is very common and the feeling will pass quickly.
3. tell the patient that his physician has ordered a medication for this and that the nurse will get it for him immediately.
4. explain that the nausea is of no particular significance but that the patient should call the nurse promptly if he vomits.

489. Of the following postoperative techniques to counteract the effects of decreased activity, which one is contraindicated for Mr. Clate?
1. Turning.
2. Coughing.
3. Ambulating.
4. Deep breathing.

490. If the nurse observes Mr. Clate carrying out the following activities on the third postoperative day, which one would be *contraindicated?*
1. Walking down the hall unassisted.
2. Lying in bed on his unoperated side.
3. Performing routines of isometric exercises.
4. Bending from the hips to pick up his slippers.

491. On the fifth postoperative day, Mr. Clate suddenly complains of a sharp pain in the operative eye and he becomes very restless. When this occurs, the nurse's action should be guided by knowledge that the postoperative complication Mr. Clate has *very likely* developed is
1. a detached retina.
2. a prolapse of the iris.
3. an extracapsular erosion.
4. an intraocular hemorrhage.

492. When preparing Mr. Clate for discharge, the nurse should stress that he maintain limited activities for a period of approximately
1. 1 to 2 weeks.
2. 2 to 4 weeks.
3. 4 to 6 weeks.

4. 10 to 12 weeks.

493. During a conversation with Mr. Clate, he says he feels "down on the world" and expresses general pessimism. The depression many older persons tend to experience is generally believed to be due to
1. fear of death.
2. loss in feelings of self-worth.
3. decreased exposure to sensory stimulation.
4. diminution in the secretion of most hormones.

494. Several weeks after discharge from the hospital, Mr. Clate receives temporary cataract glasses. When preparing Mr. Clate to use these glasses, it would be *best* for the nurse to teach him that he should
1. practice reading each day to help strengthen his eye muscles.
2. use the glasses while sitting down until he has adjusted to them.
3. hold articles for inspection at a distance of 2 to 3 feet for best focus.
4. use his unoperated eye when objects temporarily appear double until focus improves.

495. Which one of the following practices should the nurse teach Mr. Clate to use to help prevent optical distortion when cataract glasses are being worn?
1. Using one eye at a time when focusing.
2. Looking through the center of the lenses.
3. Moving the glasses lower down on the nose.
4. Moving the eyes slowly when looking to the side.

496. Which one of the following anatomical structures of the eye is without blood vessels?
1. The iris.
2. The sclera.
3. The cornea.
4. The ciliary body.

497. The lens of the eye normally functions to
1. produce aqueous humor.
2. house the rods and cones.
3. focus light rays onto the retina.
4. regulate the amount of light entering the eye.

498. Which of the following cranial nerves carries the visual impulse from the rods and cones to the brain?
1. The optic (second) nerve.
2. The oculomotor (third) nerve.
3. The trochlear (fourth) nerve.
4. The abducens (sixth) nerve.

499. When rays of light are focused in front of the retina, the person
has an eye condition known as
1. miosis.
2. myopia.
3. hyperopia.
4. presbyopia.

Mr. James Turner was admitted to the hospital after he
sustained burns of his chest, abdomen, right arm, and right leg.
The accident occurred when gasoline ignited while he was
cleaning the engine of his motorcycle.
Items 500 through 538 relate to this situation.

500. In relation to emergency care at the time of the accident, it is
generally agreed that it would have been *best* to care for Mr.
Turner's burn areas, which were moderate to severe, by
1. pouring cold water over the areas.
2. applying clean dry dressings to the areas.
3. rinsing the areas with a warm mild soap solution.
4. applying a mild antiseptic ointment to the areas.

501. The shaded areas in the diagram below indicate the burn areas
on Mr. Turner's body. Using the "Rule of Nines," approximately what percent of his body had been burned?
1. 18 percent.
2. 27 percent.
3. 45 percent.
4. 64 percent.

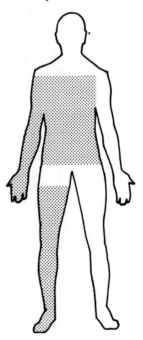

502. By which one of the following physical processes will Mr. Turner lose significant amounts of fluid from his burn areas?
   1. Diffusion.
   2. Dispersion.
   3. Evaporation.
   4. Condensation.
503. Mr. Turner is receiving intravenous fluids. When the physician orders that the nurse should regulate the rate of administering the patient's fluids, it would be *best* for her to guide action initially by observing Mr. Turner's
   1. daily weights.
   2. body temperature.
   3. hourly urinary outputs.
   4. specific gravity of urine.
504. The nurse is regulating the rate at which Mr. Turner's intravenous fluids are being administered. Which one of the following findings should serve as an *early* indication to the nurse to decrease the rate of flow?
   1. Crackling chest sounds in the patient.
   2. Distention of the patient's abdomen.
   3. A sharp increase in the patient's pulse rate.
   4. A steady increase in the patient's blood pressure.
505. The physician orders an indwelling catheter for Mr. Turner. The generally accepted *minimum* safe range for the hourly output of urine during the first few days after a burn such as Mr. Turner had is
   1. 10 to 20 ml.
   2. 30 to 70 ml.
   3. 70 to 100 ml.
   4. 100 to 150 ml.
506. Although wide variations exist, the average range for the specific gravity of urine in the absence of disease is *most commonly* stated as being between approximately
   1. 1.000 and 1.005.
   2. 1.015 and 1.025.
   3. 1.030 and 1.050.
   4. 1.050 and 1.075.
507. In addition to respiratory depression, which one of the following problems is *most likely* to occur if Mr. Turner is given narcotics in large doses for the control of pain?
   1. Suppression of urine.
   2. Camouflage of other symptoms.
   3. Depression of peripheral nerve endings.
   4. Stimulation of the central nervous system.

508. During which phase after his burn is Mr. Turner likely to experience cardiac arrhythmias when potassium losses within cells
cannot be adequately controlled?
1. During the convalescent phase.
2. During the fluid management phase.
3. During the fluid accumulation phase.
4. During the fluid remobilization phase.

509. The nurse can anticipate that the *most commonly* ordered route
for administering Mr. Turner an analgesic will be the
1. oral route.
2. rectal route.
3. intravenous route.
4. intramuscular route.

510. It is generally agreed that the *single most effective* way to help
prevent cross-contamination of Mr. Turner's wounds would
be to
1. place the patient in a private room.
2. sterilize the patient's personal care items after each use.
3. have health personnel wash their hands before and after caring for the patient.
4. use sterile disposable equipment and dressings when caring
for the patient's wounds.

511. An open method is used to care for Mr. Turner's burned chest
and abdomen while a closed method is used for his burned
extremities. Which one of the following actions should the
nurse take to help prevent discomfort caused by air currents
over Mr. Turner's chest and abdomen?
1. Keeping the patient well sedated.
2. Adding humidity to the patient's room air.
3. Supporting the patient's upper bed linens on a cradle.
4. Keeping the door and windows closed in the patient's room.

512. Which one of the following techniques should the nurse use
when bandaging Mr. Turner's hand to maintain its functional
alignment?
1. Wrapping the thumb and each finger separately.
2. Wrapping the closed fist with recurrent bandages.
3. Curving the fingers and thumb over a roll of gauze.
4. Securing the fingers to a flat well-padded handboard.

513. The physician orders that Mr. Turner receive total parenteral
nutrition (TNP) beginning on his fourth day of hospitalization.
The *primary* reason for prescribing this therapy is to help
1. correct water and electrolyte imbalances.
2. provide supplemental vitamins and minerals.
3. facilitate rest for his gastrointestinal tract.

4. assure an adequate intake of calories and proteins.

514. Mr. Turner's hyperalimentation catheter would be considered properly placed and solution may be introduced when the tip of the catheter is located in the
1. innominate vein.
2. subclavian vein.
3. superior vena cava.
4. internal jugular vein.

515. The basic component of hyperalimentation solution is *most often*
1. isotonic glucose solution.
2. hypertonic glucose solution.
3. hypotonic dextrose solution.
4. low molecular dextrose solution.

516. Which one of the following problems has been identified as the *major* complication of hyperalimentation therapy?
1. Diuresis.
2. Diarrhea.
3. Infection.
4. Air emboli.

517. The *best* information concerning Mr. Turner's ability to metabolize the hyperalimentation solution would be gained by the nurse periodically when she studies the patient's
1. urine for specific gravity.
2. blood pressure and pulse rates.
3. temperature and respiratory rates.
4. urine for the presence of glucose.

518. When changing dressings, what is the *primary* purpose for cleansing the skin around the hyperalimentation infusion catheter with ether or acetone?
1. To remove the tape.
2. To remove skin oils.
3. To sterilize the skin.
4. To anesthetize the area.

519. Which one of the following measures should the nurse use to help prevent air from being sucked into Mr. Turner's hyperalimentation catheter when it is opened during changing of the filter and intravenous tubing?
1. Instructing the patient to inhale deeply.
2. Having the patient lie on his left side.
3. Having the patient in a high Fowler's position.
4. Instructing the patient to perform the Valsalva's maneuver (bearing down).

520. The physician will very likely order a culture and sensitivity

examinations of drainage from Mr. Turner's wounds when the nurse reports that his dressings revealed a moderate amount of
1. serous stain.
2. yellow drainage.
3. serosanguineous exudate.
4. clear fluid oozing through scabs.

521. If the physician considers the following drugs for treating Mr. Turner's wound infection, which one is he *most likely* to select because of its effectiveness against the organism, *Pseudomonas aeruginosa?*
1. Erythromycin (Erythrocin).
2. Kanamycin sulfate (Kantrex).
3. Gentamicin sulfate (Garamycin).
4. Chloramphenicol (Chloromycetin).

522. Which one of the following activities should the nurse include on Mr. Turner's care plan, to be carried out approximately ½ hour prior to his daily whirlpool bath and dressing change?
1. Soak the dressings.
2. Remove the dressings.
3. Administer an analgesic.
4. Slit the dressings with a blunt scissors.

523. During his hospitalization, Mr. Turner undergoes several skin graft procedures. An important *first* step for grafting is to prepare the area where Mr. Turner will receive the graft by
1. removing dead tissue.
2. applying a local antibiotic.
3. chemically disinfecting the area.
4. scrubbing the area with distilled water.

524. Which one of the following conditions will have the *least* influence on the survival and effectiveness of Mr. Turner's skin grafts?
1. Absence of infection in the wounds.
2. Adequate vascularization in the grafts.
3. Assured immobilization of the area being grafted.
4. Potent analgesics as necessary for the relief of pain.

525. Mr. Turner demonstrates anxiety about his burns and prognosis and requires considerable emotional support. An individual is said to have received emotional support when his tensions are reduced by
1. willingly accepting advice and suggestions.
2. borrowing from the strengths of a caring person.
3. recognizing the underlying causes of his anxiety.
4. directing his strengths toward meaningful outcomes.

526. Which one of the following complications is sometimes observed

in patients with burns and appears to be the result of prolonged stress?

1. Paralytic ileus.
2. Gastric dilatation.
3. Nitrogen imbalance.
4. Gastrointestinal ulceration.

527. Mr. Turner is 25 years old. Erik Erikson, the psychologist, has general support among his peers in relation to his theory that the *primary* conflict of young adults between approximately 20 and 40 years of age is
1. autonomy versus doubt.
2. trust versus mistrust.
3. intimacy versus isolation.
4. identity versus role confusion.

528. Porcine or pigskin grafts are classified as
1. isografts.
2. xenografts.
3. autografts.
4. allografts.

529. Which one of the following types of skin grafts carries its own blood supply?
1. Free grafts.
2. Pedicle grafts.
3. Thin split-thickness grafts.
4. Thick split-thickness grafts.

530. When all extremities are severely burned, the nurse is *best* able to assess for physiological intact circulation by
1. monitoring the patient's central venous pressure.
2. observing unburned areas for color and temperature.
3. pressing skin on unburned areas and observing for capillary filling.
4. comparing pressure required to obliterate the pulse at carotid arteries with that required at the femoral arteries.

531. When burns are severe, which one of the following aspects of care should receive the *highest* priority to help prevent overwhelming infection?
1. Cleansing the wound.
2. Using antibiotic therapy.
3. Providing for new skin cover.
4. Maintaining adequate hydration.

532. An advantage of using biological dressings on burn areas is that they appear to help
1. encourage formation of tough skin.
2. provide for permanent wound closure.

3. enhance growth of epithelial tissue.

4. facilitate development of subcutaneous tissue.

533. A patient whose burn areas are being treated with dressings saturated with an aqueous solution of silver nitrate (0.5%) requires careful monitoring and prompt treatment to help prevent
1. renal failure.
2. cardiac arrest.
3. pulmonary edema.
4. electrolyte imbalance.

534. When silver nitrate is used for the care of burns, the nurse is advised to wear gloves *primarily* to prevent
1. staining of hands.
2. contact dermatitis.
3. sloughing of tissue.
4. cross-contamination.

535. When the following courses of action are possible, it is generally recommended that if one's clothing is burning, it is *best* to
1. fall to the floor and roll.
2. take off the clothing immediately.
3. remain motionless and call for help.
4. spray the clothing with fire extinguisher liquid.

536. Fluid shift in the patient with severe burns results from an increase in
1. permeability of capillary walls.
2. total volume of intravascular plasma.
3. total volume of circulating whole blood.
4. permeability of the tubules in the kidneys.

537. In which of the following locations in homes do *most* fires start?
1. Bedrooms and closets.
2. Basements and attics.
3. Garages and storage areas.
4. Living rooms and kitchens.

538. Which one of the following descriptions *best* defines the term, eschar?
1. Scar tissue in a developmental stage.
2. Burned tissue that has become infected.
3. Crust formation without a blood supply.
4. Viable living tissue with a rich blood supply.

A nursing team leader responsible for the care of post-operative surgical patients has a team conference on pain.

Items 539 through 548 pertain to information discussed at the conference.

539. The gate control theory, which deals with the pain mechanism, holds that there is a regulatory process that controls impulses reaching the cerebral cortex. This regulatory process is located in the
1. cerebellum
2. brain stem.
3. spinal cord.
4. hypothalamus.

540. Which one of the following nursing measures would be selected when caring for a patient in pain if the gate control theory was used to guide intervention?
1. Giving the patient a backrub.
2. Repositioning the patient in bed.
3. Giving the patient a prescribed analgesic.
4. Loosening a tight abdominal binder on the patient.

541. Responses to pain are directed toward improving the body's ability to
1. endure or tolerate the pain.
2. decrease the perception of pain.
3. escape or flee the source of pain.
4. divert attention form the source of pain.

542. A typical *psychic* reaction to pain is
1. crying.
2. grimacing.
3. pacing the floor.
4. experiencing anxiety.

543. An example of an impulse that is traveling along an efferent nerve route is an impulse moving from the
1. hand to the spinal cord.
2. inner ear to the cerebrum.
3. brain to the abdominal wall.
4. urinary bladder to the thalamus.

544. How high in the central nervous system does the reflex act of removing the hand immediately from a hot stove ordinarily travel?
1. To the thalamus.
2. To the spinal cord.
3. To the hypothalamus.
4. To the cerebral cortex.

545. A patient is encouraged to watch television while his dressings are changed. This method of helping a patient cope with a painful procedure illustrates nursing intervention that results in
1. relieving the source of the pain.

2. dissipating the stimulus for pain.
3. decreasing the perception of pain.
4. interfering with the pathway along which the pain impulse travels.

546. Where in the brain is pain perceived?
1. In the thalamus.
2. In the brain stem.
3. In the cerebellum.
4. In the cerebral cortex.

547. When a patient complains of pain due to a distended bladder, the type of agent causing the pain is
1. a thermal agent.
2. a chemical agent.
3. an electrical agent.
4. a mechanical agent.

548. Opioids are effective for pain relief because of their ability to
1. reduce the perception of pain.
2. decrease the sensitivity of pain receptors.
3. interfere with pain impulses traveling along sensory nerve fibers.
4. block the conduction of pain impulses along the central nervous system

Items 549 through 608 are miscellaneous items.

549. Which one of the following clinical situations does *not ordinarily* require emergency surgery?
1. Strangulated hernia.
2. Perforated peptic ulcer.
3. Gunshot wound of the chest.
4. Hemorrhoids that bleed periodically.

550. The abbreviation used to describe the quadrant of the abdomen where the surgical incision is ordinarily made for an appendectomy is
1. RUQ.
2. LUQ.
3. LLQ.
4. RLQ.

551. A middle-aged patient with well-controlled diabetes mellitus is to undergo surgery. What knowledge should form the basis upon which the nurse will plan care for this patient?
1. Glycosuria and ketoacidosis can be expected during this patient's postoperative period.
2. The patient is very likely to develop a postoperative infection and have poor healing of his wound.

3. All things being equal, the surgical risk of this patient is no greater than for a nondiabetic patient.
4. The body's demand for insulin can be expected to decrease as the patient experiences stress and apprehension.

552. Pyloroplasty is a surgical procedure done in order to
1. enlarge the pyloric opening.
2. remove the pyloric sphincter.
3. bypass the pyloric sphincter.
4. graft fundus cells to the pyloric sphincter.

553. Of the following patients, the one who is *most likely* to suffer from sensory deprivation is the patient who has had
1. chest surgery and is in a 4-bed room.
2. orthopedic surgery and is in traction.
3. eye surgery and is in a semiprivate room.
4. heart surgery and is in an intensive care unit.

554. Which one of the following nursing interventions can *best* help the patient who is experiencing sensory deprivation?
1. Darken the patient's room.
2. Discuss normal daily events.
3. Limit the patient's visitors.
4. Avoid asking the patient direct questions.

555. A patient who is to have surgery has a history of seizure activity. Which one of the following nursing measures is *contraindicated* for this patient?
1. Having the patient take his own bed bath.
2. Placing the patient through range-of-motion exercises.
3. Obtaining an oral temperature with a mercury thermometer.
4. Allowing the patient to wear his dentures while sleeping.

556. If the following notations are made by the nurse caring for a patient who had an epileptic seizure, which one would be of *least* value to the patient's physician?
1. "Patient was incontinent after the seizure."
2. "Patient was very drowsy after the seizure."
3. "Patient's pupils remained unchanged during the seizure."
4. "Patient failed to respond to painful stimuli during the clonic phase."

557. A patient has a malignancy of the prostate gland. Which one of the following blood examinations should the nurse anticipate will be ordered when the physician wishes to assess whether there has been metastasis?
1. Serum creatinine level.
2. Serum acid phosphatase level.
3. Total nonprotein nitrogen level.
4. Endogenous creatinine clearance time.

558. While a patient is convalescing following a prostatectomy, which one of the following measures should he be encouraged to use to help him regain full urinary control?
1. Taking a sitz bath twice a day.
2. Wearing a scrotal support while awake.
3. Alternately tensing and relaxing his perineal muscles.
4. Ambulating at least 10 to 15 minutes every hour while awake.

559. A patient is observed to be angry and hostile because it becomes necessary to amputate his leg. Statement A below is a correct statement. What is the relationship between statements A and B?

Statement A: It has been observed that allowing a patient independence to whatever extent is possible provides psychological benefit by helping to lessen the patient's sense of helplessness. Statement B: Since this patient's disability is permanent, it is better for the nurse to help him control his anger rather than encourage him to express it.
1. Statement B is true; statement A explains or confirms statement B.
2. Statement B is true; statement A neither helps explain nor confirm statement B.
3. Statement B is false; statement A contradicts or indicates the falsity of statement B.
4. Statement B is false; statement A neither contradicts nor indicates the falsity of statement B.

560. Emergency equipment which is recommended to be kept at the bedside of a patient who has had an amputation should include
1. a tourniquet.
2. a suture tray.
3. a transfusion set.
4. aspiration supplies.

561. Contractures in an extremity which has been partially amputated can *best* be prevented by
1. massaging the stump.
2. splinting the joint nearest the stump site.
3. placing the stump in a position of least pain.
4. placing the stump through range-of-motion exercises.

562. The bulk of the patient's weight when the patient is using conventional crutches should be borne by the
1. axillae.
2. forearms.
3. upper arms.
4. palms of the hands.

563. Which one of the following exercises is recommended to prepare

a patient for using crutches?

1. Rolling from side to side while lying in bed.
2. Placing the shoulders, elbows, and wrists through range-of-motion exercises.
3. Quadriceps drills; alternately contracting and relaxing the muscles of the thighs.
4. Push ups; while lying on the abdomen, hands near shoulders and elbows flexed, raising the body off the bed.

564. A young man was hurt while diving into shallow water and it is suspected that he has a spinal cord injury. If the following methods are available for transferring him from the beach to an ambulance, which one is preferred?

1. Placing the victim on his back on a board.
2. Placing the victim on a stretcher made with a blanket and poles.
3. Placing the victim in a sitting position on a straight-back chair.
4. Using a 3-carrier lift with the victim resting on the chest of the carriers.

565. Crutchfield tongs from which weights were hung are applied to the head of a patient who has a fracture of the cervical spine. To obtain counterweight, in what position should his bed be placed?

1. The head of the bed should be elevated.
2. The foot of the bed should be elevated.
3. The bed should be kept straight and parallel to the floor.
4. The bed should be "broken" (gatched) so that both the head and the foot of the bed will be slightly elevated.

566. If it has been determined that the area of permanent damage to the spinal cord is at the lowest end of the cervical spine (C8), which one of the following rehabilitative goals in relation to activities of daily living is *unrealistic?*

1. To walk.
2. To write.
3. To feed oneself.
4. To drive an automobile.

567. It is important that the nursing care of the patient paralyzed after a spinal cord injury be directed toward helping to prevent the four problems listed below. Most authorities are of the opinion that, of these four, it is of *prime* importance that nurses use measures to help prevent

1. constipation.
2. contractures.
3. decubitus ulcers.
4. urinary retention.

568. If a patient with a spinal cord injury suffers from spinal shock, which one of the following vital signs becomes *especially* important to monitor at frequent intervals?
1. The pulse rate.
2. The body temperature.
3. The respiratory rate.
4. The heart's electrical impulses.

569. A patient receives a general anesthesia while the surgeon performs procedures to remove a blood clot to relieve intracranial pressure. The *most likely* reason for choosing a general rather than a local anesthesia is that a general anesthesia
1. rarely depresses respirations.
2. is less painful for the patient.
3. controls fear and anxiety better.
4. presents less of an explosion hazard.

570. Arterial hypotension resulting from spinal anesthesia is due to the fact that
1. sympathetic afferent fibers are being blocked.
2. sympathetic efferent fibers are being blocked.
3. parasympathetic afferent fibers are being blocked.
4. parasympathetic efferent fibers are being blocked.

571. Epinephrine is usually added to an injectable local anesthetic because the drug helps to
1. prolong the effects of the anesthesia.
2. promote rapid absorption of the anesthesia.
3. eliminate the danger of local tissue necrosis.
4. improve muscle relaxation in the surgical area.

572. Which one of the following statements *best* describes why ether as an anesthetic agent continues to be used for many types of surgery?
1. Ether anesthesia is induced rapidly and easily.
2. Recovery from ether anesthesia is rapid and pleasant.
3. Ether has a wide margin of safety between nontoxicity and toxicity.
4. Ether produces a minimum of sympathetic nervous system stimulation.

573. Statement A below is a correct statement. What is the relationship between statements A and B?
Statement A: As the rate of metabolism decreases, the oxygen needs of the body's cells decrease.
Statement B: The patient requires less general anesthesia when hypothermia is used as a surgical adjunct.
1. Statement B is true; statement A explains or confirms statement B.

2. Statement B is true; statement A neither helps explain nor confirm statement B.
3. Statement B is false; statement A contradicts or indicates the falsity of statement B.
4. Statement B is false; statement A neither contradicts nor indicates the falsity of statement B.

574. If the objective of postoperative intravenous therapy is to replace water and electrolytes, of the following solutions, the one that *best* meets this objective is
1. normal saline 0.9%.
2. dextrose 5% in water.
3. dextrose 10% in saline.
4. lactated Ringer's solution.

575. What type of diet is generally recommended preoperatively for the malnourished patient?
1. Low carbohydrate, high protein, low vitamin.
2. Low carbohydrate, low cholesterol, low sodium.
3. High carbohydrate, high protein, high vitamin.
4. High carbohydrate, low protein, high vitamin.

576. The *most common* cause of a bunion is having
1. flat feet.
2. worn poorly fitted shoes.
3. a bone infection in the great toe.
4. had an injury with damage to the metatarsal arch.

577. A synonym for the word bunion is
1. osteoma.
2. primary gout.
3. hallux valgus.
4. Morton's neuroma.

578. Current opinion is that the cause of atherosclerosis is
1. unknown.
2. obesity.
3. sedentary lifestyle.
4. high cholesterol intake.

579. A rectal tube is used when a postoperative patient complains of abdominal distention, but the patient experiences no relief. Of the following explanations, which one offers the *best* reason for the ineffectiveness of this nursing measure?
1. The rectal tube was too large.
2. The rectal tube was inserted too far.
3. The rectal tube was too generously lubricated.
4. The rectal tube was left in place too long.

580. A Stryker frame is being used for a patient with a back injury. The advantage of a Stryker frame is that the patient

1. can turn himself without having to depend on help.
2. can be turned while keeping the spine immobilized.
3. has automatic support in a position of good anatomical alignment.
4. provides even-weight distribution so that decubitus ulcers are unlikely to develop.

581. The *primary* purpose of placing a patient on a rocking bed is to help
1. prevent decubitus ulcers.
2. facilitate breathing.
3. facilitate heart action.
4. prevent urinary retention.

582. The solution of choice for vaginal douching intended for personal hygiene purposes is a mixture of water and
1. baking soda.
2. white vinegar.
3. a mild detergent.
4. a mild antiseptic.

583. A tonometer is an instrument used to help determine whether a patient has
1. glaucoma.
2. cataracts.
3. corneal scars.
4. retinal detachment.

584. To prevent electrical shocking while bathing a patient with a temporary external pacemaker, it is *best* for the nurse to
1. place the unit and wires in a plastic bag.
2. tape the unit to a bed rail during the bath.
3. place the patient on a rubberized pad while bathing him.
4. remove other electrical devices from the patient's immediate environment.

585. In which chamber of the heart is the tip of lead from the pacemaker ordinarily placed?
1. The left atrium.
2. The right atrium.
3. The left ventricle.
4. The right ventricle.

586. Of the following symptoms, which one is *most commonly* noted when a pacemaker fails?
1. Nausea.
2. Tremors.
3. Headache.
4. Dizziness.

587. The *primary* reason for using a double balloon gastric tube to

help control bleeding from esophageal varices is that this type of tube functions to help

1. prevent intubating the duodenum.
2. create pressure on the bleeding area.
3. eliminate irritation to the bleeding area.
4. remove blood quickly from the bleeding area.

588. Consider the relationship between statements A and B below. Statement A: Suctioning a patient's airway removes oxygen, respiratory secretions, and other debris from the respiratory tract. Statement B: Humidified air helps keep respiratory secretions thin and watery so that they are easier to remove from the patient's respiratory tract.

1. Both statements A and B are false and unrelated to each other.
2. Both statements A and B are true; statement A explains or confirms statement B.
3. Both statements A and B are true; statement A neither helps explain nor confirm statement B.
4. Statement A is true and statement B is false; statement A contradicts or indicates the falsity of statement B.

589. Which of the following treatment modalities would reduce the surface tension of fat globules in the presence of a fat embolism?

1. Hypothermia.
2. Oxygen therapy.
3. Intravenous administration of ethanol.
4. Drug therapy to reduce serum cholesterol levels.

590. The *most common early* symptom of laryngeal cancer is

1. dyspnea.
2. hoarseness.
3. offensive breath.
4. excessive salivation.

591. Which one of the following symptoms is *most commonly* associated with an obstruction in the small intestine?

1. Abdominal distention.
2. Vomiting of fecal material.
3. Alteration in bowel habits.
4. Presence of mucus in the stool.

592. Which one of the following maneuvers is used to test the Babinski reflex?

1. The sole of the foot is stroked.
2. The knee is struck with a rubber hammer.
3. The elbow is struck with a rubber hammer.
4. The foot is sharply flexed so that the toes point upward toward the tibia.

593. It has been observed that problems related to the so-called empty nest syndrome among women at menopause are less severe when these women
1. have had larger than average families.
2. find purposeful activity to occupy free time.
3. are married and have not experienced divorce.
4. experience menopause in their late 40s and early 50s.

594. Which of the following nerves is *most* responsible for the proper functioning of the diaphragm?
1. The vagus nerve.
2. The phrenic nerve.
3. The thoracic nerve.
4. The thoracodorsal nerve.

595. *All* of the following vital functions of the body are regulated by centers in the medulla oblongata *except*
1. rate of respirations.
2. rate of the heartbeat.
3. maintenance of blood pressure.
4. maintenance of body temperature.

596. If a normal blood cell is placed in a hypertonic solution, the cell can be expected to
1. shrink in size.
2. divide into two cells.
3. remain unchanged in size.
4. burst from overexpansion.

597. The pressure that causes water to cross a semipermeable membrane is called
1. osmotic pressure.
2. positive pressure.
3. barometric pressure.
4. hydrostatic pressure.

598. The physical principle upon which gastric lavage operates is
1. gravity.
2. the lever.
3. the siphon.
4. air pressure.

599. When a patient is given a cool sponge bath to help reduce his temperature and alcohol is added to the water, *most* heat is transferred from the body through the phenomenon of
1. radiation.
2. conduction.
3. convection.
4. evaporation.

600. A patient with a sprained ankle has swelling at the site of the

injury. It would be *inappropriate* to apply cold to the injured area because the initial reaction of the body to applications of cold is

1. dilatation of venules.
2. constriction of arterioles.
3. increased sensitivity to pain.
4. increased capillary permeability.

601. If a patient is receiving all of the following medications, which one can the nurse expect to be discontinued several days before the patient has surgery?
1. Digoxin (Lanoxin).
2. Tolbutamide (Orinase).
3. Prednisone (Deltasone).
4. Warfarin sodium (Coumadin).

602. Which one of the following age groups generally tolerates surgery *least* well?
1. Toddlers.
2. Young adults.
3. Premature infants.
4. Middle-aged adults.

603. According to authorities on the subject, which one of the following habits, if eliminated, would cause the *greatest* reduction in the incidence of lung cancer?
1. Pipe smoking.
2. Cigar smoking.
3. Tobacco chewing.
4. Cigarette smoking.

604. In which one of the following population categories is the incidence of rheumatic fever the highest in this country?
1. Adults.
2. School age children.
3. Rural farm dwellers.
4. Immigrants to the United States.

605. The leading cause of death among persons over 45 years of age is
1. heart diseases.
2. malignant tumors.
3. cirrhosis of the liver.
4. cerebrovascular diseases.

606. According to research, between which years of life is the peak in intellectual and physical abilities reached?
1. Between 10 and 20 years of age.
2. Between 20 and 30 years of age.
3. Between 30 and 40 years of age.
4. Between 40 and 50 years of age.

607. Which one of the following age groups is the fastest growing segment in the United States today?
1. Adolescents - 10 to 20 years of age.
2. Young adults - 20 to 40 years of age.
3. Middle-aged adults - 40 to 60 years of age.
4. The elderly - over 65 years of age.
608. Which one of the following phenomena is considered to be an inevitable consequence of aging, even when health is good?
1. General intellectual decline.
2. Sudden end to sexual activity.
3. Slowing of the thought process.
4. Loss in ability to use verbal skills.

answer sheet for surgical nursing

Read each question in the examination carefully and select which one of the options is the *best* or *correct* answer. If the answer you would prefer is not given, select the one which seems *most appropriate*.

Locate on the answer sheet the number of the item you are answering. With a pencil, blacken the circle corresponding to the answer you have selected. Be sure you are recording your answer in the proper space.

	1 2 3 4		1 2 3 4		1 2 3 4		1 2 3 4
1	○○○○	18	○○○○	35	○○○○	52	○○○○
2	○○○○	19	○○○○	36	○○○○	53	○○○○
3	○○○○	20	○○○○	37	○○○○	54	○○○○
4	○○○○	21	○○○○	38	○○○○	55	○○○○
5	○○○○	22	○○○○	39	○○○○	56	○○○○
6	○○○○	23	○○○○	40	○○○○	57	○○○○
7	○○○○	24	○○○○	41	○○○○	58	○○○○
8	○○○○	25	○○○○	42	○○○○	59	○○○○
9	○○○○	26	○○○○	43	○○○○	60	○○○○
10	○○○○	27	○○○○	44	○○○○	61	○○○○
11	○○○○	28	○○○○	45	○○○○	62	○○○○
12	○○○○	29	○○○○	46	○○○○	63	○○○○
13	○○○○	30	○○○○	47	○○○○	64	○○○○
14	○○○○	31	○○○○	48	○○○○	65	○○○○
15	○○○○	32	○○○○	49	○○○○	66	○○○○
16	○○○○	33	○○○○	50	○○○○	67	○○○○
17	○○○○	34	○○○○	51	○○○○	68	○○○○

	1 2 3 4		1 2 3 4		1 2 3 4		1 2 3 4
69	○○○○	91	○○○○	113	○○○○	135	○○○○
70	○○○○	92	○○○○	114	○○○○	136	○○○○
71	○○○○	93	○○○○	115	○○○○	137	○○○○
72	○○○○	94	○○○○	116	○○○○	138	○○○○
73	○○○○	95	○○○○	117	○○○○	139	○○○○
74	○○○○	96	○○○○	118	○○○○	140	○○○○
75	○○○○	97	○○○○	119	○○○○	141	○○○○
76	○○○○	98	○○○○	120	○○○○	142	○○○○
77	○○○○	99	○○○○	121	○○○○	143	○○○○
78	○○○○	100	○○○○	122	○○○○	144	○○○○
79	○○○○	101	○○○○	123	○○○○	145	○○○○
80	○○○○	102	○○○○	124	○○○○	146	○○○○
81	○○○○	103	○○○○	125	○○○○	147	○○○○
82	○○○○	104	○○○○	126	○○○○	148	○○○○
83	○○○○	105	○○○○	127	○○○○	149	○○○○
84	○○○○	106	○○○○	128	○○○○	150	○○○○
85	○○○○	107	○○○○	129	○○○○	151	○○○○
86	○○○○	108	○○○○	130	○○○○	152	○○○○
87	○○○○	109	○○○○	131	○○○○	153	○○○○
88	○○○○	110	○○○○	132	○○○○	154	○○○○
89	○○○○	111	○○○○	133	○○○○	155	○○○○
90	○○○○	112	○○○○	134	○○○○	156	○○○○

	1 2 3 4		1 2 3 4		1 2 3 4		1 2 3 4
157	○○○○	179	○○○○	201	○○○○	223	○○○○
158	○○○○	180	○○○○	202	○○○○	224	○○○○
159	○○○○	181	○○○○	203	○○○○	225	○○○○
160	○○○○	182	○○○○	204	○○○○	226	○○○○
161	○○○○	183	○○○○	205	○○○○	227	○○○○
162	○○○○	184	○○○○	206	○○○○	228	○○○○
163	○○○○	185	○○○○	207	○○○○	229	○○○○
164	○○○○	186	○○○○	208	○○○○	230	○○○○
165	○○○○	187	○○○○	209	○○○○	231	○○○○
166	○○○○	188	○○○○	210	○○○○	232	○○○○
167	○○○○	189	○○○○	211	○○○○	233	○○○○
168	○○○○	190	○○○○	212	○○○○	234	○○○○
169	○○○○	191	○○○○	213	○○○○	235	○○○○
170	○○○○	192	○○○○	214	○○○○	236	○○○○
171	○○○○	193	○○○○	215	○○○○	237	○○○○
172	○○○○	194	○○○○	216	○○○○	238	○○○○
173	○○○○	195	○○○○	217	○○○○	239	○○○○
174	○○○○	196	○○○○	218	○○○○	240	○○○○
175	○○○○	197	○○○○	219	○○○○	241	○○○○
176	○○○○	198	○○○○	220	○○○○	242	○○○○
177	○○○○	199	○○○○	221	○○○○	243	○○○○
178	○○○○	200	○○○○	222	○○○○	244	○○○○

surgical nursing answer sheet 3

	1 2 3 4		1 2 3 4		1 2 3 4		1 2 3 4
245	○○○○	267	○○○○	289	○○○○	311	○○○○
246	○○○○	268	○○○○	290	○○○○	312	○○○○
247	○○○○	269	○○○○	291	○○○○	313	○○○○
248	○○○○	270	○○○○	292	○○○○	314	○○○○
249	○○○○	271	○○○○	293	○○○○	315	○○○○
250	○○○○	272	○○○○	294	○○○○	316	○○○○
251	○○○○	273	○○○○	295	○○○○	317	○○○○
252	○○○○	274	○○○○	296	○○○○	318	○○○○
253	○○○○	275	○○○○	297	○○○○	319	○○○○
254	○○○○	276	○○○○	298	○○○○	320	○○○○
255	○○○○	277	○○○○	299	○○○○	321	○○○○
256	○○○○	278	○○○○	300	○○○○	322	○○○○
257	○○○○	279	○○○○	301	○○○○	323	○○○○
258	○○○○	280	○○○○	302	○○○○	324	○○○○
259	○○○○	281	○○○○	303	○○○○	325	○○○○
260	○○○○	282	○○○○	304	○○○○	326	○○○○
261	○○○○	283	○○○○	305	○○○○	327	○○○○
262	○○○○	284	○○○○	306	○○○○	328	○○○○
263	○○○○	285	○○○○	307	○○○○	329	○○○○
264	○○○○	286	○○○○	308	○○○○	330	○○○○
265	○○○○	287	○○○○	309	○○○○	331	○○○○
266	○○○○	288	○○○○	310	○○○○	332	○○○○

	1 2 3 4		1 2 3 4		1 2 3 4		1 2 3 4
333	○○○○	355	○○○○	377	○○○○	399	○○○○
334	○○○○	356	○○○○	378	○○○○	400	○○○○
335	○○○○	357	○○○○	379	○○○○	401	○○○○
336	○○○○	358	○○○○	480	○○○○	402	○○○○
337	○○○○	359	○○○○	381	○○○○	403	○○○○
338	○○○○	360	○○○○	382	○○○○	404	○○○○
339	○○○○	361	○○○○	383	○○○○	405	○○○○
340	○○○○	362	○○○○	384	○○○○	406	○○○○
341	○○○○	363	○○○○	385	○○○○	407	○○○○
342	○○○○	364	○○○○	386	○○○○	408	○○○○
343	○○○○	365	○○○○	387	○○○○	409	○○○○
344	○○○○	366	○○○○	388	○○○○	410	○○○○
345	○○○○	367	○○○○	389	○○○○	411	○○○○
346	○○○○	368	○○○○	390	○○○○	412	○○○○
347	○○○○	369	○○○○	391	○○○○	413	○○○○
348	○○○○	370	○○○○	392	○○○○	414	○○○○
349	○○○○	371	○○○○	393	○○○○	415	○○○○
350	○○○○	372	○○○○	394	○○○○	416	○○○○
351	○○○○	373	○○○○	395	○○○○	417	○○○○
352	○○○○	374	○○○○	396	○○○○	418	○○○○
353	○○○○	375	○○○○	397	○○○○	419	○○○○
354	○○○○	376	○○○○	398	○○○○	420	○○○○

	1 2 3 4		1 2 3 4		1 2 3 4		1 2 3 4
421	○○○○	443	○○○○	465	○○○○	487	○○○○
422	○○○○	444	○○○○	466	○○○○	488	○○○○
423	○○○○	445	○○○○	467	○○○○	489	○○○○
424	○○○○	446	○○○○	468	○○○○	490	○○○○
425	○○○○	447	○○○○	469	○○○○	491	○○○○
426	○○○○	448	○○○○	470	○○○○	492	○○○○
427	○○○○	449	○○○○	471	○○○○	493	○○○○
428	○○○○	450	○○○○	472	○○○○	494	○○○○
429	○○○○	451	○○○○	473	○○○○	495	○○○○
430	○○○○	452	○○○○	474	○○○○	496	○○○○
431	○○○○	453	○○○○	475	○○○○	497	○○○○
432	○○○○	454	○○○○	476	○○○○	498	○○○○
433	○○○○	455	○○○○	477	○○○○	499	○○○○
434	○○○○	456	○○○○	478	○○○○	500	○○○○
435	○○○○	457	○○○○	479	○○○○	501	○○○○
436	○○○○	458	○○○○	480	○○○○	502	○○○○
437	○○○○	459	○○○○	481	○○○○	503	○○○○
438	○○○○	460	○○○○	482	○○○○	504	○○○○
439	○○○○	461	○○○○	483	○○○○	505	○○○○
440	○○○○	462	○○○○	484	○○○○	506	○○○○
441	○○○○	463	○○○○	485	○○○○	507	○○○○
442	○○○○	464	○○○○	486	○○○○	508	○○○○

	1 2 3 4		1 2 3 4		1 2 3 4		1 2 3 4
509	○○○○	531	○○○○	553	○○○○	575	○○○○
510	○○○○	532	○○○○	554	○○○○	576	○○○○
511	○○○○	533	○○○○	555	○○○○	577	○○○○
512	○○○○	534	○○○○	556	○○○○	578	○○○○
513	○○○○	535	○○○○	557	○○○○	579	○○○○
514	○○○○	536	○○○○	558	○○○○	580	○○○○
515	○○○○	537	○○○○	559	○○○○	581	○○○○
516	○○○○	538	○○○○	560	○○○○	582	○○○○
517	○○○○	539	○○○○	561	○○○○	583	○○○○
518	○○○○	540	○○○○	562	○○○○	584	○○○○
519	○○○○	541	○○○○	563	○○○○	585	○○○○
520	○○○○	542	○○○○	564	○○○○	586	○○○○
521	○○○○	543	○○○○	565	○○○○	587	○○○○
522	○○○○	544	○○○○	566	○○○○	588	○○○○
523	○○○○	545	○○○○	567	○○○○	589	○○○○
524	○○○○	546	○○○○	568	○○○○	590	○○○○
525	○○○○	547	○○○○	569	○○○○	591	○○○○
526	○○○○	548	○○○○	570	○○○○	592	○○○○
527	○○○○	549	○○○○	571	○○○○	593	○○○○
528	○○○○	550	○○○○	572	○○○○	594	○○○○
529	○○○○	551	○○○○	573	○○○○	595	○○○○
530	○○○○	552	○○○○	574	○○○○	596	○○○○

	1 2 3 4		1 2 3 4		1 2 3 4		1 2 3 4
597	○○○○	600	○○○○	603	○○○○	606	○○○○
598	○○○○	601	○○○○	604	○○○○	607	○○○○
599	○○○○	602	○○○○	605	○○○○	608	○○○○

answer sheet for surgical nursing

Read each question in the examination carefully and select which one of the options is the *best* or *correct* answer. If the answer you would prefer is not given, select the one which seems *most appropriate*.

Locate on the answer sheet the number of the item you are answering. With a pencil, blacken the circle corresponding to the answer you have selected. Be sure you are recording your answer in the proper space.

	1 2 3 4		1 2 3 4		1 2 3 4		1 2 3 4
1	○○○○	18	○○○○	35	○○○○	52	○○○○
2	○○○○	19	○○○○	36	○○○○	53	○○○○
3	○○○○	20	○○○○	37	○○○○	54	○○○○
4	○○○○	21	○○○○	38	○○○○	55	○○○○
5	○○○○	22	○○○○	39	○○○○	56	○○○○
6	○○○○	23	○○○○	40	○○○○	57	○○○○
7	○○○○	24	○○○○	41	○○○○	58	○○○○
8	○○○○	25	○○○○	42	○○○○	59	○○○○
9	○○○○	26	○○○○	43	○○○○	60	○○○○
10	○○○○	27	○○○○	44	○○○○	61	○○○○
11	○○○○	28	○○○○	45	○○○○	62	○○○○
12	○○○○	29	○○○○	46	○○○○	63	○○○○
13	○○○○	30	○○○○	47	○○○○	64	○○○○
14	○○○○	31	○○○○	48	○○○○	65	○○○○
15	○○○○	32	○○○○	49	○○○○	66	○○○○
16	○○○○	33	○○○○	50	○○○○	67	○○○○
17	○○○○	34	○○○○	51	○○○○	68	○○○○

	1 2 3 4		1 2 3 4		1 2 3 4		1 2 3 4
69	○○○○	91	○○○○	113	○○○○	135	○○○○
70	○○○○	92	○○○○	114	○○○○	136	○○○○
71	○○○○	93	○○○○	115	○○○○	137	○○○○
72	○○○○	94	○○○○	116	○○○○	138	○○○○
73	○○○○	95	○○○○	117	○○○○	139	○○○○
74	○○○○	96	○○○○	118	○○○○	140	○○○○
75	○○○○	97	○○○○	119	○○○○	141	○○○○
76	○○○○	98	○○○○	120	○○○○	142	○○○○
77	○○○○	99	○○○○	121	○○○○	143	○○○○
78	○○○○	100	○○○○	122	○○○○	144	○○○○
79	○○○○	101	○○○○	123	○○○○	145	○○○○
80	○○○○	102	○○○○	124	○○○○	146	○○○○
81	○○○○	103	○○○○	125	○○○○	147	○○○○
82	○○○○	104	○○○○	126	○○○○	148	○○○○
83	○○○○	105	○○○○	127	○○○○	149	○○○○
84	○○○○	106	○○○○	128	○○○○	150	○○○○
85	○○○○	107	○○○○	129	○○○○	151	○○○○
86	○○○○	108	○○○○	130	○○○○	152	○○○○
87	○○○○	109	○○○○	131	○○○○	153	○○○○
88	○○○○	110	○○○○	132	○○○○	154	○○○○
89	○○○○	111	○○○○	133	○○○○	155	○○○○
90	○○○○	112	○○○○	134	○○○○	156	○○○○

	1 2 3 4		1 2 3 4		1 2 3 4		1 2 3 4
157	○○○○	179	○○○○	201	○○○○	223	○○○○
158	○○○○	180	○○○○	202	○○○○	224	○○○○
159	○○○○	181	○○○○	203	○○○○	225	○○○○
160	○○○○	182	○○○○	204	○○○○	226	○○○○
161	○○○○	183	○○○○	205	○○○○	227	○○○○
162	○○○○	184	○○○○	206	○○○○	228	○○○○
163	○○○○	185	○○○○	207	○○○○	229	○○○○
164	○○○○	186	○○○○	208	○○○○	230	○○○○
165	○○○○	187	○○○○	209	○○○○	231	○○○○
166	○○○○	188	○○○○	210	○○○○	232	○○○○
167	○○○○	189	○○○○	211	○○○○	233	○○○○
168	○○○○	190	○○○○	212	○○○○	234	○○○○
169	○○○○	191	○○○○	213	○○○○	235	○○○○
170	○○○○	192	○○○○	214	○○○○	236	○○○○
171	○○○○	193	○○○○	215	○○○○	237	○○○○
172	○○○○	194	○○○○	216	○○○○	238	○○○○
173	○○○○	195	○○○○	217	○○○○	239	○○○○
174	○○○○	196	○○○○	218	○○○○	240	○○○○
175	○○○○	197	○○○○	219	○○○○	241	○○○○
176	○○○○	198	○○○○	220	○○○○	242	○○○○
177	○○○○	199	○○○○	221	○○○○	243	○○○○
178	○○○○	200	○○○○	222	○○○○	244	○○○○

	1 2 3 4		1 2 3 4		1 2 3 4		1 2 3 4
245	○○○○	267	○○○○	289	○○○○	311	○○○○
246	○○○○	268	○○○○	290	○○○○	312	○○○○
247	○○○○	269	○○○○	291	○○○○	313	○○○○
248	○○○○	270	○○○○	292	○○○○	314	○○○○
249	○○○○	271	○○○○	293	○○○○	315	○○○○
250	○○○○	272	○○○○	294	○○○○	316	○○○○
251	○○○○	273	○○○○	295	○○○○	317	○○○○
252	○○○○	274	○○○○	296	○○○○	318	○○○○
253	○○○○	275	○○○○	297	○○○○	319	○○○○
254	○○○○	276	○○○○	298	○○○○	320	○○○○
255	○○○○	277	○○○○	299	○○○○	321	○○○○
256	○○○○	278	○○○○	300	○○○○	322	○○○○
257	○○○○	279	○○○○	301	○○○○	323	○○○○
258	○○○○	280	○○○○	302	○○○○	324	○○○○
259	○○○○	281	○○○○	303	○○○○	325	○○○○
260	○○○○	282	○○○○	304	○○○○	326	○○○○
261	○○○○	283	○○○○	305	○○○○	327	○○○○
262	○○○○	284	○○○○	306	○○○○	328	○○○○
263	○○○○	285	○○○○	307	○○○○	329	○○○○
264	○○○○	286	○○○○	308	○○○○	330	○○○○
265	○○○○	287	○○○○	309	○○○○	331	○○○○
266	○○○○	288	○○○○	310	○○○○	332	○○○○

4   surgical nursing answer sheet

	1 2 3 4		1 2 3 4		1 2 3 4		1 2 3 4
333	○○○○	355	○○○○	377	○○○○	399	○○○○
334	○○○○	356	○○○○	378	○○○○	400	○○○○
335	○○○○	357	○○○○	379	○○○○	401	○○○○
336	○○○○	358	○○○○	480	○○○○	402	○○○○
337	○○○○	359	○○○○	381	○○○○	403	○○○○
338	○○○○	360	○○○○	382	○○○○	404	○○○○
339	○○○○	361	○○○○	383	○○○○	405	○○○○
340	○○○○	362	○○○○	384	○○○○	406	○○○○
341	○○○○	363	○○○○	385	○○○○	407	○○○○
342	○○○○	364	○○○○	386	○○○○	408	○○○○
343	○○○○	365	○○○○	387	○○○○	409	○○○○
344	○○○○	366	○○○○	388	○○○○	410	○○○○
345	○○○○	367	○○○○	389	○○○○	411	○○○○
346	○○○○	368	○○○○	390	○○○○	412	○○○○
347	○○○○	369	○○○○	391	○○○○	413	○○○○
348	○○○○	370	○○○○	392	○○○○	414	○○○○
349	○○○○	371	○○○○	393	○○○○	415	○○○○
350	○○○○	372	○○○○	394	○○○○	416	○○○○
351	○○○○	373	○○○○	395	○○○○	417	○○○○
352	○○○○	374	○○○○	396	○○○○	418	○○○○
353	○○○○	375	○○○○	397	○○○○	419	○○○○
354	○○○○	376	○○○○	398	○○○○	420	○○○○

	1 2 3 4		1 2 3 4		1 2 3 4		1 2 3 4
421	○○○○	443	○○○○	465	○○○○	487	○○○○
422	○○○○	444	○○○○	466	○○○○	488	○○○○
423	○○○○	445	○○○○	467	○○○○	489	○○○○
424	○○○○	446	○○○○	468	○○○○	490	○○○○
425	○○○○	447	○○○○	469	○○○○	491	○○○○
426	○○○○	448	○○○○	470	○○○○	492	○○○○
427	○○○○	449	○○○○	471	○○○○	493	○○○○
428	○○○○	450	○○○○	472	○○○○	494	○○○○
429	○○○○	451	○○○○	473	○○○○	495	○○○○
430	○○○○	452	○○○○	474	○○○○	496	○○○○
431	○○○○	453	○○○○	475	○○○○	497	○○○○
432	○○○○	454	○○○○	476	○○○○	498	○○○○
433	○○○○	455	○○○○	477	○○○○	499	○○○○
434	○○○○	456	○○○○	478	○○○○	500	○○○○
435	○○○○	457	○○○○	479	○○○○	501	○○○○
436	○○○○	458	○○○○	480	○○○○	502	○○○○
437	○○○○	459	○○○○	481	○○○○	503	○○○○
438	○○○○	460	○○○○	482	○○○○	504	○○○○
439	○○○○	461	○○○○	483	○○○○	505	○○○○
440	○○○○	462	○○○○	484	○○○○	506	○○○○
441	○○○○	463	○○○○	485	○○○○	507	○○○○
442	○○○○	464	○○○○	486	○○○○	508	○○○○

	1 2 3 4		1 2 3 4		1 2 3 4		1 2 3 4
509	○○○○	531	○○○○	553	○○○○	575	○○○○
510	○○○○	532	○○○○	554	○○○○	576	○○○○
511	○○○○	533	○○○○	555	○○○○	577	○○○○
512	○○○○	534	○○○○	556	○○○○	578	○○○○
513	○○○○	535	○○○○	557	○○○○	579	○○○○
514	○○○○	536	○○○○	558	○○○○	580	○○○○
515	○○○○	537	○○○○	559	○○○○	581	○○○○
516	○○○○	538	○○○○	560	○○○○	582	○○○○
517	○○○○	539	○○○○	561	○○○○	583	○○○○
518	○○○○	540	○○○○	562	○○○○	584	○○○○
519	○○○○	541	○○○○	563	○○○○	585	○○○○
520	○○○○	542	○○○○	564	○○○○	586	○○○○
521	○○○○	543	○○○○	565	○○○○	587	○○○○
522	○○○○	544	○○○○	566	○○○○	588	○○○○
523	○○○○	545	○○○○	567	○○○○	589	○○○○
524	○○○○	546	○○○○	568	○○○○	590	○○○○
525	○○○○	547	○○○○	569	○○○○	591	○○○○
526	○○○○	548	○○○○	570	○○○○	592	○○○○
527	○○○○	549	○○○○	571	○○○○	593	○○○○
528	○○○○	550	○○○○	572	○○○○	594	○○○○
529	○○○○	551	○○○○	573	○○○○	595	○○○○
530	○○○○	552	○○○○	574	○○○○	596	○○○○

	1 2 3 4		1 2 3 4		1 2 3 4		1 2 3 4
597	○○○○	600	○○○○	603	○○○○	606	○○○○
	1 2 3 4		1 2 3 4		1 2 3 4		1 2 3 4
598	○○○○	601	○○○○	604	○○○○	607	○○○○
	1 2 3 4		1 2 3 4		1 2 3 4		1 2 3 4
599	○○○○	602	○○○○	605	○○○○	608	○○○○

surgical nursing examination

correct answers and rationales

BREAST HEALTH CARE

1. 2. High priority should be teaching women how to examine their breasts for tumors since most tumors are discovered by women during activities of daily living. Reasons given in options 1, 3, and 4 have not been shown to be common.

2. 3. It is generally recommended that the breasts be examined during the week after menstruation. It is during this period when the breasts are least likely to be tender or swollen since the secretion of estrogen which prepared the uterus for implantation, among other things, is lowest.

3. 4. A pillow or towel under the shoulder on the side being examined elevates the chest wall. This position allows more even distribution of breast tissue over the chest wall.

4. 2. The firm connective tissue is normal. It is a supportive structure and is no cause for alarm. It is not tumorous, muscular, or glandular tissue nor tissue that changes in size due to exercise.

5. 2. Unless there is tumor growth present, the breasts are normally approximately the same size. They may vary somewhat prior to menstruation due to irregularities produced by hormones and at that time, the patient may note that her bra fits more tightly than usual.

6. 1. The ovaries are removed to eliminate the body's source of estrogen which tends to stimulate the growth of tumors.

7. 2. Of the characteristics given, the one most typical of malignant cells is that they usually grow rapidly; benign tumors gen-

erally grow slowly. Benign tumors are almost always encapsulated while malignant tumors are not. Benign tumors do not recur as a rule while malignant tumors do. Benign tumors resemble tissues whence they arise while malignant tumors are less differentiated than normal cells from which they derive.

8. 2. Men do and can have breast cancers just as women, and the cancers tend to metastasize just as in women. However, malignant tumors occur less frequently in men's breasts than in women's. Benign tumors may also attack the male breast.

9. 2. Approximately 50 percent of the malignant tumors in the breast occur in the upper outer quadrant of the breast.

10. 1. Breast cancer occurs most frequently among women who have a family history of breast cancer, are in the higher socioeconomic levels, have had a late menopause, have not had children, and have not breast fed their children.

11. 3. The women of Japan have the lowest incidence of breast cancer. The reason has not been determined.

12. 4. Paget's disease is a disease of the nipple of the breast. It attacks the lactiferous ducts that converge at the nipple.

13. 3. A symptom commonly associated with chronic cystic mastitis is breast discomfort and pain that is of a "shooting" nature. Pain is uncommon when a malignancy is present except in late stages. Options 1, 2, and 4 are not associated with chronic cystic mastitis.

RUTH MAITT

14. 1. An important nursing responsibility is preoperative teaching and the most frequently recommended guide for teaching is to tell the patient as much as she wants to know and is able to understand. Delaying discussing those things about which the patient has apprehensions is likely to aggravate the situation and cause the patient to feel distrust.

15. 3. Atropine sulfate, a cholinergic blocking agent, is given preoperatively primarily to reduce secretions in the mouth and respiratory tract. The drug does not act in ways described in the other options.

16. 3. Highest priority when receiving a patient from the operating room is to assess for airway patency. After the nurse has noted that the airway is clear and the patient is breathing well, she should proceed with other procedures, such as those given in options 1, 2, and 4.

17. 4. Lymph nodes are ordinarily removed from the axillary area when a radical mastectomy is done. In order to facilitate

drainage from the arm on the affected side, the arm should be elevated as described in option 4. Placing the arm in ways described in options 1, 2, and 3 will not promote drainage. Also, placing the arm across the chest may restrict breathing.

18. 3. A drainage tube is placed in the wound following a radical mastectomy to help remove accumulations of serum and blood in the area. The tube does not function to accomplish goals described in the incorrect options.

19. 2. The comment described in option 2 gives the patient an opportunity to express her fears and will provide the nurse with information so that she can offer the patient the type of support she needs. Options 1 and 4 are not going to help; telling her not to worry is more likely to cause her to worry more. At this point, speaking to a woman who has had breast surgery is not recommended but may be used later in her convalescing period. She needs the nurse's professional support when the dressings are first removed.

20. 4. Exercise and activity to promote the use of the arm on the affected side is recommended in order to help prevent disuse of the arm and contractures. The exercises illustrated in options 1, 2, and 3 do most to exercise the arm. The exercise illustrated in option 4 does not promote exercise for the affected arm.

21. 1. A comment that repeats what a patient has said or what a patient appears to be feeling tends to encourage the patient to talk and describe more. The comment in option 2 is likely to make the patient feel inferior and put down. She probably has the problem because she is unable to discuss it with the children. Option 3 is not offering the patient support; it ignores the problem at hand. Option 4 is belittling and is likely to intimidate the patient who will then say even less.

22. 1. A will is invalid if it can be shown that the person whose will it is has been coerced into signing it. There is nothing described in options 2, 3, and 4 that would invalidate a will.

23. 4. Option 4 offers the best suggestion the nurse could offer the patient's husband. Exercising will lose its effectiveness if another person helps move the arm. Options 2 and 3 avoid the issue and will not offer support which the husband is seeking to give his wife.

24. 3. Lotions and ointments and anything that may cause irritation to the skin (exposure to sunlight, talcum powder, adhesive, and the like) should be avoided. The area may safely be washed with water if done gently and with care.

25. 3. Of the descriptions given, the most often seen reaction of the

skin to radiation therapy is redness of the surface tissues. Dryness, desquamation, tanning, and dilatation of the capillaries are also commonly observed.

26. 3. Every effort should be made to avoid cuts, bruises, burns, and the like on the affected arm since normal circulation has been impaired. Hence, of the activities given here, working in a rose garden where she is likely to receive skin pricks, is contraindicated. The other activities are satisfactory.

27. 4. The great advantage of using a silicone prosthesis is that it is fitted to the individual. The other options do not describe silicone prostheses accurately.

28. 1. The Reach for Recovery program of the American Cancer Society is a rehabilitation program for women who have had breast surgery. It is designed to meet their physical, psychological, and cosmetic needs but does not provide funds or dressings.

CAROL SHAW

29. 2. A douche is likely to wash away secretions which are necessary for a satisfactory Pap test. Hence, it is recommended that the patient not douche for at least 24 hours prior to the test.

30. 1. Option 1 gives the patient an opening to discuss fears more and gives the nurse opportunity to better understand the patient. Options 2 and 4 make assumptions and, in the case of option 4, gives a solution without knowing the problem. Option 3 offers no support; it is a cliche type of comment.

31. 1. The Pap test is done for one purpose: to help determine cancer of the cervix.

32. 2. Although other positions may be used, the preferred position is the lithotomy position. The position offers the best visualization for examination with a speculum and is most convenient for the examiner.

33. 2. The best guide when a patient is fearful is to allow the patient opportunities to express fears. Other courses of action, such as those described in options 1, 3, and 4, will be of little avail. See also items 19 and 21.

34. 2. In many hospitals, the dietitian can make arrangements to provide Kosher food as requested; option 2 offers the nurse her best course of action in this situation. Option 1 is unlikely to help since the patient has refused other than Kosher food. Option 3 is contrary to policy. Option 4 is a threat and the patient is unlikely to be helped.

35. 2. The preparation illustrated in option 2 is best. The area that

should be shaved prior to abdominal surgery should extend from the nipples to the pubic area.

36. 1. The surgeon's signature is not a legal requirement on a consent form prior to performing a surgical procedure. Information given in option 2, 3, and 4 should appear on the operative consent form.

37. 1. Postoperatively when the patient coughs, she is most likely to experience discomfort in the incisional area. This can best be minimized by splinting the operative area with either a pillow or with her hands. The techniques described in options 2, 3, and 4 will not act to splint the incisional area.

38. 2. Hyperventilation occurs when the patient breathes too rapidly and/or deeply. He will be exhaling larger-than-normal amounts of carbon dioxide. A characteristic symptom of hyperventilation is dizziness. The signs/symptoms given in the other options are not associated with hyperventilation.

39. 1. Prednisone is a derivative of cortisone. The prolonged actions of steroids cause decreased functioning of the anterior pituitary gland which, in turn, effects the function of the adrenal glands. If the drug is discontinued abruptly, the patient may experience an adrenal crisis because the depressed pituitary does not regain complete control quickly. The conditions given in options 2, 3, and 4 are not associated with cortisone withdrawal.

40. 4. The patient needs the drug prescribed for a good night's sleep prior to surgery. Hence, the nurse should consult the physician for a proper dosage. It is not within the nurse's prerogative to change the dosage or omit giving the drug.

41. 3. The correct amount to administer is determined by using ratios as follows:
0.4 mg. : 1 ml. :: 0.3 mg. : X ml.
0.4 X = 0.3
X = ¾ or 0.75 ml. (scopolamine hydrobromide)
50 mg. : 1 ml. :: 100 mg. : X ml.
50 X = 100
X = 2 ml. (meperidine hydrochloride)
2 ml. + 0.75 ml. = 2.75 ml.

42. 1. Using a cool bedpan usually makes voiding more difficult. It is better to offer the patient a warm bedpan and use techniques described in options 2, 3, and 4 to encourage voiding.

43. 3. The area should be cleansed by moving cotton balls from an area where fewer organisms can be expected (above the meatus) toward an area where more organisms normally harbor (about the anus). This technique avoids carrying or-

ganisms from the anus toward the meatus. Moving across the meatus is not recommended since cotton balls will not then be moving along the area between the labia.

44. 2. The letter B indicates the meatus. The letter A indicates the clitoris. The letter C indicates the opening of the vagina. The letter D indicates the anus.

45. 4. When the urge to void is present but the patient only voids small amounts of urine, the nurse should suspect that the patient has retention with overflow. None of the conditions described in options 1, 2, and 3 is associated with symptoms presented in the stem.

46. 3. Moving about in bed, coughing, deep breathing, and turning are indicated for this postoperative patient. The nurse's best response to the patient's request is described in option 3. Offering to move the patient will defeat the purpose of moving in bed. A medication may releave discomfort but does not promote moving in bed. Being up an hour ago is a poor excuse to suggest resting rather than moving in bed.

47. 3. An elevated temperature on the second postoperative day is most suggestive of a respiratory tract infection. Signs of infection, if present in the wound or urinary tract, are likely to occur later in the postoperative period. So also will signs of phlebitis which is an inflammatory process in a vein.

48. 4. Serosanguineous drainage on the perineal pad is typical following a hysterectomy. The patient should be observed for signs of hemorrhage from the vagina which will produce copius bright bloody drainage. Clear serous or mucoid drainage without any bleeding is not common.

49. 3. When a dressing sticks to the wound, it is best to moisten it with sterile normal saline and then remove it carefully. Techniques described in options 1, 2, and 4 are likely to result in irritation to the skin and wound.

50. 3. Capillarity will cause the drainage to be lifted up and away from the wound when dressings are fluffed and loosely placed on the wound. Incorporating air will not help keep the dressings dry. Fluffed dressings *may* be more comfortable but that is not the primary reason for fluffing them. If drainage leaves the wound by gravity, it is likely to flow down and around the dressing onto skin which is irritating as well as uncomfortable for the patient.

51. 1. Usually, the discomforts associated with gas pains are likely to be helped when the patient ambulates. The gas will be more easily expelled with the exercise. Techniques described in

options 2, 3, and 4 are not recommended and may even aggravate the discomfort.

52. 2. Massaging the legs postoperatively is contraindicated. It may dislodge small clots of blood and cause even more serious problems. Measures described in options 1, 3, and 4 have been found beneficial to help reduce the incidence of postoperative thrombophlebitis.

53. 4. Wound opening is called dehiscence. If evisceration occurs, the nurse should cover the exposed tissues with sterile dressings moistened with sterile normal saline. The measures described in options 1, 2, and 3 are contraindicated.

54. 3. Wound dehiscence may occur at any time but it occurs most commonly approximately 6 to 8 days postoperatively.

55. 2. The primary hormone of the ovaries is estrogen and, hence, the physician will prescribe estrogen for replacement therapy for this patient.

56. 4. Option 4 describes the most accurate statement in relation to sexual relations following removal of the uterus, fallopian tubes, and ovaries. Usual sexual responses will not necessarily be reduced, sexual intercourse need not be avoided, and sexual counseling usually is unnecessary.

STEVEN JOHNSON

57. 2. For best assessment of an inguinal hernia, it is recommended that the patient be either standing or recumbent. The sitting or side-lying positions do not help the examiner to palpate for the inguinal ring.

58. 3. It is best to advise the patient to use his hearing aid just as he does at home so there will be no increased sensory loss. There is no need to remove it and he will most likely be uncomfortable without it.

59. 1. The nurse should take time to listen as the patient is given the opportunity to express his fears about surgery. Cliche responses, as described in options 2 and 4, are of little help and option 3 avoids responsibility which nurses are expected to assume. The nurse may wish to discuss the situation with the physician, but she should first further assess the patient's fears.

60. 3. The most common preoperative order for cleansing the bowels is to administer an enema. Colonic irrigations may be ordered when surgery on the intestines has been done and peristalsis is to be stimulated. Laxatives may take more hours

to work and suppositories are usually limited to rectal and lower intestinal cleansing only.

61. 3. The nurse can expect a smaller than average dosage for an elderly patient because the elderly person tends to have an increased sensitivity to most drugs. Statements made in options 1, 2, and 4 are inaccurate.

62. 2. Preoperative skin preparation is done primary to reduce the number of organisms in the operative area. The skin cannot be rendered free of organisms. Skin preparation does not improve the field of vision for the physician. The skin's defenses are not necessarily improved but when fewer organisms are present, there is less work to be done by the body to overcome their effects.

63. 1. Atropine sulfate is a cholinergic blocking substance and decreases secretions from the salivary glands. Hence, the patient should be told that he is likely to experience thirst after receiving the drug. Atropine sulfate does not influence hunger, sleepiness, or incontinence.

64. 2. Once the patient has received his preoperative medication, it is best to avoid disturbing him so that he has maximum benefit from the medication. An operative permit should be signed before a patient is medicated so that his mental lucidity is at maximum. The nurse can care for dentures after the patient has received his medication.

65. 4. The hospital's preoperative checklist is designed for health personnel so that they can be sure all preoperative preparation has been carried out as indicated and ordered. The signature of the patient is not necessary on this form. Typical items that appear on most checklists are described in options 1, 2, and 3.

66. 2. Delays of the type described in the stem tend to upset and frighten patients. Hence, it is best to stay with the patient until he can be taken to the operating room. Leaving him alone is frightening for most patients. Taking him back to his room and being with family are not restful and would be contraindicated.

67. 1. For the convenience of the anesthesiologist and in order to open the spaces between the vertebrae to the greatest extent, the patient should be on his side with his legs well flexed. The other positions described here will stand in the way of accomplishing a convenient and safe procedure.

68. 3. For the hard of hearing patient, it would be best to stand so that the patient can observe the nurse's face and the nurse should speak clearly. Usually patients can interpret expressions relatively easily and can understand with lip reading. Speaking

loudly does not help the deaf person to hear. Options 1 and 4 are generally not recommended.

69. 4. If spinal anesthesia rises too high, the patient is likely to suffer from respiratory distress since the muscles used for breathing become anesthetized. Other measures may be needed in addition to administering artificial respirations, but measures described in options 1, 2, and 3 are not indicated.

70. 1. The body's first physiological reaction when shock from fluid loss occurs is vasoconstriction. The body is using efforts to increase vascular volume and vasoconstriction will bring blood from other tissues to the vascular system. Options 2, 3, and 4 are inaccurate statements in relation to shock.

71. 2. Postoperative shock is most commonly caused by excessive bleeding. Options 1, 3, and 4 do not describe typical post-operative conditions that lead to shock.

72. 2. Since the patient's legs will be anesthetized, when he starts feeling sensations in his toes, it can be assumed that the pa-tient is recovering from spinal anesthesia. The anesthesia should not alter color of the skin. Since the patient receiving spinal anesthesia is conscious, he will not ordinarily have an airway nor will he be disoriented.

73. 2. Since this patient had a hernia repair, the patient should be catheterized on schedule to help reduce pressure on the operative area. Waiting may carry risk, even though the pa-tient's determination might help him to void.

74. 4. Experience has shown that one method that often helps pa-tients to stop hiccoughing is to apply pressure on his closed eyelids. The reason why this technique works is not clearly understood. Another method that is often successful is to have the patient rebreathe into a paper bag. Techniques described in options 1, 2, and 3 have not been found to be helpful.

75. 2. This patient should be encouraged to carry out all of the activities of daily living given here. But in order to prevent shoulders from becoming stiff ("frozen"), he should most cer-tainly be encouraged to comb his hair.

76. 3. Of the measures described here, the best one is to elevate the scrotum and place ice bags to the area intermittently. Meas-ures described in options 1, 2, and 4 are unlikely to help.

77. 2. A scrotal support is worn to help decrease local discomfort. It is of no value for conditions given in options 1, 3, and 4.

78. 3. Epididymitis is best prevented by the administration of an antibiotic.

79. 1. Postoperative atelectasis is best prevented by having the pa-

tient cough every hour or two. This is particularly important for a man of this patient's age—70 years. Elasticized stockings are used postoperatively for the prevention of thrombophlebitis. Fluids do help to liquify secretions so coughing is productive, but 1200 ml. daily is hardly of sufficient quantity to accomplish this.

80. 4. The drainage on the dressing suggests that possibly a wound infections is present. Normally, there would be no drainage. Signs/symptoms described in the first three options could normally be expected.

81. 2. It would be best for this patient to share a room with a patient with gastric ulcers who is to have medical evaluation. Since there is a possibility that a wound infection may be present, it would be contraindicated to place him with patients about to have surgery. Nor would it be recommended that he be roomed with a patient with a known infection (option 1).

82. 3. A drain is used in the patient's infected wound in order to allow adequate drainage of blood and lymph. The drain will not accomplish goals described in options 1, 2, and 4.

83. 2. The number of drops the patient should receive each minute is determined as follows:

$$\frac{50 \text{ ml.}}{30} = 1.67 \text{ ml. to be given each minute}$$

1.67×10 (drop factor) = 16 to 17 drops per minute

84. 3. The way in which the patient is likely to interpret touch in this interaction will be based on the cultural background of the patient. Touch can be interpreted as an aggressive act but this does not occur often when gentle touch is used in the nurse/patient relationship. Touch has been shown to improve communications when used effectively and it is considered to be an important part of the nurse/patient relationship.

85. 3. Infections tend to occur more frequently among elderly patients postoperatively because their cardiovascular system does not function as effectively as in younger persons. Factors given in options 1, 2, and 4 do not offer accurate reasons why wound infections tend to occur more frequently in the elderly.

86. 1. Fluid enters the vein by gravity. Hence, when the bed is lowered while the infusion bottle remains constant, the intravenous fluid will enter the vein more rapidly.

87. 1. Adipose tissue has a relatively poor blood supply. It is higher in water content than other types of tissue but this is not the basic reason for increased incidence of infection in fatty tissues.

88. 4. The body's response is to provide more white blood cells to fight infection. Infection does not effect blood findings given in options 1, 2, and 3.
89. 3. A "clean catch" urine specimen is obtained in a sterile container. The other options describe recommended procedure.
90. 2. It is generally recommended that a specimen of urine obtained at approximately midstream be used since it best reflects the consistency of the urine in the bladder. The first portion may contain organisms washed from about the meatus. It is difficult to know when the last portion of urine is leaving the bladder.
91. 3. The average normal range for the specific gravity of urine is generally given as between 1.010 and 1.030.
92. 4. Normal urine does not contain protein and hence, in this situation, should be judged as being abnormal. The average normal pH of urine is generally considered to be between 4.8 and 7.5. An occasional cast and two white blood cells would not be judged as being abnormal.
93. 3. When kidney function is not adequate, the wastes of protein metabolism accumulate in the blood. Studying the level of the blood urea nitrogen (BUN) helps assess the quality of kidney function. The examinations described in options 1, 2, and 4 will not help assess kidney function.
94. 4. Studies have shown that the most frequent cause of postoperative bladder infections is bladder catheterization. As a result of these findings, nurses are urged to use measures to assist patients to void in order to minimize the use of catheterization. Encouraging ambulation and encouraging an adequate fluid intake are two recommended measures to assist patients to void.
95. 3. Coffee and cola drinks, both of which ordinarily contain caffeine, will not help prevent constipation. However, measures described in options 1, 2, and 4 are recommended for helping to maintain normal elimination.
96. 4. Peanut butter is a rich source of protein. Foods given in options 1, 2, and 3 are not high in protein content.
97. 4. In general, the elderly patient does not exercise and have as much activity as young persons and, hence, energy requirements decrease. Therefore, caloric needs for the elderly are less than for younger persons. Regardless of age, persons need protein, calcium, and vitamins in their diets for health and well-being.
98. 1. A visiting nurse service provides skilled nursing care for patients at home. An extended care facility is one that provides services after hospitalization but before the patient is ready for

discharge home. The two organizations listed in options 3 and 4 do not provide home care.

MADELEINE CRAWFORD

99. 4. A KUB ordinarily requires no preparation since it is simply an x-ray examination done usually while the patient lies on his back. A KUB does not involve the use of radiopaque substances.

100. 2. Residual urine in the calyces of kidneys predisposes to nephritis and, hence, an obstruction that causes urine to accumulate in the kidneys requires prompt treatment. The factors mentioned in options 1 and 4 do not play a role in the development of nephritis when an obstruction in this urinary tract is present. Impaired circulation in this case is a secondary factor.

101. 2. Examining the urine for acetone level will not assist to find renal calculi. Measures described in options 1, 3, and 4 are recommended procedures.

102. 2. The tourniquet should be removed as soon as the needle is in the vein. Until then, the tourniquet keeps the vein distended so that it is more visible and easier to enter. Once the needle is in the vein, the tourniquet should be removed before applying tape so that fluid will start to enter the vein promptly.

103. 2. It would be best to avoid using an area on the inner aspect of the elbow. Once a vein higher up on the arm has been damaged, veins lower in the arm cannot be used. Therefore, recommended procedure is to use veins low on the arm or on the hand so that, should the vein be damaged, veins higher on the arm are still available for use.

104. 3. When circulatory overload occurs, the lungs become congested with fluid. This sign is best assessed with a stethoscope. The patient has maximum space for respiratory efforts when in a semisitting position. The positions given in the other options will not help relieve respiratory distress.

105. 2. The drug of choice is aluminum hydroxide. This agent reacts with hydrochloric acid to form aluminum chloride as well as other compounds, one other being aluminum phosphate which is then eliminated through the intestines. For this reason, it is often used in the management of patients who tend to form phosphate-type kidney stones.

106. 4. The smooth muscles in the urinary tract contract in order to attempt to move the stone along, with excruciating pain resulting. A patient with renal colic usually requires a narcotic drug for relief of the severe pain.

107. 3. The pain of renal colic has been observed to be referred most often to the bladder area and the genitalia.

108. 3. The nephrons are located in the medulla and cortex of the kidneys. The hilus is a depression where the vessels enter the kidney. The pelvis is a saclike structure that receives urine from all parts of the kidney from the calyces which are cup-shaped extensions of the sac. The capsule is a fibrous tissue which forms the covering of the kidney.

109. 2. The adrenal gland is a mushroom-shaped structure which sits on top of the kidney.

110. 1. When adrenal failure occurs, because the body will be in short supply of epinephrine, the patient's blood pressure is likely to fall.

111. 4. In order to use techniques that present the least likelihood of causing an infection in the urinary tract, it is recommended that a urine specimen be obtained as described in option 4. This technique makes it unnecessary to open the drainage system to the air, as techniques described in the first three options do. Also, a specimen taken from the tubing better reflects present urinary constituents. Other methods permit mixing with sediment.

112. 2. It is recommended that tape to hold the drainage tube in place be securely fastened to the patient's thigh. Taping it to the gown or to bed linen will likely cause tension on the tube when the patient moves about in bed. Taping it to the lower abdomen does not secure the tube as well to prevent tension.

113. 2. A patient with paralytic ileus is ordinarily ordered to have nothing by mouth since contents leaving the stomach cannot move along the intestinal tract. Orders described in options 1, 3, and 4 are typical for a patient with paralytic ileus.

114. 1. Evidence that peristalsis is occurring can be noted when the patient passes flatus. Bowel sounds may be heard by auscultation. Peristalsis is difficult to palpate and hence, a poor method to assess bowel activity. Thirst is related to dehydration, not to peristalsis.

115. 3. When a patient is lying in bed, drainage from a nephrectomy dressing following the force of gravity can most often be noted by examining the bottom bed linen. The top dressing may appear dry while blood seeps down and onto the bed linens. The bladder drainage will not necessarily contain blood when the patient hemorrhages from the wound.

116. 1. The greatest danger when a patient has thrombophlebitis is that a clot may break loose and travel to a vital organ, as the lungs, heart or brain. The results then can be grave. Cere-

brovascular accident is not related to emboli formation from thrombophlebitis. The conditions given in options 2 and 4 are of less significance than pulmonary emboli.

117. 4. Heparin sodium is the agent of choice of those given here since it delays the blood clotting time. Vitamin K hastens blood clotting. Vitamin B$_{12}$ and folic acid do not influence blood clotting.

118. 1. Warfarin sodium is an anticoagulant, as is heparin sodium. Warfarin sodium acts more slowly than heparin and hence, is generally prescribed for continued therapy while heparin is used for immediate and emergency-type therapy.

119. 2. For routine analysis of urine specimens, it is recommended that approximately 70 to 100 ml. of urine be collected.

120. 2. Low milk intake is not associated with the development of urinary calculi. Conditions given in options 1, 3, and 4 have been found to predispose to calculi. Persons living in the so-called stone belts of the United States tend to have a higher incidence of stones; these areas include the southwest, the southeast, and the Great Lakes basins.

121. 1. The accumulation of uric acid in the blood, which is characteristic of patients with gout, predisposes to the formation of kidney stones. The conditions given in options 2, 3, and 4 have not been observed to predispose to kidney stones.

122. 2. Normal urine is acid but upon standing, becomes alkaline. The color will not change unless it becomes darker as a result of water evaporation in which case the specific gravity will increase. Several hours will not change odor appreciably.

123. 4. Polycystic disease is hereditary. The conditions given in options 1, 2, and 3 are not considered hereditary in nature.

ELIZABETH WALKER

124. 4. It has been observed that serious physical illnesses have originated from psychological problems. While emotional support is important, it is ordinarily not sufficient to "treat" most psychosomatic illnesses. Options 1 and 3 are inaccurate statements.

125. 1. Studying ureterovesical valve reflux is done to determine the amount of urine that enters the ureters from the bladder. Ureteral catheterization is necessary to determine how much urine leaves each kidney. Residual urine is urine remaining in the bladder after voiding and can be determined by catheterization after voiding. Urine escaping involuntarily from the opening of the urethra is called incontinence.

126. 2. Radiopaque dye is used when a cystogram is done. In order to

avoid diluting the dye which would make visualizations more difficult, the patient's fluid intake should be restricted prior to the examination.

127. 2. Abdominal discomfort after a cystogram is best relieved by having the patient take a sitz bath. Measures described in the other three options are not indicated.

128. 2. The primary reason for taking an x-ray before needle biopsy of the kidney is to determine the exact location of the kidney. This knowledge will assist the physician in the placement of the needle.

129. 1. Occasionally, there is bleeding at the site of needle entry in the kidney. Hence, the patient should be observed for hemorrhaging. The conditions given in the other three options are not associated with needle biopsy of the kidney.

130. 3. The nurse assisting during a surgical procedure should anticipate that the physician will use clamps to help control bleeding during the procedure. Other measures may also be used but clamps are of primary importance.

131. 4. The urine causes some local irritation on the intestine and hence, the patient with an ileal conduit can be expected to excrete urine that contains mucus. Pus, feces, or blood in the urine would be abnormal signs.

132. 3. Following surgery for urinary diversion, it will be important to prevent abdominal distention. Hence, it is common for the patient to be ordered to have continuous gastric suction postoperatively. Suction is not used for this patient for any of the reasons described in options 1, 2, and 4.

131. 1. The elderly patient often becomes disoriented when he is removed from a familiar environment. It is recommended that the patient be helped to understand where she is. Option 2 is not likely to help orient the patient. Options 3 and 4 are likely to increase a sense of isolation and aloneness and will not help orient the patient.

134. 4. If the collecting device becomes too full, it is likely to fall from the skin. Since there is a free exit from the ileal conduit, conditions given in options 1, 2, and 3 are not likely to occur should the collecting device fill. Rather, the device will overflow.

135. 1. In order to prevent leakage, it is best to insert a small gauze wick into the stoma which will absorb the urine. Options 2, 3, and 4 are contraindicated.

136. 3. For cleansing purposes, it has been found that it is best to use water and detergent or soap.

137. 3. It has been found that a distilled vinegar solution acts as a

good deodorizing agent after the collecting device has been cleansed well with soap and water. Salt solution does not deodorize. Ammonia and bleaching agents may damage the device and they do not deodorize.

138. 4. Cranberry juice is noted to help increase urine acidity.

139. 3. The patient's skin can be protected with karaya powder which is least irritating and most protective of skin. Ointments are contraindicated. Baking powder and cornstarch have been used by some patients but they have not been found to be as effective as karaya powder.

140. 4. The thigh is recommended when the patient complains of discomfort when the collecting device is worn on the abdomen. It is not oridinarily recommended for other reasons.

GLORIA DUNN

141. 1. The patient's pain is most probably caused by spasms of smooth muscles in the biliary tract. Nitroglycerine acts to relax smooth muscles. It does not act in ways described in options 2, 3, and 4.

142. 1. The purpose of using a tourniquet before introducing needle for intravenous therapy is to distend the vein. See also item 102.

143. 1. When bile is not reaching the intestines, the feces will not contain bile pigments. Hence, the characteristic color of the stool is gray or putty color. A black stool is most characteristic of occult blood.

144. 4. An obstruction of the common bile duct prevents bile from entering the gastrointestinal tract. An absence of bile in the tract prevents absorption of vitamin K. Vitamin K is necessary for the formation of prothrombin. Prothrombin deficiency results in delayed clotting of the blood.

145. 4. All of the foods given in these options are relatively high in fat content except roast beef and tapioca pudding.

146. 2. If the patient is allergic to seafoods or iodine, he may have an allergic reaction to iopanoic acid which contains iodine. Anaphylaxis is possible.

147. 1. Water is the only recommended substitute for milk for this patient the evening before she is to have a cholecystogram. The patient is ordinarily NPO or on fluid restriction the morning of the examination.

148. 2. The suffix, -otomy, refers to an incision into. Choledocho- refers to the common bile duct. Choledochotomy means an incision into or an opening of the common bile duct.

149. 2. Oral fluids and food are withheld prior to surgery when the

patient has general anesthesia primarily in order to help prevent nausea and vomiting. When these occur during surgery, there is great danger that the patient may aspirate.

150. 1. The muscle into which the nurse will inject the medication is the gluteus medius muscle. The rectus femoris muscle is on the anterior aspect of the thigh. The gluteus maximum muscle is located in the buttock; it is called the dorsogluteal site. The vastus lateralis muscle is located on the anterolateral aspect of the thigh.

151. 3. A T tube is used to help prevent spillage of bile into the peritoneum and it also helps to provide patency of the duct. Suggested reasons for its use in the other three options are incorrect.

152. 2. The best way to record T tube drainage is to record it separately on the output record. If it is added to other output, the amount of drainage is difficult to ascertain. The patient's total intake will be in error if drainage is subtracted from it.

153. 1. In order to offer the patient the most support and comfort, the scultetus binder should be applied by wrapping it from the bottom to the top.

154. 4. The primary purpose for using blow bottles is to maximize respiratory ventilation. There may be some circulatory stimulation and strengthening of abdominal muscles but these are not the primary purposes for using blow bottles.

155. 2. The signs described in the stem suggest that the fluid is infiltrating. The only solution is to discontinue the infusion and prepare to inject another vein. Continuing to allow fluids to enter the patient will likely cause further tissue injury. Irrigating the needle will not overcome infiltration and it is a contraindicated procedure.

156. 4. All of the drugs given here are classified as tranquilizers. However, only prochloperazine is effective to help prevent nausea and vomiting. It is believed to act by blocking the effects of emetic chemicals upon the chemoreceptor zone.

157. 2. Paralytic ileus is manifested by a lack of bowel sounds when auscultation is used. None of the other signs given in wrong options is typical of paralytic ileus.

158. 1. In order to facilitate passage of the nasogastric tube, the patient should be placed preferably in a sitting up position with his neck hyperflexed. This straightens the anatomical passageway to the stomach to the greatest extent. Other options described here will not accomplish this goal.

159. 2. It is contraindicated to irrigate the tube and then to observe for the return of fluid. If the tube is not in the stomach, fluid will

be aspirated. Techniques described in options 1, 3, and 4 are recommended to determine whether the tube is in the stomach.

160. 4. Neostigmine methylsulfate is a typical anticholinesterase agent. It increases transmission from cholinergic nerves to smooth and skeletal muscles. In this case, the desired action is stimulation of peristalsis.

161. 4. Anticholinesterase drugs act by prolonging the effect of acetylcholine at the myoneural junction.

162. 4. Replacement therapy, when a patient has nasogastric suction, has as its main purpose maintenance of fluid and electrolyte balance.

163. 2. When irrigating solution does not return via the nasogastric tube, it should be recorded as intake. This is important in order to have an accurate intake record.

164. 1. The nasogastric tube causes discomfort because of the local irritation. This can best be helped by having the patient use anesthetic lozenges as indicated. Measures described in the other three options are not likely to help reduce discomfort.

165. 3. The Miller-Abbott, Cantor, and Harris tubes are mercury-weighted tubes. The weight helps facilitate passage of the tubes into the duodenum.

166. 1. Patients with disorders of the biliary tract usually find that foods high in fat content produce nausea. A diet high in carbohydrates and proteins is recommended. Normal mineral and vitamin requirements should be maintained.

167. 1. Gallbladder disease has its highest incidence among obese women, usually past 40 years of age and multiparous.

168. 2. The gallbladder and biliary tract normally store, transport, and concentrate bile but do not secrete bile. Secretion of bile occurs in the liver.

169. 3. Bile salts are the physiologically active part of bile. They increase fat solubility and break up fat into tiny particles. Lecithin and cholesterol exist in bile and serve to keep the water-soluble cholesterol in solution, thus preventing stone formation. Bilirubin is a pigment and is carried to the liver for excretion by bile.

170. 4. The sphincter of Oddi controls the passage of bile and pancreatic enzymes into the duodenum. The point at which the common bile duct and the pancreatic duct join is called the ampulla of Vater. The pyloric sphincter is at the distal end of the stomach, and controls entry of stomach contents to the duodenum. The common bile duct is formed when the right and left hepatic and the cystic ducts join.

171. 3. Cholecystokinin causes the gallbladder to contract and empty itself. It plays no role in processes described in options 1, 2, and 4.

ROBERT SHELLY

172. 2. The primary reason for taking an apical-radial pulse in this patient is to determine the pulse deficit. When there is a difference in the number of beats per minute, the pulse deficit is likely to be a sign of possible atrial fibrillation.

173. 1. Although all options describe valuable nursing measures to support a patient preoperatively, allowing the patient time to express his fears has the most potential for decreasing anxieties concerning impending surgery.

174. 3. Baseline information should be ascertained first when beginning a teaching program for a patient. One piece of baseline information is to learn what the patient already knows. Learning can be stifled when the patient is subject to teaching which is a repeat of previous knowledge. Options 2 and 4 are unnecessary and contraindicated. The goal of teaching should be determined *with* the patient. Terms should be defined but extensive use of medical terminology is generally not advised.

175. 3. Alternating tourniquets are utilized for circulatory overload but are very unlikely to be used for this patient. Devices described in options 1, 2, and 4 are very likely to be used.

176. 2. An endotracheal tube which passes through the mouth or nose into the trachea, prevents the patient from being able to speak while it is in place. No incision is necessary to insert it. The patient will not be required to lie quietly on his back while the tube is in place but will need frequent position changes. The tube will be removed postoperatively when respiration is free of difficulties.

177. 1. A chest tube will not help prevent hemorrhaging. The primary purpose for chest tubes here is to re-establish negative intrathoracic pressure, thereby promoting lung re-expansion. Options 2, 3, and 4 are additional goals which can be accomplished with chest tubes.

178. 2. Because of the nature of his illness, the patient's usual role at home as father and breadwinner will have to change, at least temporarily. A change in role often is accompanied by withdrawal and concern. It is unlikely that this patient's behavior is caused by factors given in options 1, 3, and 4.

179. 1. Most drugs have to be discontinued prior to heart surgery. However, complete rest is desired. Hence, the nurse should

question the order that would discontinue a drug acting as a sedative which in no way affects the cardiovascular system except indirectly as a result of added rest.

180. 1. As body temperature lowers, metabolism decreases in the body. Body tissues therefore require less blood to survive adequately. Shivering does the opposite to the metabolic activity and is to be avoided. Shivering is not necessarily contraindicated prior to heart surgery for reasons given in options 2, 3, and 4.

181. 3. For best access to the heart, the incision is made over the sternum as a midline thoracotomy.

182. 1. The ball-in-cage is most commonly used to replace a diseased mitral valve. All parts except for the ball are covered with dacron, thus permitting invasion of location tissue to seal the structure in the heart.

183. 1. Heparin acts to delay clotting of the blood and is, hence, referred to as an anticoagulant. However, the patient is subject to hemorrhaging when an anticoagulant is being used. The drug is not associated with complications given in options 2, 3, and 4.

184. 4. The patient's blood leaves the body via the superior and inferior vena cava and ordinarily re-enters the body via the femoral or the ascending artery when the patient is on a cardiopulmonary bypass machine. The machine stimulates the action of the left ventricle and provides for oxygenation of blood.

185. 3. The drug of choice to counteract heparin sodium is protamine sulfate. Warfarin sodium is an anticoagulant, as heparin is. Vitamins A and C do not influence blood clotting.

186. 4. Bearing down against a closed glottis can best be prevented by instructing the patient to avoid holding his breath during activity. For example, the patient should be cautioned against bearing down when having a bowel movement or when moving himself about in bed. Techniques described in options 1, 2, and 3 will not help prevent using the Valsalva's maneuver.

187. 4. The illustration in option 4 illustrates premature ventricular contractions. Option 1 illustrates ventricular tachycardia. Option 2 illustrates atrial fibrillation. Option 3 is essentially normal heart rhythm.

188. 4. The solution to this problem is as follows:
1000 mg. : 500 ml. :: 3 mg. : X ml.
1000 X = 1500

$$X = \frac{1000}{500} = 1.5 \text{ ml. of solution should be given each minute}$$

1.5 ml. × 60 (microdrops) = 90 microdrops should be given each minute

189. 2. Typical side effects of a reaction to lidocaine hydrochloride include drowsiness, light headedness, and dizziness. The symptoms given in options 1, 3, and 4 are not associated with toxicity to lidocaine hydrochloride.

190. 3. The dorsalis pedis pulse can best be determined at site C. Areas either below or above this site do not offer a good area for palpating the pulse.

191. 2. The quality of peripheral circulation can be assessed by checking the patient's feet for color and warmth. If color is pink and the feet feel warm, peripheral circulation can be assessed as satisfactory. Techniques described in the wrong options will not help assess circulation in the feet.

192. 3. For this patient, CVP was monitored primarily in order to assess the heart's ability to receive and pump blood. CVP may be used for assistance in assessing the patient's cardiovascular status but in this situation, its use to determine blood volume is not of primary concern.

193. 3. When a chest tube slips out, the nurse should take immediate steps to prevent air from entering the chest cavity which may cause collapse of the lung. Hence, her first course of action in this case is to place a closed hand over the chest opening. Then, a petrolatum dressing may be placed over the area. Actions described in options 1 and 4 will not help prevent air from entering the chest cavity.

194. 4. A characteristic sign of pulmonary congestion is the development of rales which can be heard with auscultation. Rales are not indicative of conditions described in options 1, 2, and 3.

195. 2. Prothrombin is produced in the liver and normally found in the blood. For prothrombin to be manufactured, vitamin K must be present in the liver to act as a catalyst. When the prothrombin time is longer than normal (above approximately 40 to 50 percent), the patient is subject to hemorrhage. A prolonged prothrombin time helps prevent emboli. It will not influence conditions described in options 3 and 4.

196. 4. See item 195.

197. 4. The tension of each turn when elastic bandages are applied to the lower extremities should be equal. Unnecessary and uneven overlapping of turns should be avoided to prevent undue

and uneven pressure. Bony prominences are generally best protected with padding but should be covered (ankles) in order to provide good support to the veins of the legs. An extremity should be bandaged toward the trunk to avoid congestion in the distal part of the leg and foot. The bandage should not cover the toes in order that they may be observed to assess peripheral circulation.

198. 1. Although all measures described here will help to decrease the incidence of wound infections, most authorities hold that washing of the nurse's hands before dressing wounds is of prime importance in helping to reduce the incidence of wound infections.

199. 3. Every effort should be made to prevent stagnation of blood in the lower extremities during the postoperative period. Having the knees flexed by using a gatched bed or by placing pillows under the knees promotes stagnation of blood and, hence, is contraindicated. The practice may well play a role in conditions described in options 1 and 4 but they are of lesser importance than preventing venous congestion.

200. 4. According to Erikson's theory, middle-aged adults are usually most concerned with generativity versus stagnation. Option 1 describes typical concerns of young adults. Option 2 describes most common concerns of the elderly person. Option 3 describes the major concern of most school age children.

201. 1. Although all suggested measures described in these options may assist the patient to adjust to less intensive care, it is of prime importance to convey to the patient that the nurse is still assessing him frequently. This can best be done by observing the technique described in option 1.

202. 3. There is no evidence that neglecting to have health care is an inherited trait. However, options 1, 2, and 4 accurately describe reasons why many persons do neglect to obtain health care.

203. 1. Option 1 illustrates poor body mechanics. Stretching and twisting place the nurse's body in poor alignment and strains muscles. Option 2 illustrates the proper way to pick up an object from the floor; the nurse stoops and prevents strain on his back muscles while using the long and strong muscles in the legs to return to the standing position. Option 3 illustrates working at a proper level; the nurse neither stretches, stoops, nor twists in this position. Option 4 brings the line of gravity closer to the nurse's base of support, thus improving balance and reducing strain on arm muscles.

204. 2. Elasticized stockings should be removed daily in order to

inspect and bathe the legs. Evidence of irritation or poor circulation should be noted. Elasticized stockings should be laundered regularly; they are reusable. They stay in place without support and garters would be contraindicated in any case because they tend to promote venous stasis. Elasticized stockings should be put on the first thing in the morning before getting out of bed in order to avoid congestion that may occur once the patient has been walking about.

205. 4. When mitral stenosis is present, the left atrium has difficulty emptying its contents into the left ventricle. Hence, since there is no valve to prevent backward flow into the pulmonary vein, the pulmonary circulation is under pressure. Functioning of the aorta, the right atrium, and the superior vena cava are not immediately influenced by mitral stenosis.

206. 2. Most patients with mitral stenosis have a history of having had rheumatic fever. Conditions given in the wrong options do not predispose to mitral stenosis.

207. 4. Revascularization is done when arteriosclerotic heart disease results in poor blood supply to heart muscle. Cardiac arrhythmias are due to faulty impulse conduction in the heart and are not ordinarily treated surgically. Congestive heart failure is usually handled medically by employing methods that will help the efficiency of the left ventricle. Congenital anomalies are often treated surgically but bypass procedures are not indicated.

208. 3. The general population holds great respect for the importance of the heart and it is generally believed this accounts for many expressions that include the word, heart. There is no evidence to support the statement described in option 2. Nor are options 1 and 4 believed to be related to the use of the word in many everyday expressions.

BERNARD CARTER

209. 3. Tomography provides for visualization of sections of the lung from various planes. Floroscopy affords study of pulmonary motion. The bronchial tree is examined by bronchograms. A biopsy would be necessary to study the thickness of membranes in the lungs.

210. 3. In this patient, cytologic examination was done to determine the presence of malignant cells. It is a study of cells the body sheds and is used when a malignancy is suspected.

211. 1. Because the throat has been anesthetized for the bronchoscopy, if the patient takes fluids before the anesthesia has worn off, he is most likely going to choke because he will not have

regained control of his epiglottis. Coughing, vomiting, and sneezing are unlikely to occur.

212. 4. Lung surgery when a malignancy is present usually entails removing large parts of lung tissue. Hence, preoperative evaluation of pulmonary function is done to help determine whether the surgical procedure will leave enough functioning lung tissue to sustain life. Function tests will not help determine factors given in options 1, 2, and 3.

213. 4. Tidal air refers to the volume of air that is inhaled and exhaled with one normal respiration. Residual air describes air that remains in the lungs after a forced expiration. Inspiratory reserve is the amount of air, in excess of tidal, that can be inhaled by the deepest possible inspiration. Expiratory reserve is the amount of air, in excess of tidal, that can be exhaled by the greatest possible exhalation.

214. 4. IPPB therapy is ordinarily used to increase total ventilation. However, preoperatively, it is most often used to clear the patient's airway to the greatest extent possible.

215. 1. The patient described here is most probably suffering from hyperventilation because he is breathing too rapidly. His body is ridding itself of carbon dioxide in excessive amounts.

216. 3. The primary reason for using radiation therapy preoperatively for this patient is to help minimize the risk of metastasis. In some instances, the tumor will also shrink with this type of therapy but this is less likely to be the reason for using radiation treatments. The therapy will not alleviate symptoms nor depress the formation of red blood cells.

217. 1. The dosage is larger than normal. The average preoperative dosage for an adult for atropine sulfate is between 1/200 and 1/50 grain (0.3 to 1.2 mg.), the average dosage being 1/120 grain (0.5 mg.). Patients scheduled for chest surgery very often are given more than the *average* dose of atropine sulfate because of the importance of minimizing respiratory secretions but not as much as 1/6 grain.

218. 3. The muscle transsected is the latissimus dorsi.

219. 3. When oxygen is given by nasal cannula at the rate of 3 liters per minute, the percentage of oxygen the patient will receive will be approximately 32 percent.

220. 1. The best way to assess whether tracheal suctioning is indicated is to auscultate breath sounds. If mucus and debris is accumulating, the breath sounds will be noisy. Techniques described in options 2, 3, and 4 are not effective for determining whether suctioning is necessary.

221. 1. It is particularly important that this patient keep a clear airway. Suctioning will help but the chief reason for using suctioning postoperatively is to encourage the patient to cough. This is the most effective way to remove large amounts of mucus and mucus plugs.

222. 3. Hypoxia occurs during suctioning when the suctioning is so extensive as to remove too much oxygen from the respiratory tract. Hence, prior to suctioning, oxygenating the patient for several minutes is recommended. While factors described in options 1, 2, and 4 are important also, hypoxia will be best prevented by oxygenation.

223. 1. Normal CVP readings range between 5 and 12 cm. of water. Lower than normal readings suggest that the patient has had loss of fluids. A higher than average reading is likely to mean hypervolemia or poor cardiac contractibility. There is no information given here that suggests the pressure gauge is out of order.

224. 3. CVP catheters are not ordinarily used for administering a blood transfusion. There is too much danger of the blood clogging the tube. However, the CVP catheter may be used for procedures described in options 1, 2, and 4.

225. 3. Of the effects given, the most undesirable result of the indiscriminate use of morphine sulfate is that it acts to depress the respiratory center. It may decrease mental alertness but this would not be contraindicated for this patient during the first day or two postoperatively. It will not increase blood pressure nor inhibit the secretion of mucus. An additional problem in the indiscriminate use of morphine sulfate is that of addiction.

226. 4. It would be best to medicate this patient prior to turning him. It is essential that he keep a clear airway and have maximum ventilation and hence, it would be best not to medicate him before coughing and deep-breathing routines. Range-of-motion exercises are ordinarily not uncomfortable and, hence, medication would not be indicated.

227. 3. Closing the glottis is accomplished by bearing down. Techniques described in options 1, 2, and 4 will not close the glottis. Closing the glottis before starting a cough strengthens the cough which for this patient is especially important to raise debris in the respiratory passages. See also item 186.

228. 2. If the patient is to receive 60 ml. in an hour's time, he should receive 1 ml. in each minute's time. With a drop factor of 15, the patient should receive 1×15, that is 15 drops per minute.

229. 4. There are 480 ml. of whole blood in one unit. If the patient is to receive 60 ml. each hour, it will take 8 hours to infuse one unit of blood ($\frac{480}{60}$ = 8 hours).

230. 1. Too rapid infusion of blood, or any intravenous fluid, is likely to cause pulmonary edema. Conditions given in the wrong options are not related to rapid infusion.

231. 2. The amount of chest drainage this patient had in the 4-hour period was 250 ml. (350 ml. − 100 ml. = 250 ml.)

232. 1. The chest tubes serve two purposes; to help remove air from the pleural space and to help remove drainage from the chest cavity. When this is accomplished, the lung has room to re-expand following chest surgery. The upper anterior catheter ordinarily should return air which is being forced from the pleural cavity as the lung expands. Drainage can be expected to return from the lower posterior tube. It is normally serosanguineous fluid that accumulates in the lower part of the pleural space.

233. 3. Option 3 illustrates the correct setup for a one bottle closed chest drainage system. Air is allowed to escape freely from the bottle but since the tube from the patient is under water, no air will enter the pleural cavity.

234. 1. Since the tube from the patient is under water, there is a water seal. This prevents return flow of air and fluid into the pleural space. The mechanisms described in the wrong options do not accomplish this goal.

235. 2. "Stripping" the chest tubes is done primarily in order to keep the tubes patent. The "stripping" should be done by moving the fingers along the tube *away* from the patient and *toward* the drainage bottle in order not to force debris into the patient's chest cavity.

236. 2. The equivalent of 100.4° F. on the Celsius scale is 38.0° C. The formula to convert Fahrenheit to Celsius is as follows: subtract 32° and multiply by 5/9.
100.4 − 32 = 68.4; 68.4 × 5/9 = 38.0° C.

237. 3. it has been noted that the body temperature is lowest early in the morning and highest in late afternoon and early evening hours. An inversion of this has been noted for persons who sleep during the day and work at night.

238. 1. Mercury in the bulb of a mercury thermometer expands when heated. Options 2, 3, and 4 are inaccurate statements.

239. 2. Worry usually is defined as mild anxiety. Worry ordinarily can be identified and expressed as a concern while anxiety usually is associated with a feeling of indefiniteness and not

being able to state what its cause is. Options 1, 3, and 4 do not differentiate worry from anxiety and are inaccurate.

240. 1. Intermittent bubbling is normal when chest drainage with a water seal is working properly. The bubbling occurs with the patient's expirations.

241. 2. The bottles when a closed drainage system is used should always be kept below the level of the patient's chest. Drainage by gravity is thus maintained and drainage from the bottle will not return to the chest cavity.

242. 3. Clamps should be readily available and in view when a patient has chest drainage. They are not used as frequently as once was the case but there are times when clamps are necessary. For example, tubes may be double clamped to locate a source of malfunctioning of the apparatus. Occasionally, they may be used when transporting a patient. If air drainage has been occurring, clamping the tubes may cause tension pneumothorax.

243. 3. The most frequent wound care following removal of a chest tube is to cover it with petrolatum gauze and cover this with dry sterile dressings. The petrolatum gauze directly over the wound serves as an air tight seal to prevent air leakage or movement of air in either direction. Bandages or straps are not generally used directly over wounds. Mesh gauze would allow air movement.

244. 2. Fluctuation of the water level in the long glass tube is related to the patient's inspirations and expirations. When the fluctuations ceased on this patient's fifth postoperative day, the most probable cause was that the patient's lung had re-expanded.

245. 2. The physician will most likely order that the x-ray examination of the chest be done to confirm that the lung has indeed re-expanded. The other courses of action are unnecessary once it has been established that the lung has re-expanded. If it has not, then there may be need for other action, as being sure the tube is patent.

246. 1. Bottle A will receive drainage from the patient. Bottle B provides a water seal so that air cannot enter the patient's chest cavity. Bottle C is attached to a suction motor and helps provide better drainage.

247. 3. The pressure regulator bottle is labeled C in the diagram. See item 246.

248. 4. The proper procedure would be to disconnect the tube leading to the suction motor from the setup (bottle C). Using techniques described in options 1, 2, or 3 would cause air to enter the patient's chest cavity.

249. 4. It is generally contraindicated to place the patient in the Trendelenburg's position. The abdominal organs tend to shift upward and give the lungs less space in which to expand and function at their best. This position also interferes with gravitational drainage forces. The positions described in options 1, 2, and 3 are not contraindicated.

250. 3. To encourage movement in the shoulder, the patient should be encouraged to raise his arm on the affected side over his head. Exercises as described in the wrong options will not exercise the shoulder.

251. 2. It would be best to recommend that this patient contact the American Cancer Society which is a volunteer organization devoted to research and public education in relation to malignant diseases. Other organizations mentioned here have interests in malignant diseases but are not committed as the American Cancer Society is.

252. 1. Smoking immobilizes and destroys cilia in the respiratory passages. The cilia normally function to help the respiratory tract rid itself of debris taken in with breathing. While smoking influences other respiratory structures also, it is the cilia which are concerned chiefly with keeping the passages clean.

253. 1. An early sign of bronchogenic cancer is a hacking cough. Other symptoms, such as those described in options 2, 3, and 4, are later symptoms.

254. 1. Screening for bronchogenic cancer is best done by chest x-rays. The examinations described in options 2, 3, and 4 may be used to assist with diagnosis but are not ordinarily used for screening purposes.

255. 3. Although longer intervals have usually been recommended in the past, habitual smokers are encouraged to have screening examinations at least every 6 months. This recommendation started when statistics revealed the high incidence of lung cancer among smokers.

256. 2. Option 2 describes a current trend in relation to smoking. More teenagers than in the past are starting to smoke each year (option 1). When tar and nicotine levels were reduced in cigarettes, the habitual smoker tended to smoke more rather than fewer cigarettes (option 3). There continues to be an increase in the number of smokers in the general population although certain categories of people have a decreased number of smokers. For example, the total number of physicians who smoke has decreased markedly over the past decade.

257. 3. When a secondary tumor is present, tumor cells of the primary

tumor have spread to the organ in question. Options 1, 2, and 4 are inaccurate statements.

258. 2. Cells lining the bronchioles are ciliated columnar epithelial cells. Simple squamous cells line blood and lymph vessels. Stratified squamous epithelial cells are numerous in the epidermis of the skin. Cuboidal glandular cells are found in the thyroid gland and in kidney tubules.

GLENN HOPKIN

259. 1. Antacids containing magnesium salts tend to predispose to diarrhea. The bicarbonates are associated with flatulence. Bloody stools and abdominal cramping would be unusual symptoms associated with antacids.

260. 3. Aluminum and calcium compounds used as antacids tend to cause constipation. Symptoms described in options 1, 2, and 4 are not associated with the administration of antacids.

261. 3. Certain drugs have been found to be ulcerogenic. The salicylates, such as aspirin, are among them. In some individuals, they cause sufficient irritation to stomach mucosa so that bleeding may occur. The types of agents given in options 1, 2 and 4 are not associated with ulcers.

262. 2. When an ulcer perforates, the first symptom the patient has is sharp abdominal pain. Other signs/symptoms given here may occur but they will be later signs/symptoms of perforation.

263. 2. A jejunumotomy is a surgical procedure which joins the jejunum to the stomach, thus bypassing the duodenum. The ileum is distal to the jejunum. The cardiac sphincter will not be bypassed but the pyloric sphincter will be. The anastomosis is ordinarily made somewhere in the area of the fundus of the stomach.

264. 4. Innervation to produce symptoms of anxiety is carried by the autonomic division of the nervous system. It is also referred to as the visceral system since it supplies the internal organs. The cerebrospinal, or voluntary, nervous system connects the central nervous system with structures of the body wall. It is also referred to as the somatic system. The brain and the spinal cord make up the central nervous system which includes the nerves that connect this system to the body wall and with viscera.

265. 1. It is normal for the drainage from gastric suction to appear brown in color during the first 12 to 14 hours after surgery. This is due to digested blood in the content being removed. Green, yellow, and cloudy white would not be typical during this period.

266. 4. The indiscriminate use of gastric suction will result in electrolyte imbalances since electrolytes are being removed through the use of suction. If they are not replaced, along with adequate fluids, the patient will suffer both electrolyte and fluid imbalances. Renal failure is not associated with gastric suction. Gastric suction will ordinarily help to prevent paralytic ileus and abdominal distention.

267. 3. In order to relax abdominal muscles and provide for maximum respiratory and cardiovascular functioning it is best to have this patient assume a low semisitting position.

268. 3. The respiratory center is very sensitive to levels of carbon dioxide in the body. When it accumulates, respirations become deep. This is the body's effort to rid itself of excessive carbon dioxide. Inhalations of carbon dioxide used postoperatively are often given to help improve ventilation but these inhalations will not be of particular help to accomplish goals described in the wrong options.

269. 3. For the patient who is having gastric suctioning, fluids and electrolytes are ordinarily supplied with intravenous therapy. Hyperalimentation would not be usual. Patients having gastric suction are not given fluids or food by mouth since they will be returned via the suctioning tube. Furthermore, fluids given by mouth would tend to wash out the stomach which would result in even greater problems with electrolyte imbalance.

270. 1. Normal saline is the solution of choice. Since it is an isotonic solution, it will not disturb electrolyte balances as distilled water or soda bicarbonate solutions may. Antiseptic solutions are not recommended.

271. 3. In order to avoid misunderstandings concerning words used when recording, it is best to describe observations precisely without using medical terminology or judgmental words (option 1). Hence, option 3 describes the amount of drainage in a way so that there is little likelihood of misunderstanding. Comparisons with previous descriptions, as in options 2 and 4, are meaningless unless the reader knows the amount with which the observer is making a comparison.

272. 4. The discomfort of a sore throat associated with gastric tube is most often due to local irritation, although if dehydration is present, it may aggravate the symptom. An infection or chemical irritation is very unlikely. See also item 164.

273. 3. Normal adult values for blood level of potassium are within a range of approximately 3.5 and 5 mEq./L. Hence, this patient's potassium level is within normal range.

274. 2. Following partial removal of the stomach, the patient is aware of being unable to accommodate even average size meals. However, the patient should be taught that the stomach will likely accommodate larger meals in time. It is most unlikely that the stomach will become even smaller (option 1). Tolerance for spicy foods is an individual matter; most persons with peptic ulcers find they do not tolerate them well but are likely to tolerate them better after the surgical procedure. A sphincter will not develop at the site of the anastamosis.

275. 2. Eructating small amounts of food after eating is usually due to taking too much food with each meal. Factors given in options 1, 2, and 4 are less likely to cause this condition.

276. 3. A characteristic symptom of the "dumping syndrome," faint-

277. 4. ness, is believed due to the rapid distention of the jejunum after eating and the removal of water from the general circulation in order to dilute carbohydrates and electrolytes in preparation for absorption. Persons with this condition have learned that symptoms are less likely to occur when they restrict their intake of high carbohydrate foods and salt.

278. 2. Following a gastrectomy, patients may develop signs/symptoms similar to those of pernicious anemia because of the low supply of intrinsic factor. This factor is lacking in stomach secretions in the patient who has pernicious anemia. The intrinsic factor is not related to conditions described in options 1, 3, and 4.

279. 2. Gastrin is a hormone produced by cells in the pyloric portion of the stomach mucosa. When it enters the bloodstream, it is carried to glands in the fundus and body of the stomach where it stimulates the production of gastric juices. The secretions described in options 1, 3, and 4 are not related to the production of gastric juices.

280. 4. Hydrochloric acid converts pepsinogin, which is an inactive form of pepsin, to pepsin. Ptylin is found in saliva and it begins the digestion of carbohydrates. Secretin is a duodenal secretion which indirectly influences the duodenal pH. Cholecystokinin is a duodenal secretion that works to dispatch bile to the duodenum.

281. 2. Of the factors given here, duodenal ulcer is most closely associated etiologically with persons under emotional stress.

CARL SHORT

282. 2. Of the breakfast foods given, the one lowest in residue is Rice Krispies.

283. 1. For best visualization of the rectum and sigmoid colon, the

lower colon should be empty when performing a sigmoidoscopy. Usually this is most effectively accomplished by giving the patient an enema an hour or so before the examination. Having the patient fast, giving a liquid diet, and using a laxative the evening before examination are not as effective for emptying the lower colon.

284. 4. Castor oil breaks down in the intestines to form ricinoleic acid. This acid acts to irritate nerve endings in the intestinal mucosa which produces evacuation. Mineral oil is a laxative that acts to soften and lubricate the stool. Saline cathartics, such as magnesium sulfate and citrate, act to increase the volume of intestinal contents, thus stimulating evacuation.

285. 4. Following a barium enema, the physician is most likely to write an order for a cathartic. This is done to assist with the expulsion of the barium because if it is retained, it predisposes to constipation and fecal impaction.

286. 3. Meat residue, especially meat that is eaten rare, such as beef, may lead to a false positive result when the stool specimen is examined for blood. A high iron intake may cause the stool to appear black, as do certain dark green vegetables, but these factors will not lead to false positive readings. Options 2 and 4 are situations that do not lead to false positive results.

287. 2. The reason for giving the patient chemical agents prior to surgery for an abdominoperineal resection and colostomy is to reduce the bacterial count in the colon. By so doing, the likelihood of infection postoperatively in the operative areas is reduced.

288. 3. Since the reason for giving the drug is to reduce the bacterial count in the intestinal tract, the drug of choice is one that is poorly absorbed from the gastrointestinal wall. This characteristic is true of succinylsulfathiazole.

289. 3. When there is a choice, the preferred site for a permanent colostomy is in the lower portion of the descending colon. The colon normally absorbs large quantities of water. Hence, when the colostomy is as near the end of the colon as possible, the colostomy is easier to manage since the stool will be near its normal consistency.

290. 2. Site B illustrates the splenic flexure. It is so named since it is that part of the colon which lies nearest the spleen.

291. 2. The solution of choice when administering blood in a tandem setup is a 0.9 percent saline solution. This solution is isotonic and least likely to upset fluid and electrolyte balances.

292. 4. The symptoms this patient presented are suggestive of an allergic reaction to the blood. The nurse's first course of

action should be to stop administering the blood immediately. The physician then should be notified. The symptoms given in the stem do not suggest that infiltration is occurring nor that the blood is being given too rapidly.

293. 4. This patient should not have his knees resting over a blanket roll. The roll can cause constriction of blood vessels and predispose to thrombophlebitis. Measures described in options 1, 2, and 3 are recommended procedures to help prevent thrombophlebitis and pulmonary congestion.

294. 3. The sign that indicates the patient's colostomy is open and ready to function is passage of gas from it. When this occurs, gastric suction is ordinarily discontinued. The patient is then allowed to start taking food and fluids by mouth. Signs described in options 1, 2, and 4 are not criteria for judging whether gastric suction is or is not necessary.

295. 4. Vanilla ice cream is not considered to be a clear liquid. Beef broth, apple juice, and tea with sugar are classified as clear liquids. Sherbert is considered to be a clear liquid in many health agencies.

296. 2. It would be best to prepare the patient for the sight of his colostomy by showing him pictures of a colostomy. Measures described in options 1, 3, and 4 are recommended but will do less for preparing the patient for the appearance of his colostomy.

297. 4. The purpose of the colostomy irrigation on this patient's fifth postoperative day is to stimulate peristalsis. It is not done to flush the colon. Stimulating peristalsis so that the colon will empty naturally is an early step in working toward controlling elimination from a colostomy. There is no sphincter to control elimination from the colostomy.

298. 1. The abdominal cramping that may occur during a colostomy irrigation is due to stimulation of the colon by the irrigating fluid. The best course of action is to stop allowing fluids to enter the colon until the cramping subsides. Options 3 and 4 will not help to stop cramping. There is no need to remove the tube since this will mean having to re-insert it again when the irrigation is continued.

299. 2. When the colostomy irrigation is carried out properly, there is no need for the nurse to wear gloves since her hands should not become contaminated with feces. If she wears gloves, the patient is likely to feel that he is "unclean," "infectious," or "undesirable." Measures described in options 1, 3, and 4 are recommended.

300. 2. When the patient asks about supplies used for his dressings,

the patient demonstrates that readiness may be occurring in relation to his participating in his own care. Options 1, 3, and 4 indicate behavior that avoids the subject of his colostomy.

301. 1. Of the preparations given, zinc oxide is the preparation of choice. The colostomy drainage is likely to be irritating and, hence, a preparation that adheres well and offers good protection, such as zinc oxide, is preferred.

302. 1. The most effective way to cleanse the operative area well and to bring moisture and heat to the area simultaneously is to have this patient use sitz baths. Most patients find the sitz baths to be comfortable and relaxing as well.

303. 2. Experience has shown that it is best to adjust the diet of a patient with a colostomy in a manner that best suits the patient. No standard formula, such as those described in the wrong options, work as well. Diets described in options 1 and 4 are not recommended. The diet suggested in option 3 may well be best for *some* patients.

304. 4. An ileostomy empties the intestines before water absorption has had a chance to occur. Hence, the stool is liquid in nature and control of bowel evacuation is an unrealistic goal for most patients. Options 1, 2, and 3 describe realistic goals for patients who have had an ileostomy.

305. 2. Antimetabolites have chemical structures similar to nutrients that cells need to grow and reproduce. These anticancer drugs keep the malignant cells from using natural nutrients which interferes with their proper nutrition. Options 1, 3, and 4 are inaccurate statements in relation to antimetabolite drugs.

306. 1. Fluorouracil is often toxic to bone marrow, the result being that the white blood cells decrease in number and the patient becomes susceptible to infection. In view of the patient's elevated temperature, the nurse should notify the physician since very often it becomes necessary to discontinue the drug therapy. Giving the patient a cool bath may be comfortable but will not overcome toxicity. There is more need for a blood count than a urine culture.

307. 1. The primary purpose of reverse (protective) isolation is to reduce the spread of organisms from sources outside his environment to the patient. In this case, the patient is being protected from organisms to the greatest extent possible rather than being isolated so that organisms from him do not spread to other persons and things.

308. 2. Common chemotherapeutic agents used in the care of patients with malignancies often affect hair follicles causing the patient to lose his hair. This often influences the patient's self-

concept and body image and requires skilled, supportive intervention measures.

309. 1. Antineoplastic drugs have a disadvantage in that they often fail to distinguish between tumor and normal cells. Statements in options 2, 3, and 4 do not tend to occur.

310. 4. See item 306. Cytotoxic drugs often cause depression of bone marrow functioning. Other toxic symptoms may occur but this sign is most common.

311. 1. The word, thrombocytopenia, means that the platelet count is low. By definition, none of the other terminology given here is applicable.

312. 4. When the patient has reached the stage of accepting his imminent death, he is likely to be at peace and contented. It is during this stage that the patient appears to wish more privacy in order to be alone with his thoughts. During earlier stages, the patient needs the support of others and will often experience feelings of isolation when he is ignored or left alone.

313. 4. The patient's body temperature is usually elevated but he feels cool when central nervous system deterioration is present. The signs/symptoms given in options 1, 2, and 3 are not typically associated with central nervous system deterioration.

314. 3. Making a statement that indicates a time period, such as given in option 4, or avoiding the question, as in options 1 and 2, could give the family member false hope or reflect an attitude of not caring. A direct honest response will be received more readily.

315. 4. It is generally believed that the last sense to leave the body as death approaches is the sense of hearing. This offers a guide to health personnel; even though the patient appears unconscious, he may still be hearing what is said.

316. 1. It is generally recommended that the family may be taken to an area of privacy where they can be alone for a while. Option 2 may not be contraindicated in some situations although when death occurs, the family is not usually ready to discuss what should be done for at least a while. Option 3 describes behavior that may only add to the family's grief. It is unlikely that the family is ready to handle personal items at the time death occurs. It would be best for the nurse to wait until the family makes a request rather than suggesting doing something as specific as behavior described in option 4.

317. 4. Developing awareness usually results in anger. The anger can be turned inward, which causes depression, or outward and demonstrated as aggressive behavior.

318. 2. The most common reason why terminally ill patients are often avoided by health personnel is best described in option 2. Family members may help with care but should not be expected to assume the nurse's responsibility to provide it. The dying patient often requires maximum amounts of care. While every patient has the right to die in dignity, ignoring the patient will not accomplish this goal.

319. 1. Statistics show that most malignancies of the lower gastrointestinal tract arise from the sigmoid and rectum.

320. 4. Of the examinations given here, x-rays using contrast media provide the most conclusive evidence when a tumor exists. The examinations given in options 1, 2 and 3 may be used to assist with diagnosis but are not as conclusive as an x-ray examination with contrast media.

321. 1. Bacteria in the large bowel are necessary for the synthesis of vitamin K, thiamin, riboflavin, vitamin B_{12}, folic acid, biotin, and nicotinic acid. These bacteria do not play a role in actions described in options 2, 3, and 4.

322. 2. The cephalic stage of digestion stimulates the secretion of gastric juices but does not influence activity described in the wrong options.

323. 3. The act of defecation is stimulated primarily by the distention of the rectum with fecal matter. Toxins have not been found to be present to stimulate defecation. Relaxation of the anal sphincter occurs after the urge to have a bowel movement is present and the person allows relaxation of the sphincter. Phenol has not been found to stimulate defecation.

HILDA TOWE

324. 1. In order to obtain an accurate basal metabolism rate, the patient should not receive any medication before the examination. Preparations described in options 2, 3, and 4 are commonly observed.

325. 1. Normal BMR values are between -15 and $+15$. A BMR of $+15$ or above is considered to be a sign of hyperthyroidism. A value of -15 or below is usually considered to be a sign of hypothyroidism.

326. 1. The patient is likely to have a falsely elevated PBI and ^{131}I uptake test results if he has taken any drugs containing iodine within the past month or so. Estrogens can also cause falsely elevated results. These two tests are used to evaluate thyroid functioning.

327. 3. Iodine is excreted in the urine, as is radioactive iodine. The patient should save her urine for the 24-hour period and bring

it with her for laboratory analysis. Preparations described in options 1, 2, and 4 are not indicated for this test.

328. 2. Palpation, inspection, and auscultation are used when examining the thyroid gland; percussion is not.

329. 2. Exophthalmus is characterized by protrusion of the eyeballs. The signs/symptoms described in options 1, 3, and 4 are not associated with this condition.

330. 4. When exophthalmus is present, the eyelids tend not to close completely during sleep. Hence, it is recommended that the eyelids be taped shut in order to prevent drying of the eyeballs. Measures described in options 1, 2, and 3 are not recommended.

331. 1. Fine hand tremors are common when hyperthyroidism is present. The symptoms given in options 2, 3, and 4 are more typical of hypothyroidism.

332. 1. Amenorrhea is very likely to be present in the patient with hyperthyroidism while other symptoms given in the wrong options are not.

333. 3. It can be expected that the patient will have a more rapid and exaggerated response when the deep tendon reflex is tested.

334. 1. The patient should be taught to report the symptoms if she experiences a sore throat, general malaise, fever, rash, or jaundice. These symptoms of drug reaction usually mean that the drug must be discontinued. The symptoms given in options 2, 3, and 4 are not associated with reactions to propylthiouracil.

335. 2. The only option which satisfactorily explains this patient's behavior is given in option 2. Options 1, 3, and 4 are not associated with hyperthyroidism.

336. 1. The best guideline when caring for a patient with hyperthyroidism is to provide an environment that promotes maximum physical and mental rest. A private room located in an area where the patient has privacy and quietness is best. When the room is near the noise and activity of the nurses station, the patient is likely to be disturbed.

337. 1. Potassium iodide is frequently administered preoperatively because the drug helps to decrease the size and vascularity of the thyroid gland. The drug does not act to accomplish goals described in options 2, 3, and 4.

338. 3. It is suggested that a saturated solution of potassium iodide be well diluted with milk, water, or juice prior to administration to help disguise the strong unpleasant bitter taste. Also, it could be very irritating to mucosa if taken in an undiluted state.

339. 1. The preparation is a saturated solution which means that if

exposed to air for a period of time, it will evaporate readily. The nurse in this situation found everything as she had left it 45 minutes earlier. Hence, her most accurate assumption should be that which is described in option 1.

340. 3. There are 9 calories in every Gram of fat and 4 calories in every Gram of protein and carbohydrate. The total number of calories in this patient's diet is determined as follows:

$4 \times 300 = 1200$ calories in carbohydrate.
$4 \times 150 = 600$ calories in protein.
$9 \times 150 = 1350$ calories in fat.

Total   3150 calories in the daily diet.

341. 4. Option 4 offers an accurate description of the patient for a friend concerned about the patient's condition. It does not offer confidential information. The wrong options do not offer the friend support.

342. 1. Instructions distributed with injectable diazepam warn that it not be mixed or diluted with other solutions or drugs and that it is not to be added to intravenous fluids. Injectable diazepam is described as a colorless crystalline compound, insoluble in water.

343. 3. For a woman of this patient's size, it would be best to select a 22-gauge by 1½-inch needle. A 1-inch needle is too short to reach deep muscular tissue easily. There is no need to use needles as large as 19 or 20 gauge; the larger needle is likely to cause more trauma and discomfort than the smaller needle.

344. 3. A danger when surgery is performed on the thyroid gland is that injury to the laryngeal nerve may occur because of their close anatomical locations. Asking the patient to speak helps evaluate whether injury has occurred. Consciousness can be assessed to a degree by asking the patient to speak but in this case, this is not the primary reason for doing so.

345. 3. Morphine sulfate tends to depress the respiratory center. Hence, before administering the drug, the respiratory rate should be checked and the drug should be withheld if the rate is as low as 12 or below. Pupil size will decrease when morphine is used indiscriminately and usually indicates poisoning.

346. 1. This patient's symptoms are typical of respiratory distress. The cause may be edema, hemorrhage, laryngeal nerve damage, or tetany. The first course of action is to start oxygen therapy in this situation.

347. 1. Following a thyroidectomy, the patient is most often placed in the Fowler's position. The dressings are rather bulky. To check for hemorrhage, it is best to slip the hand behind the

patient's neck and check for blood on the back of the neck and bed linens. Considerable bleeding can have occurred if options 1, 3, and 4 are used for checking for bleeding.

348. 1. It is unlikely that a cutdown tray will be necessary for this patient. However, the items described in options 2, 3, and 4 are advised to be ready for immediate use. See item 346.

349. 2. Tetany may occur if the parathyroid glands are accidently removed during surgery. An early symptom of tetany is a tingling sensation in the fingers.

350. 2. The patient with tetany is suffering from hypocalcemia. It is treated by administering preparations of calcium.

351. 2. In order to afford the most comfort and security, it is best to support the head by placing both hands behind the head while moving into the sitting position. The techniques described in options 1, 3, and 4 will not accomplish these goals.

352. 1. In order to minimize scarring on the suture line, it is generally recommended that the patient apply cold cream or petrolatum over the suture line daily. The other techniques described here have not been shown to be effective to accomplish this goal.

353. 3. Typical signs of hypothyroidism include consistent weight gain and increasing fatigue. The symptoms described in options 1, 2, and 4 are not typical of hypothyroidism.

354. 3. When hyperthyroidism progresses without abatement, the heart literally "races itself to death," due to excess thyroxin in the system.

355. 2. The thyroid gland receives its stimulus from the thyroid-stimulating hormone (TSH) which is released by the anterior pituitary gland. Because of many body functions related to its proper functioning, the pituitary gland is often referred to as the "target" or "master" gland.

PETER HOYT

356. 1. The best way to assess for a distended bladder is for the nurse to check for a rounded swelling above the pubis. This swelling is the distended bladder rising above the pubis into the abdominal cavity.

357. 3. For best examination of the prostate gland, it is generally recommended that the patient stand while leaning over the edge of the examining table with his body bent at approximately a right angle to his hips. It is convenient for the operator and allows best access for digital examination of the prostate.

358. 4. It is unlikely that this patient will report having a urinary

stream of greater force than usual. Symptoms described in options 1, 2, and 3 are typical when the prostate is enlarged.

359. 2. Lubricating the catheter well decreases friction along the urethra and, hence, reduces irritation of urethral tissues. Since the urethra of the male is tortuous, a liberal amount of lubrication is advised to make passage of the catheter as easy as possible.

360. 3. Rapidly emptying an overdistended bladder may cause hypotension and shock due to the sudden changes of pressure within the abdominal viscera. Renal collapse is not likely, nor are signs/symptoms described in options 2 and 4.

361. 3. When a patient has a history of urinary retention, hydrone-phrosis is likely to develop as a result of the gradual backing up of stagnant urine into the pelvis of the kidneys. There are no true sphincters at the ureteral openings in the bladder so that sufficient pressure will cause the urine to back up.

362. 2. While there is helpful information in all of the options given here, the description given in option 2 will be most helpful to the admitting nurse. The information is exact, objective, and concise. There is no subjective terminology that could be judged differently by various people.

363. 4. An IVP will provide visualization of the ureters, the kidneys, and the bladder. It will not produce visualization of the urethra.

364. 3. Normal BUN range is between approximately 5 and 23 mg. per 100 ml. of whole blood. This patient's BUN is above normal by a sufficient amount which suggests that some renal damage has occurred. However, the finding does not suggest acute renal failure nor does the BUN reflect the acid-base balance of the body.

365. 1. Residual urine is defined as that amount of urine which remains in the bladder after voiding.

366. 1. The primary reason for taping in the manner illustrated is to prevent pressure at the penoscrotal angle. Research studies have found that with prolonged pressure on the angle, following catheter removal strictures have developed.

367. 2. It is generally agreed that bladder infections that occur when a patient has an indwelling catheter are due to an infection that ascends from the urethra and into the bladder. Hence, of highest priority is to give catheter care that includes meticulous cleansing of the area around the urethral meatus.

368. 3. The presence of red and white blood cells in the urine is most typical of urinary tract infection. The finding is not characteristic of conditions given in options 1, 2, and 4.

369. 4. The sensitivity test has one purpose: to assist the physician to select a drug to which the microorganisms found in the patient's urine are susceptible.

370. 1. An untoward effect to a drug is viewed usually as an idiosyncratic or abnormal or peculiar reaction. It is an unusual effect that can be a reverse of the expected or an under-response to the desired action. It is generally agreed that chloral hydrate produces a natural sleep and the patient can be awakened easily. The best choice in this case to explain the untoward reaction is described in option 1.

371. 3. It has been observed that the most common preoperative problem, among those mentioned here, among elderly patients is lower than normal total blood volume. This predisposes to postoperative problems since a low blood volume often leads to shock even when relatively small amounts of blood are lost during the surgical procedures.

372. 1. The number of minims to administer can be determined as follows:

50 mg. : 1 ml. :: 30 mg. : X ml.

$50 X = 30$

$X = \frac{3}{5}$ of 1 ml.

There are approximately 15 minims in each milliliter.

$\frac{3}{5}$ of 15 = 9 minims. The patient will receive this amount. 15 minims − 9 minims = 6 minims, the amount the nurse will discard.

373. 1. For continuous irrigation, the lumen marked A should be used.

374. 2. The lumen marked B should be used for the outflow of urine and irrigating solution. The lumen marked C is used for inflating the balloon which will hold the catheter in the bladder.

375. 3. The rate at which solution is entering the bladder should be increased when the drainage has become a brighter red color. The color indicates the presence of blood. Increasing the flow of irrigating solution helps flush the catheter well so that clots do not plug the catheter. There is no reason to increase the flow when situations described in options 1 and 2 are present. Increasing the flow would be contraindicated if the situation described in option 4 is present.

376. 3. The best explanation for the patient's feeling the urge to void is that it is caused by the catheter and possibly some bladder spasms. Explanations offered in options 1, 2, and 4 are less likely to be accurate.

377. 2. Ordinarily, when an indwelling catheter is removed, the pa-

tient experiences some dribbling incontinence. This is normal and temporary. The problem usually resolves itself as perineal muscles are strengthened through exercises.

378. 2. Bethanechol chloride is a cholinergic drug. It acts to increase the tone and motility of the urinary and gastrointestinal tract smooth muscles. It is frequently used when the bladder tone is lacking and there is inability to completely empty the bladder. All other options are related to urinary tract infections. By administering this drug to the patient, it is hoped that infections will be prevented.

379. 4. Alternately flexing and relaxing the quadriceps femoris muscles help the patient prepare for ambulation. The exercise is frequently referred to as quadriceps drills or sets. The exercises described in option 1, 2, and 3 will not effectively prepare muscles that are important for walking.

380. 1. A vasectomy is frequently performed at the time of the prostatectomy in order to decrease urinary tract infections and epididymitis. This procedure helps prevent retrograde spread of infection from the prostatic urethra through the vas and into the epididymis.

381. 2. It has been found that older men tend to believe that it is normal to have to live with some urinary problems.

382. 4. Despite many advantages, the transurethral resection has at least one disadvantage; it is the surgical procedure that most often requires having surgery again to remove tissue. This has not been found to be the case when other surgical approaches are used to perform a total prostatectomy.

383. 3. The prostate gland serves one purpose: it produces a secretion that helps in the nourishment and passage of the sperm. The gland does not function in ways described in options 1, 2, and 4.

384. 1. When paralysis of vasomotor nerves occurs when spinal anesthesia is used, the patient is likely to develop hypotension. Oxygen, blood, and drug therapy are used to overcome hypotension.

385. 4. Of those given, the most common postoperative complication associated with a prostatectomy is circulatory collapse and shock. Hemorrhage is the frequent cause of the complications.

FLORENCE HILL

386. 3. The dosage of a drug is related to many factors. In the case of hydromorphone hydrochloride, the drug is very potent and, hence, a small dose is indicated. Factors described in options 1, 2, and 4 do not apply to this drug.

387. 2. When selecting the needle for this patient, the size of the patient's arm should be considered first. The viscosity of the solution helps determine appropriate needle diameter. The dosage to be given does not influence length of needle.

388. 2. Since the patient is not due for additional medication for another 2 hours, it is best to try to control pain with other measures. Giving the patient a back massage is the best procedure to follow, of those offered here. This nursing measure is based on the gate control theory. The stimulation of large cutaneous nerve fibers appears to close the gating mechanism, thus reducing the perception of pain.

389. 4. The leg on the affected side following a hip fracture is characteristically shorter, adducted, and rotated externally.

390. 1. The term, crepitation, is used to describe the grating sensation produced when broken bone fragments are rubbed against each other. Ossification refers to the depositing of lime salts and the formation of bone. Proliferation refers to growth by the multiplication of cells. Consolidation refers to the conversion of a substance into a solid mass.

391. 1. In order to prevent external rotation of the patient's leg, it is best to support the leg in its proper anatomical position by supporting it with sandbags. They should be placed along the entire length of the thigh and lower leg. The devices described in options 2, 3, and 4 will not help prevent external rotation.

392. 3. The intertrochanteric area of the femur is that area identified in the illustration at site C.

393. 1. Tolbutamide is one of the sulfonylureas. It acts as a hypoglycemic by stimulating the production of insulin.

394. 1. Diabetic acidosis is caused by an inadequate amount of insulin in the body. This causes decreased utilization of carbohydrates and increased breakdown of fat and protein. The number of ketone bodies increases as the result of rapid fat breakdown.

395. 4. There are various advantages to the use of a pin for the internal fixation of a fractured hip. However, the procedure is especially favored for older patients since it makes earlier postoperative ambulation possible.

396. 3. The primary reason for applying suction to the tube placed in the patient's wound is to prevent fluid from accumulating in the wound. This greatly enhances wound healing and helps prevent abscess formation.

397. 2. When insulin is administered intravenously, the insulin of choice is crystalline zinc insulin, or regular insulin. This is the only unmodified form of insulin. All other insulins have

been modified to alter their rate of absorption from subcutaneous tissues.

398. 2. By placing the feet apart, the nurses will have a wide base of support and increased stability of the body when moving a patient. The techniques given in options 1, 3, and 4 will not provide the best body stability nor will they allow the nurses to use their longest and strongest muscles effectively.

399. 2. Of the measures given here, the only one which will help the patient from having flexion of the hip is to place the patient on a mattress that has bedboards under it. A trapeze helps the patient to help herself move in bed. An alternating pressure mattress is used primarily to help prevent decubitus ulcers. Using a footboard helps prevent footdrop.

400. 2. The manufacturers of enemas using hypertonic solution recommend the knee-chest position whenever possible. However, this patient cannot assume the position because of her fracture. She should also not lie on her affected right side. Hence, the position of choice for this patient is to have her lie in a left lateral position.

401. 3. A pillow was placed between the patient's legs while she was lying on her side to help prevent adduction of the thighs. By so doing, the hip is in proper alignment and does not adduct. Dislocation of the hip can occur if the leg on the affected side is allowed to adduct.

402. 3. Nerve damage may be indicated by the presence of any of the following "P's": pain, pallor, pulselessness, paresthesia, and paralysis. Porosis (bone cavitation) is not indicative of peripheral nerve damage.

403. 4. In order to help keep the patient in the best possible alignment when sitting in a chair following surgery for a hip fracture, a high-backed straight chair with arm rests is recommended. Soft, low, and swivel chairs do not promote good body alignment nor good security.

404. 1. Crossing the legs causes adduction of the hips and following hip surgery, this may result in a dislocation of the operated hip. Hence, the patient should not cross her legs. Elevating the legs, flexing the ankles, and extending the knees are not necessarily contraindicated.

405. 1. Every precaution should be used to prevent wound infection. Using sterile gloves and wearing a mask are recommended. However, wearing a gown is not ordinarily indicated.

406. 3. Many elderly patients are simply not strong enough to use crutches; nor is their coordination sufficiently adequate to make crutch-walking safe. Factors mentioned in options 1, 2,

and 4 *may* influence the ability to learn crutch-walking but are not observed to be as important as factors given above.

407. 2. The patient should support her weight with her hands when crutch-walking, not in her axilla which may cause nerve damage. In preparation for hand weight-bearing, the patient should be taught to squeeze a rubber ball in order to strengthen her hands. The activities described in options 1, 3, and 4 will not help strengthen her hands.

408. 4. Constipation is associated with the use of codeine sulfate but not with the other drugs given here.

409. 4. Psyllium hydrophilic mucilloid stimulates peristalsis by increasing the bulk within the intestinal tract. It absorbs water and produces a gelatinous-type material.

410. 3. If bulk-producing laxatives containing fibers, seeds, and granules are taken without a sufficient amount of water, they may pick up just enough moisture in the esophagus to swell and cause an obstruction.

411. 2. A diet that is low in roughage tends to leave so little residue that there is little mechanical stimulus for peristalsis. Hence, of the foods given here, it is best to recommend that the patient include bran cereals in order to help overcome constipation caused by a low residue diet.

412. 1. The best way to determine bone healing is to assess by follow-up x-ray studies. The factors given in options 2, 3, and 4 will do little to assess bone healing.

413. 2. Scatter rugs have been found to be a source of danger in the home, especially for older persons who are unsure of their walking.

414. 4. Important constituents of bone tissue are phosphorus and calcium. In order to help determine skeletal metabolic activity, of the tests given, determination of serum and urine calcium and phosphorus levels will be of most help while the other tests given here will provide little if any information for this particular assessment.

415. 4. Infection in the bone is referred to as osteomyelitis. Osteolysis refers to a softening of the bone. Osteomalacia is due to vitamin D deficiency; its symptoms are similar to rickets. The bones are soft and become deformed with relative ease. Demineralization of bone tissue is called osteoporosis.

416. 2. Muscles are attached to bones with tendons. Fascia is a layer of fibrous tissue that supports organs and muscles. A ligament consists of tough fibrous tissue that articulates bones. Cartilage is nonvascular connective tissue; it appears in the earlobes and nose.

417. 3. The patient with a herniated disc is least likely to complain of poor muscle coordination but is very likely to complain of symptoms given in options 1, 2, and 4.

418. 3. Hyperextension of the spine will occur when the patient lies on her abdomen. The patient with a herniated disc is most comfortable when lying an any of the positions described in options 1, 2, and 4.

419. 4. The myelogram uses a radiopaque dye as a contrast media.

420. 2. In order to reach the disc, the surgeon will need to remove a portion of the involved vertebra's posterior arch.

421. 2. A spinal fusion uses a bone graft.

422. 4. It is recommended that the patient's head be placed on a small pillow. Lowering the head of the bed may help drainage from the mouth but many patients have increased amounts of vomiting when the head is lowered. At this point, an airway is not indicated and will prevent good drainage from the mouth. There is no need for a blow on the chest and this technique may injure the patient.

423. 4. A disadvantage of many drugs that decrease nausea and vomiting is that they tend to cause the blood pressure to drop below normal.

424. 4. In order to inject into the thickest part of the deltoid muscle, site D is recommended.

425. 2. Human serum albumin serves the same function as plasma when used intravenously.

426. 4. In order to help bring peripheral blood into the central system, the patient in shock is best placed in the position illustrated in option 4. The Trendelenburg's position, as illustrated in option 1, was usually recommended in the past but it was found to decrease respiratory expansion and impair cardiac output.

427. 3. When glomerular filtration is impaired, the typical sign is a decreased urinary output. The pH level of the urine is not necessarily affected when shock initially occurs.

428. 4. In order to rid itself of excessive carbon dioxide, the body responds by causing deep and rapid respirations. The mechanisms given in options 1, 2, and 3 are not typical of metabolic acidosis.

429. 3. The intravenous therapy is very unlikely to be discontinued when a patient who has experienced shock has responded to therapy. The vein should be kept open, should further therapy become necessary. Rather, the rate of flow will be decreased since the circulating blood volume has improved

sufficiently to relieve the condition of shock and overload is to be avoided.

430. 2. Of the measures given, the one that is most likely to help relieve the discomfort of abdominal distention is to insert a rectal tube. The tube should be used for short periods of time since the tube should act as a stimulant for peristalsis. Leaving it in place indefinitely defeats this goal.

431. 4. Neostigmine bromide acts to stimulate peristalsis by its effects on the smooth muscles in the intestinal tract. Psyllium hydrophilic mucilloid helps to relieve constipation and constipation predisposes to distention. However, the first choice for relatively early relief of distention is to use the neostigmine bromide. Codeine sulfate and diazepam may relieve discomfort and worry but will not relieve the condition causing it.

432. 1. It is much easier to lift a patient from the bed when she is lying near the edge of the bed rather than in the middle of the bed. The least amount of effort will be used by the carriers if the patient is slid to the edge of the bed rather than lifted to the position. Techniques described in options 2, 3, and 4 will place extra and unnecessary strain on the carriers.

433. 3. It is best for the nurse to rest the patient on her hip after she has formed a wide base of support by separating her feet. This maneuver is relatively easy and can be maintained until help is available. Having the patient close her eyes is unlikely to relieve her symptoms of fainting. Maneuvering the patient to the floor requires considerable strength and the technique may result in injury to the patient. This patient cannot use the technique described in option 4 since she recently had back surgery.

434. 1. It is best for the patient to place her feet flat on the floor. This ordinarily provides the greatest comfort since it places no strain on the operative area. If the patient is allowed to choose her own position, she may choose one that places strain on her back. The nurse should serve as the teacher and explain that placing the feet flat on the floor is recommended.

435. 2. The brace should be applied before the patient is out of bed and before she places weight on her legs and back. The brace should be placed on the bed while the patient is on her side. She should then be rolled onto the brace. Hyperextension of the back following back surgery is contraindicated.

436. 2. Experience has shown that it is best to have the patient wear a thin cotton shirt under the brace. Using padding may increase pressure points. Lubricating and powdering the skin

under the brace does not provide the best protection for the
skin from irritation by the brace.

437. 1. Following back surgery, the patient should keep her back in
straight alignment. Hence, squatting to the floor is not contraindicated. Activities described in options 2, 3, and 4 are
ordinarily contraindicated because of the possibility of back
strain and twisting.

JOHN MARLEN

438. 3. For this unmarried gentleman, it would be best to obtain
permission for treatment from a responsible relative.

439. 1. Of highest priority for this patient is to be sure that his airway
is patent. Other measures can wait until the nurse is sure the
patient is able to breathe properly.

440. 4. Passive immunity for tetanus will be provided by tetanus
antitoxin. The other agents given here will provide active
immunity because they stimulate the body to produce its own
antibodies.

441. 4. Tetanus antitoxin is manufactured from horse serum. It
should not be given if the patient has a history of an allergic
reaction to horse serum until further consultation with the
physician.

442. 2. Tetanus immunity is specific for the prevention of lockjaw.
The etiological agent for lockjaw is Clostridium tetani. Gas
gangrene is usually caused by Clostridium perfringens; an
antitoxin is available. Tetany is a muscular contraction and
not a disease. Meningitis may be caused by many different
organisms and is usually treated with the help of drugs.

443. 4. The pulse pressure is determined by subtracting the diastolic
pressure from the systolic pressure. This patient's admission
pulse pressure was 44. Option 4 describes a pulse pressure of
60 and is greater than the patient's initial pressure.

444. 3. The respiratory center is located in the medulla oblongata
which is area C in the illustration.

445. 4. As the cranial content is increased within the bony cranial
frame, the thermal regulatory center is compressed resulting
in uncontrolled elevated temperature. Signs given in the
other options are typical of the condition.

446. 3. The foramen magnum is a large opening in the skull through
which the spinal cord communicates with the brain. It is
through this opening that the brain will herniate if intracranial
pressure progresses markedly.

447. 1. The area where an extradural hematoma has developed is best
depicted as site A in the illustration.

448. 1. Visual acuity is least significant when assessing for intracranial pressure. Assessments given in options 2, 3, and 4 are important.

449. 4. Pupil accommodation is controlled by the oculomotor nerve. The optic nerve is the nerve of vision. The acoustic nerve is concerned with hearing and equilibrium. The olfactory nerve is concerned with the sense of smell.

450. 3. Cerebrospinal fluid will have a positive glucose reaction; mucus will not.

451. 1. It would be least helpful to suggest that the family and friends of this patient wait at home. Options 2, 3, and 4 offer supportive measures and are recommended.

452. 1. Manitol is a diuretic. It helps to decrease intracranial pressure by its dehydrating effects. The drug is acting in the desired manner when the urinary output is increasing. Although goals described in options 2, 3, and 4 *may* be desired, this drug is not being used to accomplish these effects.

453. 4. To help this patient become oriented after a period of unconsciousness, it would be best for the nurse to explain where the patient is and why he is there. The comments described in options 1, 2, and 3 may be helpful for the nurse to determine the patient's mental orientation.

454. 2. Option 1 requires coordination as well as motor ability. Option 3 shows motor ability but not strength that the nurse can measure. Option 4 indicates sensory ability. Only option 2 can show comparative strength.

455. 1. It would be best to wrap the patient's hands in washcloths when he became restless while regaining consciousness. The measures described in options 2, 3, and 4 place a restraint on the patient which tends to increase activity and thus, intracranial pressure.

456. 4. Swallowing is least likely to increase intracranial pressure but sneezing, coughing, and vomiting are likely to increase intracranial pressure.

457. 3. The primary reason for using a cuffed tracheostomy tube is that it prevents air from escaping around it, thus facilitating ventilation. It *may* be more difficult to dislodge than an uncuffed tube but it is no more easy to clean and suction than an uncuffed tube. The patient is unable to speak with either an uncuffed or cuffed tube.

458. 1. The most important procedure to follow when a patient's tracheostomy tube is dislodged is to keep the airway patent. This can best be accomplished by opening the trachea with a hemostat.

459. 3. When suctioning is being used, the suction removes not only debris but also oxygen. It is recommended that suctioning be done for short periods in order to avoid depriving the patient of necessary oxygen. It is also often recommended that the patient be oxygenated prior to suctioning.

460. 2. For the reason described in item 459, it is generally recommended that suctioning be used for no longer than 10 to 15 seconds at one time.

461. 4. When the vagus nerve is stimulated (its pathway is along the back of the throat), the heart rate decreases. Prolonged suctioning could cause cardiac arrest for this reason.

462. 2. The recommended technique is to use a *sterile* catheter for *each* suctioning.

463. 3. The cuff on the tracheostomy tube decreases blood circulation to that part of the trachea. Hence, in order to prevent tissue trauma due to lack of circulation, it is recommended that the pressure in a cuffed tracheostomy tube be released for a few minutes at regular intervals.

464. 4. All observations described here will help to assess whether airway suctioning has been effective. However, hearing clear breath sounds during auscultation of the patient's chest is the most accurate method for assessing.

465. 2. The least appropriate procedure described here is to change the tracheostomy tube every other day. Ordinarily, the tracheostomy tube is changed by the physician and requires changing at less frequent intervals than two days.

466. 1. Whenever oxygen is administered, it should be humidified in order to decrease the viscosity of respiratory secretions. Oxygen given without added humidity will cause drying of the secretions and of the mucus membranes also. Humidified oxygen does not serve purposes described in the other options.

467. 4. The course of action recommended when humidity collects in the mechanical ventilator's tubing is to empty the fluid from the tubing and reconnect it again. Excessive water condensation in the tubing may impair the ventilator's proper functioning. The humidity is necessary to prevent irritation and drying of respiratory passages. It is not recorded.

468. 4. There are two parameters of particular significance in this patient's blood findings. The pCO_2 is below normal, normal being between approximately 35 and 45. The pH is in the alkaline range, normal being between 7.35 and 7.45. The bicarbonate level is somewhat elevated, normal being approximately 24. The patient is in respiratory alkalosis since the

alkaline pH is due to respiratory causes. It is probably due to the patient's hyperventilating and he would profit from using a slower rate of respirations.

469. 3. The normal range of the pH of arterial blood is between 7.35 and 7.45

470. 2. The degree of acidity or alkalinity of the blood involves the relationship between the cation, hydrogen, and the anion, hydroxyl.

471. 2. Diabetes insipidus is due to a deficiency in the antidiuretic hormone (ADH). The condition may occur in conjunction with head injuries as well as with other disease conditions. When the hormone is deficient, the patient excretes large amounts of highly diluted urine. This can be assessed by studying the specific gravity of urine samples.

472. 3. The air mattress is used primarily to relieve pressure on body parts. It helps prevent decubitus ulcers.

473. 2. Many nurses are finding that having the patient wear ankle high tennis shoes helps prevent footdrop. The shoes are worn periodically, that is, on 2 hours and off 2 hours. Another effective and more tradional technique is to place the patient's feet against a footboard to prevent footdrop. The measures described in options 1 and 3 are not indicated to help prevent footdrop. Even though using a cradle to keep linens off the patient's feet relieves pressure that tends to place the feet in footdrop position, in itself, the cradle will not prevent foot-drop. The patient's feet would still need support.

474. 3. To prevent external rotation of the hips, trochanter rolls alongside the patient's legs from the ilium to midthigh are recommended. Using sandbags from the knees to the ankle will not effectively support the hips in proper alignment. Op-tions 1 and 4 describe measures that also will not prevent hip rotation.

475. 3. The patient will not be in proper body alignment if his left arm rests on the mattress with the elbow flexed. This positioning of the arm pulls the left shoulder out of good alignment and by so doing, restricts respiratory movements. The positioning described in options 1, 2, and 4 are recommended.

476. 2. Decubitus ulcers are caused by pressure in an area which in turn, decreases circulation to that area. The poorly oxygen-ated tissues then tend to break down, causing a decubitus ulcer. The primary reason for massage is to improve circula-tion in the area. The massage may help relax muscles and may allow the skin to dry but these are of lesser importance in this instance.

477. 1. The knees are the least likely area for developing decubitus ulcers although it is possible for ulcers to develop there also.

478. 3. Meperidine hydrochloride is a narcotic. After receiving 100 mg. intramuscularly, it is very likely that the patient will be lethargic an hour later as a result of this drug.

SIDNEY CLATE

479. 3. All of the measures are of importance when planning this patient's postoperative care. However, since his eyesight is impaired and he will be wearing eyepatches postoperatively, it is of prime importance that he be well oriented to his physical surroundings.

480. 4. The patient with cataracts characteristically complains of blurred vision and hazy appearance of objects he views. The other options do not describe characteristic symptoms of cataracts.

481. 2. The exact cause of cataracts is not clearly understood but current theory is that it may possibly be related to changes in metabolism in the lenses of the eyes.

482. 3. O.D. (oculis dexter) refers to the right eye. O.S. (oculis sinister) refers to the left eye. O.U. (oculis uterque) refers to both eyes.

483. 2. When used topically, such as in eyedrops, phenylephrine hydrochloride acts to cause dilatation of the pupil and constriction of the blood vessels.

484. 1. Cyclopentolate hydrochloride produces cyclopegia, that is, paralysis of the ciliary muscles. By paralyzing the muscles, less movement of the eye will occur during the surgical procedure.

485. 2. Placing pressure against the nose at the inner angle of the closed eye prevents the drug from entering the lacrimal system where it would be absorbed into the general circulatory system. Eyedrops should be placed in the lower conjunctival sac which will help to prevent conditions given in options 1, 3, and 4.

486. 1. In order to help this patient and give him necessary support, it is best for the nurse to give the patient an opportunity to further express his feelings. She can then better plan nursing intervention and the patient has had an opportunity to vent his emotions. Comments posed in the other three options will not accomplish these goals as effectively.

487. 3. Patients with both eyes patched often will demonstrate symptoms of sensory deprivation unless steps are taken to prevent it. Of the options given here, the best choice is to

provide frequent verbal and physical stimulation. Options 1, 2, and 4 are likely to aggravate the situation since they decrease, not increase, sensory stimulation.

488. 3. Vomiting is contraindicated for the patient who has had cataract surgery. It tends to increase intraocular pressure which can lead to complications.

489. 2. Any activity that is likely to cause stress on the eye and increased intraocular pressure should be avoided. Activities such as coughing, sneezing, crying, straining, and the like, are contraindicated. The activities given in options 1, 3, and 4 are indicated and will not influence intraocular pressure.

490. 4. Bending from the hips to pick up slippers is contraindicated since this is likely to cause increased intraocular pressure. See also item 489. Activities described in options 1, 2, and 3 are not contraindicated.

491. 4. Pain and restlessness should suggest to the nurse that the patient may be suffering from intraocular hemorrhage. On the fifth postoperative day or so, hemorrhage is most likely to occur because at this time, granulation tissue is highly vascular and capillaries are very fragile.

492. 3. In order to give the eye ample time to heal and keep intraocular pressure at a minimum, generally patients should be instructed to limit activities for a period of about 4 to 6 weeks.

493. 2. Many older persons have been observed to feel that they have lost value and suffer with loss of feelings of self-worth. When this occurs, these people will almost always show signs of depression.

494. 2. Adjusting to the use of cataract glasses usually takes some
495. 2. time. Several suggestions have been found helpful. It is best to start wearing these glasses while sitting down because of the distortion in vision they create. Clear vision is best through the center of the lenses of these glasses. The patient should be taught to turn his head for lateral vision rather than try to use the periphery of the lenses. They should be worn at all times when awake. Colors of objects may be distorted in the operated eye.

496. 3. The cornea is composed of dense connective tissue. There are no blood vessels present in the cornea.

497. 3. The lenses of the eye focus light rays onto the retina. Accommodation is the process of bringing light rays into focus from both near and far objects. The aqueous humor is secreted from the ciliary bodies. The retina houses the rods and cones. The iris regulates the amount of light entering the eye.

498. 1. The optic nerve carries visual impulses from the eye to the

brain. The oculomotor, trochlear, and abducens nerves are concerned with movements of the eye.

499. 2. Rays focused in front of the retina result in myopia, or near-sightedness. When the rays are focused in back of the retina, hyperopia or farsightedness is present. The lenses tend to lose their elasticity with age, a condition known as presbyopia. This condition requires persons to wear bifocals for comfort while seeing; the glasses are making the adjustments which the lenses are no longer able to do. Miosis refers to constriction of the pupil.

JAMES TURNER

500. 1. Once a burn has occurred, the recommended emergency treatment is the application of cold. This helps relieve pain and also diminishes tissue damage. Measures described in options 2, 3, and 4 are contraindicated and may lead to further tissue damage.

501. 3. Using the "Rule of Nine" as a guide, this patient has sustained a burn of approximately 45 percent of his body.

502. 3. The burn victim loses much body fluid by the process of evaporation. The capillaries dilate and there is increased capillary permeability at the site of the burn. Plasma seeps out into the burned tissue and evaporation causes fluid loss.

503. 3. The best way to guide action in relation to the rate of flow of intravenous fluids being given to the burn victim is to observe hourly urine outputs. If output is low, the patient is under-hydrated. As the patient becomes hydrated, urinary output will increase. Many persons prefer CVP monitoring to regulate fluid administration. However, in this situation, it was not used and so the hourly output would provide the best information.

504. 1. An early sign that should alert the nurse to decreasing the rate of intravenous flow is hearing crackling chest sounds. This sign indicates pulmonary congestion.

505. 2. Most authorities indicate a minimum safe range for the hourly urine output to be between about 30 and 70 ml. If the output falls below this range, the situation requires immediate assessment and evaluation.

506. 2. The normal specific gravity is usually considered to be between about 1.015 and 1.025 or 1.030.

507. 2. Narcotics in large doses when pain is severe tends to camouflage the patient's symptoms. He is also usually not sufficiently alert mentally to report symptoms he does note. This adds to the difficulty of accurately assessing the patient.

508. 3. The fluid accumulation phase, or shock phase, occurs during

the first 48 hours after major burns. Extensive trauma to cells causes the release of potassium into extracellular spaces and the patient will then show signs of potassium excess.

509. 3. A severely burned patient will ordinarily receive analgesics intravenously. This assures immediate absorption. The patient is often unable to tolerate drugs orally. The rectal route is the least desirable in terms of effective absorption. The intramuscular route is often difficult to use because of the patient's condition.

510. 3. Many precautionary measures are ordinarily used when caring for the burn victim. However, authorities agree that the single most effective way to prevent infection is to have health personnel wash their hands carefully and thoroughly before and after all care.

511. 3. When the open method of wound care is used, bed linens should be kept off the wounds. To prevent air drafts over the burn areas, it is best to place a cradle on the bed and drape bed linens over the cradle. Other measures given here would not accomplish this task.

512. 3. When bandaging the hand, care should be taken to prevent two body surfaces from touching and also to maintain functional body alignment by placing the fingers and thumb over a roll of gauze or bandage roll.

513. 4. Gastric dilatation and paralytic ileus commonly occur when a patient is severely burned. Hence, oral fluids and foods are contraindicated. Parenteral hyperalimentation is an effective method for supplying the body with nutrients, and especially protein which the burn victim ordinarily needs in larger than average amounts.

514. 3. The superior vena cava is preferred since it is a large rapid-flow vein and the concentrated solution will dilute rapidly. The superior vena cava is generally entered via the right or left subclavian vein.

515. 2. The solution introduced when TPN is used is hypertonic.

516. 3. The major complication associated with TPN is infection. Hence, it is of utmost importance to observe rigid aseptic techniques when caring for the patient and when handling the equipment and dressings related to the TPN therapy.

517. 4. The urine should be examined for glucose. If the patient is not metabolizing the nutrients well, glucose tends to be found in the urine.

518. 2. Skin oils tend to harbor organisms. Hence, it is recommended that ether or acetone be used to remove these oils since these two agents break down bacteria cell walls.

519. 4. When the catheter is open, air may enter in sufficient quan-

tities to produce a fatal air embolism. Using the Valsalva's maneuver causes increased intrathoracic pressure and helps prevent air from entering the system.

520. 2. Yellow drainage suggests the presence of organisms and hence, when it appears, a sensitivity test and culture are most likely to be ordered.

521. 3. Gentamicin sulfate has been found to be particularly effective for treating pseudomonas infections.

522. 3. Removing dressings which will expose sensitive nerve endings to air is very painful. Hence, most persons advise administering analgesics prior to major painful dressing changes to provide for more patient comfort.

523. 1. The first step before beginning skin grafts is to be sure the area receiving grafts is free of dead and necrotic tissue. If this is not done, the graft is unlikely to take and may become infected.

524. 4. The use of analgesics for the control of pain will not influence graft survival and effectiveness. Factors noted in options 1, 2, and 3 will influence the graft.

525. 2. Emotional support has been described in many ways. The best definition indicates that the person needing support receives it by using the strengths of a caring person. This is different, it can be noted, from allowing venting of emotions. Patients very often reject advice and suggestions.

526. 4. Gastrointestinal ulceration is often observed following severe burns. The ulcers are referred to as Curling's ulcers. The other complications given here are not generally stress-related, as Curling's ulcers are.

527. 3. The young adult is ordinarily concerned with resolving intimacy and isolation. Autonomy versus doubt is a conflict usually observed in toddlers. Trust versus mistrust is a conflict of babyhood. Identity versus role confusion is a conflict of youth.

528. 2. Grafts made from animal tissues or from other species are called xenografts. An isograft is a graft taken from a person other than the patient, such as an identical twin. An autograft is one taken from the patient himself. The term, allograft, is used interchangeably with homograft, meaning that skin taken from cadavers of the same species is used.

529. 2. A pedicle graft carries its own blood supply. The other grafts given here are free grafts and depend on the recipient site for nourishment.

530. 3. The best way to assess physiological circulation in this case is to press skin on unburned areas and observe for capillary

filling. Central venous pressure may be necessary but for monitoring hemodynamic parameters.

531. 3. Many measures are used to help prevent overwhelming infection but of highest priority is to provide a new skin cover. Other aspects given in options 1, 2, and 4 are also involved but do not have highest priority.

532. 3. Biological dressings serve many purposes, one of which is that they enhance growth of epithelial tissues. They also prevent loss of water and protein, decrease pain, increase mobility, and help prevent infection.

533. 4. Silver nitrate solutions tend to upset electrolyte balance. Sodium and potassium in particular are lost into the dressings.

534. 1. Silver nitrate stains everything with which it comes in contact. The nurse is advised to use gloves to protect her hands from staining.

535. 1. Emergency action when the clothes are on fire is to roll on the floor. This helps to smother the fire and extinguish it.

536. 1. The capillary walls become permeable and fluid is lost with relative ease.

537. 4. It has been determined that most fires in the home start in living rooms and kitchens.

538. 3. Eschar is dead tissue, heavily contaminated with bacteria, and without a blood supply. It is tissue that sloughs.

CONFERENCE ON PAIN

539. 3. According to the gate control theory, the regulatory process is located in the spinal canal.

540. 1. Stimulating cutaneous fibers tends to close the gate. Hence, giving the patient a back rub when pain is present uses the gate control theory.

541. 3. Responses to pain are directed toward the body's ability to escape or flee the source of pain. The body's responses are typical of the fight-or-flight phenomenon.

542. 4. A typical psychic reaction to pain is experiencing anxiety. The other responses given here are autonomic (crying) or skeletal (grimacing and pacing) responses to pain.

543. 3. Efferent nerve routes carry impulses from the central nervous system to an effector. An efferent nerve carries an impulse from the brain to the abdomen. The impulses given in options 1, 2, and 4 are traveling along afferent nerves, that is, they are traveling from the periphery to the central nervous system.

544. 2. A reflex response travels to and from the spinal cord—it does not travel to higher centers in the central nervous system.

545. 3. In this example, the patient's attention is diverted. This

technique decreases the patient's perception of his pain. Distraction does not function in ways described in the wrong options.

546. 1. Pain perception is located in the thalamus.
547. 4. The cause of pain when the bladder is distended is a mechanical agent. A thermal agent is one that causes pain due to heat, as in the case of a burn. A chemical agent causes irritation, such as a burn caused by an acid. An electrical agent involves electrical shock.
548. 1. The opioids relieve pain by reducing the perception of pain. They do not function in ways given in options 2, 3, and 4.

MISCELLANEOUS ITEMS

549. 4. Hemorrhoids that bleed periodically do not constitute an emergency situation. Options 1, 2, and 3 describe emergency situations.
550. 4. The appendix is located in the right lower quadrant of the abdomen. The letters, RLQ, are often used to designate this area. RUQ refers to the right upper quadrant. LUQ refers to the left upper quadrant. LLQ refers to the left lower quadrant.
551. 3. A middle-aged person with well-controlled diabetes has no more surgical risk than a nondiabetic patient. The statements made in options 1, 2, and 4 are not necessarily accurate.
552. 1. A pyloroplasty is a surgical procedure done in order to enlarge the pyloric opening. It is commonly preformed on newborns with pyloric stenosis.
553. 4. The patient in an intensive care unit often suffers from sensory deprivation. Sensory deprivation is due to a lack of sensory input as well as a change in the quality of sensory input. The patient in an intensive care unit is subject to monotonous, continuous noises of equipment, and he has few if any normal social contacts. Hence, this patient will frequently suffer from sensory deprivation.
554. 2. Discussing normal daily events with a patient subject to sensory deprivation is helpful. The experience offers a social-like relationship that provides sensory input which is a welcomed relief from the usual monotony of the unit. Options 1, 3, and 4 suggest measures that tend to increase sensory deprivation.
555. 3. A patient subject to seizure activity should have his temperature taken by a route other than oral when a mercury glass thermometer is used. There is danger of breaking a ther-

mometer of this type in his mouth if a seizure occurs while taking his oral temperature.

556. 4. The patient will not normally respond to painful stimuli during the clonic phase of an epileptic seizure. Hence, reporting this information would be of least value. However, observations described in options 1, 2, and 3 are of value to the physician.

557. 2. The serum acid phosphate level frequently increases when a malignancy extends outside of the prostatic capsule. The other examinations given here are not diagnostic of metastasis.

558. 3. To help regain urinary control, the patient should be taught to alternately tense and relax the perineal muscles. This exercise may be performed as many as 20 or 30 times every hour.

559. 4. It has been found that allowing the patient to express his anger is more helpful than trying to help him control it. Anger as an emotional expression does not have the equivalent psychological benefit that patients experience when they develop independence after periods of illness.

560. 1. A tourniquet should be available when caring for a patient who has had an amputation. The tourniquet will be used to control bleeding should it occur from the stump postoperatively. The equipment listed in options 2, 3, and 4 is not ordinarily required by a patient who has had an amputation.

561. 4. Range-of-motion exercises should be started early after an amputation in order to help avoid contracture deformities. Splinting the joint may prevent contractures but may also result in an ankylosis ("frozen joint") and is contraindicated.

562. 4. The palms of the hands should bear the bulk of the weight when crutch-walking. If the weight is borne by the axillae, damage to nerves may result.

563. 4. In order to strengthen arm muscles, push ups as described in options 3 are recommended. The exercises described in options 1, 2, and 3 may play important roles in the care of a patient prior to ambulation but they will not strengthen arm muscles.

564. 1. When a spinal cord injury is believed to be present, the patient should be transported in such a way that there is least movement (turning, twisting, bending) of the back. Injury to the cord may be increased if the back is not held straight and firmly. Of the available methods to transport this patient, placing him on a board is the method of choice since it best accomplishes the goal described above.

565. 1. When Crutchfield tongs are used, counterweight will be obtained by the weight of the patient's body. In order to prevent

pulling the patient up in bed and against the head board, the head of the bed should be elevated.

566. 1. A patient with permanent damage to the spinal cord at C8 will not be able to walk but is capable of learning to write, feed himself, and drive a car.

567. 3. Pressure sores are especially difficult to treat in a patient with a spinal cord injury and can endanger the life of the patient. Hence, preventing decubitus ulcers is of prime importance when caring for a patient with spinal cord injury. The conditions given in options 1, 2, and 4 are not necessarily life-threatening but nursing efforts should be directed toward preventing them.

568. 2. The parts of the body below the injury are paralyzed and flaccid and the reflexes are absent. Since sympathetic activity is blocked, the patient will not perspire in that part of the body. Hence, the patient should be watched especially carefully for onset of fever when he is suffering with spinal shock. The blood pressure will fall when spinal shock is present.

569. 3. A general anesthesia controls fear and anxiety since the patient is unconscious. Options 1, 2, and 4 are inaccurate statements, except that respiratory depression is not common when general anesthesia is well administered.

570. 1. With spinal anesthesia, sympathetic afferent fibers to a region of the body have been blocked. Therefore, constrictor impulses to veins in that region are blocked and there is diminished return of blood to the heart. This results in a decrease in arterial blood pressure.

571. 1. Epinephrine when used with an injectable local anesthesia prolongs the effects of the anesthesia. Since epinephrine causes vasconstriction, the anesthesia is absorbed slowly and there is also likely to be less bleeding in the area.

572. 3. The primary reason for the continued use of ether as an anesthesia is that it has a wide margin of safety between nontoxicity and toxicity. It rarely produces cardiovascular complications. It also produces good muscle relaxation. However, it is explosive and recovery is ordinarily accompanied with unpleasant symptoms.

573. 1. Hypothermia decreases the rate of metabolism and, hence, the body then requires less oxygen. Therefore, less general anesthesia is required if hypothermia is used prior to or as an adjunct to a surgical procedure.

574. 4. Lactated Ringer's solution contains several electrolytes—sodium, potassium, calcium, chloride, and lactate, for example. Solutions described in options 1 and 2 do not conatin electrolytes; option 3 contains only one electrolyte.

575. 3. Preoperatively, the malnourished patient needs a high caloric diet with high carbohydrate, protein, and vitamin content to help prevent complications and promote wound healing.

576. 2. Bunions are most often caused by improperly fitted shoes. A short shoe is the usual culprit. Conditions given in the other options do not predispose to bunions.

577. 3. The synonym for bunion is hallux valgus. An osteoma is a tumor composed of bone. Primary gout is a painful inflammation of joints, usually those in the great toe. Morton's neuroma is a type of tumor which contains nervelike cells.

578. 1. Despite much research, the cause of atherosclerosis is unknown. However, it is believed that a high level of cholesterol is related to the disease and obesity and lack of activity appear to predispose to it.

579. 4. The rectal tube provides an exit for flatus but it also acts to stimulate the colon to contract. If the tube is left in too long, the responsiveness of the colon is reduced. It is generally recommended that the tube not be left in place for periods of longer than 20 minutes.

580. 2. The advantage of the Stryker frame is that the patient can be turned while keeping the spine immobilized. A patient cannot turn himself on a Stryker frame and it does not automatically support the body in good anatomical alignment. The patient on this frame still needs care to avoid pressure sores since the weight is not distributed in a way so that decubitus ulcers are unlikely to develop.

581. 2. The rocking bed has a motor which causes the bed to rock rhythmically up and down. The motor is set to correspond with the patient's respirations. By shifting abdominal organs, the diaphragm is helped to move up and down, thereby facilitating breathing.

582. 2. In order to help maintain the normal acid environment in the vagina, a douche with a white vinegar solution is recommended by many gynecologists. The other agents given here *may* by necessary (an antiseptic if an infection is present) or at least may not be contraindicated. But the vinegar solution is the one of choice for personal hygiene purposes.

583. 1. The tonometer measures intraocular pressure. It is used to help in diagnosing glaucoma. Instruments are not ordinarily used to diagnose cataracts, corneal ulcers, or retinal detachment, other than using the ophthalmoscope.

584. 1. It is important that no currents reach the pacemaker since they could cause ventricular fibrillations. The environment must be electrically safe. Protecting the unit and wires in a plastic bag while giving the patient a bath will help prevent currents

from reaching the unit. Such currents would travel especially well on the wet skin surface.

585. 4. The tip of the catheter is placed in the apex of the right ventricle which is muscular (thicker than the atrial wall) and there is less tendency for the lead to become dislodged or rupture through the wall in this location.

586. 4. Common symptoms of pacemaker failure which the patient should be taught to report immediately include dizziness, fainting, change in pulse rate, palpitations, and chest pain. Symptoms given in options 1, 2, and 3 are not associated with pacemaker failure.

587. 2. The double balloon gastric tube is used in order to create pressure on the bleeding areas in the esophagus. Once the tube is in the stomach, the balloon is inflated and pulled toward the cardiac sphincter. The balloon creates the pressure on the varices.

588. 3. Both statements are true. However, suctioning does not explain the reason for using humidified air for patients with respiratory problems.

589. 2. Oxygen has been found to reduce the surface tension of fat globules in the presence of a fat embolism. Other types of therapy, as described here, will not help decrease fat emboli.

590. 2. The most common symptom of laryngeal cancer is hoarseness that does not respond to usual therapy.

591. 2. Obstruction in the small intestines will produce vomiting of fecal material. Reverse peristalsis brings the material up to the stomach and it is then vomited.

592. 1. If the lateral aspect of the sole of the foot is stroked, the toes will normally contract and be drawn tightly together. This is referred to as the Babinski reflex. A positive Babinski reflex usually indicates meningeal irritation.

593. 2. Women who experience feelings of worthlessness or say their usefulness has ceased are suffering from what is often called the "empty nest" syndrome. It is best prevented and treated by helping the person find purposeful activity to occupy free time.

594. 2. The phrenic nerve is a branch of the cervical plexus. It supplies motor fibers to the diaphragm. If it is injured, respirations will be affected.

595. 4. The temperature regulating center is located in the hypothalamus. Rates of respiration and heartbeat and maintenance of blood pressure are regulated by centers in the medulla oblongata.

596. 1. When a normal blood cell is placed in a hypertonic solution,

fluid from the cell will leave the cell and enter the solution. The result is that the cell will shrink in size. This is referred to as crenation. If the cell was placed in a hypotonic solution, fluid would enter the cell and the cell would eventually burst. This is referred to as hemolysis.

597. 1. The passage of a solvent through a semipermeable membrane is referred to as osmosis.

598. 3. Gastric lavage uses the principle of a siphon. The stomach contents are emptied by the use of a syringe or bulb device. A partial vacuum is created in the bulb or syringe and the pressure of the contents in the stomach forces the contents to seek the area of a partial vacuum.

599. 4. Alcohol has a low vaporization point. Alcohol added to water when giving the patient a cool sponge bath causes evaporation to occur more rapidly. The heat necessary for evaporation comes from the patient's body.

600. 2. The initial reaction of the body to cold is vasoconstriction. If edema is already present, cold is contraindicated. When an ankle sprain occurs, cold is indicated beftre swelling occurs to help prevent edema.

601. 4. Wafarin sodium is an anticoagulant. Therefore, in order to prevent excessive bleeding, a patient about to have surgery should discontinue the use of the medication. Digoxin is a digitalis preparation used to strengthen the heart beat. Tolbutamide is an oral hypoglycemic. Prednisone is a cortisone derivative used usually as an antiinflammatory agent. It would be most unlikely that any of these three drugs would be discontinued before surgery.

602. 3. Of the age groups given here, premature infants tolerate surgery least well.

603. 4. Lung cancer deaths could be reduced markedly, according to most authorities, by eliminating the cigarette-smoking habit. There are harmful aspects to any use of tobacco but cigarette smoking is most often linked to lung cancer.

604. 2. The incidence of rheumatic fever is highest among school age children. See also item 206.

605. 1. The leading cause of death among persons over 45 years of age is heart diseases. Malignant neoplasms rank second. Cerebrovascular diseases rank third. Cirrhosis of the liver ranks approximately last.

606. 2. According to research, the peak of intellectual and physical abilities is reached between the ages of 20 and 30.

607. 4. The fastest growing segment of the population, in relation to age, is the elderly, that is, persons over 65 years of age. It has

been predicted that there will be 16 percent more people over 65 years of age in 1980 than there were in 1970.

608. 3. The thought process slows with advancing age. Older persons are perfectly capable of learning but it takes a little longer. Intelligence survives intact and older persons in good health do not lose judgment, their ability to think abstractly, or their knowledge. Sexual activity need not necessarily end with advancing age.

obstetric nursing

Ms. Julie Anderson, a nurse and a childbirth educator, is preparing and reviewing material for classes she is conducting for a group of pregnant women and their husbands. Items 1 through 73 pertain to these classes.

Items 1 through 17 pertain to the anatomy, physiology, and genetics of human reproduction.

1. When during the menstrual cycle do most women ovulate?
    1. During the menstrual period.
    2. Shortly before the menstrual period.
    3. Shortly following the menstrual period.
    4. Approximately 2 weeks before the beginning of the menstrual period.
2. When the ovum is expelled from the graafian follicle, it is next received by the
    1. ovary.
    2. vagina.
    3. uterus.
    4. fallopian tube.
3. The anatomical structure in which fertilization of the ovum normally occurs is the
    1. uterus.
    2. corpus luteum.
    3. fallopian tubes.
    4. graafian follicle.
4. The uterus receives its blood supply directly from the uterine artery and from the
    1. iliac artery.
    2. ovarian artery.

3. hypogastric artery.

4. uterosacral artery.

5. Which one of the following hormones stimulates ovulation and the development of the corpus luteum?

1. Estrogenic hormone.

2. Luteinizing hormone.

3. Adrenocorticotropic hormone.

4. Follicle-stimulating hormone.

6. For approximately how many hours after ovulation does the ovum normally remain viable?

1. 1 to 2 hours.

2. 3 to 6 hours.

3. 10 to 12 hours.

4. 22 to 26 hours.

7. For approximately how long a period of time is the sperm capable of fertilizing the ovum?

1. 12 to 24 hours.

2. 24 to 48 hours.

3. 2 to 3 days.

4. 3 to 7 days.

8. In approximately how many days after conception does the fertilized ovum normally implant itself in the uterine wall?

1. 3 days.

2. 7 days.

3. 11 days.

4. 15 days.

9. The placenta is formed by a fusion of the chorionic villi and the

1. decidua vera.

2. chorion laeve.

3. decidua basalis.

4. chorion frondosum.

10. Which one of the following statements does *not* describe a function of the placenta?

1. The placenta acts to bring maternal blood directly to the fetal circulatory system.

2. The placenta acts as an organ to provide nourishment between the mother and the fetus.

3. The placenta acts as a gland producing hormones which affect both the mother and the fetus.

4. The placenta acts as a barrier to prevent certain substances from entering the fetal circulation.

11. The bluish discoloration of the vaginal mucosa, which is a presumptive sign of pregnancy, is called

1. Babcock's sign.

2. Chadwick's sign.
3. Goodell's sign.
4. Hegar's sign.
12. An early sign of pregnancy is present when, upon manual manipulation, the examiner feels the walls of the lower uterine segment to be
1. nodular.
2. softened.
3. elongated.
4. thickened.
13. The purplish streaks that sometimes appear on the breasts and abdomen during pregnancy are called
1. alveoli.
2. chloasma.
3. linea nigra.
4. striae gravidarum.
14. The nurse's discussion of the discoloration and enlargement of the areola during pregnancy should be based on knowledge that these changes are
1. without significance in relation to physical health.
2. more pronounced when the fetus is a male.
3. more common in blondes than brunettes.
4. related to an allergic response of the body.
15. The genetic information in the chromosomes is carried in a part of the cell known as
1. golgi apparatus.
2. endoplasmic reticulum (ER).
3. ribonucleic acid (RNS).
4. deoxyribonucleic acid (DNA).
16. The number of chromosomes in each mature sperm or ovum is
1. 4.
2. 12.
3. 23.
4. 45.
17. The presence of a Y chromosome in the fertilized ovum means that the resulting infant will be a
1. boy.
2. girl.
3. mongoloid.
4. hemophiliac.

Items 18 through 23 pertain to fetal development.

18. In the fetus, the foramen ovale allows blood to bypass the
1. left ventricle.

2. coronary sinus.

3. superior vena cava.

4. pulmonary circulatory system.

19. The nurse teaches that the umbilical cord contains blood vessels, the total number normally being

1. two arteries and one vein.

2. one vein and one artery.

3. two veins and one artery.

20. Which organ in the mother's body acts to *detoxify* the waste products of the fetus?

1. The spleen.

2. The liver.

3. The lungs.

4. The kidneys.

21. A father asks when the fetal heartbeat begins. At approximately what age does the anatomical structure in the fetus that eventually becomes the heart normally begin to beat?

1. 1 month.

2. 2 month.

3. 3 months.

4. 4 months.

22. The nurse speaks about how the fetus is nourished. The name of the blood vessel in which the oxygen content is highest in the fetus is the

1. aorta.

2. umbilical vein.

3. pulmonary artery.

4. inferior vena cava.

23. Although research to date has had certain contradictory conclusions, the *most* consistent finding is that, when compared with nonsmokers, mothers who smoke during an entire pregnancy tend to produce infants that

1. are anemic.

2. have lower birth weights.

3. are prone to develop breathing difficulties.

4. have a higher rate of congenital anomalies.

Items 24 through 50 pertain to certain dietary considerations and to some of the common discomforts of pregnancy.

24. One mother states that she prefers skim milk to whole milk. Which one of the following nutrients is deficient in unfortified skim milk?

1. Calcium.

2. Protein.

3. Vitamin A.
4. Riboflavin.
25. When whole milk is fortified, the vitamin added to the milk before it is marketed is vitamin
1. A.
2. B.
3. C.
4. D.
26. Folic acid deficiency during pregnancy can be avoided by including foods in the diet that are high in folic acid content, one food being
1. asparagus.
2. peaches.
3. eggs.
4. milk.
27. Of the following food constituents, the one which *most* pregnant women need supplementary amounts of is
1. iron.
2. calcium.
3. potassium.
4. vitamin C.
28. An inadequate diet during pregnancy is generally believed to be a contributing factor in *all* of the following conditions *except*
1. prematurity.
2. preeclampsia.
3. abortion and stillbirth.
4. placenta previa and placenta abruptio.
29. The physician ordered one mother to have a diet that contains 70 Gm. of protein each day. How many calories will the protein contribute to her daily diet?
1. 140 calories.
2. 210 calories.
3. 280 calories.
4. 350 calories.
30. The nurse teaches the mothers that, of the following factors, the one that contributes *most* to the discomfort of hemorrhoids is
1. lifting heavy objects.
2. taking long automobile rides.
3. having frequent constipation.
4. having sexual intercourse late in pregnancy.
31. Of the following solution, which one is *most often* recommended for women at home when wet compresses are used to relieve the discomfort of hemorrhoids?
1. Witch hazel solution.

2. Table salt solution.

3. Boric acid solution.

4. Soda bicarbonate solution.

32. In relation to constipation, the nurse should teach that it is *best* for the patient to

1. use a glycerin suppository as necessary.

2. increase the amounts of roughage and liquids in her diet.

3. increase the amount of rest and sleep in her daily living.

4. use a mild laxative, such as Milk of Magnesia, as necessary.

33. If one of the women complain of some vaginal discharge and local itching, the nurse should advise her to

1. report the symptoms to her physician.

2. refrain from having sexual intercourse.

3. take a mild acid douche under low pressure.

4. take an alkaline douche under low pressure.

34. Of the following suggestions that the nurse could offer, which one is *least often* recommended to help prevent flatulence during pregnancy?

1. Avoiding foods that tend to produce gas.

2. Eating small amounts of food at one time.

3. Taking a little soda bicarbonate in water as necessary.

4. Establishing the habit of having a daily bowel movement.

35. The nurse explains that frequency of urination is common during the first 3 months of pregnancy because of

1. anxiety about labor and delivery.

2. changes in the water and electrolyte balance.

3. pressure on the bladder from the enlarging uterus.

4. increased hydrostatic pressure in the bladder.

36. The nurse should teach that heartburn is due to

1. an increase in peristaltic action.

2. a displacement of the stomach by the uterus.

3. an increase in the secretion of hydrochloric acid.

4. a backflow of stomach contents into the esophagus.

37. Heartburn can often be prevented if, before a meal, the patient eats or drinks a

1. pat of butter.

2. few sips of tea.

3. teaspoon of lemon juice.

4. teaspoon of soda bicarbonate.

38. Which one of the following suggestions is *most helpful* in relieving early morning nausea when it occurs?

1. Use a liquid diet for breakfast.

2. Eat a little dry food before arising.

3. Sip a glass of milk before breakfast.

4. Drink a carbonated beverage before arising.

39. Cramps in the legs during pregnancy are believed to be caused by an increased absorption of
    1. iron.
    2. calcium.
    3. phosphorus.
    4. vitamin B.

40. Of the following measures for relieving discomfort due to leg cramps, the one that is *most effective* is
    1. walking until the cramp disappears.
    2. alternately flexing and extending the leg.
    3. lying flat in bed with the legs extended and elevated.
    4. pushing upward on the toes and downward on the knee.

41. Which one of the following positions in bed is likely to be *most helpful* in relieving the discomfort of varicosities of the vulva?
    1. Lying flat in bed on the abdomen.
    2. The back-lying position with the legs elevated on pillows.
    3. The semisitting position with the knees somewhat flexed.
    4. The side-lying position with the hips elevated on a pillow.

42. Which one of the following exercises has been found to be *most helpful* in relieving backaches during pregnancy?
    1. Sit-ups.
    2. Leg-lifts.
    3. Knee-bends.
    4. Pelvic-rock.

43. The nurse teaches that varicose veins often occur during pregnancy due to
    1. a decrease in normal cardiac output.
    2. an increase in maternal blood volume.
    3. an interference with venous return from extremities.
    4. a constriction in the blood vessel walls in extremities.

44. Of the following practices, which one is *contraindicated* because of a possible problem with varicose veins?
    1. Wearing sandals.
    2. Wearing no stockings.
    3. Wearing round garters.
    4. Wearing a garter belt.

45. One woman with varicose veins was advised to place her legs upright against the wall several times a day. The purpose of this procedure is to help
    1. strengthen the valves in the veins.
    2. increase the muscle tone of the legs.
    3. facilitate drainage from the extremities.
    4. decrease the supply of blood through the arteries.

46. Statement A below is a correct statement. What is the relationship between statements A and B?

Statement A: Weakened veins can usually function more effectively when their walls are supported.

Statement B: When an extremity is being bandaged because of varicosities, bandaging should start at the distal end of the extremity and be worked toward the trunk of the body.

1. Statement B is true; statement A explains or confirms statement B.
2. Statement B is true; statement A neither helps explain nor confirm statement B.
3. Statement B is false; statement A contradicts or indicates the falsity of statement B.
4. Statement B is false; statement A neither contradicts nor indicates the falsity of statement B.

47. Statement A below is a correct statement. What is the relationship between statements A and B?

Statement A: Blood flow through tissues is decreased by applying excessive pressure on blood vessels.

Statement B: When applying an elastic bandage to the leg because of varicose veins, the entire foot, including the toes, should be wrapped.

1. Statement B is true; statement A explains or confirms statement B.
2. Statement B is true; statement A neither helps explain nor confirm statement B.
3. Statement B is false; statement A contradicts or indicates the falsity of statement B.
4. Statement B is false; statement A neither contradicts nor indicates the falsity of statement B.

48. One of the women asks the nurse about the brown discoloration across her nose and cheeks. Which one of the following statements most accurately reflects current opinion concerning such skin discolorations?

1. It is best to see her physician since discolorations may be potentially serious and may require treatment.
2. It is best to do nothing since discolorations usually disappear and are without clinical significance.
3. Exposure to sunlight frequently helps to fade the discolored areas.
4. Most discoloration will fade when her physician prescribes an antihistamine drug for her.

49. Which one of the following statements *best* describes current opinion concerning pregnant women traveling by automobile?

1. It is recommended that seat belts be worn over the abdomen.
2. It is recommended that periodic rest periods be taken while traveling by automobile.
3. It is recommended that traveling by automobile be avoided during pregnancy.
4. It is recommended that automobile travel be limited to 1- or 2-hour trips.
50. One woman tells the nurse that she wants to nurse her baby but says she has inverted nipples. She asks what she can do during pregnancy to alleviate the problem. Of the following suggestions, which one is *most likely* to help?
1. Pull out the nipples daily with the fingers.
2. Wear a brassiere that is cut open at the nipples.
3. Brush the nipples lightly with a terry cloth towel.
4. Wear a breast shield that exerts mild suction on the nipples.

Items 51 through 73 pertain to late pregnancy, labor, and delivery.

51. The nurse explains that late in pregnancy, showers rather than tub baths are usually recommended. Which one of the following statements provides the *best* rationale for this recommendation?
1. Bath water is likely to introduce bacteria from the body into the vagina.
2. A change in the center of gravity of the mother predisposes her to accidental falls when using a tub.
3. Sitting in warm water increases the frequency of Braxton-Hicks contractions.
4. The shower spray provides necessary stimulation of the skin for optimal elimination of wastes.
52. Lightening, which the nurse explains as a typical sign of approaching labor, is *best* defined as
1. intermittent painless contractions.
2. settling of the fetal head into the pelvis.
3. loss of weight that occurs just prior to the onset of labor.
4. shortening of the cervix that occurs prior to the onset of true labor.
53. It is theorized that an increase in *all* of the following secretions in the body plays a role in initiating the onset of labor *except* for secretions of
1. relaxin.
2. oxytocin.
3. progesterone.
4. fetal corticosteroids.

54. The major distinction between true labor and false labor is that when true labor is present, the patient will demonstrate
   1. an increase in vaginal discharge.
   2. discomfort with uterine contractions.
   3. regular and rhythmic uterine contractions.
   4. progressive dilatation of the cervix with effacement.
55. The nurse explains that effacement means a normal change during labor which is described as
   1. a decrease in the length of the cervical canal.
   2. an increase in the opening of the cervical canal.
   3. relaxation of perineal musculature.
   4. contraction of abdominal musculature.
56. The unit of measure commonly used to describe effacement is a
   1. decimal.
   2. percentage.
   3. centimeter.
   4. fingerbreadth.
57. The nurse teaches that systematic abdominal palpation, commonly called Leopold's maneuvers, is used *primarily* to help
   1. determine the fetal position.
   2. turn the fetus in the uterus.
   3. ease the fetus lower into the pelvis.
   4. estimate the position of the placenta.
58. The patient will be more comfortable and the results more accurate when the patient is prepared for Leopold's maneuvers by having her
   1. empty her bladder.
   2. lie on her left side.
   3. hyperventilate for a short time.
   4. avoid eating immediately before the examination.
59. Which one of the following techniques should the nurse use to help prevent contractions of the patient's abdominal muscles when the nurse begins utilizing Leopold's maneuvers?
   1. Have the patient extend her legs flat on the bed.
   2. Palpate with her hands flat on the patient's abdomen.
   3. Use her fingers to palpate an outline of the fetal body.
   4. Have the patient take quick breaths when beginning the procedure.
60. The nurse explains that flexion of the fetal head during labor is important because the more the head is flexed, the
   1. straighter is the plane of delivery.
   2. greater is the long axis of the fetus.
   3. smaller is the diameter of the skull entering the pelvis.
   4. more directly the fontanel is aligned with the cervical opening.

61. The nurse discusses presentation, which is *best* defined as the
    1. part of the cervix that first becomes dilated during labor.
    2. relationship of the head of the fetus to the maternal pelvis.
    3. part of the fetal body that can be felt at the opening of the cervix.
    4. relationship between the long axis of the mother and the long axis of the fetus.
62. The nurse teaches that the fetus normally goes through a sequence of maneuvers during labor. When the head will be born first, the normal sequence is
    1. descent, flexion, external rotation, and extension.
    2. engagement, external rotation, flexion, and expulsion.
    3. internal rotation, descent, engagement restitution, and expulsion.
    4. descent, flexion, internal rotation, extension, and external rotation.
63. As the head of the fetus approaches delivery, if the phrase, "station plus one" is used, it means that the head is 1
    1. centimeter above the ischial spines.
    2. centimeter below the ischial spines.
    3. fingerbreadth above the ischial spines.
    4. fingerbreadth below the ischial spines.
64. When the nurse describes approaching birth, she uses the term crowning, which is *best* defined as the
    1. accommodation of the fetal head to the pelvic shape.
    2. elongation of the fetal head at the ischial spines.
    3. first appearance of the fetal head at the vaginal opening.
    4. encircling of the largest diameter of the fetal head by the vulvar ring.
65. The amniotic fluid and sac serve *all* of the following functions *except* that of
    1. helping to dilate the cervix.
    2. cleansing the birth canal.
    3. protecting the fetus from injury.
    4. providing the fetus with immune bodies.
66. Which one of the following designations accurately describes the position of the baby during delivery when its face is directed toward the physician's left hand and the mother's sacrum?
    1. L.O.A. (Left occipito-anterior).
    2. L.O.P. (Left occipito-posterior).
    3. R.O.A. (Right occipito-anterior).
    4. R.O.P. (Right occipito-posterior).
67. A mother asks how much blood she will lose during delivery. The maximum blood loss during the third stage of labor that is

considered to be within normal limits is approximately
1. 100 ml.
2. 300 ml.
3. 500 ml.
4. 700 ml.

68. A mother pregnant for the first time (primipara) asks how long labor will last. The nurse should base her response on knowledge that the average length of time a primipara is in labor is approximately
1. 6 hours.
2. 14 hours.
3. 22 hours.
4. 30 hours.

69. The circulatory changes that normally occur in the infant at the time of birth are initiated by
1. the birth process.
2. pulmonary ventilation.
3. cutting of the umbilical cord.
4. change in environmental temperature.

70. Dystocia is *best* defined as
1. a difficult labor.
2. a multiple delivery.
3. continuous uterine contractions.
4. diminished strength of contractions.

71. Questions arise in the class concerning twins. The term dizygotic refers to twins who have
1. developed from two ova and two sperms.
2. been born several hours apart from each other.
3. developed physically at different rates from each other.
4. developed in one amnion and have one chorion.

72. Which one of the following statements describes a generally accepted reason for the relatively *infrequent* use of hypnosis in obstetrics?
1. Hypnosis has proven to be too time-consuming to use.
2. Hypnosis has been proven ineffective for most vaginal deliveries.
3. There are relatively few health personnel adequately prepared to train patients to use hypnosis.
4. There are relatively few patients who are willing to give consent for the use of hypnosis.

73. It has been observed that if implantation occurs in one of the fallopian tubes, the time during pregnancy when the tube will generally rupture is during the
1. first 3 months.

2. third or fourth months.
3. fourth or fifth months.
4. fifth or sixth months.

Ms. Ruth Fielding was admitted to the labor suite of a hospital in early labor. She was accompanied by her husband. They explained to the nurse that they had attended Lamaze classes.
Items 74 through 121 pertain to this situation.

74. The *major* purpose of education for childbirth is to
    1. experience childbirth without pain.
    2. minimize the use of medication during labor.
    3. experience labor and delivery without fear.
    4. prepare the couple for approaching childbirth.

75. To which one of the following books should couples be referred if they wish to study the Lamaze method of preparing for childbirth?
    1. *Awake and Aware; Participating in Childbirth Through Psychoprophylaxis*, Irwin Chabon (New York: Delacorte Press, 1969).
    2. *Childbirth Without Fear: The Original Approach to Natural Childbirth*, Grantly Dick-Read (New York: Harper & Row Publishers, Ed. 4, 1972).
    3. *Husband-Coached Childbirth*, Robert A. Bradley (New York: Harper & Row Publishers, Rev. ed., 1974).

Ms. Fielding experienced difficulty in attaining muscular relaxation and decided to use the procedure of biofeedback to assist her. She used galvanic skin responses (GSR) and electromyelograph (EMG) sensors in her training.

76. Which one of the following normal responses of the body to anxiety is measured by the galvanometer?
    1. Increased muscular tension.
    2. Increased amounts of perspiration.
    3. Increased feelings of helplessness.
    4. Increased gastrointestinal secretions.

77. The EMG is used in biofeedback to measure
    1. blood pressure.
    2. brain patterns.
    3. level of anxiety.
    4. muscular tension.

78. Which one of the following statements *best* describes the con-

cept upon which techniques of biofeedback are based?
1. Modification of biological functions can be attained by voluntary means.
2. Maintenance of the body's homeostasis is achieved by self-regulation.
3. Interpretation of the body state is achieved by monitoring responses to stimuli.
4. Regulation of vital signs is attained under the direction of the therapist.

79. When the Lamaze method of preparing for childbirth is taught, the type of respirations the pregnant woman uses during early labor is moderately paced and effortless with
1. abdominal breathing.
2. deep chest breathing.
3. diaphragmatic breathing.
4. shallow chest breathing.

80. Ms. Fielding tells the nurse that she has found effleurage to be effective for helping her "keep on top of the contractions." Effleurage means a type of massage that consists of
1. deep kneading of muscular tissues.
2. light stroking on the skin's surfaces.
3. secure grasping of muscular tissues.
4. punctuated tapping on the skin's surfaces.

81. According to the gate control theory concerning pain, where in the body is the gating mechanism located?
1. In the spinal cord.
2. In reticular fibers.
3. In the cerebral cortex.
4. In cutaneous nerve fibers.

82. According to the gate control theory, a *closed* gate means that the individual will experience
1. pain.
2. no pain.
3. reduced pain.

83. Ms. Fielding has been taught to use personalized concentration points or ideas to promote muscular relaxation during labor. These points or ideas serve as a
1. projection for pain.
2. distraction from pain.
3. rationalization for pain.
4. counterirritant for pain.

84. Early in labor, Ms. Fielding expresses fear that she will have a "back labor." What is the position of the fetus when "back labor" occurs?
1. Chin-caudal.

2. Sacral-anterior.
3. Shoulder-ventral.
4. Occipito-posterior.
85. Which one of the following positions is being used increasingly for the relief of pain when a mother has "back labor"?
1. Lying on either side (Sims's position).
2. Assuming a crawling position (up-on-all-fours position).
3. Lying on the back with the head of the bed somewhat elevated (semi-Fowler's position).
86. The pain characteristically associated with "back labor" is caused by
1. unusual stretching of the uterosacral ligaments.
2. unusual sensitivity of pain receptors in the back.
3. pressure of the fetal head on the maternal sacrum.
4. pressure of the fetal shoulder on the maternal pubic bone.
87. At the beginning of Ms. Fielding's labor, a moderate increase in the amount of bloody vaginal discharge ("show") should be assessed by the nurse as an indication of
1. coagulation defect.
2. increased cervical dilatation.
3. rupture of the fetal membranes.
4. premature separation of the placenta.
88. The nurse notes fluid on the pad under Ms. Fielding's hips and uses nitrazine paper to determine whether it was amniotic fluid or urine. This test is based on the fact that normally
1. urine is acidic and amniotic fluid is alkaline.
2. amniotic fluid contains protein and urine does not.
3. urine contains glucose and amniotic fluid does not.
4. amniotic fluid contains meconium and urine does not.
89. The nurse checks Ms. Fielding's blood pressure *between* contractions *primarily* because
1. the blood pressure normally increases during a contraction.
2. the blood pressure is normally erratic during a contraction.
3. a patient is unable to cooperate sufficiently with the procedure during a contraction.
4. the procedure interferes with techniques the patient has been taught to use during a contraction.
90. The physician orders that Ms. Fielding have only fluids during labor, his *primary* reason *most likely* being that
1. the patient's appetite can be expected to be poor.
2. the digestive process is normally slower during labor.
3. solid foods tend to cause nausea and vomiting during labor.
4. the body normally has a sufficient store of energy to make eating solid foods during labor unnecessary.
91. The nurse should assess that Ms. Fielding is *most probably*

hyperventilating when she complains of
1. feeling warm.
2. having a headache.
3. shortness of breath.
4. tingling in her fingers.
92. Which one of the following actions should the nurse take to help Ms. Fielding overcome the effects of hyperventilation?
1. Have her breathe into a paper bag.
2. Have her breathe rapidly and shallowly.
3. Have her take several whiffs of oxygen.
4. Have her breathe with forceful expirations.
93. Which one of the following acid-base imbalances is Ms. Fielding likely to experience when she hyperventilates extensively?
1. Metabolic acidosis.
2. Metabolic alkalosis.
3. Respiratory acidosis.
4. Respiratory alkalosis.
94. Which one of the following conditions in the fetus will result if Ms. Fielding's hyperventilation is prolonged?
1. Acidosis.
2. Alkalosis.
3. Hypoglycemia.
4. Hypocalcemia.
95. If Ms. Fielding attempts to bear down with contractions during the first stage of labor, the *most likely* result is that the cervix will
1. prolapse.
2. become swollen.
3. dilate too rapidly.
4. efface too rapidly.
96. Ms. Fielding vomits and her arms and legs begin to shake. She says, "I can't take it! I can't take it!" Which one of the following actions is *most appropriate* for the nurse to take at this time?
1. Ask her husband to leave the labor room.
2. Notify the physician of her condition.
3. Give her an analgesic and review breathing techniques with her.
4. Explain that her symptoms are typical of this phase of labor.
97. Most practicing obstetricians will order a patient having her first baby to be transferred to the delivery room when
1. effacement has been completed.
2. the cervix is 7 to 8 cm. dilated.
3. the top of the baby's head becomes visible.

4. the patient feels strong urges to bear down.

98. After delivery, it would be *best* for the nurse to remove Ms. Fielding's legs from the stirrups and lower them together slowly in order to help prevent the patient's having
   1. leg cramps; rapid extension of muscle tissue predisposes to cramping.
   2. shortness of breath; the body's respiratory system needs time to adjust to the change in position.
   3. fainting sensations; the body's vascular system needs time to compensate for the change in position.
   4. nerve damage; rapid extension of nerves in the popliteal spaces predisposes to nerve tissue damage.

99. Approximately 10 minutes after delivery, Ms. Fielding experiences a chill. Which one of the following actions is *most* appropriate for the nurse to take?
   1. Catheterize the patient.
   2. Take the patient's temperature.
   3. Cover the patient with additional blankets.
   4. Notify the physician of the patient's condition.

100. According to research, it appears *most likely* that a mother's care of her newborn infant is set in motion when the mother first
   1. hears her baby cry.
   2. breast feeds her baby.
   3. has examined her baby for defects.
   4. has eye-to-eye contact with her baby.

101. To instill a medication properly into Baby Fielding's eyes, where in the eye should the medication be placed?
   1. On the cornea.
   2. At the inner canthus.
   3. At the outer canthus.
   4. In the lower conjunctival sac.

102. Which one of the following methods is the easiest way to get an infant to open his eyes for inspection?
   1. Place the infant in an upright position.
   2. Place the infant under an overhead light.
   3. Pull down on the lower eyelid with the thumb.
   4. Separate the eyelids with the thumb and forefinger.

103. Which one of the following biological preparations is *not* an appropriate prophylactic agent for ophthalmia neonatorum?
   1. Silver nitrate 1%.
   2. Oxytetracycline (Terramycin) ointment.
   3. Gentian violet.
   4. Penicillin drops.

104. Baby Fielding is ordered to have an injection of phytonadione

(Aqua-MEPHYTON) 0.5 ml. intramuscularly. Which one of the following muscles if *most often* recommended as the *best* one to use when the nurse injects the medication?

1. Deltoid muscle.
2. Gluteus medius muscle.
3. Gluteus maximus muscle.
4. Vastus lateralis muscle.

105. Which one of the following signs reported by the nurse assisted the physician to diagnose that Baby Fielding has thrush?

1. Green liquid stools.
2. Tremors of the hands.
3. White patches in the mouth.
4. Red rash on the abdomen.

106. Baby Fielding is circumcized. Following a circumcision, the *most common* protection used to cover the penis is a sterile dressing that is imbedded with

1. petrolatum.
2. talcum powder.
3. an antibiotic ointment.
4. benzalkonium chloride (Zephiran).

107. The nurse observes a small amount of bright red bleeding from the circumcision site. Of the following actions, which is the *most appropriate* for the nurse to take first?

1. Notify the physician of the bleeding.
2. Do nothing since a small amount of bleeding is usual.
3. Apply gentle pressure to the area with a sterile gauze pad.
4. Secure the diaper so that there is pressure on the bleeding area.

108. The nurse should teach Ms. Fielding to cleanse the circumcision site with cotton balls and

1. mild soap.
2. warm water.
3. hexachlorophene (pHisoHex).
4. benzalkonium chloride (Zephiran).

109. If a circumcision is being performed as a rite of the Jewish religion, the nurse should anticipate that preferably the procedure should be attended by

1. the mother.
2. the physician.
3. several close relatives.
4. a quorum of adult males.

110. Ms. Fielding uses rooming-in. The rooming-in method of caring for newborns has been developed on the principle that rooming-in

1. allows for easier supervision of the baby.
2. eliminates the necessity of having a routine for the mother and baby.
3. provides opportunities for developing a positive relationship between the mother and baby.
4. decreases the cost of administering care since it requires fewer skilled personnel.

111. Ms. Fielding tells the nurse that her baby spits up a small amount of milk after each feeding. Which one of the following measures is *most likely* to help decrease regurgitation?
1. Diluting the formula offered to the baby.
2. Giving small amounts and increasing the frequency of feeding him.
3. Placing the baby on his right side with his head elevated after feeding him.
4. Placing the baby on his abdomen after he has been fed and rubbing his back slightly.

112. The cause of regurgitation is believed to be due to the fact that an infant has
1. a poorly developed cardiac sphincter.
2. a small stomach in relation to his total size.
3. slow peristaltic action when compared with an older child.
4. a proportionately longer gastrointestinal tract when compared with an older child.

113. When Ms. Fielding signs her baby's birth certificate, she asks the nurse why it has to be completed. Which one of the following statements is an accurate answer to her question?
1. It is a record required by the hospital.
2. It is a record required by the physician.
3. It is a souvenir furnished by the hospital.
4. It is a legal document required by the state.

114. When the nurse accidently bumps the bassinet, Baby Fielding throws out his arms and legs and begins to cry. The reflex Baby Fielding is demonstrating is called the
1. Moro reflex.
2. stepping reflex.
3. Babinski's reflex.
4. knee jerk reflex.

115. Ms. Fielding is assisted to the bathroom for the first time following delivery. The *safest* way for the nurse to assist Ms. Fielding is to have the
1. patient hold onto the nurse's arm.
2. nurse hold onto the patient's arm.
3. nurse walk immediately behind the patient, ready to grasp the

patient if necessary.

4. patient walk next to the nurse, ready to grasp the nurse if necessary.

116. Which one of the following exercises is *most frequently* recommended for women soon after they have delivered?
    1. Alternately rolling from one side to the other.
    2. Alternately tensing and relaxing the muscles of the perineum.
    3. While on the abdomen, lifting the upper torso by flexing and extending the elbows.
    4. While in the sitting position, encircling the arms around flexed knees and rocking back and forth on the buttocks.

117. If progress is normal, on Ms. Fielding's second postpartal day, the nurse should anticipate that she will observe the patient to have a vaginal discharge called lochia
    1. serosa.
    2. rubra.
    3. alba.

118. If the Fielding home allows the parents to place their infant's bassinet in any of the following locations in a room, where would it be *best* to place it?
    1. Near a window.
    2. Near the room's source of heat.
    3. Against a wall that divides two rooms.
    4. Against a wall with a southern exposure.

119. Ms. Fielding was approximately 10 pounds overweight when she became pregnant. It is generally recommended that an appropriate weight gain for her during pregnancy should be
    1. the same as for any other pregnant woman.
    2. the amount that results when she satisfies her normal appetite.
    3. approximately 1 pound a week limited to the last half of her pregnancy.
    4. 10 pounds less than the commonly recommended gain of 20 to 25 pounds during pregnancy.

120. According to the authority, Grantly Dick-Read, which one of the following factors is the chief cause of the pain women describe during a normal labor?
    1. Fear.
    2. Guilt.
    3. Anxiety.
    4. Ignorance.

121. The LeBoyer method of delivery is based on the belief that the quality of life is improved when there is
    1. provision for including the father during labor and delivery.
    2. provision for a homelike atmosphere during labor and delivery.

3. utilization of techniques to give the newborn considerate and gentle care.
4. utilization of the fewest medications possible by the mother during labor and delivery.

Ms. Mary Ann Young consulted her physician after missing two menstrual periods. She was found to be pregnant.

Items 122 through 151 pertain to her prenatal care, her labor and delivery, and to the care of her baby.

122. Since July 13 was the first day of Ms. Young's last menstrual period, her estimated date of delivery, according to Naegele's rule is
1. March 6.
2. March 20.
3. April 6.
4. April 20.

123. While the nurse is preparing Ms. Young for her pelvic examination, she says, "I'm afraid of these visits to the doctor." Which one of the following responses would be *best* for the nurse to make?
1. "You have a very fine physician who will take excellent care of you."
2. "Nearly all mothers have some fears but there is really no need to worry."
3. "Please tell me more about what you mean when you say you are afraid."
4. "I will explain each part of the procedure while the doctor is examining you."

124. Which one of the following measures by the nurse will help Ms. Young to relax during her pelvic examination?
1. Having her bear down slightly.
2. Helping her to breathe normally.
3. Having her grasp the nurse's hand snugly.
4. Conversing with her to distract her attention.

125. One advantage of an immunological test, when compared with a biological test, is that an immunological pregnancy test
1. is more accurate.
2. provides an answer more quickly.
3. uses urine rather than a blood sample.
4. provides positive evidence of pregnancy.

126. Ms. Young's history indicates that she has been well. Which one of the following laboratory examinations could be omitted from Ms. Young's antepartal care at this time without jeopardizing the health of the patient or fetus?

1. Blood urea nitrogen level.
2. Serological test for syphilis.
3. Blood type and Rh determinations.
4. Hemoglobin and hematocrit determinations.

127. During Ms. Young's first visit to her physician's office, it is likely that *all* of the following signs of pregnancy will be present *except*
1. an increase in the size of the uterus.
2. a softening of the lower uterine segment.
3. being able to feel the outline of the fetus.
4. a purplish discoloration of the vaginal mucosa.

128. In keeping with current thinking, what advice is Ms. Young's physician *most likely* to give the patient concerning weight gain during pregnancy?
1. She should gain at least 10 pounds.
2. She should gain 12 to 14 pounds.
3. She should gain 20 to 30 pounds.
4. She may gain as much as results from satisfying a normal appetite.

129. If Ms. Young enjoyed all of the following activities, which one should she be taught to discontinue at about the beginning of her seventh month of pregnancy?
1. Walking.
2. Swimming.
3. Gourmet cooking.
4. Horseback riding.

130. Late in pregnancy, Ms. Young says sexual intercourse is uncomfortable because of her large abdomen. Which one of the following responses is *best* for the nurse to make to Ms. Young?
1. "You should not be uncomfortable. Let's discuss it with your physician."
2. "Tell your husband why you are finding it uncomfortable. He will understand and not insist."
3. "Intercourse is safe but try alternate positions, such as side-lying with your husband at your back."
4. "This is nature's way of saying it is time to stop having intercourse until after the baby is born."

131. Ms. Young sees her physician at 4-week intervals until the 30th week of pregnancy, at 2-week intervals between her 30th and 36th week, and each week from the 36th week until delivery. This visitation schedule should suggest to the nurse that Ms. Young
1. has developed a complication which the physician wishes to

follow closely.
2. is progressing normally and is being seen by her physician at typical intervals.
3. has not followed instructions concerning her care and needs more teaching and supervision.
4. needs frequent visits prior to delivery because of her apprehension about labor and giving birth.

132. When Ms. Young is admitted to the hospital in early active labor, the following signs are present: cervix 3 cm. dilated with effacement nearing completion; presenting part at a minus 1 station. In view of these findings, which one of the following actions should the nurse take *first?*
1. Do a perineal preparation for delivery.
2. Prepare the delivery room for delivery.
3. Prepare to administer an intravenous infusion.
4. Check the patient's blood pressure and the fetal heart rate.

133. Ms. Young asks how long she will be in labor. *All* of the following factors will influence the length of her labor *except*
1. size of the placenta.
2. mental attitude of the mother.
3. position of the fetus in utero.
4. resistance of maternal soft tissues.

134. A tap water enema is ordered for Ms. Young. If Ms. Young is able to be placed in any of the positions below, which one is considered *best* when administering the enema?
1. Lying on her back.
2. Lying on either side.
3. Sitting on a bedpan or toilet.

135. The nurse encounters resistance while she is inserting the rectal tube for the enema. Which one of the following actions is *most* helpful in overcoming the resistance?
1. Exerting persistent, gentle pressure.
2. Inserting the tube further during a contraction while the anus dilates.
3. Instructing the patient to relax while taking a few deep and slow breaths.
4. Withdrawing the tube slightly while letting a small amount of the solution enter.

136. While the nurse administers the enema, Ms. Young has a contraction. Which one of the following actions is *most appropriate* for the nurse to take at this time?
1. Clamp the tubing.
2. Continue as before.
3. Remove the rectal tube.

4. Slow the flow of solution.

137. Most authorities recommend that the optimal temperature for the enema solution is between approximately
    1. 85° F. to 95° F. (29.5° C. to 35° C.).
    2. 95° F. to 105° F. (35° C. to 40.5° C.).
    3. 105° F. to 115° F. (40.5° C. to 46.1° C.).
    4. 115° F. to 125° F. (46.1° C. to 51.7° C.).

138. A nurse is observed to be taking the following actions while shaving Ms. Young's perineal area prior to delivery. Which one of the actions is *inappropriate?*
    1. Holding the skin taut while shaving.
    2. Moving the razor from the pubic area toward the anus.
    3. Moving the razor with as long a stroke as is possible.
    4. Moving the razor opposite from the direction in which the hair grows.

139. Immediately following the birth of Ms. Young's baby, the nurse should carry out *all* of the following procedures on the baby *except*
    1. clearing the airway.
    2. removing the cord clamp.
    3. applying identification.
    4. putting drops in the baby's eyes.

140. Which one of the following signs indicates that Ms. Young's placenta has detached from the uterine wall?
    1. The cord lengthens outside of the vagina.
    2. The mother complains of pain low in her back.
    3. There is a noticeable relaxation in the abdominal wall.
    4. The uterus falls below the level of the symphysis pubis.

141. Ms. Young had spinal anesthesia for her delivery. Unlike the patient who has had general anesthesia, the nurse should plan a several hour delay for Ms. Young's first
    1. meal.
    2. voiding.
    3. ambulation.
    4. nursing of her baby.

142. To help reduce anxiety and worry during the puerperium, it is important that the nurse take into account all of the factors given below. However, it is generally recommended that the nurse be *especially* alert to the mother's having
    1. sufficient rest.
    2. adequate food intake.
    3. diversional activities.
    4. visitors as agency policy allows.

143. Ms. Young wears hard contact lenses and plans to take a nap.

Which one of the following statements describes the *most often* recommended precaution concerning sleep and the wearing of hard contact lenses?

1. The lenses should be removed before sleep.
2. The lenses should be moistened before sleep.
3. The lenses should be left in place without special care.
4. The lenses should be moistened immediately upon awakening.

144. The nurse noted that, for about 2 hours after birth, Baby Young was awake and alert and he startled and cried easily. Respirations at times rose to 70 per minute and his heart rate on two occasions was 180 per minute. He then slept quietly for about 1½ hours, wakened with a start, and cried and waved his arms. He choked, gagged, and regurgitated some mucus. Of the following actions, which one would be *best* for the nurse to take?

1. Call the physician; the baby appears to have hypoglycemia.
2. Place the baby in an incubator; his signs suggest that he needs humidity and well-oxygenated air to breathe.
3. Change the baby's position and aspirate mucus as necessary; the signs he presents are normal.
4. Wrap the baby carefully in a blanket and feed him; he appears hungry and needs to be protected from injuring himself.

145. Which one of the following observations, if noted in Baby Young, should be reported to the physician promptly?

1. The nurse is unable to retract the foreskin.
2. The infant does not pass meconium during the first 12 hours.
3. The infant regurgitates some mucus after the first two feedings.
4. The nurse is unable to insert the rectal thermometer for more than ½ inch.

146. Baby Young weighed 8 pounds and 1 ounce (3.66 kg.) at birth and at 3 days of age, he weighs 7 pounds and 12 ounces (3.52 kg.). In view of baby Young's weight change, the nurse *appropriately* assesses that

1. he be given an intravenous solution to prevent further weight loss and dehydration.
2. he be switched from breast feedings to bottle feedings since his mother's milk appears to be inadequate.
3. his weight loss should be evaluated and that he be transferred to a pediatric unit for further study.
4. his weight loss is within normal limits and that nothing special need be done at this time.

147. Two days after delivery, the nurse assessed Baby Young's umbil-

ical cord as being normal when she noted that
1. the stump was dark and dry.
2. there was an odor from the umbilical stump.
3. there was redness around the umbilical stump.
4. some bleeding and moisture appeared at the umbilical stump.

148. At 3 days of age, Baby Young is jaundiced and laboratory findings indicate an indirect bilirubin of 8 mg. percent. The nurse should anticipate that the physician will *most likely* order
1. vitamin K.
2. phototherapy.
3. an exchange transfusion.
4. continuation of previous care.

149. Ms. Young is being given home-going instructions concerning the care of her baby. Which one of the following signs, if exhibited by the baby, should she be taught to report to her physician promptly?
1. He has hiccups and sneezes.
2. He has frequent green stools.
3. He yawns and sighs frequently.
4. He spits up part of his feedings.

150. Ms. Young asks when she can start omitting her baby's night feeding. It is *best* to teach her to omit it when her baby
1. starts eating solid foods.
2. begins sleeping through the night.
3. gains more than approximately ½ pound each week.
4. has increased his birth weight by approximately one-half.

151. What should Ms. Young be taught about thumb sucking?
1. The baby is comforting himself.
2. The baby is most likely underfed.
3. The baby's arms should be restrained when put to bed.
4. The baby is likely to develop a deformed jaw unless the habit is broken early.

Ms. Helen Pearson is pregnant for the first time. There is question about whether her pelvis is adequate for normal vaginal delivery.

Items 152 through 171 pertain to this situation.

152. The *most important* measurement for helping to determine whether the pelvis is adequate for normal vaginal delivery is the
1. oblique diameters.
2. diagonal conjugate.
3. transverse diameter.

4. intertuberous diameter.

153. *All* of the following statements about the pelvic inlet are true *except*
   1. the widest diameter of the inlet is the transverse diameter.
   2. the pelvic inlet must be larger than normal in order to deliver twins vaginally.
   3. when the anteroposterior diameter is normal, the inlet is assumed to be of adequate size.
   4. the minimum normal measurement for the anteroposterior diameter is 11 cm.

154. The physician orders roentgenologic studies of Ms. Pearson's pelvis (pelvimetry). Which one of the following statements in relation to preparing Ms. Pearson for pelvimetry is *most accurate?*
   1. A tap water enema usually is ordered prior to doing pelvimetry.
   2. Fluids and food are usually restricted for 4 to 6 hours prior to doing pelvimetry.
   3. A mild analgesic is usually ordered to be given immediately before doing pelvimetry.
   4. It is unusual that the patient will require any special preparation prior to doing pelvimetry.

155. When the physician orders roentgenologic studies for Ms. Pearson, she asks the nurse about the dangers of having the examination. The nurse's response should be guided by knowledge that
   1. these studies are most dangerous during labor and delivery.
   2. any unfavorable reaction to these studies is temporary and affects the mother only.
   3. modern technique makes these studies a relatively safe procedure when they are done late in pregnancy.
   4. physicians now tend to recommend these studies to determine precise pelvic measurements for most women pregnant for the first time.

156. Which one of the following statements is the *best guide* for the nurse when she explains the procedure to Ms. Pearson?
   1. Several flat-plate x-ray pictures of the pelvis are taken from different angles.
   2. A laminogram (planogram) is done so that the pelvis can be viewed from three dimensions.
   3. A contrast dye is injected while a series of flat-plate x-ray pictures are taken of the pelvis.
   4. Floroscopy is used so that the pelvis can be viewed continuously for a period of time.

157. Ms. Pearson's physician elects to perform a cesarean section. When the nurse takes the consent (permit) form to the Pearsons for signing, Mr. Pearson says, "I'll sign it. I always take care of our business affairs." Which one of the following responses would be *most appropriate* for the nurse to make in this situation?
1. "Is that all right with you, Ms. Pearson?"
2. "All right, Mr. Pearson. You may sign right here."
3. Thank you, Mr. Pearson, but the patient must also sign her consent form."
4. "Just a minute. I will have to ask the doctor if that is all right with him."

158. Factors that affect the legality of the consent to an operative procedure include *all* of those given below *except*
1. age of the patient.
2. occupation of the witness.
3. ability of the patient to read.
4. medications the patient has received.

159. Immediately following delivery of the placenta, the physician orders that oxytocin (Pitocin) be added to the intravenous solution Ms. Pearson is receiving. The physician's rationale for ordering the drug is that it helps to
1. hasten blood clotting.
2. stimulate milk production.
3. induce uterine involution.
4. promote relaxation of the abdominal wall.

160. General anesthesia was used for the cesarean section. Adverse effects of general anesthesia in obstetrics generally include *all* of the following phenomena *except*
1. a delay in the production of breast milk.
2. an increased likelihood of uterine atony and excessive bleeding.
3. a delay in the onset of spontaneous respirations in the infant.
4. a greater lag in maternal feelings than when no anesthesia is used.

161. Ergonovine maleate (Ergotrate maleate) is ordered for Ms. Pearson as follows: 0.2 mg. orally 4 times a day for 2 days. The nurse should plan to withhold the medication until she has consulted with the physician when she notes that the patient has
1. uterine cramping.
2. an irregular pulse rate.
3. excessive vaginal bleeding.
4. an elevated blood pressure.

162. To be prepared for possible problems when caring for Baby Pearson, the nurse should be guided by knowledge that, when compared with babies born vaginally, babies born by cesarean section tend to have an increased incidence of
1. convulsions.
2. hypoglycemia.
3. umbilical cord infections.
4. respiratory distress syndrome.

163. Identification was provided for Baby Pearson immediately after her birth. Which one of the following techniques is the *most reliable* way to identify the baby?
1. Taking footprints of the baby.
2. Taking a photograph of the baby.
3. Placing a wristlet on the baby.
4. Tattooing the baby with ultraviolet.

164. After determining that Ms. Pearson's fundus is firm and in the midline, the nurse ambulates the patient for the first time after delivery. A moderate amount of lochia gushes from the patient's vagina. Of the following courses of action, it would be *best* for the nurse to
1. put the patient to bed and notify the physician.
2. help the patient to lie down in bed and massage her fundus until it is firm.
3. administer the next dose of ergonovine maleate to the patient immediately.
4. continue to ambulate the patient and explain that the gush was caused by pooling of discharge in the vagina.

165. Ms. Pearson should turn and deep breathe regularly following her cesarean operation *primarily* in order to help prevent
1. adhesions.
2. subinvolution.
3. postpartal infection.
4. respiratory congestion.

166. When Ms. Pearson is changing her baby's diaper, she questions the nurse about some red-tinged drainage from the baby's vagina. Of the following responses, which one would be the *most accurate* for the nurse to make?
1. "The cause of vaginal bleeding in newborns is unknown. I'll report it to your physician."
2. "I don't know what it is but since it is such a small amount, I doubt that it can be serious."
3. "Sometimes baby girls have a small amount of vaginal bleeding due to hormones received from the mother."
4. "Vaginal bleeding in newborns is caused by a temporary

bleeding problem. I'll check to see whether your baby has received a medication for it."

167. On Ms. Pearson's fifth postpartal day, the physician asks the nurse to remove every other suture from the patient's abdominal incision. Of the following responses, which one is the *most appropriate* for the nurse to make?
   1. "I'll do it if you stand right here and watch me."
   2. "Sorry, Dr. Brown, that's the physician's responsibility."
   3. "All right. I'll do it as soon as I gather the necessary supplies."
   4. "I'll ask a student nurse to do it. She hasn't had a chance to remove sutures yet."

168. On her fifth postpartal day, Ms. Pearson says she is afraid she is losing her milk because the baby has been eating every 4 hours and now is crying to be fed every 2 hours. Which one of the following statements is the *most likely* reason for the baby's need for more frequent feedings?
   1. The baby is becoming more alert and active.
   2. The mother no doubt had a decrease in her milk supply.
   3. The patient is most likely not allowing the baby enough time to suck with each feeding.
   4. The baby is in a temporary growth spurt and requires more frequent feedings for the time being.

169. Ms. Pearson had been crying and says she thinks she was having "normal postpartal blues." She asks if this would decrease her milk supply. Of the following responses, which one is the *most appropriate* for the nurse to make?
   1. "Yes, it could, but it's highly unlikely."
   2. "Do you think your milk supply is decreasing?"
   3. "No; postpartal blues do not affect the milk supply."
   4. "Are you worried about the effects of the postpartal blues?"

170. The purposes for Ms. Pearson's being taught exercises during the postpartal period are similar to the purposes for using
   1. rooming-in.
   2. breast feeding.
   3. early ambulation.
   4. analgesics during labor.

171. Ms. Pearson tells the nurse she expects her husband to participate more in learning how to care for the baby so they will both do things the same way. Which one of the following responses is *most appropriate* for the nurse to make?
   1. "That's an unreal expectation, don't you think?"
   2. "This seems important to you. Could you tell me more about it?"

3. "We're all different and need to be allowed to be ourselves."
4. "Men are slower to do these things. He will help more at home, I'm sure."

Ms. Jean Tallon was admitted to the hospital for delivery. She will have saddle block anesthesia. She is receiving fluids intravenously.

Items 172 through 175 pertain to this situation.

172. The recommended position for Ms. Tallon during the administration of the anesthetic agent is the
    1. sitting position.
    2. side-lying position.
    3. knee-chest position.
    4. back-lying position with the knees flexed.

173. If it is noted that Ms. Tallon's blood pressure is falling following the administration of the anesthesia, which one of the following actions should the nurse take *first?*
    1. Turn the patient on her side.
    2. Raise the legs of the patient.
    3. Increase the intravenous flow rate.
    4. Administer the prescribed vasopressor drug.

174. A common complaint following saddle block anesthesia is a headache. Which one of the following nursing measures is recommended for helping to prevent the headache?
    1. Darkening the patient's room.
    2. Elevating the patient's legs.
    3. Increasing the patient's fluid intake.
    4. Placing the patient in a semisitting position.

175. Which one of the following statements offers the nurse her *best* guide as she prepares to discuss anesthesia with patients such as Ms. Tallon?
    1. Most women demand and, hence, usually need anesthesia during delivery.
    2. Each patient requires individual help and instruction concerning the use of anesthesia.
    3. Patients generally accept their physician's advice about anesthesia without question.
    4. Relatively few women need anesthesia during delivery when prenatal education discourages its use.

Ms. Doris Benet, who is pregnant for the third time and has had two normal deliveries, is in active labor. Her condition

and that of the fetus have been good since admission to the hospital. Suddenly she calls, "Nurse, the baby is coming."
Items 176 through 183 pertain to this situation.

176. When the nurse responds to Ms. Benet's call, which one of the following observations should the nurse make *first?*
1. Inspect the perineum.
2. Time the contractions.
3. Obtain the blood pressure.
4. Auscultate for fetal heart rate.

177. It appears that delivery of the baby is imminent and that it will take the physician about 5 minutes to reach the hospital. Of the following actions, which one is *most appropriate* for the nurse to take?
1. Have the patient pant to delay the delivery.
2. Hold the patient's legs together to delay delivery.
3. Administer the ordered prn analgesic immediately.
4. Prepare a clean area upon which to deliver the baby.

178. When the head of the baby is at the vaginal opening, which one of the following actions is *most appropriate* for the nurse to take?
1. Support the perineum by exerting pressure around the vaginal opening.
2. Control delivery of the head by exerting gentle pressure against the head.
3. Assist the fetus farther into the vagina by exerting pressure on the fundus.
4. Hold the head back until such time as one contraction will deliver the baby entirely.

179. In relation to a contraction, when is the *best time* to deliver the head?
1. Between contractions.
2. At the end of a contraction.
3. At the peak of a contraction.
4. At the beginning of a contraction.

180. Which one of the following statements is *most likely* to assist Ms. Benet to remain calm and cooperative during the delivery?
1. "The baby is coming. Just relax and everything will be fine."
2. "Even though the baby is coming, the doctor will be here very soon so there is no need for worry."
3. "The baby is coming. I will explain what is happening and tell you what to do as we go along."
4. "There is no need for concern. Most babies could be born safely without the assistance of a doctor."

181. After the baby is delivered, what should the nurse do in relation to the umbilical cord?

1. Cut it.
2. Clamp it.
3. Leave it untouched.
4. Wrap it in normal saline.

182. In relation to the delivery of the placenta, which one of the following actions is *most appropriate* for the nurse to take?
1. Have the patient bear down.
2. Massage the fundus for a few minutes.
3. Wait for signs of placental separation before taking any action.
4. Exert a gentle pull on the cord until the placenta begins to appear at the vaginal orifice.

183. Which one of the following complications is *least likely* to be associated with a precipitate delivery?
1. Ruptured uterus.
2. Cerebral trauma to the baby.
3. Tears of the umbilical cord.
4. Laceration of the maternal soft tissues.

Ms. Peggy Miller is entering her fourth month of pregnancy and has had "morning sickness" during the first 3 months. She calls her physician's office nurse to report that her "morning sickness" has reached the point that she has not been able to "keep anything down for 3 days."
Items 184 through 193 pertain to this situation.

184. When the nurse receives the call, of the following suggestions, it would be *best* for her to recommend that Ms. Miller
1. take sips of carbonated beverages.
2. come to the physician's office that day.
3. go to the hospital for admission immediately.
4. eat saltine crackers before arising in the morning.

185. Because Ms. Miller has been unable to retain food, her body has been using reserve fat tissues. Consequently, which one of the following substances, not normally found in the urine, can the nurse anticipate will be present when Ms. Miller's urine is examined?
1. Glucose.
2. Protein.
3. Albumin.
4. Acetone.

186. The acid-base imbalance Ms. Miller is *most likely* to experience if her vomiting continues unchecked is
1. metabolic acidosis.
2. respiratory acidosis.
3. metabolic alkalosis.
4. respiratory alkalosis.

187. Excessive vomiting will result in the body's having a deficit of the electrolyte
   1. calcium.
   2. potassium.
   3. bicarbonate.
   4. organic acid.
188. When excessive vomiting occurs, the kidneys assist in maintaining the body's acid-base balance by retaining larger than normal amounts of the ion
   1. sodium.
   2. sulfate.
   3. hydrogen.
   4. bicarbonate.
189. Ms. Miller is admitted to the hospital. If the nurse observes that the patient has the following symptoms, which one would be *least indicative* of dehydration?
   1. Scanty urine.
   2. Poor skin turgor.
   3. Puffiness about her eyelids.
   4. Oral temperature of 99.5°F. (37.5°C.).
190. The physician orders that Ms. Miller receive 1000 ml. of intravenous fluid in each 8-hour period. If the intravenous equipment has a drop factor of 15, how many drops per minute should be administered?
   1. 15 to 16 drops.
   2. 20 to 21 drops.
   3. 31 to 32 drops.
   4. 40 to 41 drops.
191. When intravenous fluids are administered continuously over a period of time, it is generally recommended that the tubing be changed every
   1. 8 hours.
   2. 24 hours.
   3. 36 hours.
   4. 72 hours.
192. Thiamine (vitamin B₁) is added to Ms. Miller's intravenous solution because the thiamine acts to help
   1. control vomiting.
   2. metabolize carbohydrates.
   3. improve kidney filtration.
   4. correct an acid-base imbalance.
193. The respirations of a patient whose carbonic acid is in excess are characteristically
   1. slow and deep.
   2. rapid and deep.

3. slow and shallow.

4. rapid and shallow.

Ms. Theresa Enoc, a 26-year-old Pima Indian, lives on a reservation in southern Arizona. She is a Class B diabetic and has been admitted to the hospital at 37 weeks of gestation for induction of labor.

Items 194 through 211 pertain to this situation.

194. To understand factors that are likely to influence Ms. Enoc's care, it is important for the nurse to know that *all* of the following statements about American Indians are true *except*

1. most American Indians who live on reservations live in poverty.

2. infant death rates among American Indians are much higher than those among Caucasians.

3. maternal death rates among American Indians are much higher than those for the United States as a whole.

4. since American Indians are eligible for free health services, most receive at least adequate health care.

195. Which one of the following physiological changes that normally occur during pregnancy complicates determination of Ms. Enoc's need for insulin?

1. A decrease in the secretion of insulin.

2. A decrease in the renal threshhold for glucose.

3. An increase in the carbon dioxide content of the plasma.

4. An increase in the peripheral utilization of carbohydrates.

196. Prior to the induction of labor, an oxytocin challenge test is performed. The following pattern is noted:

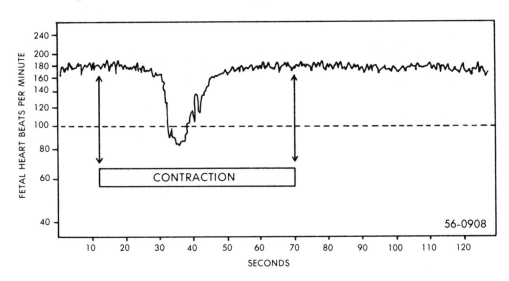

56-0908

This pattern should be interpreted to mean that, in relation to the fetal heart rate, there is
1. normal slowing during a contraction.
2. late deceleration after a contraction.
3. early deceleration before a contraction.
4. variable deceleration during a contraction.

197. The physician orders 1000 ml. of 5% dextrose in water to be given intravenously, with 1000 ml. of 5% dextrose in water containing 10 units of oxytocin (pitocin) given by the "piggyback" method. One advantage of administering drugs intravenously using this method is that it is
1. impossible for the flow rate to be increased accidently.
2. impossible for the patient to reach the tubing and adjust the flow rate.
3. possible to determine exactly how much drug the patient is receiving.
4. possible to stop administering the drug at any time and the vein remains open.

198. The physician could have ordered that the oxytocin be administered with an infusion pump. An advantage for using an infusion pump is that it
1. delivers exact amounts of the drug intravenously.
2. overcomes venous resistance and allows a rapid infusion rate.
3. reduces nursing time because the nurse does not have to monitor the infusion.
4. acts as a regulator to synchronize infusion rate and rate of uterine contractions.

199. During the oxytocin infusion, the physician is called to his office 2 miles from the hospital. The American College of Obstetricians and Gynecologists recommends that in such cases, the nurse should
1. slow the intravenous rate to approximately 5 drops per minute.
2. continue as when the physician was present and stay with the patient.
3. alternately discontinue and restart the infusion every 5 to 6 minutes.
4. turn off the infusion of oxytocin until the physician returns from his office.

200. During the intravenous infusion of oxytocin, Ms. Enoc has a strong contraction which lasts about 90 seconds. Of the following courses of action, the one that would be *most appropriate* for the nurse to take at this time would be to
1. turn the patient onto her left side.
2. take the patient to the delivery room.

3. continue with the patient's plan of care as ordered.

4. reduce the rate at which the oxytocin has been given.

201. When prostaglandins are used to induce labor, it is important for the nurse to know that, when compared with oxytocin, the onset of uterine effect when prostaglandins are used is
1. slower.
2. more rapid.
3. unpredictable.
4. approximately the same.

202. Which one of the following routes of administration is *inappropriate* for prostaglandins?
1. Oral.
2. Vaginal.
3. Intravenous.
4. Intramuscular.

203. Determining need for analgesia during Ms. Enoc's labor is made more difficult because a characteristic of the American Indian culture is that Indians
1. seldom exhibit external symptoms of pain.
2. refuse to be examined vaginally by males.
3. wail in labor as part of a religious ritual.
4. moan loudly as an expression of their emotions.

204. When Ms. Enoc is about 5 cm. dilated, the physician ruptures her membranes. The fetal head is high in the pelvis. The *most important* nursing action after the patient's membranes have been artificially ruptured is to
1. auscultate for fetal heart rate.
2. position the patient on her left side.
3. determine the patient's blood pressure.
4. be prepared for a precipitate delivery.

205. Even though in good condition at birth, babies of diabetic mothers must be watched closely because they are prone to develop
1. paralytic ileus.
2. hyperbilirubinemia.
3. respiratory distress.
4. intracranial bleeding.

206. At 1½ hours of age, Baby Girl Enoc's blood sugar level is 45 mg. per 100 ml. and at 2 hours of age, the blood sugar level is 25 mg. per 100 ml. This change in blood sugar is *most likely* due to
1. a reaction to the stresses of labor and the period of increased activity following delivery.
2. an interruption in the source of glucose and a continued high production of insulin by the baby.

3. an increase in the production of urine that occurs when the kidneys are ridding the body of excess glucose.
4. a physical response of the body that normally occurs during transition from intrauterine to extrauterine life.

207. The nurse can anticipate that moderate hypoglycemia in the early newborn period is usually treated by giving the infant
1. oral glucose.
2. intravenous glucose.
3. subcutaneous insulin.
4. an oral hypoglycemic agent.

208. The period of hypoglycemia observed in many infants of diabetic mothers will almost always correct itself as soon as the baby
1. receives milk rather than colostrum from the breast.
2. establishes regular feedings of glucose water or milk.
3. begins normal intestinal and urinary excretory functions.
4. excretes the insulin that crossed the placenta while in utero.

209. The *most probable* reason for Baby Girl Enoc's weighing more than the average newborn is that
1. girl babies tend to be larger than boy babies at birth.
2. the mother miscalculated her expected date of confinement.
3. the mother gained more weight during pregnancy than most mothers do.
4. babies of diabetic mothers tend to weigh more than babies of nondiabetic mothers.

210. Baby Enoc was born with two lower teeth which were removed 2 days after birth. The *primary* reason for removing the teeth was that they may
1. be aspirated.
2. become decayed.
3. interfere with sucking.
4. injure the mother's nipples.

211. Ms. Enoc has symptoms of hypoglycemia several times during the first 3 days postpartum. Of the following statements, which one does *not* support this phenomenon?
1. There is a withdrawal of the effect of the fetal pancreas.
2. There is conversion of some blood glucose into mammary lactose.
3. There are significant changes in the amount of the mother's physical activity.
4. There are endocrine and metabolic changes associated with the termination of pregnancy.

Ms. Joan Carter, who has previously delivered two non-viable fetuses, is now at approximately 28 weeks of gestation.

The physician performs an amniocentesis and orders the following tests of the fluid: L/S ratio; orange-staining cells; osmolality; creatinine concentration, and bilirubin level.
Items 212 through 245 pertain to this situation.

212. What is the color of normal amniotic fluid in a pregnancy near term?
    1. Pink, with a small amount of blood.
    2. Light green, with meconium staining.
    3. Clear, with flecks of vernix caseosa.
    4. Yellow, with urine voided by the fetus.
213. The *most common* preparation for amniocentesis requires that the patient should
    1. have an enema.
    2. empty her bladder.
    3. have her abdomen shaved.
    4. have nothing by mouth for approximately 4 hours.
214. Ms. Carter asks the nurse about the significance of the tests that were ordered by the physician. The nurse's explanation concerning the L/S (lecithin/sphingomyelin) ratio should be based on the knowledge that these substances are the major components of surfactant which functions in the infant to
    1. regulate the heart rate.
    2. prevent coagulation defects.
    3. maintain expansion of the lungs.
    4. stimulate the respiratory center.
215. The nurse's explanation concerning the orange-staining cells should be based on knowledge that increasing numbers of orange-staining cells indicate that the fetus
    1. is in distress.
    2. is nearing maturity.
    3. has a congenital defect.
    4. has a chromosomal abnormality.
216. As the fetus matures, osmolality of amniotic fluid decreases because the fetus
    1. excretes increasing amounts of urine.
    2. digests increasing amounts of metabolites.
    3. excretes increasing amounts of metabolites.
    4. swallows increasing amounts of amniotic fluid.
217. The nurse correctly explains that the concentration of creatinine in amniotic fluid is an indirect measure of the ability of the fetus to adapt to extrauterine life because creatinine
    1. increases as the liver matures and secretes it.
    2. decreases as the fetus swallows and metabolizes it.

3. increases as the fetal kidneys mature and excrete it.

4. decreases as the size of the fetus increases and absorbs it.

218. The optic density of bilirubin in amniotic fluid is a measure of fetal maturity because as the fetus matures, bilirubin is
1. absorbed by the skin.
2. excreted by the kidneys.
3. metabolized by the liver.
4. retained in the gastrointestinal tract.

219. It is generally recommended for safety reasons that an amniocentesis performed for the purpose of diagnosing chromosomal abnormalities *not* be done until the age of the fetus is at least
1. 3 to 4 weeks.
2. 7 to 8 weeks.
3. 15 to 16 weeks.
4. 19 to 20 weeks.

220. Many authorities believe that an amniocentesis should be done to detect chromosomal abnormalities in order to
1. satisfy the patient's curiosity.
2. prevent birth of a defective baby.
3. take remedial action before it is too late to correct the fault.
4. assist the parents if they wish to initiate adoption procedures.

221. The nurse should teach Ms. Carter that, if the following symptoms occur following her amniocentesis, the one she should report to her physician promptly is
1. nausea.
2. vaginal bleeding.
3. frequent voiding.
4. abdominal tenderness.

222. Labor contractions began the day after Ms. Carter has the amniocentesis. Her physician orders that she should receive an intravenous solution of ethyl alcohol and 5% glucose in water in order to try to stop labor. Which of the following signs/symptoms are common undesirable side effects of this treatment?
1. Nausea, vomiting, and mental confusion.
2. Abdominal cramping, diarrhea, and excessive perspiration.
3. Headaches, elevated blood pressure, and a rapid pulse rate.
4. Muscle spasms, double vision, and a rapid respiratory rate.

223. When labor continues, the alcohol solution is stopped. Ms. Carter becomes very uncomfortable and asks why she cannot have a medication for pain. The nurse's response should be based on knowledge that during premature labor, analgesics tend to
1. stop the labor.

2. depress the infant.
3. hasten the delivery.
4. react with the alcohol.

224. The nurse should anticipate that outlet forceps may be used during Ms. Carter's delivery *primarily* in order to help
   1. hasten delivery.
   2. prevent perineal tears.
   3. protect the baby's head from trauma.
   4. assist the mother in her efforts to expel the fetus.

225. The physician requests that Ms. Carter's labor contractions be monitored with a tokodynamometer (external monitor). The optimal placement of the tokodynamometer disc is over the area of greatest
   1. body size of the fetus.
   2. discomfort during a contraction.
   3. circumference of the mother's abdomen.
   4. uterine displacement during a contraction.

226. When the monitor has been in place for about 2 hours, the nurse notes that the pattern of contractions recorded by the monitor has changed from a regular wave pattern to an almost flat pattern. Which one of the following actions should the nurse take *first?*
   1. Notify the physician.
   2. Administer oxygen to the patient.
   3. Turn the patient on her left side.
   4. Adjust the placement of the tokodynamometer.

227. A Doppler (ultrasound) probe was used to monitor the fetal heart rate. The *best* placement of the transducer is on the mother's abdomen and located
   1. near the mother's umbilicus.
   2. approximately 2 inches above the symphysis pubis.
   3. over the area where fetal heart tones are best heard.
   4. approximately midway between the mother's umbilicus and the symphysis pubis.

228. The major advantage of monitoring the fetal heart rate electronically, when compared with obtaining the rate with a fetoscope, is that an electronic monitor
   1. records the actual heart rate.
   2. takes less nursing time to use.
   3. causes less discomfort to the mother.
   4. determines beat-to-beat variabilities.

229. What is the normal range of the fetal heart rate in beats per minute?
   1. 80 to 120 beats.

2. 100 to 140 beats.

3. 120 to 160 beats.

4. 140 to 180 beats.

230. When Ms. Carter is about 5 cm. dilated, the physician ruptures the membranes and applies an internal monitor. For which one of the following complications should the nurse be *especially* alert when internal monitoring of uterine contractions is being done?

1. Intrauterine infection.

2. Amniotic fluid embolism.

3. Perforation of the uterus.

4. Detachment of a low-lying placenta.

231. Ms. Carter tells the nurse she is afraid to move because of the internal monitor. Which one of the following responses would be *most appropriate* for the nurse to make to Ms. Carter?

1. "Lying on your back is the best position. You won't need to move."

2. "You may lie in any position that is comfortable. I will help you turn now."

3. "Don't worry. The physician has attached the wires of your monitor very securely."

4. "We turned you to your left side which is the best position. Lie quietly but you may flex and extend your legs."

232. During a uterine contraction, the nurse can expect that, under normal conditions, the contractions will cause the fetal heart rate to

1. increase.

2. change by decreasing and increasing.

3. remain the same as it was prior to the contraction.

233. Of the following conditions, all of which cause a decrease in the fetal heart rate, which one is the *least* ominous?

1. A knot in the cord.

2. Prolapse of the cord.

3. Uteroplacental insufficiency.

4. Pressure on the fetal head by the cervix.

234. Ms. Carter is delivered of a premature baby. Which one of the following actions is *inappropriate* when using a bulb syringe to suction the mouth and nose of the newborn?

1. Suction the mouth first.

2. Keep the baby's head lower than his body.

3. Compress the bulb before insertion.

4. Stimulate the baby to cry before suctioning.

235. Current opinion holds that, within the first 10 minutes after birth,

deep suctioning of the nasopharynx carries the danger of
1. injuring tender mucous membranes.
2. abolishing the infant's normal efforts to clear mucus.
3. stimulating the vagus nerve which causes a slow heartbeat.
4. removing too much carbon dioxide which causes respiratory distress.

236. Baby Carter did not breathe spontaneously so oxygen is given by a mask attached to a hand-operated bag. In which one of the following positions should the baby be placed while being given oxygen?
1. On his abdomen with the head to the side.
2. On his side with the neck slightly flexed.
3. On his back with the neck slightly extended.

237. Of the following observations, the one that indicates *best* that the oxygen is being administered properly is when the nurse notes that, with each compression of the bag, the baby's
1. chest rises.
2. abdomen rises.
3. heart rate increases slightly.
4. respiratory efforts to breathe offer resistance.

238. External heart massage becomes necessary for Baby Carter. Which one of the following techniques is *incorrect?*
1. Cardiac massage is alternated with ventilation.
2. The midsternum is compressed with the heel of the hand.
3. The heart is compressed approximately 120 times per minute.
4. The downward displacement of the chest wall is no more than 1 inch.

239. After the respirations and heartbeat were established, the infant was placed in an oxygen hood. Which one of the following actions is *unnecessary* when administering oxygen by the hood method?
1. Humidifying the air.
2. Covering the baby's eyes.
3. Deflecting the oxygen from the baby's head.
4. Measuring the oxygen concentration in the hood.

240. The percentage of oxygen in normal room air is approximately
1. 10 percent.
2. 20 percent.
3. 30 percent.
4. 40 percent.

241. If the baby develops retrolental fibroplasia, the child will *most likely* be
1. deaf.
2. mute.

3. blind.

4. mentally retarded.

242. Which one of the following actions is *least likely* to be helpful to the parents of a baby transported to a neonatal center for premature infants to receive intensive care?
   1. Encouraging the parents to call or visit the neonatal center.
   2. Allowing the parents to see and touch the baby before transport.
   3. Allowing the parents to participate in as much of the care as possible.
   4. Reporting the positive aspects of the baby's condition rather than the negative aspects.

243. Baby Carter is being fed by gavage. If the catheter passed for gavage entered the trachea rather than the stomach, which one of the following observations will the nurse note when she places the end of the catheter under water?
   1. The baby will cry.
   2. The level of the water will drop.
   3. The catheter will be forced out of the water.
   4. Air bubbles will appear at regular intervals.

244. All of the following observations in a premature infant are important. Which one should take *highest* priority in terms of planning his care?
   1. Skin eruptions.
   2. Frequent crying.
   3. Cyanosed extremities.
   4. Respiratory difficulties.

245. Which one of the following emotional feelings does a mother who has given birth to a premature baby *usually* demonstrate *first?*
   1. Fear.
   2. Guilt.
   3. Anger.
   4. Dependency.

Ms. Marilyn O'Brian has been told by her physician that her baby may be affected by hemolytic disease of the newborn. She was admitted to the hospital for study and care. Items 246 through 266 pertain to this situation.

246. Which one of the following combinations of blood types is *most likely* to produce hemolytic disease of the newborn?
   1. O− mother and A+ father.
   2. A+ mother and A− father.

3. O− mother and B− father.
4. O+ mother and O− father.

247. Hemolytic disease of the newborn due to Rh sensitivity is *rarely* a problem in a first pregnancy because
1. the first baby is usually Rh negative.
2. most women today are immunized against the Rh factor.
3. the mother's blood is able to neutralize antibodies formed in the first pregnancy.
4. antibodies are not ordinarily formed until there is exposure to an antigen.

248. The *most common* cause of sensitization to the Rh factor is
1. deficiency of immunoglobins.
2. delivery of an Rh positive baby.
3. transfusion with improperly matched blood types.
4. pregnancy with an Rh negative baby.

249. Which one of the following effects of hemolysis due to Rh sensitization is *rarely* present at the time of birth?
1. Edema.
2. Anemia.
3. Jaundice.
4. Heart failure.

250. Antibody titers may be done during pregnancy to monitor the severity of Rh sensitization. What specimen is used to determine the antibody titer?
1. Fetal blood.
2. Amniotic fluid.
3. Maternal urine.
4. Maternal blood.

251. Which one of the following tests is done to determine the presence of antibodies?
1. Direct Coombs'.
2. Indirect Coombs'.
3. Direct bilirubin.
4. Indirect bilirubin.

252. A direct Coombs' test is done on the cord blood to detect the presence of
1. fetal red cells in the maternal serum.
2. maternal red cells in the fetal circulation.
3. antigens coating the mother's red blood cells.
4. antibodies coating the baby's red blood cells.

253. Ms. O'Brian's fetus is found to be severely affected by hemolytic disease and an intrauterine transfusion is planned. The *primary* reason for an intrauterine transfusion is to
1. remove excess bilirubin.

2. replace destroyed red blood cells.

3. dilute maternal antibody concentration.

4. serve as a focus for maternal antibodies.

254. Labor is induced for Ms. O'Brian at 32 weeks of gestation, and an exchange transfusion is planned for immediately after delivery. When this procedure is performed, which one of the following actions is *legally* considered to be a nursing responsibility?

1. Cross-matching the blood.

2. Having the equipment ready.

3. Getting the consent form signed.

255. The nurse can anticipate that the vein which will *most likely* be used to give Baby O'Brian the exchange transfusion is the

1. femoral vein.

2. jugular vein.

3. temporal vein.

4. umbilical vein.

256. Infection is a potential complication of Baby O'Brian's exchange transfusion. Which one of the following signs is the *least* reliable when the nurse assesses the baby for signs of infection?

1. Lethargy.

2. A poor sucking reflex.

3. An elevated temperature.

4. Redness around the umbilicus.

257. Intravenous albumin is ordered for Baby O'Brian. How will albumin help to reduce the baby's blood bilirubin level?

1. Bilirubin production is prevented by maintaining high levels of blood albumin.

2. Bilirubin binds to albumin and is transported to the liver for eventual excretion.

3. Albumin combines with enzymes and couples with bilirubin which can then be excreted.

4. Albumin acts as a catalyst to convert bilirubin to biliverdin which can then be excreted.

258. The reasons for giving Baby O'Brian an exchange transfusion include relieving the baby's anemia and

1. replenishing the body's white blood cells.

2. restoring the blood's antigen-antibody balance.

3. lowering the blood's concentration of bilirubin.

4. replacing Rh negative blood with Rh positive blood.

259. Which organ in the body is *most* subject to damage when hemolytic disease remains uncontrolled?

1. The brain.

2. The liver.
3. The spleen.
4. The kidneys.
260. Which one of the following precautions should be observed when Baby O'Brian is ordered to receive phototherapy?
1. The eyes should be patched.
2. The genitalia should be covered.
3. Oxygen therapy should be withheld.
4. An unhealed naval should be covered.
261. Baby O'Brian's condition deteriorates and death appears imminent. The parents are both Roman Catholic and a priest of the church is not available to baptize the baby. Which one of the following statements *most accurately* reflects the tenets of the Roman Catholic church concerning who may properly baptize this infant, assuming the individual has the intent of doing what the church desires?
1. It would be acceptable only if one of the parents performed the baptism.
2. It would be acceptable only if the person performing the baptism was a Roman Catholic.
3. It would be acceptable only if the person performing the baptism had been baptized.
4. It would be acceptable for anyone to baptize this infant regardless of his religious beliefs.
262. Ms. O'Brian asks to see the baby after it dies. Which one of the following statements offers the nurse the *best* guide for answering the mother's request?
1. She should be allowed to view the body but only if the fetus was physically normal.
2. She should not be allowed to view the body since seeing the baby may precipitate postpartal depression.
3. She should be allowed to view the body since this has been found to help complete the grieving process.
4. She should not be allowed to view the body since it is the nurse's responsibility to protect patients from unnecessary trauma.
263. An autopsy is to be performed on the body. Who may *legally* give permission for the autopsy to be done?
1. The priest.
2. The parents.
3. The physician.
4. The hospital lawyer.
264. Ms. O'Brian asks how she should tell her 4-year-old son about the death of the baby. Of the following responses, which one is

the *most appropriate* for the nurse to make?
1. "What do you think he knows now?"
2. "Tell him God took the baby to heaven."
3. "Explain to him that death is a long sleep."
4. "Don't you think he is too young to understand what happened?"

265. An antibody is *best* defined as
1. a chemical substance that initiates an allergic reaction.
2. an albumin substance produced by white blood cells that acts as a phagocytic agent.
3. a chemical substance that is a nonspecific antagonist to protein substances.
4. a protein substance that reacts with specific other proteins to maintain homeostasis.

266. An antigen is *best* defined as a substance that acts to
1. produce an immune response in the body.
2. initiate an allergic response by the body.
3. protect the body against a specific disease.
4. stimulate the body's production of histamine.

Ms. Becky Andrew is 17 years old, unmarried, and pregnant. She has been receiving prenatal care at a clinic. At present, she has early signs of preeclampsia.
Items 267 through 292 pertain to this situation.

267. Which one of the following descriptions is *most typical* of the father of a baby whose mother is an unmarried adolescent?
1. An older man who has taken advantage of an adolescent.
2. A younger boy with whom she has engaged in sexual experimentation.
3. One of many with whom the adolescent has had a series of casual relationships.
4. A member of the adolescent's peer group with whom she has had a relationship over a period of time.

268. The two *most commonly* seen problems among pregnant adolescents are preeclampsia and
1. hypoglycemia.
2. gestational diabetes.
3. excessive weight gain.
4. iron deficiency anemia.

269. The nurse plans to discuss diet with Ms. Andrew. She should emphasize that during pregnancy, there is an increased need for *all* of the following food constituents *except*
1. iron.

2. protein.
3. calcium.
4. vitamin D.

270. Of the following considerations, the one that would be *least* important when the nurse instructs Ms. Andrew on her nutritional needs is that of her
   1. marital status.
   2. likes and dislikes.
   3. stage of development.
   4. religious and ethnic background.

271. At the nurse's request, Ms. Andrew records her typical daily menu as follows:

Breakfast: one doughnut.
Lunch: hamburger, french fries, and a cola drink.
Dinner: garden salad with dressing, spaghetti with meatballs, and garlic bread.

Which one of the following supplements to the above menu would provide the necessary nutrients for Ms. Andrew for one day?
   1. One glass of milk with each meal, one egg, one serving of green beans, one orange, and one apple.
   2. One milkshake, one serving of meat, one banana, and two slices of bread with two pats of butter.
   3. One glass of milk with each meal and one at bedtime, one dish of custard, one serving of liver, one apple, and one banana.
   4. One glass of milk with each meal, two eggs, two slices of bread with two pats of butter, one apple, and one serving of carrots.

272. Of the following symptoms, the one that is *typical* of preeclampsia is
   1. abdominal cramping.
   2. swelling of the fingers.
   3. increased urinary output.
   4. intermittent bloody spotting.

273. Of the following signs, the one that is typical of preeclampsia and which Ms. Andrew's health practitioners are *most likely* to note is
   1. mental confusion.
   2. a slow, bounding pulse.
   3. an elevated blood pressure.
   4. an elevated blood urea nitrogen (BUN).

274. The signs/symptoms of preeclampsia are caused by increased
   1. plasma proteins with an increase in glomerular filtration.
   2. aldosterone production with an increase in fluid retention.

3. circulating blood volume and decreased respiratory vital capacity.

4. vascular constriction with a decrease in renal and uterine circulation.

275. Common complications of preeclampsia that effect the fetus include *all* of the following problems *except*

1. stillbirth.

2. prematurity.

3. congenital anomalies.

4. small baby in relation to gestational age.

276. Ms. Andrew calls the nurse at the clinic one morning and states she has had a headache for 2 days. She says she is nauseated and, therefore, does not want to take aspirin. She asks the nurse to recommend something for her. Of the following responses, which one would be *best* for the nurse to make?

1. "Take one of the new buffered aspirin. It isn't as likely to upset your stomach."

2. "I think the doctor needs to see you today. Could you come to the clinic this morning?"

3. "We can't prescribe on the phone. I will make an appointment for you to see the doctor."

4. "I'll have your doctor phone a prescription for you to your pharmacy. You can pick it up sometime later today."

277. Because of her preeclampsia, Ms. Andrew is admitted to the hospital. If the following choices are available, which room would be *most appropriate* for the patient?

1. A room that is brightly lighted and close to the nurses' station.

2. A room in the labor suite where the patient can be transferred quickly for delivery.

3. A room where the patient will have quietness and where personnel can observe her frequently.

4. A room on a surgical unit where the patient can be transferred quickly to the operating room for an emergency cesarean.

278. Ms. Andrew's hourly urine output is monitored. Of the following actions, which one should the nurse take when she notes that for 2 consecutive hours, the patient's output was 17 ml. and 15 ml.?

1. Continue with the present regimen of care.

2. Apply warmth over the patient's kidney areas.

3. Notify the patient's physician of the observation.

4. Encourage the patient to take more fluids by mouth.

279. The physician orders that Ms. Andrew have a low salt diet. Planning an adequate diet when low sodium intake is important is complicated to the *largest extent* by the fact that most

foods that are low in sodium are usually also
1. expensive.
2. unpalatable to most women.
3. low in vitamin and mineral content.
4. low in essential amino acid content.

280. In an effort to promote diuresis, an infusion of hypertonic glucose is started for Ms. Andrew. Of the following signs/symptoms that may occur during the infusion, *all* should be reported to the physician immediately *except*
1. a headache.
2. noisy gurgling respirations.
3. urinary output of 100 ml. per hour.
4. central venous pressure above 12 cm. of water.

281. A 24-hour urine specimen is analyzed daily for estriol levels. The *primary* reason for studying Ms. Andrew's urinary estriol level is to help
1. assess the condition of the fetus.
2. determine the severity of preeclampsia.
3. evaluate the patient's kidney functioning.
4. estimate when the onset of labor can be expected.

282. Of the following equipment, the *least important* apparatus to keep in Ms. Andrew's room would be
1. a vaginal speculum.
2. a padded tongue blade.
3. a tourniquet and an airway.
4. several sterile syringes and needles.

283. If Ms. Andrew complains of all of the following symptoms, which one should suggest to the nurse that the patient may be about to have a convulsion?
1. Feeling very warm.
2. Being unable to void.
3. Having epigastric pain.
4. Feeling fetal movements.

284. The physician orders magnesium sulfate for Ms. Andrew. Careful administration of this drug is required because of the likelihood of its impairing the proper functioning of the
1. excretory system.
2. endocrine system.
3. respiratory system.
4. pulmonary blood system.

285. The antidote for magnesium sulfate is
1. calcium gluconate.
2. potassium bicarbonate.
3. levallorphan (Lorfan).

4. nalorphine hydrochloride (Nalline).

286. During labor, the two *primary* goals of Ms. Andrew's care are to
1. lessen edema and reduce blood pressure.
2. prevent convulsions and deliver the baby safely.
3. increase urinary output and limit kidney damage.
4. sedate the patient and decrease reflex excitability.

287. Ms. Andrew has one convulsion before she delivers. Once she is delivered of the baby, which one of the following statements *most accurately* describes her prognosis for having additional convulsions?
1. There is little likelihood that the patient will have additional convulsions.
2. The possibility of having additional convulsions is great for an indefinite period of time.
3. The possibility of having additional convulsions is great for at least the first week after delivery.
4. The possibility of having additional convulsions is great for at least the first 48 hours after delivery.

288. At what height can the nurse expect Ms. Andrew's uterus to be approximately 12 hours after delivery when progress of involution is normal?
1. Slightly above the level of the umbilicus.
2. Midway between the umbilicus and the symphysis pubis.
3. Barely palpable above the upper margin of the symphysis pubis.
4. No specific height; there is great individual variation among patients.

289. When the nurse checks Ms. Andrew's fundus about 24 hours after delivery, she notes that it is to the right of the midline. Which one of the following conditions is the *most likely* cause for this finding?
1. Constipation.
2. Uterine atony.
3. Urinary retention.
4. Retention of blood clots.

290. Which one of the following positions is the *most appropriate* for the nurse to recommend to Ms. Andrew to help in the involution of her uterus?
1. Flat on her back.
2. Flat on her abdomen.
3. In a semisitting position.
4. On her side with her knees flexed.

291. The nurse observes Baby Andrew gagging on mucus and becoming cyanotic after a feeding. Of the following measures, the

first one the nurse should take is to
1. start mouth-to-mouth breathing.
2. administer a little 100% oxygen.
3. raise the infant's head and pat him on the back.
4. clear the infant's airway with gravity or suction.

292. Ms. Andrew plans to place her baby for adoption but requests to hold and feed the baby while she is hospitalized. Of the following responses, which is the *most appropriate* for the nurse to make?
1. "All right, Ms. Andrew. We will bring the baby to you for his next feeding."
2. "We'll ask your mother if she thinks that is a good idea. She knows you better than we do."
3. "It is not a good idea to hold and feed the baby. It will be that much harder to give it up to other parents."
4. "We will ask your social worker the next time she visits. Policies concerning your request vary among agencies."

Ms. Andrea Nicol, gravida II, para I, is at approximately 37 weeks of gestation. She was admitted to the labor suite of the hospital with a diagnosis of possible placenta previa.
Items 293 through 317 pertain to this situation.

293. After helping Ms. Nichol to bed upon admission, the nurse's *most appropriate* action would be to
1. perform a vaginal examination.
2. give the patient a cleansing enema.
3. shave the patient's abdomen and perineal area.
4. check the fetal heart tones and the mother's blood pressure.

294. A differential diagnosis between placenta previa and placenta abruptio was made at the time of admission. Of the following symptoms, the one that is *most typical* of placenta abruptio is
1. lack of pain.
2. a rigid abdomen.
3. early rupture of the amnion.
4. lack of uterine contractions.

295. A complication of placenta abruptio is hypofibrinogenemia. One *typical late* sign of this condition is
1. blurred vision.
2. a tendency to bleed.
3. an elevated blood pressure.
4. a tendency to form excess scar tissue.

296. The *most typical* symptom of placenta previa is
1. painless bleeding.

2. a boardlike abdomen.

3. intermittent pain with spotting.

4. a dull aching pain in the lower abdominal quadrants.

297. The physician diagnoses Ms. Nichol as having placenta previa and orders a sonogram for her. The patient begins to cry when she is told of the procedure. Of the following statements that the nurse could make to the patient, which one is *most appropriate?*

1. "There is nothing to worry about. You won't feel a thing."

2. "Sound waves are used to determine the location of the placenta. It is a painless and safe procedure."

3. "Please try to stop crying. We need your cooperation during the procedure which is necessary to save your baby."

4. "A dye is injected and serial x-ray pictures are taken to determine the size of the fetus. The only thing you will feel is the insertion of the needle to inject the dye."

298. After 3 days of bed rest in the hospital, Ms. Nichol is discharged and told to remain in bed until the onset of labor. Ms. Nichol's husband works and she has a 2-year-old child. After assessing that Ms. Nichol needs assistance at home, which one of the following courses of action would be *most appropriate* for the nurse to take?

1. Exploring with the patient the kinds of assistance that are available to her.

2. Suggesting that the patient's mother come to stay until after the baby is born.

3. Suggesting that her husband take a leave of absence from work until the baby is born.

4. Telling the patient that bed rest seems difficult under the circumstances but that she should rest as much as possible.

299. Ms. Nichol is admitted to the hospital in labor 10 days later and a vaginal delivery is accomplished. A pudendal block was used. For this type of anesthesia, into which tissues is the anesthetic administered?

1. Through the sacrospinous ligament into the posterior areolar tissue.

2. Through the peridural space via the sacral hiatus into the dural space.

3. Through the vaginal mucosa into the tissue surrounding the paracervical nerves.

4. Through the subcutaneous tissues into the levator ani muscle midway between the anus and the ischial tuberosities.

300. A pudendal block is given *primarily* because it acts on the mother to

1. relax the cervix in order to prevent the mother from bearing down too soon.
2. reduce pain perception during the first stage of labor in order to help the mother relax.
3. reduce the strength of contractions in order to relieve undue pressure on the presenting part.
4. reduce pain reception during the second stage of labor in order to help keep the mother comfortable.

301. Ms. Nichol delivers a male infant over a midline episiotomy with a first-degree laceration. Which one of the following anatomical structures is involved when a first-degree laceration is present?
1. The cervix.
2. The levator ani muscle.
3. The perineal body.
4. The vaginal mucosa.

302. Baby Nichol had an Apgar score of 8 at 1 minute, and 10 at 5 minutes. These Apgar scores are accurately assessed when the baby's condition is judged to be
1. poor.
2. fair.
3. good.
4. critical.

303. The nurse obtains Baby Nichol's temperature rectally shortly after birth. The first temperature of a newborn is usually taken rectally *primarily* in order to
1. stimulate the vagus nerve.
2. ascertain patency of the rectum.
3. stimulate the passage of meconium.
4. obtain the most accurate temperature reading.

304. Approximately how long after birth can the nurse anticipate it will take Baby Nichol to stabilize his temperature?
1. 2 hours.
2. 8 hours.
3. 16 hours.
4. 24 hours.

305. According to research, which one of the following statements concerning the relationship of the rectal and axillary temperatures of an infant immediately following birth is *most accurate?*
1. The axillary temperature and the rectal temperature are approximately the same.
2. The axillary temperature is approximately 1 degree lower than the rectal temperature.

3. The axillary temperature is approximately 1 degree higher than the rectal temperature.
4. No assumption can be made about one temperature based on knowledge of the other.

306. Ms. Nichol is given ergonovine maleate (Ergotrate) 0.2 mg. intramuscularly in the delivery room after the delivery of the placenta. On admission to the recovery room, her blood pressure is 152/86 and her pulse rate is 74. Of the following courses of action, which one should the nurse take when she observes these signs?
1. Notifying the physician immediately.
2. Continuing to monitor the vital signs every 15 minutes.
3. Administering the prescribed antihypertensive medication.
4. Rechecking the vital signs with a different sphygmomanometer.

307. The recovery room nurse notes that Ms. Nichol's fundus is "boggy." Of the following actions, which would be the *most appropriate* for the nurse to take?
1. Notifying the physician.
2. Elevating the foot of the bed.
3. Massaging the patient's fundus.
4. Administering the analgesic the physician ordered.

308. When Ms. Nichol is unable to void, the nurse prepares to catheterize her. Resistance to the catheter is felt when it reaches the internal sphincter. Of the following courses of action, which one would be *most appropriate* for the nurse to take?
1. Removing the catheter and waiting about an hour before trying again.
2. Pulling the catheter back about ½ inch before trying to move it inward again.
3. Allowing the labia to fall into place and then gently moving the catheter inward again.
4. Asking the patient to breathe through her mouth while rotating the catheter before moving it inward again.

309. On Ms. Nichol's second postpartal day, the nurse notes a large ecchymotic area to the right of the perineum which was due to the pudendal block anesthesia. Which one of the following nursing measures would be *most appropriate* in this situation?
1. Applying an ice bag to the perineum.
2. Continuing with the patient's usual care.
3. Increasing the number of sitz baths from three to six each day.
4. Consulting the physician about whether he wishes to evacuate the hematoma.

310. Ms. Nichol is to take her first shower since delivery. The nurse should stay nearby while the patient showers *primarily* because the patient is likely to
   1. chill.
   2. vomit.
   3. faint.
   4. hemorrhage.
311. On the second postpartal day, Ms. Nichol begins to cry because she feels constipated and her baby will not eat. Of the following judgments, it would be *most appropriate* for the nurse to assess the patient as experiencing the
   1. "taking in" phase of childbearing and exhibiting typical signs of sleep hunger.
   2. "taking hold" phase of childbearing and reacting to her feelings of inadequacy and dependency.
   3. "postpartal blues" phase of childbearing and possibly needing the help of psychological counseling.
   4. "let down" phase of childbearing and needing help to take the responsibility for caring for her bady.
312. The night nurse finds Ms. Nichol drenched in perspiration. The nurse should explain to the patient that the condition
   1. is common and due to a temporary increase in sweat gland activity.
   2. will subside quickly if the patient limits her water intake for a few days.
   3. will be called to her physician's attention since excessive perspiration in the early puerperium is unusual.
   4. is often an early sign of infection and her physician will most likely order an antibiotic for her in the morning.
313. Ms. Nichol complains of afterpains while nursing the baby. The nurse should explain to her that these pains are caused by
   1. blood loss during delivery.
   2. retention of small placental tags.
   3. excessive stretching of the uterus.
   4. release of oxytocin during nursing.
314. Ms. Nichol is afraid her 2-year-old daughter will be jealous of the baby and asks the nurse for help. Of the following suggestions, which one is *most appropriate* for the nurse to make?
   1. "Divide your time equally between the two children."
   2. "Ignore any signs of jealousy to diminish the behavior."
   3. "Give your undivided attention to your daughter several times a day."
   4. "Keep the children apart to prevent your daughter from harming the baby."

315. Ms. Nichol asks what kind of behavior changes are normal in a 2-year-old when a new baby is brought home. Of the following possible responses, which one is *most accurate* for the nurse to make?
1. "A 2-year-old will most likely ignore the baby until it is old enough for her to play with."
2. "A 2-year-old will most likely assume a 'big sister' attitude and try to be 'mother's little helper.'"
3. "A 2-year-old will most likely ignore the mother and later display regressive behavior, such as wanting a bottle."
4. "A 2-year-old will most likely learn to depend on her father for meeting emotional needs and tend to ignore her mother."

316. Ms. Nichol asks about postpartal exercises. Which one of the following types of exercises is the *best* to use the first few days after delivery?
1. Leg-lifts.
2. Knee-bends.
3. Partial sit-ups.
4. Perineal contractions.

317. When Ms. Nichol is 4 weeks postpartum, the physician recommends that she use the knee-chest position twice a day for 2 to 3 minutes. Which one of the following sketches *best* illustrates the correct knee-chest position?

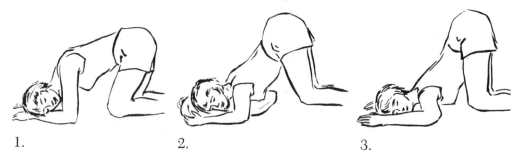

1.   2.   3.

Ms. Laurie Becker, who does not have a physician, was admitted to the hospital in early labor. She delivered a 6 pound, 4 ounce baby after an 8-hour uneventful labor. Ms. Becker told the nurse upon admission that she has been using heroin for the past 2 years.

Items 318 through 323 pertain to this situation.

318. When the nurse learned that Ms. Becker has been using heroin, which one of the following actions should she have taken?
1. Informed the police; using heroin is illegal.
2. Informed the head nurse; she is responsible for taking the next steps.

    3. Informed the physician who was called to deliver Ms. Becker; heroin addiction affects care.

    4. Informed no one; the information the nurse learned is confidential.

319. In the immediate postpartal period, the behavior Ms. Becker will *most likely* demonstrate is

    1. fatigue and drowsiness.

    2. euphoria and hyperactivity.

    3. nervousness and inability to sleep.

    4. depression and wanting to withdraw.

320. Approximately when after birth can the nurse anticipate that Ms. Becker's baby will demonstrate symptoms of heroin withdrawal?

    1. Within the first day.

    2. During the third day.

    3. During the fifth day.

    4. During the seventh day.

321. Ms. Becker should be taught that the effects of heroin addiction may be noticeable in her baby for as long as approximately

    1. 72 hours.

    2. 2 weeks.

    3. 8 weeks.

    4. 4 months.

322. Which one of the following signs related to crying will Ms. Becker's baby *most likely* demonstrate when she is having symptoms of heroin withdrawal?

    1. No cry.

    2. A weak cry.

    3. A shrill cry.

    4. A constant cry.

323. Which one of the following medications can the nurse anticipate the physician will use for Baby Becker during the period of withdrawal from heroin?

    1. Levallorphan (Lorfan).

    2. Nalorphine hydrochloride (Nalline).

    3. Meperidine hydrochloride (Demerol).

    4. Chlorpromazine hydrochloride (Thorazine).

       Ms. Malissa Mason has had three abortions because of an incompetent cervical os.
    Items 324 through 328 pertain to this situation.

324. Because of the nature of Ms. Mason's abortions, they would be classified as

    1. induced.

    2. clinical.

3. spontaneous.

4. therapeutic.

325. When during pregnancy do *most* abortions of the type Ms. Mason had occur?
   1. During the first trimester.
   2. During the second trimester.
   3. During the third trimester.

326. Ms. Mason's second abortion was incomplete and she continued to bleed after passing the fetus. The nurse should anticipate that the nature of treatment the physician *most likely* ordered at that time was that the patient
   1. have a dilatation and curettage.
   2. be given oxytocin intravenously.
   3. have her fundus massaged and kneaded.
   4. be given progesterone intramuscularly.

327. To maintain another pregnancy, the physician performed a cerclage procedure, using the modified Shirodkar technique. The technique helps prevent cervical relaxation and dilatation by
   1. removing the lowest cervical segment.
   2. reflecting the lower cervix back upon itself.
   3. encircling the cervical os with a suture-type material.
   4. closing the cervical os by suturing its edges together.

328. Ms. Mason became pregnant again after having the cerclage procedure. She is admitted to the hospital before term in an early stage of labor. Although the physician will be interested in knowing about all of the following signs, the nurse should anticipate that he will be *especially* interested in the patient's
   1. vital signs.
   2. state of hydration.
   3. vaginal discharge: amount and type.
   4. contractions: quality and frequency.

A nurse is performing a physical assessment on Baby Girl Harris who is approximately 24 hours old.
Items 329 through 350 pertain to this situation.

329. At what time in relation to her feedings would it be *best* to assess Baby Harris's physical condition?
   1. Midway between her feedings.
   2. Immediately after she has a feeding.
   3. Immediately before she is to have a feeding.
   4. The time of her feeding is unimportant.

330. Baby Harris was born after approximately 39 weeks of gestation and weighed 7 pounds, 8 ounces at birth. When compared

with her length of gestation, her body weight is *most accurately* assessed as

1. small.
2. large.
3. average.

331. The nurse measures the circumference of the head and chest. If Baby Harris is normal, it would be *typical* to find that when the two measurements are compared, the head will be

1. larger than the chest.
2. smaller than the chest.
3. the same size as the chest.

332. The nurse notes some molding of Baby Harris's head. Molding is *best* defined as

1. a normal condition due to bacteria in the birth canal.
2. a normal condition due to overriding of cranial bones.
3. an abnormal condition due to a scalp infection.
4. an abnormal condition due to excessive pressure on the cranium.

333. The anterior fontanel is normally shaped as a

1. circle.
2. square.
3. diamond.
4. triangle.

334. An effective way for the nurse to evaluate the patency of Baby Harris's nostrils is to

1. insert a catheter through each nostril.
2. cover the mouth and auscultate the chest on each side.
3. observe for ciliary movements within each of the nostrils.
4. occlude one nostril at a time and observe for respiratory effort.

335. Which one of the following findings, if noted by the nurse while listening to Baby Harris's chest, should be reported promptly for further investigation?

1. Heart murmur.
2. Expiratory grunt.
3. Heart rate of 156 beats per minute.
4. Respiratory rate of 40 breaths per minute.

336. The nurse assesses Baby Harris's tonic neck reflex. Which one of the following statements *best* describes movement when the tonic neck reflex is normal and when the baby is on her back?

1. She is able to touch her chin on the acromial process of either shoulder.
2. She resists pull on her arms and does not move her chin beyond the point of her elbows.

3. She turns her head to her left side, extends all of her extremities, and then promptly relaxes them.
4. She turns her head to her left side, extends her left extremities, and flexes her right extremities.

337. Bruises from the use of forceps during delivery are noted on Baby Harris's cheeks. In relation to the care of these bruises, it is *most typical* that they will require
1. no special type of treatment.
2. cleansing with an antiseptic daily until healed.
3. applying an antibiotic ointment daily until healed.
4. covering the area with a sterile dressing until healed.

338. Ms. Harris expressed concern when she noted that her baby's eyes were crossed. The nurse should explain that strabismus in a newborn is judged to be
1. normal; the eyes drift until the infant can see.
2. normal; there is a lack of eye muscle coordination in newborns.
3. abnormal; the eye muscles are of unequal strength and will probably need surgical intervention to correct.
4. abnormal; the condition is common in prematurely born infants, but full-term infants ordinarily can focus their eyes well.

339. If Baby Harris is typical of *most* newborns, the color of her eyes will be
1. blue or gray.
2. gray or black.
3. blue or brown.
4. brown or black.

340. The nurse notes a white cheeselike substance in Baby Harris's body creases. This substance is
1. milia.
2. lanugo.
3. smegma.
4. vernix caseosa.

341. The nurse inspects Baby Harris's palms. Which one of the following findings in relation to creases is *most often* associated with chromosomal abnormalities?
1. Many creases across the palm.
2. Absence of creases on the palm.
3. A single crease across the palm.
4. Two large creases across the palm.

342. Which one of the following organs is the nurse *least likely* to be able to palpate during her examination of Baby Harris?
1. The liver.
2. The spleen.

3. The kidneys.

4. The thyroid gland.

343. The bottom of Baby Harris's feet are examined. Which one of the following statements about creases would be *typical* of a newborn?

1. There are no creases on the bottom of the feet.

2. There are creases in the area under the heals only.

3. There are creases spread over the entire bottom of the feet.

4. There are creases in the area forward of the transverse arch only.

344. Which one of the following observations in relation to Baby Harris's cord should be reported to the physician promptly?

1. The cord stump is bluish and dry.

2. The area at the base of the cord stump is moist.

3. The cord clamp and cord dressing have been removed.

345. Baby Harris's anterior fontanel will normally close when she reaches the age of approximately

1. 2 to 3 months.

2. 6 to 8 months.

3. 12 to 18 months.

4. 20 to 24 months.

346. Baby Harris's posterior fontanel will normally close when she reaches the age of approximately

1. 2 to 3 weeks.

2. 2 to 3 months.

3. 6 to 8 months.

4. 12 to 18 months.

347. The nurse notes that Baby Harris's hands and feet have changed from a pink to a bluish color during the examination. Appropriate action for the nurse to take in relation to this finding is to

1. wrap the baby warmly.

2. massage his extremities.

3. report the change to the physician promptly.

4. administer oxygen to the baby promptly.

348. Which one of the following senses is believed to be *most highly* developed at birth?

1. Smell.

2. Touch.

3. Taste.

4. Hearing.

349. Observations have tended to illustrate that the amount of crying a newborn infant does is *most often* related to the

1. difficulty of the delivery.

2. length of time the mother was in labor.

3. method of feeding and dressing the baby.

4. kind and amount of comforting the baby receives.

350. What is the approximate range of hemoglobin in a normal newborn at birth?

1. 5 to 10 Gm. per 100 ml. of blood.

2. 10 to 15 Gm. per 100 ml. of blood.

3. 15 to 20 Gm. per 100 ml. of blood.

4. 20 to 25 Gm. per 100 ml. of blood.

Ms. Barbara Henderson decided when she was 4 months pregnant to breast feed her baby. She discusses this with the nurse in her physician's office during her pregnancy and later after her delivery.

Items 351 through 367 pertain to this situation.

351. Ms. Henderson says, "I am worried that I will not be able to nurse my baby because my breasts are so small." Which one of the following statements offers the nurse the *best* guide when she responds to the patient's comment?

1. The size of the breasts does not influence the ability to nurse a baby.

2. Women with small breasts tend to produce less milk than women with large breasts.

3. The woman's belief in her ability to nurse is less important than the size of the breasts.

4. The baby is able to grasp the nipples more easily when the breasts are small than when they are large.

352. Ms. Henderson asks what she can do to prepare for nursing the baby. The nurse should teach her that it would be *best* to

1. do nothing special since the breasts prepare themselves for nursing.

2. wash her breasts three times a day and follow that with a lanolin massage.

3. brush her nipples lightly with a rough towel and roll her nipples daily.

4. apply alcohol to her nipples daily in order to toughen them for nursing.

353. During her sixth month of pregnancy, Ms. Henderson calls the nurse because she notes fluid leaking from her nipples. The nurse should explain to her that

1. this is colostrum and indicates her breasts are being readied for nursing.

2. her milk has come in early and she should pump her breasts until the baby is born.

3. she should come to the office since her physician will most likely prescribe a medication for this.
4. she should limit her salt intake since most likely she is retaining fluids which results in the discharge.

354. Ms. Henderson delivers a normal baby. The nurse teaches Ms. Henderson that she should *not* take medications while she is lactating unless the physician prescribes them. The rationale for this advice is that many drugs
1. have been found to suppress milk production.
2. have been found to depress the baby's appetite.
3. are excreted in breast milk and, hence, will affect the baby.
4. tend to delay normal involution and, hence, predispose to postpartal infections.

355. Which one of the following food constituents is *especially* important for the lactating mother to have in larger amounts than the nonlactating mother?
1. Fats.
2. Proteins.
3. Vitamin K.
4. Carbohydrates.

356. When compared with Ms. Henderson's fluid intake prior to pregnancy, most authorities would recommend that while lactating she should
1. increase her fluid intake in order to foster the production of milk.
2. decrease her fluid intake in order not to dilute the quality of her milk.
3. satisfy her normal appetite for fluids since there seems to be no relationship between fluid intake and lactation.

357. Which one of the following actions will *most likely* stimulate the baby to open his mouth to grasp the nipple when Ms. Henderson starts to nurse him?
1. Pinching his toes gently.
2. Rubbing his back with her hand.
3. Brushing the nipple across his lips.
4. Stroking his cheeks with her fingers.

358. Ms. Henderson asks the nurse how often she should bubble her baby while feeding it. The nurse's response should be guided by the fact that
1. babies eat more if they are bubbled frequently.
2. babies fed on demand rarely need to be bubbled.
3. proper techniques of nursing eliminate the need for bubbling.
4. breast-fed babies usually do not swallow as much air as bottle-fed babies.

359. Although variations exist, approximately how long is the average nursing period of a baby who has become well accustomed to nursing?
   1. 5 minutes.
   2. 10 minutes.
   3. 20 minutes.
   4. 30 minutes.
360. Ms. Henderson tells the nurse that her nipples are sore from the baby's nursing. Which one of the following measures would be *least likely* to alleviate the soreness?
   1. Wearing a breast binder.
   2. Alternating the breasts for feeding.
   3. Applying a nipple cream after each feeding.
   4. Exposing the nipples to the air after each feeding.
361. Which one of the following measures is generally considered to be *most important* when treating a lactating mother who has breast engorgement?
   1. Emptying the breasts regularly.
   2. Wearing a supportive brassiere.
   3. Applying ice bags to the breasts.
   4. Administering an analgesic medication.
362. The so-called let-down sensation which is brought on when milk from the mammary cells is carried to the nipples of the nursing mother is regulated by the hormone
   1. oxytocin.
   2. prolactin.
   3. thyrotropin.
   4. parathormone.
363. The nurse teaches Ms. Henderson how to express milk manually. The proper method for manual expression includes using the thumb and forefinger to
   1. alternately compress and release the nipple.
   2. alternately compress and release the breast at the edge of the areola.
   3. slide forward from the edge of the areola toward the end of the nipple.
   4. roll the nipple between the fingers while exerting a gentle pull on the nipple.
364. Of the following practices, the one which has been found to be *most effective* in helping maintain an adequate milk supply is to
   1. feed the baby at regular intervals.
   2. empty the breasts at each feeding time.
   3. refrain from substituting a formula feeding for a breast feeding.

4. allow the baby to nurse for specific amounts of time with each feeding.

365. Ms. Henderson asks the nurse how she will stop producing milk when she wishes to wean the baby. The nurse's response should be based on knowledge that the
    1. milk supply will diminish as the baby nurses less.
    2. physician usually orders a medication to suppress lactation.
    3. wearing of a tight breast binder usually is effective to suppress lactation.
    4. milk supply normally diminishes at approximately 4 to 6 months after delivery.

366. If she is interested, which one of the following organizations would be *best* able to give Ms. Henderson information about breast feeding?
    1. The LaLeche League.
    2. The American Red Cross.
    3. The Childbirth Education Association.
    4. The American Society for Psychoprophylaxis in Obstetrics.

367. Of the following illnesses, the one which appears to have the *least* relationship to breast feeding is
    1. breast cancer.
    2. thrombophlebitis.
    3. prolapse of the uterus.
    4. late postpartal hemorrhage.

A nurse is preparing to discuss formula preparation with a group of postpartal mothers.

Items 368 through 379 pertain to material the nurse discussed.

368. Which of the following food constituents is poorly tolerated by infants, making dilution of whole milk necessary when preparing formula?
    1. Fats.
    2. Minerals.
    3. Proteins.
    4. Carbohydrates.

369. When preparing formula for an infant, commercial premodified milks are diluted in order to have approximately the same number of calories per ounce as does human milk, which, on the average, is approximately
    1. 10 calories.
    2. 20 calories.
    3. 30 calories.
    4. 40 calories.

370. When using evaporated milk to prepare an infant's formula, most physicians prescribe that one of the following food constituents be added, that one being
    1. fat.
    2. protein.
    3. minerals.
    4. carbohydrate.

371. Which one of the following combinations of vitamins is contained in *most* vitamin preparations for infants?
    1. B, C, and E.
    2. A, D, and K.
    3. B, D, and K.
    4. A, C, and D.

372. Which one of the following babies is *least likely* to have supplemental vitamins prescribed for him?
    1. Baby Aner, breast fed.
    2. Baby Trove, 2% cow's milk formula.
    3. Baby Noone, evaporated milk formula.
    4. Baby Cahen, commercial premodified milk formula, such as Similac.

373. Which one of the following factors appears to have the *most* influence on the number of calories infants require for normal growth and development?
    1. The sex of the infant.
    2. The infant's birth weight.
    3. The amount of the infant's activity.
    4. The type of feeding, that is, breast or formula.

374. As a *general* rule, approximately how many calories each day per pound of weight are required by newborns in order to maintain normal growth and development?
    1. 20 to 25 calories.
    2. 30 to 35 calories.
    3. 40 to 45 calories.
    4. 50 to 55 calories.

375. Which one of the following methods is *most often* recommended for enlarging the holes in a feeding nipple?
    1. Piercing the hole with a toothpick.
    2. Piercing the hole with a hot needle.
    3. Cutting the hole with sharp scissors.
    4. Cutting the hole with a sharply pointed knife.

376. When the terminal method of sterilization is used, it is *generally* recommended that, after boiling the bottles of formula, the sterilizer should be removed from the heat and the lid left on until the sterilizer is cool enough to touch in order to help

prevent
1. contamination by bacteria.
2. formation of a large curd.
3. separation of the formula into layers.
4. formation of a film on top of the formula.

377. Sterilizing items by boiling them is discussed. The nurse should teach that the time needed to sterilize by boiling at high altitudes will need to be increased because, in contrast to areas near sea level, in mountainous areas the
1. conduction of heat is lowered.
2. atmospheric pressure is greater.
3. boiling point of water is lower.
4. oxygen content in the air is less.

378. When using the terminal method of sterilization, how many minutes, *minimum*, do *most* authorities recommend that bottles of formula be boiled?
1. 15 minutes.
2. 25 minutes.
3. 35 minutes.
4. 45 minutes.

379. When teaching mothers how to care for the nipples after bottle feeding their infants, the nurse explains that it is *best* to
1. wash the nipples as soon after use as possible.
2. rinse the nipples under hot running water after use.
3. boil the nipples for a short period before handling them.
4. soak the nipples in a mild disinfectant before washing them.

Ms. Janet Brown, whose physician determined that she was approximately 17 weeks pregnant, was admitted to the hospital for an abortion by saline injection.
Items 380 through 390 pertain to this situation.

380. Preparation prior to injection of the saline solution includes having Ms. Brown
1. drink fluids to fill the bladder which will help push the uterus out of the pelvic cavity.
2. empty her bladder which will help avoid perforating the bladder during insertion of the needle.
3. restricted to nothing by mouth (NPO) which will help decrease nausea and vomiting during the delivery.
4. prepared with a perineal shave which will help decrease the chance of infection following delivery.

381. Which one of the following possible responses by the nurse would be *most accurate* when Ms. Brown asks how much pain

there will be and what anesthetic she will receive?

1. "The pain will be moderate; your physician will most likely give you a spinal anesthetic."
2. "The pain will be mild; to control it, you will receive an injection with a pain-relieving medication."
3. "The pain will be rather severe; a short-lasting but general anesthetic will be used so that you will be asleep during the procedure."
4. "There will be some pain when the needle perforates the abdominal wall; your physician will use a local anesthetic to help control the pain."

382. If some of the saline solution inadvertently enters the vascular system, which of the following signs/symptoms are *most likely* to occur?

1. Chills, generalized perspiration, vomiting, and an elevated blood pressure.
2. Flushing of the face, slow pulse rate, and tingling sensations in the hands and feet.
3. Dry mouth, ringing in the ears, rapid pulse rate, feeling hot, and a severe headache.
4. Constriction of the pupils, a low blood pressure, general apprehension, and shortness of breath.

383. Following the saline injection, Ms. Brown says, "I can still feel it moving. What is wrong?" The nurse's response should be guided by knowledge that the patient's sensation is

1. normal; the sensation is almost always noticeable in patients who feel guilt about having an abortion.
2. normal; the movement will stop in approximately an hour when the fetus dies.
3. abnormal; the movement indicates that the patient is likely to hemorrhage and the physician should be notified.
4. abnormal; the sensation indicates that possibly an insufficient amount of saline solution was injected and the physician should be notified.

384. Eighteen hours after the saline injection, Ms. Brown begins to have mild contractions which increase in intensity, duration, and frequency. Of the following nursing interventions, which would be the *most appropriate* for the nurse to take at this time?

1. Administering an analgesic as ordered, spending some time with the patient, and explaining what is happening.
2. Doing frequent vaginal examinations and taking the patient to the delivery room when she is about 8 cm. dilated.
3. Telling the patient that it will soon be over and that she need

not feel guilty since she chose to have an abortion which is
entirely legal.
4. Giving the patient some time alone, letting her think about her
condition, and then helping her understand that she is the one
who requested the abortion.

385. Ms. Brown calls the nurse when she begins feeling rectal pressure. Which one of the following nursing measures should
the nurse take *first?*
1. Transferring the patient to the delivery room.
2. Staying with the patient until the fetus is expelled.
3. Calling the physician to assist with the patient's delivery.
4. Telling the patient that the fetus is still not nearly ready for
delivery.

386. Which one of the following courses of action should the nurse
take *first* when the placenta is not expelled immediately after
delivery of the fetus?
1. Clamp the cord and remove the fetus.
2. Prepare the patient for surgical removal of the placenta.
3. Knead the patient's abdomen until the placenta is expelled.
4. Exert slight pull on the cord to help dislodge the placenta.

387. Ms. Brown is ordered to receive testosterone enanthate and
estradiol valerate (Deladumone) *primarily* because they help
to
1. aid uterine involution.
2. prevent breast engorgement.
3. relieve abdominal discomfort.
4. prevent conception for about 6 weeks.

388. Ms. Brown calls the clinic 2 days after discharge to report that
she has passed three large blood clots. Her temperature was
101° F. (38.3° C.) the day before, 100° F. (37.7° C) this morning,
and she is having abdominal pain. Of the following courses of
action, it would be *best* for the nurse to advise the patient to
1. take 10 grains of aspirin and get extra rest in bed.
2. stay in bed and call the next day if her temperature goes up
again.
3. go to the hospital immediately since she is in danger of hemorrhaging.
4. come to the clinic that afternoon for an examination by her
physician.

389. Ms. Brown's abortion was a legal act because of a 1973 ruling
made by the
1. Conference of State Governors.
2. Association of Federal Judges.
3. Supreme Court of the United States.

4. Attorney General of the United States.

390. When during pregnancy does terminating the pregnancy carry the *least* amount of risk to the mother?
1. From the time of fertilization to 4 weeks of gestation.
2. Between the 8th and 12th weeks of gestation.
3. Between the 16th and 20th weeks of gestation.
4. Between the 20th and 24th weeks of gestation.

Ms. Helen Olson has a 26-month-old child and a 7-month-old child. She consulted her physician after missing two menstrual periods and when pregnancy was confirmed, she burst into tears and cried, "I can't take it! I can't take it!" Items 391 through 396 pertain to this situation.

391. Of the following courses of action, which one would be *best* for the nurse to take in this situation?
1. Explaining to Ms. Olson that she will adjust sooner than she realizes to pregnancy.
2. Holding Ms. Olson's hand while remaining silent and listening as she is speaking.
3. Asking Ms. Olson why she feels upset and unhappy about being pregnant for the third time.
4. Telling Ms. Olson that most women are unhappy when they first learn they are pregnant again.

After talking with her husband, Ms. Olson decided to have an abortion. The physician used dilatation and suction curettage and performed the procedure under general anesthesia. The administration of intravenous solution was begun during the procedure. The postprocedure orders include the following: Methylergonovine maleate (Methergine) 0.2 mg. orally t.i.d. Dextropropoxyphene (Darvon) 50 mg. q 4 h., prn.

392. Which one of the following nursing measures is *most appropriate* to take during the period immediately following the procedure?
1. Massaging the fundus as necessary.
2. Observing the patient for vaginal bleeding.
3. Discontinuing the intravenous therapy as soon as the patient awakens from anesthesia.
4. Preparing to catheterize the patient if she has not voided within approximately 1 hour after awakening.

393. Fifteen minutes after Ms. Olson receives her first dose of methylergonovine maleate, she complains of moderately se-

vere abdominal cramping. Of the following courses of action, it would be *best* for the nurse to
1. call the physican.
2. ambulate the patient.
3. administer the analgesic.
4. plan to administer an antidote.
394. Ms. Olson receives human anti-D globulin (RhoGAM) before her discharge from the hospital, the purpose being to help prevent the patient from
1. becoming Rh negative.
2. developing Rh sensitivity.
3. developing AB antigens in her blood.
4. becoming pregnant with an Rh positive fetus.
395. The nurse makes an error on Ms. Olson's record. In addition to identifying herself on the record, which one of the following procedures is *legally* acceptable for correcting the error?
1. Erasing the error carefully and making the correction.
2. Drawing a line through the error and adding the correction.
3. Copying the sheet of the record with corrections and destroying the sheet in error.
396. Approximately how old are most women who decide to terminate pregnancies with an abortion?
1. Between 15 and 24 years of age.
2. Between 25 and 29 years of age.
3. Between 30 and 39 years of age.
4. Between 40 and 45 years of age.

Ms. Janet Adamer, who is 21 years old, plans to be married in 2 months. She visits a planned parenthood agency for contraceptive information.
Items 397 through 408 pertain to this situation.

397. According to research, when an ideal situation exists, the *shortest* time it takes for the sperm to reach the ovum is approximately
1. 1 to 5 minutes.
2. 20 to 30 minutes.
3. 45 to 55 minutes.
4. 65 to 75 minutes.
398. Biological preparations used as oral contraceptives will help prevent Ms. Adamer from becoming pregnant by
1. destroying ova.
2. destroying sperm.
3. inhibiting ovulation.
4. preventing implantation.

399. *Common* side effects for *most* oral contraceptives include
   1. nausea, edema, and breast tenderness.
   2. thrombophlebitis, amenorrhea, and vomiting.
   3. blurred vision, hypertension, and headaches.
   4. abdominal cramping, excessive bleeding, and intermenstrual spotting.
400. If Ms. Adamer forgets to take her contraceptive pill one day, she should be instructed to
   1. take two pills as soon as she remembers that she missed taking the one pill.
   2. wait until menstruation occurs and then start the next series of pills.
   3. take it as soon as she remembers and take the next pill at the regular time.
   4. take the next pill at the regular time without compensating for the missed pill.
401. When a condom is used for contraceptive purposes and lubrication seems necessary, which one of the following lubricants is *least appropriate* to use?
   1. Water.
   2. Saliva.
   3. Petrolatum.
   4. Contraceptive jelly.
402. If Ms. Adamer wishes to use a contraceptive cream and wishes to douche after intercourse, what is the *minimum* number of hours she should be taught to wait before douching?
   1. 3 hours.
   2. 5 hours.
   3. 8 hours.
   4. 12 hours.
403. Ms. Adamer inquires about an intrauterine device (IUD). By which one of the following mechanisms is the IUD thought to prevent conception?
   1. It suppresses ovulation.
   2. It depresses production of progesterone.
   3. It prevents sperm from entering the fallopian tube.
   4. It prevents the implantation of the fertilized ovum.
404. When, in relation to a menstrual period, is the optimal time to insert an IUD?
   1. During a menstrual period.
   2. Immediately after a menstrual period.
   3. Immediately before a menstrual period.
   4. Midway between menstrual periods.
405. If Ms. Adamer uses a diaphragm, for effective contraception, the

recommended *minimum* length of time to wait after intercourse before she should remove her diaphragm is

1. 1 hour.
2. 6 hours.
3. 12 hours.
4. 24 hours.

406. Ms. Adamer is taught the relationship between basal temperatures and fertility. The following diagram illustrates one woman's basal temperature chart.

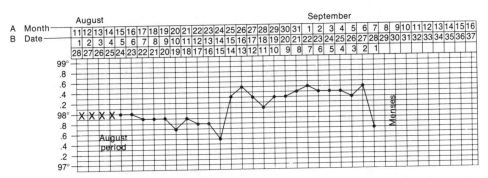

On what two dates in August is this woman *most likely* to be ovulating and, hence, *most* fertile?

1. On August 20 and 21.
2. On August 22 and 23.
3. On August 24 and 25.
4. On August 25 and 27.

407. When should a woman who is obtaining her basal temperatures take her temperature?

1. Every morning after breakfast.
2. Every evening before retiring.
3. Every afternoon between 3 and 4 o'clock.
4. Every morning upon awakening and before arising.

408. Which one of the following conditions will result in a woman's being infertile?

1. Absence of an ovary.
2. A dilated hymenal ring.
3. Occluded fallopian tubes.
4. An obstructed Bartholin's gland duct.

Items 409 through 456 are miscellaneous items.

409. The following four men are being studied for homologous artificial insemination; that is, semen from the husband will be given to his wife. Which one of the four is *least likely* to be

advised to use this procedure?
1. Mr. Brown who has hypospadias.
2. Mr. White who has undescended testicles.
3. Mr. Black who has premature ejaculations.
4. Mr. Green who has difficulty maintaining an erection.
410. According to the National Research Council, how many Grams of protein is the average pregnant woman encouraged to include in her daily diet?
1. By 55 Gm.
2. By 65 Gm.
3. By 80 Gm.
4. By 85 Gm.
411. If the nurse notes that the physician has made the following observations on four different multigravida women, the nurse should anticipate that a cesarean operation will *least likely* be ordered for the patient whose record states
1. "Breech presentation present."
2. "Status of fetus high in pelvis."
3. "Transverse presentation is apparent."
4. "Engagement occurred one week before admission."
412. Of the following considerations, which one is *most important* to guide the nurse in planning the care of a pregnant patient with heart disease?
1. The size of the heart.
2. The etiology of the heart disease.
3. The functional capacity of the heart.
4. The degree of pulmonary complications.
413. Which one of the following situations is used to confirm the presence of eclampsia?
1. The fetus dies.
2. The mother has a convulsion.
3. The placenta separates prematurely.
4. There is hemorrhaging into the mother's retina.
414. Common factors that predispose to toxemias during pregnancy include
1. malnutrition, hypotension, and multiparity.
2. habitual abortion, anemia, and placenta previa.
3. diabetes, vascular disease, and multiple pregnancy.
4. essential hypertension, an incompetent cervix, and obesity.
415. Which one of the following organisms is the cause of the vaginal infection which has the *most serious* consequences for the mother?
1. *Candida albicans.*
2. *Neiserria gonorrhoeae.*

3. Trichomonas vaginalis.

4. Beta hemolytic streptococcus.

416. A physician performs an amniotomy before the fetal head is well engaged. The complication he will expect the nurse to observe for carefully is

1. injury to the fetus.

2. prolapse of the cord.

3. change in the position of the fetus.

4. pressure of the fetus on the maternal vena cava.

417. One of the complications of abruptio placenta is hypofibrinogenemia. Of the following biological preparations, the nurse can anticipate that the physician is *most likley* to order that a patient with this condition receive

1. heparin.

2. vitamin K.

3. estriol (Theelol).

4. folic acid (Folvite).

418. For which one of the following patients in labor would a cleansing enema most certainly be *contraindicated?*

1. Ms. Bord, a primigravida, 5 cm. dilated, membranes ruptured.

2. Ms. Tast, multigravida, 6 cm. dilated, fetal heart tones 126.

3. Ms. Wolk, primigravida, 3 cm. dilated, bright red vaginal bleeding.

4. Ms. Farr, multigravida, 4 cm. dilated, contractions every 3 minutes lasting 45 seconds.

419. A patient complained of pain and was given meperidine hydrochloride (Demerol) 50 mg. intravenously. After the drug is administered, delivery appears imminent. Which one of the following medications should the nurse anticipate the physician is *most likely* to prescribe for the mother in order to help prevent the depressing effects of the meperidine on the infant?

1. Sodium bicarbonate.

2. Epinephrine (Adrenaline).

3. Caffeine sodium benzoate.

4. Nalorphine hydrochloride (Nalline).

420. If a patient displays all of the following symptoms during her first stage of labor, which one should the nurse report to the physician immediately?

1. Vomiting.

2. Bearing down.

3. Expelling a mucous plug.

4. Tonic contracted uterus.

421. A nurse is preparing equipment for a breech delivery. Which one of the following pieces of equipment should she have in

readiness for the physician's use?

1. Traction bar.
2. DeLee forceps.
3. Piper forceps.
4. Luikart Simpson's forceps.

422. Of the following four patients, the nurse can anticipate that the one with the *least* need for using obstetrical forceps during delivery will *most probably* be a
1. multigravida with rheumatic heart disease.
2. multigravida who is a gestational diabetic.
3. primigravida with a fetus at 32-weeks gestation.
4. multigravida with the fetus in the breech position.

423. Of the following actions, which one should the nurse take *first* if the cord has prolapsed?
1. Turning the mother onto her left side.
2. Reporting the fetal heart rate to the physician immediately.
3. Replacing the cord very slowly with a sterile-gloved hand.
4. Pushing upward on the presenting part with a sterile-gloved hand.

424. Which one of the following complications is *frequently* associated with the delivery of twins?
1. Vaginal tears.
2. Puerperal infection.
3. Rupture of the uterus.
4. Postpartal hemorrhage.

425. A patient has delivered her tenth baby. Which one of the following postpartal complications is she *more likely* to have than a woman who has delivered only 1 or 2 babies?
1. Uterine atony.
2. Vaginal hematoma.
3. Urinary infection.
4. Puerperal infection.

426. If a mother complains of afterpains while she is breast feeding her baby, the nurse should explain that the pain is due to the fact that
1. milk is forming too rapidly.
2. the baby is grasping the nipple too firmly.
3. milk production is insufficient for the baby's needs.
4. the uterus is stimulated to contract by the release of oxytocin.

427. The *major* cause of genetic malformation syndromes is thought to be
1. fusion of chromatids.
2. mutation of a single gene.
3. expression of a dominant trait.

4. absence of adequate deoxyribonucleic acid (DNA).

428. Down's syndrome is believed to be a condition *most probably* caused by a
1. chromosome abnormality.
2. metabolic abnormality.
3. failure in the development of the thymus gland.
4. failure in the development of the adrenal glands.

429. Which one of the following statements about Down's syndrome is *lacking* in scientific support?
1. Persons with Down's syndrome are especially susceptible to infections.
2. Down's syndrome has proven difficult to diagnose at the time of birth.
3. Treatment for curing Down's syndrome has met with little success to date.
4. Down's syndrome occurs more frequently in babies born of mothers over approximately 35 years of age.

430. The well-being of a fetus carried more than 2 weeks postterm may be compromised because the
1. umbilical cord begins to atrophy.
2. fetal nutritional requirements decrease.
3. placental function begins to deteriorate.
4. fetus causes undue pressure on the umbilical cord.

431. Which one of the following conditions is *least likely* to be present in the postmature infant?
1. Long, thin body.
2. Cracked, dry skin.
3. Meconium staining.
4. Long, molded head.

432. The *most important* determiner of the effects of drug-induced malformations of the fetus is the
1. amount of the drug the mother took.
2. length of time the mother took the drug.
3. amount of sensitivity the mother has for the drug.
4. stage of embryonic development when the drug was taken.

433. A score of 3 or less, obtained by using the Apgar Scoring Chart for evaluating newborn infants, indicates that
1. emergency measures are indicated.
2. no special type of care is needed.
3. special care is needed but it is not urgent in nature.
4. a scoring error has been made and assessment of the infant should be repeated.

434. Which one of the following criteria differentiates cephalhematoma from a caput succedaneum?

1. The size of the swelling.
2. The area of involvement.
3. The period of time required for absorption.
4. The kind of trauma at the time of delivery.

435. When a baby born after 37 weeks of gestation is 2 hours old, the nurse notes an increased respiratory rate and tremors of the hands and feet. These signs are *most likely* a manifestation of
1. hypothermia.
2. hypocalcemia.
3. hypoglycemia.
4. respiratory distress syndrome.

436. Which one of the following conditions, if observed in a newborn baby, should be reported to the physician promptly?
1. Cephalhematoma.
2. Erythema toxicum.
3. Caput succedaneum.
4. Impetigo neonatorum.

437. At 4 hours of age, a newborn infant took ½ ounce of glucose water eagerly which he regurgitated with mucus about 5 minutes later. When put to breast for the first time, he sucked briefly and then fell asleep. The nurse accurately assesses the baby's behavior as being
1. normal; many babies regurgitate mucus soon after delivery and are sleepy during the first few feedings.
2. normal; however, the mother should consider bottle feeding since the baby took the bottle better than the breast.
3. abnormal; the baby was experiencing the effects of analgesia given to the mother during labor.
4. abnormal; vomiting and drowsiness may indicate that the baby has increased intracranial pressure from delivery trauma.

438. Which one of the following conditions in the fetus is present *most frequently* when there are less than the normal number of umbilical cord vessels present?
1. A dead fetus.
2. A malnourished fetus.
3. A fetus with Rh negative blood.
4. A fetus with congenital anomalies.

439. *All* of the following observations are normal in a newborn who is 2 hours old *except*
1. dark stools.
2. irregular respirations.
3. persistent and shrill cry.
4. beginning cyanosis in the hands and feet.

440. Respiratory distress syndrome of the newborn (hyaline mem-

brane disease) is caused by the body's inability to secrete
1. ptylin.
2. surfactant.
3. vasopressin.
4. aldosterone.

441. For which one of the following reasons is vitamin K *usually* administered to newborns?
1. Newborns have no intestinal bacteria.
2. Newborns are susceptible to avitaminosis.
3. Hemolysis of the fetal red blood cells destroys vitamin K.
4. The newborn's liver is incapable of producing sufficient vitamin K.

442. A newborn has aspirated meconium and an endotracheal intubation is to be done. In addition to suctioning and administering oxygen, the nurse should be prepared to assist with
1. lavaging the airway.
2. inserting chest tubes.
3. using cardiac massage.
4. performing a tracheostomy.

443. Which one of the following hazards exists when a newborn has aspirated meconium?
1. The meconium predisposes to an antigen-antibody reaction.
2. The meconium will be absorbed and create a blood chemistry imbalance.
3. The meconium provides nutrients for bacterial growth in the respiratory systems.
4. The meconium acts as an irritant and eventually produces ulceration of mucous membranes.

444. It has been demonstrated that retrolental fibroplasia is *most likely* to develop when a premature infant's care has included the indiscriminate use of
1. oxygen.
2. vitamin K.
3. blood transfusions.
4. respiratory stimulants.

445. A patient was referred to a neurologist by her obstetrician. The neurologist called the hospital for a copy of the patient's record. Who may *legally* give permission for a copy of the record to be sent to the neurologist?
1. The patient.
2. The neurologist.
3. The obstetrician.
4. The medical librarian.

446. A newspaper reporter calls a hospital to ask about a pregnant

woman injured in an accident. Which one of the following items of information may the nurse tell the reporter without danger of legal problems?

1. The patient's age.
2. The patient's diagnosis.
3. The patient's treatment.
4. The extent of the patient's injuries.

447. A nurse wishes to investigate the relationship between the time of admission to a hospital and the length of labor. She wishes to gather data from patients' records. From whom must she obtain written consent for the use of these records?

1. The patient.
2. The physician.
3. The medical librarian.
4. A hospital representative.

448. A nurse notes that she incorrectly read a physician's order and gave 1½ grains of a medication instead of ½ grain. Of the following courses of action, which should the nurse take *first*?

1. Record the error.
2. Notify the physician.
3. Administer an antidote.
4. Check the patient's condition.

449. In 2 weeks' time, a registered nurse and a licensed practical nurse are scheduled to be the only nursing personnel on night duty on a unit where patients who have had voluntary abortions are hospitalized. The registered nurse is opposed to voluntary abortions; the licensed practical nurse is not opposed. Under these circumstances, which one of the following courses of action is *best* for the registered nurse to take?

1. State her opposition to voluntary abortions to her supervisor and request another assignment.
2. Care for the patients who have had voluntary abortions but explain her opposition to the procedure to them.
3. Accept the assignment but have the licensed practical nurse care for patients who have had voluntary abortions.
4. Accept the assignment and care for patients who have had voluntary abortions as a responsibility to persons needing her nursing skills.

450. According to official statistics that report maternal deaths in the United States, how many live births are used when describing maternal death rates?

1. 100.
2. 1000.
3. 10,000.

4. 100,000.

451. The *most frequent* cause of maternal deaths during childbirth is
    1. sepsis.
    2. toxemia.
    3. asphyxia.
    4. hemorrhage.

452. The *greatest single* factor for decreasing maternal deaths during the past 3 decades is *most often* credited to
    1. improved antenatal care.
    2. fetal monitoring during labor.
    3. the use of analgesia during delivery.
    4. medical supervision of care during the puerperium.

453. According to official statistics that report infant deaths in the United States, how many live births are used when describing infant mortality rates?
    1. 100.
    2. 1000.
    3. 10,000.
    4. 100,000.

454. Infant mortality rates include the death of infants up to the age of
    1. 1 week.
    2. 1 month.
    3. 6 months.
    4. 1 year.

455. Most infant deaths occur in the United States when the age of the infant is between
    1. birth and 7 days.
    2. 7 and 14 days.
    3. 1 and 2 months.
    4. 2 and 4 months.

456. The cause of most neonatal deaths in the United States is
    1. prematurity.
    2. atelectasis.
    3. birth injuries.
    4. congenital malformations.

answer sheet for obstetric nursing

Read each question in the examination carefully and select which one of the options is the *best* or *correct* answer. If the answer you would prefer is not given, select the one which seems *most appropriate*.

Locate on the answer sheet the number of the item you are answering. With a pencil, blacken the circle corresponding to the answer you have selected. Be sure you are recording your answer in the proper space.

	1 2 3 4		1 2 3 4		1 2 3 4		1 2 3 4
1	○○○○	18	○○○○	35	○○○○	52	○○○○
2	○○○○	19	○○○○	36	○○○○	53	○○○○
3	○○○○	20	○○○○	37	○○○○	54	○○○○
4	○○○○	21	○○○○	38	○○○○	55	○○○○
5	○○○○	22	○○○○	39	○○○○	56	○○○○
6	○○○○	23	○○○○	40	○○○○	57	○○○○
7	○○○○	24	○○○○	41	○○○○	58	○○○○
8	○○○○	25	○○○○	42	○○○○	59	○○○○
9	○○○○	26	○○○○	43	○○○○	60	○○○○
10	○○○○	27	○○○○	44	○○○○	61	○○○○
11	○○○○	28	○○○○	45	○○○○	62	○○○○
12	○○○○	29	○○○○	46	○○○○	63	○○○○
13	○○○○	30	○○○○	47	○○○○	64	○○○○
14	○○○○	31	○○○○	48	○○○○	65	○○○○
15	○○○○	32	○○○○	49	○○○○	66	○○○○
16	○○○○	33	○○○○	50	○○○○	67	○○○○
17	○○○○	34	○○○○	51	○○○○	68	○○○○

	1 2 3 4		1 2 3 4		1 2 3 4		1 2 3 4
69	○○○○	91	○○○○	113	○○○○	135	○○○○
70	○○○○	92	○○○○	114	○○○○	136	○○○○
71	○○○○	93	○○○○	115	○○○○	137	○○○○
72	○○○○	94	○○○○	116	○○○○	138	○○○○
73	○○○○	95	○○○○	117	○○○○	139	○○○○
74	○○○○	96	○○○○	118	○○○○	140	○○○○
75	○○○○	97	○○○○	119	○○○○	141	○○○○
76	○○○○	98	○○○○	120	○○○○	142	○○○○
77	○○○○	99	○○○○	121	○○○○	143	○○○○
78	○○○○	100	○○○○	122	○○○○	144	○○○○
79	○○○○	101	○○○○	123	○○○○	145	○○○○
80	○○○○	102	○○○○	124	○○○○	146	○○○○
81	○○○○	103	○○○○	125	○○○○	147	○○○○
82	○○○○	104	○○○○	126	○○○○	148	○○○○
83	○○○○	105	○○○○	127	○○○○	149	○○○○
84	○○○○	106	○○○○	128	○○○○	150	○○○○
85	○○○○	107	○○○○	129	○○○○	151	○○○○
86	○○○○	108	○○○○	130	○○○○	152	○○○○
87	○○○○	109	○○○○	131	○○○○	153	○○○○
88	○○○○	110	○○○○	132	○○○○	154	○○○○
89	○○○○	111	○○○○	133	○○○○	155	○○○○
90	○○○○	112	○○○○	134	○○○○	156	○○○○

2　obstetric nursing answer sheet

	1 2 3 4		1 2 3 4		1 2 3 4		1 2 3 4
157	○○○○	179	○○○○	201	○○○○	223	○○○○
158	○○○○	180	○○○○	202	○○○○	224	○○○○
159	○○○○	181	○○○○	203	○○○○	225	○○○○
160	○○○○	182	○○○○	204	○○○○	226	○○○○
161	○○○○	183	○○○○	205	○○○○	227	○○○○
162	○○○○	184	○○○○	206	○○○○	228	○○○○
163	○○○○	185	○○○○	207	○○○○	229	○○○○
164	○○○○	186	○○○○	208	○○○○	230	○○○○
165	○○○○	187	○○○○	209	○○○○	231	○○○○
166	○○○○	188	○○○○	210	○○○○	232	○○○○
167	○○○○	189	○○○○	211	○○○○	233	○○○○
168	○○○○	190	○○○○	212	○○○○	234	○○○○
169	○○○○	191	○○○○	213	○○○○	235	○○○○
170	○○○○	192	○○○○	214	○○○○	236	○○○○
171	○○○○	193	○○○○	215	○○○○	237	○○○○
172	○○○○	194	○○○○	216	○○○○	238	○○○○
173	○○○○	195	○○○○	217	○○○○	239	○○○○
174	○○○○	196	○○○○	218	○○○○	240	○○○○
175	○○○○	197	○○○○	219	○○○○	241	○○○○
176	○○○○	198	○○○○	220	○○○○	242	○○○○
177	○○○○	199	○○○○	221	○○○○	243	○○○○
178	○○○○	200	○○○○	222	○○○○	244	○○○○

	1 2 3 4		1 2 3 4		1 2 3 4		1 2 3 4
245	○○○○	267	○○○○	289	○○○○	311	○○○○
246	○○○○	268	○○○○	290	○○○○	312	○○○○
247	○○○○	269	○○○○	291	○○○○	313	○○○○
248	○○○○	270	○○○○	292	○○○○	314	○○○○
249	○○○○	271	○○○○	293	○○○○	315	○○○○
250	○○○○	272	○○○○	294	○○○○	316	○○○○
251	○○○○	273	○○○○	295	○○○○	317	○○○○
252	○○○○	274	○○○○	296	○○○○	318	○○○○
253	○○○○	275	○○○○	297	○○○○	319	○○○○
254	○○○○	276	○○○○	298	○○○○	320	○○○○
255	○○○○	277	○○○○	299	○○○○	321	○○○○
256	○○○○	278	○○○○	300	○○○○	322	○○○○
257	○○○○	279	○○○○	301	○○○○	323	○○○○
258	○○○○	280	○○○○	302	○○○○	324	○○○○
259	○○○○	281	○○○○	303	○○○○	325	○○○○
260	○○○○	282	○○○○	304	○○○○	326	○○○○
261	○○○○	283	○○○○	305	○○○○	327	○○○○
262	○○○○	284	○○○○	306	○○○○	328	○○○○
263	○○○○	285	○○○○	307	○○○○	329	○○○○
264	○○○○	286	○○○○	308	○○○○	330	○○○○
265	○○○○	287	○○○○	309	○○○○	331	○○○○
266	○○○○	288	○○○○	310	○○○○	332	○○○○

4   obstetric nursing answer sheet

	1 2 3 4		1 2 3 4		1 2 3 4		1 2 3 4
333	○○○○	355	○○○○	377	○○○○	399	○○○○
334	○○○○	356	○○○○	378	○○○○	400	○○○○
335	○○○○	357	○○○○	379	○○○○	401	○○○○
336	○○○○	358	○○○○	480	○○○○	402	○○○○
337	○○○○	359	○○○○	381	○○○○	403	○○○○
338	○○○○	360	○○○○	382	○○○○	404	○○○○
339	○○○○	361	○○○○	383	○○○○	405	○○○○
340	○○○○	362	○○○○	384	○○○○	406	○○○○
341	○○○○	363	○○○○	385	○○○○	407	○○○○
342	○○○○	364	○○○○	386	○○○○	408	○○○○
343	○○○○	365	○○○○	387	○○○○	409	○○○○
344	○○○○	366	○○○○	388	○○○○	410	○○○○
345	○○○○	367	○○○○	389	○○○○	411	○○○○
346	○○○○	368	○○○○	390	○○○○	412	○○○○
347	○○○○	369	○○○○	391	○○○○	413	○○○○
348	○○○○	370	○○○○	392	○○○○	414	○○○○
349	○○○○	371	○○○○	393	○○○○	415	○○○○
350	○○○○	372	○○○○	394	○○○○	416	○○○○
351	○○○○	373	○○○○	395	○○○○	417	○○○○
352	○○○○	374	○○○○	396	○○○○	418	○○○○
353	○○○○	375	○○○○	397	○○○○	419	○○○○
354	○○○○	376	○○○○	398	○○○○	420	○○○○

obstetric nursing answer sheet   5

	1 2 3 4		1 2 3 4		1 2 3 4		1 2 3 4
421	○○○○	430	○○○○	439	○○○○	448	○○○○
422	○○○○	431	○○○○	440	○○○○	449	○○○○
423	○○○○	432	○○○○	441	○○○○	450	○○○○
424	○○○○	433	○○○○	442	○○○○	451	○○○○
425	○○○○	434	○○○○	443	○○○○	452	○○○○
426	○○○○	435	○○○○	444	○○○○	453	○○○○
427	○○○○	436	○○○○	445	○○○○	454	○○○○
428	○○○○	437	○○○○	446	○○○○	455	○○○○
429	○○○○	438	○○○○	447	○○○○	456	○○○○

answer sheet for obstetric nursing

Read each question in the examination carefully and select which one of the options is the *best* or *correct* answer. If the answer you would prefer is not given, select the one which seems *most appropriate*.

Locate on the answer sheet the number of the item you are answering. With a pencil, blacken the circle corresponding to the answer you have selected. Be sure you are recording your answer in the proper space.

	1 2 3 4		1 2 3 4		1 2 3 4		1 2 3 4
1	○○○○	18	○○○○	35	○○○○	52	○○○○
2	○○○○	19	○○○○	36	○○○○	53	○○○○
3	○○○○	20	○○○○	37	○○○○	54	○○○○
4	○○○○	21	○○○○	38	○○○○	55	○○○○
5	○○○○	22	○○○○	39	○○○○	56	○○○○
6	○○○○	23	○○○○	40	○○○○	57	○○○○
7	○○○○	24	○○○○	41	○○○○	58	○○○○
8	○○○○	25	○○○○	42	○○○○	59	○○○○
9	○○○○	26	○○○○	43	○○○○	60	○○○○
10	○○○○	27	○○○○	44	○○○○	61	○○○○
11	○○○○	28	○○○○	45	○○○○	62	○○○○
12	○○○○	29	○○○○	46	○○○○	63	○○○○
13	○○○○	30	○○○○	47	○○○○	64	○○○○
14	○○○○	31	○○○○	48	○○○○	65	○○○○
15	○○○○	32	○○○○	49	○○○○	66	○○○○
16	○○○○	33	○○○○	50	○○○○	67	○○○○
17	○○○○	34	○○○○	51	○○○○	68	○○○○

	1 2 3 4		1 2 3 4		1 2 3 4		1 2 3 4
69	○○○○	91	○○○○	113	○○○○	135	○○○○
70	○○○○	92	○○○○	114	○○○○	136	○○○○
71	○○○○	93	○○○○	115	○○○○	137	○○○○
72	○○○○	94	○○○○	116	○○○○	138	○○○○
73	○○○○	95	○○○○	117	○○○○	139	○○○○
74	○○○○	96	○○○○	118	○○○○	140	○○○○
75	○○○○	97	○○○○	119	○○○○	141	○○○○
76	○○○○	98	○○○○	120	○○○○	142	○○○○
77	○○○○	99	○○○○	121	○○○○	143	○○○○
78	○○○○	100	○○○○	122	○○○○	144	○○○○
79	○○○○	101	○○○○	123	○○○○	145	○○○○
80	○○○○	102	○○○○	124	○○○○	146	○○○○
81	○○○○	103	○○○○	125	○○○○	147	○○○○
82	○○○○	104	○○○○	126	○○○○	148	○○○○
83	○○○○	105	○○○○	127	○○○○	149	○○○○
84	○○○○	106	○○○○	128	○○○○	150	○○○○
85	○○○○	107	○○○○	129	○○○○	151	○○○○
86	○○○○	108	○○○○	130	○○○○	152	○○○○
87	○○○○	109	○○○○	131	○○○○	153	○○○○
88	○○○○	110	○○○○	132	○○○○	154	○○○○
89	○○○○	111	○○○○	133	○○○○	155	○○○○
90	○○○○	112	○○○○	134	○○○○	156	○○○○

	1 2 3 4		1 2 3 4		1 2 3 4		1 2 3 4
157	○○○○	179	○○○○	201	○○○○	223	○○○○
158	○○○○	180	○○○○	202	○○○○	224	○○○○
159	○○○○	181	○○○○	203	○○○○	225	○○○○
160	○○○○	182	○○○○	204	○○○○	226	○○○○
161	○○○○	183	○○○○	205	○○○○	227	○○○○
162	○○○○	184	○○○○	206	○○○○	228	○○○○
163	○○○○	185	○○○○	207	○○○○	229	○○○○
164	○○○○	186	○○○○	208	○○○○	230	○○○○
165	○○○○	187	○○○○	209	○○○○	231	○○○○
166	○○○○	188	○○○○	210	○○○○	232	○○○○
167	○○○○	189	○○○○	211	○○○○	233	○○○○
168	○○○○	190	○○○○	212	○○○○	234	○○○○
169	○○○○	191	○○○○	213	○○○○	235	○○○○
170	○○○○	192	○○○○	214	○○○○	236	○○○○
171	○○○○	193	○○○○	215	○○○○	237	○○○○
172	○○○○	194	○○○○	216	○○○○	238	○○○○
173	○○○○	195	○○○○	217	○○○○	239	○○○○
174	○○○○	196	○○○○	218	○○○○	240	○○○○
175	○○○○	197	○○○○	219	○○○○	241	○○○○
176	○○○○	198	○○○○	220	○○○○	242	○○○○
177	○○○○	199	○○○○	221	○○○○	243	○○○○
178	○○○○	200	○○○○	222	○○○○	244	○○○○

obstetric nursing answer sheet 3

	1 2 3 4		1 2 3 4		1 2 3 4		1 2 3 4
245	○○○○	267	○○○○	289	○○○○	311	○○○○
246	○○○○	268	○○○○	290	○○○○	312	○○○○
247	○○○○	269	○○○○	291	○○○○	313	○○○○
248	○○○○	270	○○○○	292	○○○○	314	○○○○
249	○○○○	271	○○○○	293	○○○○	315	○○○○
250	○○○○	272	○○○○	294	○○○○	316	○○○○
251	○○○○	273	○○○○	295	○○○○	317	○○○○
252	○○○○	274	○○○○	296	○○○○	318	○○○○
253	○○○○	275	○○○○	297	○○○○	319	○○○○
254	○○○○	276	○○○○	298	○○○○	320	○○○○
255	○○○○	277	○○○○	299	○○○○	321	○○○○
256	○○○○	278	○○○○	300	○○○○	322	○○○○
257	○○○○	279	○○○○	301	○○○○	323	○○○○
258	○○○○	280	○○○○	302	○○○○	324	○○○○
259	○○○○	281	○○○○	303	○○○○	325	○○○○
260	○○○○	282	○○○○	304	○○○○	326	○○○○
261	○○○○	283	○○○○	305	○○○○	327	○○○○
262	○○○○	284	○○○○	306	○○○○	328	○○○○
263	○○○○	285	○○○○	307	○○○○	329	○○○○
264	○○○○	286	○○○○	308	○○○○	330	○○○○
265	○○○○	287	○○○○	309	○○○○	331	○○○○
266	○○○○	288	○○○○	310	○○○○	332	○○○○

	1 2 3 4		1 2 3 4		1 2 3 4		1 2 3 4
333	○○○○	355	○○○○	377	○○○○	399	○○○○
334	○○○○	356	○○○○	378	○○○○	400	○○○○
335	○○○○	357	○○○○	379	○○○○	401	○○○○
336	○○○○	358	○○○○	480	○○○○	402	○○○○
337	○○○○	359	○○○○	381	○○○○	403	○○○○
338	○○○○	360	○○○○	382	○○○○	404	○○○○
339	○○○○	361	○○○○	383	○○○○	405	○○○○
340	○○○○	362	○○○○	384	○○○○	406	○○○○
341	○○○○	363	○○○○	385	○○○○	407	○○○○
342	○○○○	364	○○○○	386	○○○○	408	○○○○
343	○○○○	365	○○○○	387	○○○○	409	○○○○
344	○○○○	366	○○○○	388	○○○○	410	○○○○
345	○○○○	367	○○○○	389	○○○○	411	○○○○
346	○○○○	368	○○○○	390	○○○○	412	○○○○
347	○○○○	369	○○○○	391	○○○○	413	○○○○
348	○○○○	370	○○○○	392	○○○○	414	○○○○
349	○○○○	371	○○○○	393	○○○○	415	○○○○
350	○○○○	372	○○○○	394	○○○○	416	○○○○
351	○○○○	373	○○○○	395	○○○○	417	○○○○
352	○○○○	374	○○○○	396	○○○○	418	○○○○
353	○○○○	375	○○○○	397	○○○○	419	○○○○
354	○○○○	376	○○○○	398	○○○○	420	○○○○

	1 2 3 4		1 2 3 4		1 2 3 4		1 2 3 4
421	○○○○	430	○○○○	439	○○○○	448	○○○○
422	○○○○	431	○○○○	440	○○○○	449	○○○○
423	○○○○	432	○○○○	441	○○○○	450	○○○○
424	○○○○	433	○○○○	442	○○○○	451	○○○○
425	○○○○	434	○○○○	443	○○○○	452	○○○○
426	○○○○	435	○○○○	444	○○○○	453	○○○○
427	○○○○	436	○○○○	445	○○○○	454	○○○○
428	○○○○	437	○○○○	446	○○○○	455	○○○○
429	○○○○	438	○○○○	447	○○○○	456	○○○○

obstetric nursing examination

correct answers and rationales

CHILDBIRTH CLASSES

1. 4. It has been found that ovulation occurs approximately 2 weeks before menstruation begins. Stated in another way, it has been found that menstruation occurs approximately 2 weeks after ovulation.

2. 4. The ovum is extruded into the peritoneal cavity. The fimbricated ends of the fallopian tube draw it by movement of the cilia into the fallopian tube.

3. 3. Fertilization normally occurs in the fallopian tubes. If for some reason the fertilized ovum does not pass on into the uterus, the condition is known as an ectopic or tubal pregnancy.

4. 2. The uterus receives its blood supply from the uterine and the ovarian arteries. The ovarian artery is a branch of the aorta. It enters the broad ligament and supplies the ovary with blood while its main stem makes its way to the upper margin of the uterus.

5. 2. The anterior lobe of the pituitary gland releases gonadotropins. There are two principle gonadotropins; the luteinizing hormone (LH) which is concerned with ovulation and the development of the corpus luteum, and the follicle-stimulating hormone (FSH) which stimulates development of the follicle. Estrogen, among other things, brings about a thickening of the endometrium. Adrenocorticotropic hormone (ACTH) is concerned with the body's response to stress.

6. 4. It has been found that the ovum normally remains viable for approximately 22 to 26 hours. This is significant for fertility studies and for conception control.

7. 4. Studies have shown that the sperm is capable of fertilizing the ovum for as long as 3 to 7 days, and possibly even longer. Although millions are normally discharged into the vagina at the time of intercourse, it is estimated that only thousands reach the uterus and fewer still eventually reach the fallopian tubes.

8. 2. The fertilized ovum remains in the fallopian tube about 3 days and in the uterus about 4 days until it implants itself in the uterine wall.

9. 3. The chorionic villi and decidua basalis fuse to become the placenta. The decidua vera is also a layer of the decidua, but neither it nor the decidua capsularis is in direct contact with the ovum. The chorionic frondosum is that part of the chorionic villi that fuses with the decidua basalis. The chorionic laeve is that part of the chorionic villi which does not fuse with the decidua basalis; it degenerates and finally almost disappears.

10. 1. Option 1 is an incorrect statement since the mother and fetus have separate, independent circulatory systems and there is no direct interchange of fetal and maternal blood in the placenta.

11. 2. The stem defines Chadwick's sign. Goodell's sign is a softening of the cervix and is also a presumptive sign of pregnancy. Hegar's sign is a softening of the lower uterine segment and is considered a sign of pregnancy. There is a Babcock's test, but it is unrelated to pregnancy.

12. 2. The lower uterine segment will feel soft. See item 11.

13. 4. These streaks are called striae gravidarum and are often referred to as "stretch marks." Chloasma is often called the "mask of pregnancy" since it occurs usually on the face; the spots on the skin are yellowish-brown. Linea nigra refers to dark lines that are usually found mostly on the abdomen. Alveoli are air vesicles in the lungs.

14. 1. Discoloration and enlargement of the areola are without significance and generally disappear after delivery. Options 2, 3, and 4 are inaccurate statements in relation to the phenomenon described in the stem.

15. 4. That part of the cell which carries genetic information has been found to be the DNA. The golgi apparatus is a network of rods in the cytoplasm and is thought to be related to secretory activity. The endoplasmic reticulum consists of membranes interconnected and arranged to form a tiny network of

canals. RNA is formed from DNA and is part of a system that enables DNA to control the manufacture of protein.

16. 3. Each mature sperm or ovum contains 23 chromosomes.

17. 1. Each body cell contains 22 pairs of autosomes and one pair of sex chromosomes (total—46). Male cells normally contain one X and one Y chromosome. Hemophilia is inherited as a sex-linked characteristic. Down's syndrome (mongoloid) is due to a chromosomal abnormality.

18. 4. The foramen ovale allows blood to bypass the pulmonary circulatory system. Since the fetus receives oxygen from the mother's circulation, only enough blood to supply the lung tissue circulates through the fetal lungs. After birth when the lungs are functioning, the foramen ovale normally closes.

19. 1. The umbilical cord normally consists of two arteries and one vein. A single umbilical artery is associated with congenital anomalies.

20. 2. The organ that acts to detoxify wastes is the liver. The lungs and kidneys eliminate wastes but do not detoxify. The spleen plays no role in the elimination of wastes.

21. 1. The tube that eventually becomes the heart in the fetus begins to pulsate and propel blood near the end of the first lunar month.

22. 2. Oxygenated blood flows through the umbilical vein to the fetus; blood leaving the fetus to return to the placenta travels through the umbilical arteries.

23. 2. Research has demonstrated that babies born of mothers who smoke have lower than average birth weights. Other factors given here have not been found to be associated with smoking.

24. 3. Vitamin A is deficient in unfortified skim milk. The other constituents of milk are not changed when the fat content of milk is reduced.

25. 4. Fortified whole milk is fortified with vitamin D. Fortified skim milk is often fortified with both vitamins A and D. See item 24.

26. 1. Of the foods given here, asparagus has the highest content of folic acid.

27. 1. Of the constituents given here, most pregnant women require extra amounts of iron.

28. 4. An inadequate diet may predispose to the conditions given in options 1, 2, and 3. The causes of placenta previa and placenta abruptio are unknown but are not considered related to dietary insufficiencies or indiscretions.

29. 3. Each Gram of protein contributes 4 calories; hence, 70 Grams of protein will contribute 280 calories to the diet.

30. 3. While several factors may contribute to the discomfort of

hemorrhoids, being constipated frequently contributes most to discomfort.

31. 1. Witch hazel is the most often recommended agent of those given since it acts as an astringent and helps shrink swollen tissues. The other agents in solution may provide some comfort but will not act as astringents.

32. 2. It is best to increase the amounts of roughage and liquids in the diet to help prevent constipation. The use of suppositories and laxatives can easily become habit forming and should be used only as necessary when diet alone has not controlled the problem.

33. 1. There is normally an increased vaginal discharge during pregnancy, but local itching is associated with infections, such as those due to Trichomonas vaginalis or gonorrhea. The best advice to give this mother is that she discuss the vaginal discharge with her physician. It may be of a serious nature and require treatment. Douches are not often prescribed during pregnancy. Intercourse may be contraindicated, depending on the cause of the discharge and the discomfort associated with it.

34. 3. Options 1, 2, and 4 are recommended to help prevent flatulence. It is not recommended that soda bicarbonate be used since it will not influence flatulence; also, the high sodium content may contribute to edema.

35. 3. Frequent urination is common early in pregnancy because of the pressure of the enlarging uterus on the urinary bladder. The symptoms ordinarily subside when the uterus rises out of the pelvis and into the abdominal cavity.

36. 4. Heartburn is due to reverse peristalsis which carries stomach contents into the distal end of the esophagus. This results in a burning sensation which is usually referred to as heartburn.

37. 1. Fats tend to decrease the secretion of gastric acids. Therefore, eating a small amount of butter or taking some cream will often help prevent heartburn. If heartburn is already present, the butter or cream will not help the situation and may even aggravate it.

38. 2. Eating some dry carbohydrate food, such as a cracker or toast, seems to be effective for most women who complain of early morning nausea. For a few people, taking fluids has been successful but only when the fluids were hot.

39. 3. It is generally believed that increased absorption of phosphorus, which upsets the calcium/phosphorus ratio, causes leg cramps which some women experience during pregnancy.

Calcium pills may be prescribed to help regain the proper balance.

40. 4. The measure that has been found to be most effective is described in option 4. Keeping the legs warm and elevated as much as possible are good preventive measures.

41. 4. The recommended position is described in option 4. The other positions will not allow for maximum drainage away from the vulva to help decrease venous congestion in the varicosities.

42. 4. The pelvic-rock, which seems to help strengthen back muscles, has been found to help many women who complain of backaches during pregnancy. The exercise is done as follows: while in a sitting position with hands on hips, alternately "tuck" the buttocks under and then relax. The exercises described in options 1, 2, and 3 are too strenuous to perform during pregnancy for most women.

43. 3. The enlarging uterus places pressure on blood vessels carrying blood to and from the legs. Interference with the venous return from the extremities predisposes to varicose veins. Options 1, 2, and 4 are inaccurate statements.

44. 3. Wearing round garters interferes with venous return from the legs, and hence, contributes to the formation or aggravation of varicose veins.

45. 3. The practice of elevating the legs in the manner described enhances venous return and, hence, decreases venous stasis and relieves varicosities.

46. 2. The manner of bandaging the leg is correctly described. However, the reason is not described in statement A. An extremity is bandaged toward the trunk of the body to avoid congestion and impaired circulation in the distal part.

47. 4. Statement B is a false statement. The toes should not be covered when bandaging an extremity so that they will be visible to determine that circulation is adequate.

48. 2. The discolorations described (chloasma—see item 13) usually disappear and are without clinical significance. Options 1, 3, and 4 are inaccurate statements in relation to these discolorations of the skin.

49. 2. Experience has shown that even long auto trips do not seem contraindicated unless the pregnant woman is experiencing complications. However, regular rest is advised. During the rest period, it is important to walk to encourage circulation that becomes sluggish during long periods of sitting. Option 1 is contraindicated. Traveling as described in options 3 and 4 is not contraindicated.

50. 4. There are breast shields now available that provide suction on the nipples. These have been found to be more effective than measures described in options 1, 2, and 3 when nipples are inverted.

51. 2. Tub baths were not recommended in the past for a variety of reasons, at least one of which is described in option 1. However, in recent years, showers are recommended primarily because of the danger of falling when using a tub as the mother's center of gravity changes during pregnancy.

52. 2. Lightening is defined as the settling of the fetal head into the pelvis. It usually occurs a week or two before delivery. Intermittent painless contractions are called Braxton-Hicks sign.

53. 3. Progesterone is believed to decrease uterine contractability and its level has been observed to drop late in pregnancy. Simultaneously, estrogen which has the opposite effect on the muslces of the uterus, increases. The combination of these two hormones, one decreased and the other increased, is an often accepted theory concerning the initiation of labor. Relaxin acts in the body to relax the pelvic ligaments and the cervix which helps to make passage of the fetus easier through the birth canal. The fetal corticosteroids increase as the fetus matures and many believe these steroids may play a part in triggering labor.

54. 4. Although regular and rhythmic contractions may be observed in both false and true labor, when true labor is present, there is a progressive dilatation of the cervix with effacement. Symptoms described in options 1, 2, and 3 may occur in both false and true labor.

55. 1. Effacement refers to thinning and shortening of the cervix. Options 2, 3, and 4 are not related to effacement.

56. 2. Effacement is described in terms of percentage and denotes the amount by which the cervix has shortened.

57. 1. Leopold's maneuvers consist of four maneuvers in which the abdomen is systematically palpated in order to determine the position of the fetus.

58. 1. The patient should empty her bladder before the nurse palpates the abdomen. This increases the patient's comfort and makes palpation a more accurate procedure.

59. 2. The nurse should palpate by placing her hands flat on the abdomen. The patient should have her knees flexed to help relaxation of abdominal muscles. Using fingers is likely to cause muscular contractions. Option 4 will be of no particular value.

60. 3. The suboccipito-bregmatic diameter is the smallest diameter

of the fetal head. When the head is well flexed, the smallest part of the head enters the pelvis first.

61. 3. Presentation is defined as that part of the infant's body that lies nearest the internal os. It is the part of the body which can be felt by the hand at the opening of the cervix. When the presenting part is known, the relationship between the long axis of the baby's body and that of the mother can be determined.

62. 4. The correct sequence of maneuvers through which the fetus proceeds occurs in the order described in option 4.

63. 2. The ischial spines are used as landmarks to determine the position of the head and are called "stations." Status plus one describes the fetal head when it has passed 1 centimeter below the ischial spines. If the phrase, "station minus one" had been used, the fetal head would have been 1 centimeter above the ischial spines.

64. 4. Crowning is the word used to describe the encircling of the largest diameter of the fetal head by the vulvar ring. The fetal head may be observed at the vaginal opening before crowning has been accomplished.

65. 4. The amniotic fluid does not provide the fetus with immune bodies.

66. 1. The left occipito-anterior position (L.O.A.) is described in the stem. The occipital position is considered most favorable for both mother and infant and L.O.A. is preferred.

67. 3. In a normal delivery, a total blood loss of approximately 500 ml. is generally considered to be within normal but at the high end of normal range.

68. 2. The average length of time a primigravida is in labor is approximately 14 hours. The first stage of labor lasts about 12½ hours; the second stage, about 1¼ hours; and the last stage, about 10 to 15 minutes.

69. 2. As soon as the baby starts to ventilate, circulatory changes occur in the infant. Factors described in options 1, 3, and 4 are not credited for changes in the infant's circulatory system.

70. 1. Dystocia is defined as a difficult labor. It may also be prolonged or painful.

71. 1. Dizygotic, or fraternal, twins develop from two ova and two sperms. They may be of the same sex but their chances of resembling each other are no greater than that of any brother and sister. Identical, or monozygotic, twins are called identical twins and develop from a single ovum.

72. 3. There are few experts adequately prepared to administer hypnosis. Options 1, 2, and 4 are inaccurate statements.

73. 1. Rupture when a tubal pregnancy is present is early in pregnancy, during the first 3 months.

RUTH FIELDING

74. 4. The major purpose for education for childbirth is to prepare the couple for approaching childbirth. This preparation may result in at least some of the benefits described in options 1, 2, and 3, but these options do not describe the *major* purpose.
75. 1. The Lamaze method of preparing for childbirth is best described in Irwin Chabon's book. The other two books describe the Bradley and the Dick-Read methods.
76. 2. Of the responses given here, the galvanometer is able only to measure amounts of perspiration.
77. 4. Of those given, the EMG is able only to measure muscular tension.
78. 1. The concept upon which biofeedback depends is best described in option 1. Options 2, 3, and 4 are not true of biofeedback.
79. 4. Moderately paced, effortless, and shallow chest breathing is used. This type of breathing affords greatest relaxation and comfort.
80. 2. The term effleurage is used to describe light stroking of the skin.
81. 1. According to the gate control theory, the gating mechanism is in the spinal cord, perhaps in the substantia gelatinosa.
82. 2. A closed gate means no pain since pain impulses cannot be transmitted to the brain. An open gate results in the opposite phenomenon.
83. 2. Personalized concentration points or ideas serve as distraction for pain. They play no role in options 1, 3, and 4.
84. 4. Back labor, which occurs in about 25 percent of women, occurs when the fetus is in the occipito-posterior position. With each contraction, the occiput presses against the mother's sacrum to cause the discomfort of back labor.
85. 2. The up-on-all-fours position has been found to help many mothers with back labor. The position may even help to rotate the head to the anterior position. The position likely to give the least comfort is lying flat in bed.
86. 3. See item 84.
87. 2. "Show" normally occurs when there is an increase in cervical dilatation. Option 1 is unrelated to "show." Rupture of the fetal membranes will result in the escape of amniotic fluid. Premature separation of the placenta is usually accompanied by frank bleeding.

88. 1. Nitrazine paper becomes darker in color in the presence of an alkaline substance.
89. 1. The blood pressure normally increases during a contraction. The statements in options 2, 3, and 4 are inaccurate.
90. 2. The digestive process is normally slower during labor and, hence, solids are generally withheld. It is not unusual to experience nausea and vomiting late in the first stage of labor; if the patient has eaten, this offers a hazard if general anesthesia is used during delivery.
91. 4. Of the symptoms given here, the most common symptom of hyperventilation is a tingling sensation in the fingers.
92. 1. The symptoms of hyperventilation are due to excess carbon dioxide elimination from the body. Hence, rebreathing into a paper bag increases the intake of carbon dioxide during respirations. Options 2 and 3 and possibly 4 also describe measures that may aggravate the condition.
93. 4. The carbon dioxide insufficiency that occurs during hyperventilation will lead to respiratory alkalosis.
94. 1. The fetus will have acidosis when the mother hyperventilates. Levels of calcium and glucose in the blood will not be influenced.
95. 2. The first stage of labor consists of uterine contractions which are involuntary. Hence, it does not help for the mother to bear down during this stage. Bearing down before the cervix is dilated completely is likely to produce swelling of the cervix and contribute to the difficulty of labor.
96. 4. The symptoms described are typical of this state of labor. There is no need for action described in options 1, 2, and 3.
97. 3. Although practices may vary, most obstetricians will ask that the mother having her first child be brought to the delivery room when the top of the head becomes visible. Amount of effacement and dilatation and the strength of urges to bear down are less accurate methods for determining when delivery will occur. The delivery of the first baby takes longer. A multigravida would most probably be transferred to the delivery room when she is at 7 to 8 cm. dilated.
98. 3. Removing the legs from stirrups slowly helps prevent fainting sensations. Lowering the legs will increase blood flow to the extremities; if the legs are moved rapidly, the sudden demand for blood will cause fainting sensations.
99. 3. A chill at this time is not uncommon. There is no need to call the physician; catheterization is not indicated by a chill. If the patient has a change in temperature, it will take some time for this to occur.

100. 4. Findings illustrate that it is eye-to-eye contact which releases the maternal caretaking responses. Options 1, 2, and 3 are important for the mother but are not believed responsible for starting the maternal responses.

101. 4. A medication placed in the eye is best instilled into the lower conjunctival sac. Much of the medication is likely to be lost if placed in the inner or outer canthus. The medication may irritate and damage the cornea if placed on it.

102. 1. It has been found the most effective position in which to place the infant so that he will open his eyes is the upright position. The other methods described here are likely to result in the infant's closing his eyes.

103. 3. Gentian violet is not used as a prophylactic agent for ophthalmia neonatorum. The other agents are.

104. 4. The vastus lateralis muscle is most frequently recommended for intramuscular injections in the newborn. The muscle affords best tissue and least likelihood of injuring other structures.

105. 3. Thrush is an infection caused by *Candida albicans*. The characteristic sign of the infection is the appearance of white patches in the mouth.

106. 1. Although many persons no longer recommend dressings following circumcisions, those who do recommend using petrolatum in sterile dressings most often. Powder is not indicated because of its drying and caking effects. The other agents are not recommended.

107. 3. If bleeding occurs, most authorities recommend that the nurse first apply gentle pressure on the circumcision with sterile gauze. Bleeding is not common and, when it occurs, it requires attention. Applying pressure with the diaper does not allow the nurse to observe whether bleeding has stopped. It becomes necessary to notify the physician when bleeding cannot be stopped with conservative nursing measures.

108. 2. The most often recommended procedure is to cleanse the circumcision with no more than cotton balls and warm water. Other methods of care may become necessary if complications occur.

109. 4. A quorum of adult males is desirable. However, such a quorum is not necessary in order for the procedure to be recognized as a religious circumcision.

110. 3. Rooming-in helps provide opportunities for developing a positive relationship between the mother and her infant. Options 1, 2, and 4 are inaccurate statements in relation to rooming-in.

111. 3. Regurgitation occurs as a result of imperfect control of the stomach's cardiac sphincter which is poorly developed in the newborn. The recommended position, as described in option 3, promotes the emptying of the stomach toward the pyloric sphincter. Options 1 and 2 will not help and option 4 may aggravate the condition. Frequent bubbling of the infant during feedings is also often recommended.
112. 1. See item 111.
113. 4. State law requires that each baby have a birth certificate for registration purposes. The information contained on the certificate is used in various ways, one of which is for the compilation of vital statistics.
114. 1. The reflex described in the stem is called the Moro, or startle, reflex. The stepping or dancing reflex is demonstrated when the baby takes small steps when held upright with his feet touching a surface. The Babinski's reflex is demonstrated when, upon stroking the sole of the feet, the toes extend instead of flexing. The knee jerk reflex occurs when, upon striking at the knee, the lower leg automatically rises.
115. 2. The safest way is for the nurse to hold onto the patient's arm in an arm-in-arm manner. This method gives the nurse the best opportunity to provide support, should the patient need it.
116. 2. The most frequently recommended exercise soon after delivery is for the mother to alternately contract and relax muscles in the perineum. This improves muscle tone at the orifice of the vagina, urethra, and rectum and helps reduce congestion in the pelvic region.
117. 2. The vaginal discharge that normally occurs for approximately 3 days after delivery is called rubra because it contains mostly blood. The discharge then becomes more serous and watery and is called serosa. Toward about the tenth day after delivery, the discharge becomes thinner, scanty, and almost without color; it is called alba.
118. 3. Heat radiates from a baby's body toward any area that is cooler. If the bassinet is placed against an outside wall or window, the baby will have difficulty maintaining his body temperature. Or if placed near a source of heat, the infant may become too warm. The newborn's temperature regulating center is not as well developed as that of an adult.
119. 1. It is generally recommended that pregnant women be allowed to gain as much as 20 to 25 pounds during pregnancy. Underweight women may safely gain even more. It is no longer recommended that weight reduction programs be undertaken during pregnancy. Option 2 does not offer a good guide if

normal appetite results in eating considerably less, or more, than would be healthful for the mother.

120. 1. Grantly Dick-Read believes that, from his observation, the greatest cause of pain during labor is fear.

121. 3. The quality of life may be improved by any of the methods described here. But Dr. LeBoyer promotes utilizing every technique possible to give the newborn infant considerate and gentle care, including a quiet dimly lighted delivery room and a warm soothing bath immediately after delivery.

MARY ANN YOUNG

122. 4. Using Naegele's rule, count back 3 calendar months from the first day of the last menstrual period; in this patient's case, that would be April 13. Then add 7 days; in this patient's case, that would be April 20.

123. 3. Option 3 gives the patient a chance to describe her feelings and while listening to them, the nurse may find nursing intervention measures to assist the patient. Options 1 and 2 offer the patient no help and ignore the problem at hand. Option 4 focuses on the procedure which may or may not be related to the patient's fears.

124. 2. Helping the patient to breathe normally tends to help the patient to relax. Options 1 and 3 could result in more tension. Option 4 is unlikely to help the tense patient.

125. 2. The immunological pregnancy test provides a very fast answer and eliminates the need for using animals. It does not provide positive evidence of pregnancy. Blood samples are not used for biological testing.

126. 1. Blood tests described in options 2, 3, and 4 are still essential even though the patient has been well. However, a BUN, which helps evaluate kidney function, would not be essential at this time.

127. 3. Signs described in options 1, 2, and 4 are early signs of pregnancy. It would be unrealistic to expect to feel the outline of the fetus at this time.

128. 3. In recent years, a weight gain of 20 to 25 or 30 pounds is believed best. Limiting the weight gain as much as indicated in options 1 and 2 is no longer advised since, contrary to what was once believed, limiting the weight gain does not appear to decrease the incidence of toxemias and may deprive the fetus of nutrients it needs. Option 4 may or may not be indicated, depending on the amount of weight gain that results when satisfying normal appetite.

129. 4. The more strenuous exercises, such as horseback riding, are ordinarily contraindicated late in pregnancy.

130. 3. In certain positions, intercourse may well be uncomfortable late in pregnancy. The best advice is offered in option 3. Option 4 is an inaccurate statement. Option 2 is usually unrealistic and unnecessary.

131. 2. The most realistic evaluation of this patient's visitation schedule is that she is progressing normally and is being seen by her physician at typical intervals. As delivery approaches, physicians choose to see patients more frequently and there is no evidence that situations as described in options 1, 3, and 4 exist.

132. 4. This patient is not near enough to time of delivery to carry out procedures given in options 1, 2, and 3 before first taking the patient's blood pressure and checking the fetal heart rate.

133. 1. The size of the placenta has no relationship to the length of labor. Factors described in options 2, 3, and 4 can influence the length of labor.

134. 2. The most often recommended position for the patient receiving an enema is to place her on either side. Lying on the back is generally uncomfortable and awkward for administering the enema. Sitting up is contraindicated because the solution tends to pool in the rectum and the results are not likely to be satisfactory.

135. 4. It may be dangerous to apply pressure because of possible injury to mucosa. The best procedure is as described in option 4; the tube may be resting against a fold in the mucosa and this technique often will help overcome the difficulty. Options 2 and 3 are unlikely to be of help.

136. 1. The best procedure is to stop the flow of solution until the contraction subsides. Downward pressure of the fetus during a contraction forms resistance to the inflow of the enema solution and the mother needs to concentrate on relaxing during the contraction.

137. 3. The recommended temperature of the solution for an enema is between 105° F. and 115° F. (40.5° C. and 46.1° C.). Enemas using hypertonic solution are ordinarily given at room temperature.

138. 4. Actions described in options 1, 2, and 3 are correct. Shaving should be done by moving the razor in the same direction as the hair grows.

139. 2. Options 1, 3, and 4 describe procedures which should be carried out immediately following the birth of the baby. The cord clamp should not be removed until the cord is dry enough

so that no bleeding will occur when it is removed. This is usually in about 24 hours.

140. 1. The most reliable sign that the placenta has detached from the uterine wall is observing the cord lengthen outside of the vagina. Signs/symptoms described in options 2, 3, and 4 are not related to placental separation.

141. 3. Spinal anesthesia results in a paralysis of the lower part of the body. After its effects have worn off, it is generally recommended that the patient remain in bed to help prevent postanesthesia headaches. This anesthesia should not interfere with meals, voiding, or nursing of the baby.

142. 1. Following delivery, mothers are usually tired. However, the excitement of having the baby and helping with its care tends to interfere with normal rest and sleep. Sleep deprivation is sometimes associated with postpartal depression. Hence, the nurse should be especially alert to helping the mother avoid fatigue by getting sufficient rest.

143. 1. It is recommended that hard contact lenses be removed before sleep.

144. 3. The baby's signs are normal for his age. He appears to be regurgitating and choking on mucus, which is common also for his age. Recommended procedure is best described in option 3.

145. 4. Options 1, 2, and 3 describe normal findings in a newborn. Being unable to insert a rectal thermometer suggests that the infant's anus may be imperforated and the finding should be reported to the physician promptly.

146. 4. Newborns tend to lose weight, about 5 to 10 percent of their birth weight, for the first few days. This is very likely due to inadequate nourishment since the breasts are still not secreting milk and due to excess fluid losses. In this case, nothing need be done since the infant's weight loss is within normal.

147. 1. The normal cord stump appears dark and dry 2 days after delivery. Odor, redness, bleeding, and moisture suggest complications.

148. 4. The bilirubin findings are within normal range for a newborn and, hence, the physician is likely to continue with usual care. Physiological jaundice in the newborn is believed due to an increase in serum bilirubin as a result of breakdown of red blood cells, also normal in the newborn, since the concentration of red blood cells is especially high during fetal life and drops after birth.

149. 2. The only abnormal sign among these options is frequent green stools. The mother should be instructed to report this promptly should it occur.

150. 2. The most frequently recommended guide in relation to night feedings is to omit them when the baby sleeps through the night. The guides given in options 1, 3, and 4 are unreliable.

151. 1. A thumb-sucking baby is comforting himself. Options 2, 3, and 4 are inaccurate statements in relation to thumb sucking.

HELEN PEARSON

152. 2. The diagonal conjugate is the distance between the sacral prominence and the lower margin of the symphysis pubis. If the measurement is below 11.5 cm., there is danger that the pelvic inlet is too small for vaginal delivery. The other measurements are also significant but not as important in relation to delivery as the diagonal conjugate.

153. 2. Twins are normally delivered separately and usually each is smaller than the average baby at birth. Hence, the incorrect statement is option 2, since the pelvic inlet could be normal in size and twins could still be safely delivered.

154. 4. Ordinarily, the patient does not require any preparation, such as described in options 1, 2, and 3, prior to pelvimetry. The procedure should be explained to the patient.

155. 3. The statement in option 3 is a true statement in relation to roentgenologic studies. Options 1, 2, and 4 are inaccurate statements in relation to these studies.

156. 1. Option 1 is the only accurate statement. Planograms and floroscopy are not done for pelvimetry examinations nor is a dye injected.

157. 3. Preparation for a cesarean section is similar to preparation for any abdominal surgery. A consent must be given by the patient. Another person may not sign for the patient, unless the patient is unable to sign for herself, in which case only certain designated persons may do so legally.

158. 2. The occupation of the witness to the signing of a permit is unnecessary information and does not affect the legality of the permit. However, the factors given in options 1, 3, and 4 must be taken into consideration. Minors cannot sign permits. The patient should be able to read—or if she cannot, the consent form must be read to the patient so that she is certain of what she is signing. Also the patient should not be under the influence of medications that may influence reasoning.

159. 3. Oxytocics are drugs that act on the smooth muscle of the uterus to increase its tone and motility. Hence, oxytocin was ordered to induce uterine involution. This drug has no effect on blood clotting or abdominal musculature. It does not influence milk production but does stimulate the milk let-down.

160. 1. Following a general anesthetic, the patient requires special care because of typical effects described in options 2, 3, and 4. A general anesthesia does not influence milk production.
161. 4. This ergot alkaloid produces contraction of the smooth muscles in the uterus. In this instance, it was ordered to promote involution. An adverse effect is vasoconstriction with an accompanying increase in blood pressure. If an increased blood pressure occurs, the physician should be notified.
162. 4. Respiratory distress syndrome has been noted to be somewhat more common among babies born by cesarean operations when compared with babies born vaginally. Conditions described in options 1, 2, and 3 are not associated with cesarean births.
163. 1. Taking the baby's footprints is the safest method of identification. It provides a permanent record. Photographs are of little help for permanent purposes. Wristlets may be lost. Tattooing the baby with ultraviolet is temporary.
164. 4. It can be expected that the lochia will increase when the patient is first ambulated. If bright red bleeding continues, the patient should be put to bed. Massaging the fundus is not indicated since the lochia is normal. A medication is also not indicated in this situation.
165. 4. Turning and deep breathing is used postoperatively to help prevent respiratory congestion. These activities are not associated with the prevention of conditions described in options 1, 2, and 3.
166. 3. It is believed that the estrogenic hormone causes slight vaginal bleeding in the newborn. It is normal and to be expected and, hence, actions described in options 1, 2, and 4 are not indicated.
167. 2. It is the physician's responsibility to remove sutures. The nurse may place herself in legal jeopardy if she takes over this responsibility, even when the physician is at hand.
168. 1. As the newborn becomes more alert and active, he will need more to eat. Increasing the infant's eating will help stimulate the mother's milk production. Options 3 and 4 describe unlikely reasons for demanding more food.
169. 2. Option 2 encourages the mother to explain more about what she believes may be occurring. Options 1 and 3 are very unlikely to satisfy the mother and are not necessarily true. Option 4 gives the mother an opportunity to answer "yes" or "no" and, hence, gives the nurse little information on how to proceed further.
170. 3. Both exercises and early ambulation help to prevent complica-

tions, some examples being emboli formation, respiratory congestion, urine retention, and constipation. They serve no purpose in relation to options 1, 2, and 4.

171. 2. Only option 2 gives the patient encouragement to speak more of her concerns. Option 1 tends to put the patient down. Options 3 and 4 are pat answers and do not afford the nurse an opportunity to learn more about the patient.

JEAN TALLON

172. 1. Saddle block anesthesia is injected into the lumbar area. The patient should be in the sitting position so that the anesthesia will fall lower in the spinal canal. If it rises to the thoracic area, the patient may experience respiratory distress.

173. 2. When the blood pressure falls, the patient's legs should be elevated. The position brings additional blood to the central circulation. This action should be taken first. Actions described in options 3 and 4 *may* be taken but first, the patient's legs should be elevated.

174. 3. Postspinal headache may be due to a drop in spinal fluid pressure when spinal fluid is lost at the site of injection. Fluid intake should be increased. It is also generally recommended that the patient remain flat in bed on her back following spinal anesthesia to help reduce the likelihood of headache.

175. 2. Options 1, 3, and 4 are not necessarily true. Each patient needs individual counseling in relation to the use of anesthesia during delivery.

DORIS BENET

176. 1. If the birth of the baby is indeed imminent, the nurse should first inspect the perineum to see whether crowning has occurred. If the mother is not ready to deliver, the nurse might use actions described in options 2, 3, and 4.

177. 4. Options 1, 2, and 3 describe action that is contraindicated when birth is imminent. The nurse should immediately prepare a field for delivery of the baby.

178. 2. It would be most appropriate for the nurse to control the delivery of the head. Options 3 and 4 describe inappropriate delivery and may lead to complications. The perineum is protected when the head is gently delivered. The head should not be held back!

179. 1. In order to protect the perineum, it is best to deliver the head between contractions.

180. 3. Option 3 offers an accurate description of what is occurring.

The cliché, "Everything is fine," is of little value and may arouse suspicion. Option 2 offers a statement that may not be accurate and the mother may become suspicious. Option 4 tends to be derogatory of the physician.

181. 2. There is no hurry to cut the cord. The best procedure is simply to clamp it until such time as it is convenient to cut it. Options 3 and 4 may present difficulty for the infant.

182. 3. The best course of action is to wait for sign of placental separation. Pulling on the cord before the placenta is detached may cause an eversion of the uterus. Once separation occurs, the patient can be asked to bear down. After delivery of the placenta, the fundus may be massaged.

183. 1. Complications that occur with a precipitate delivery are described in options 2, 3, and 4. Rupture of the uterus is associated with difficult deliveries and a precipitate delivery is an "easy" delivery.

PEGGY MILLER

184. 2. Since this patient has not retained nourishment for 3 days, it would be best to recommend that she come to the physician's office that day. After 3 days, it is late to recommend actions described in options 1 and 4. The patient may need hospitalization, but this is best determined after examination. Early morning nausea usually occurs during the first trimester. When vomiting persists into the second trimester, it is more serious in nature.

185. 4. When fat is burned in the body without the presence of carbohydrates, combustion does not go on to completion. Improper fat metabolism results in acetone and diacetic acid in the urine.

186. 3. Unchecked vomiting may produce metabolic alkalosis because the loss of acid from the stomach leaves the body with a relative excess of alkali.

187. 2. Gastrointestinal secretion losses from vomiting, as well as from diarrhea and excessive suctioning, will result in loss of potassium.

188. 3. Hydrogen is retained by the kidneys in the form of carbonic acid when metabolic alkalosis is present. In this situation, the kidneys are functioning in a compensatory manner.

189. 3. Options 1, 2, and 4 describe common signs of dehydration. Puffiness about the eyelids is a sign of water retention.

190. 3. The number of drops the patient should receive each minute is determined as follows:

$$\frac{1000 \text{ ml.} = 125 \text{ ml. to be given each hour}}{8 \text{ hours}}$$

$$\frac{125 \text{ ml.} \times 15 \text{ (drop factor)}}{60 \text{ (minutes)}} = \frac{1875}{60} = \text{approximately 31 to 32 drops per minute}$$

191. 2. It is generally recommended that the tubing be changed every 24 hours in order to decrease the likelihood of infection.

192. 2. Thiamine is converted to a coenzyme that plays an important part in carbohydrate metabolism. It has not been found effective for the relief of conditions described in the other options.

193. 2. As the carbonic acid content increases, the lungs work to rid the body of carbon dioxide through an increased rate and depth of respirations.

THERESA ENOC

194. 4. Options 1, 2, and 3 are true statements in relation to the American Indian. However, most Indians are not receiving adequate health care despite the services available to them.

195. 2. Glycosuria, because of a lowered renal threshhold for sugar, and lactosuria are common in pregnancy. Thus, insulin requirements cannot be based solely on the finding of glucose in the urine. The placenta secretes a hormone which is an insulin antagonist. The carbon dioxide content of the plasma is not related to insulin determination.

196. 1. This electronic evaluation of the fetal heart rate shows normal slowing of the fetal heart rate during a contraction.

197. 4. The "piggy back" method of administering a drug allows one to stop administering the drug while still keeping the vein open. The method makes it possible to estimate only approximately how much of the drug has been administered. Options 1 and 2 are inaccurate statements in relation to the "piggy back" method of administering drugs.

198. 1. The infusion pump allows one to deliver exact amounts of a drug intravenously. Options 2, 3, and 4 are inaccurate statements in relation to an infusion pump.

199. 4. The recommended procedure is as described in option 4. The administration of pitocin is a hazardous procedure and the physician should be in attendance to provide immediate intervention if necessary.

200. 4. Oxytocin acts to produce contractions of the uterus. When the

contraction described in the stem occurred, it would have been best to reduce the rate at which the drug was being administered. Despite the contraction's strength and length, the patient is not necessarily ready for delivery.

201. 1. Prostaglandins act more slowly than oxytocin. Another reported advantage of prostaglandins is that they do not have the antidiuretic effects of oxytocin.

202. 4. The intramuscular injection of prostaglandins is contraindicated. Prostaglandins are very irritating to tissues and, hence, there is no preparation of this agent for intramuscular use.

203. 1. The American Indian characteristically does not exhibit symptoms of pain. Although tribal and individual characteristics differ, most American Indians try to be polite and stoic and accept the procedures performed on them in the hospital.

204. 1. Since the fetal head was high in the pelvis, the nurse should auscultate the fetal heart rate. As amniotic fluid gushes out, the cord may prolapse. This is more likely if the fetal head is not engaged. A drop in the heart rate suggests fetal distress which may be caused by pressure of the head on the umbilical cord. The umbilical cord may have started to prolapse at the time the membranes were ruptured.

205. 3. Of the conditions given here, babies born of diabetic mothers most often tend to develop respiratory distress.

206. 2. Glucose crosses the placenta but insulin does not. Hence, a high blood sugar in the mother will cause a high blood sugar in the fetus. This causes the fetus to produce more insulin. At birth, the infant loses its source of glucose from the mother but has a continued high production of insulin which often results in a drop in blood sugar in the newborn.

207. 1. The usual practice is to give the infant oral glucose. Options 2, 3, and 4 describe unlikely procedures. Options 3 and 4 would also tend to aggravate the situation.

208. 2. Option 2 has been observed frequently. Regular feedings with glucose as necessary, along with the milk, are important. Establishing excretory functioning plays no role in the control of hypoglycemia. Insulin does not cross the placenta.

209. 4. The combination of glucose and insulin is responsible for the increased size of infants of diabetic mothers. Boy babies tend to weigh more than girl babies; option 1 is inaccurate. Miscalculations do not influence weight. Option 3 presents a less likely reason than option 4, which has been well demonstrated.

210. 1. The primary danger when teeth are present at the time of birth

is that they may become dislodged and the infant may aspirate them.

211. 3. Options 1, 2, and 4 support the statement in the stem; option 3 does not. The mother's activity has most probably been less during these first 3 days of postpartum. Increases in exercise and activity are more likely to cause hypoglycemia since they tend to increase insulin production.

JOAN CARTER

212. 3. The amniotic fluid is described as being a clear, alkaline fluid, flecked with vernix caseosa when the fetus is near term. The appearance of blood or meconium in the fluid is considered to be abnormal and may indicate complications. There may be urine in the fluid but this would not color the fluid yellow.

213. 2. In order to help avoid the danger of puncturing a full bladder, the patient should void in preparation for amniocentesis. Preparation described in options 1, 3, and 4 are not ordinarily indicated.

214. 3. Surfactant acts to help eliminate the stickiness of alveolar tissues in the lung. This allows for expansion of the lungs. Insufficient amounts of surfactant predisposes to respiratory distress in the newborn.

215. 2. When amniotic fluid is mixed with a stain for fat, squamous cells from the fetus will take up the stain and appear orange. These cells increase with maturity of the fetus.

216. 1. Osmolality refers to the proportion of solutes in a solution. As the solvent (in this case, urine) is increased, the osmolality decreases. Amniotic fluid early in pregnancy is isotonic.

217. 3. The concentration of creatinine in amniotic fluid increases with maturity of the fetal kidneys. Maturity of the kidneys increases their ability to excrete creatinine.

218. 3. Because of the maturation of the fetal liver, the concentration of bilirubin in the amniotic fluid decreases toward term since the fetus swallows amniotic fluid and metabolizes the bilirubin. Studies of bilirubin in the amniotic fluid also help to evaluate a fetus in Rh sensitization.

219. 3. Until the fetus is 15 to 16 weeks old, the amniotic fluid level is such that an amniocentesis is not considered safe.

220. 2. Studies to detect chromosomal abnormalities are most frequently done in order that parents may be assisted in deciding whether pregnancy should be interrupted. Option 1 is not advised because there are some dangers associated with the procedure. The fault cannot be corrected even though noted

early in pregnancy (option 3). Adoption is not an issue when defects are found to be present.

221. 2. Some abdominal cramping may occur following amniocentesis. However, if there is vaginal bleeding or leakage of fluid, the mother should be taught to go to bed and call her physician promptly.

222. 1. The symptoms described in option 1 are most often noted when a patient is receiving alcohol intravenously. It will be noted that the symptoms are not unlike those that occur when alcohol in sufficient quantities is taken orally.

223. 2. Analgesics are often withheld because of the effects on the infant. The preterm infant is frequently compromised and cannot tolerate the depressing effects of an analgesic. Analgesics will not produce results described in option 1, 3, and 4.

224. 3. The preterm baby's skull is soft and forceps may be used to protect the brain during delivery.

225. 4. During external monitoring, as the uterus contracts, the abdominal wall rises and presses against the transducer. This movement is transmitted into an electrical current which is then recorded. The tokodynamometer should be placed where uterine displacement during contractions is greatest for best results.

226. 4. It is possible that the transducer has slipped out of place. See item 225 for a description of placement. The first course of action would be for the nurse to adjust the placement of the tokodynamometer.

227. 3. Since the fetal heart rate is being monitored, the best placement of the Doppler is over the area where the best, sharp fetal heart tones are heard. They may not necessarily be best heard in areas described in options 1, 2, and 4.

228. 4. The major advantage for monitoring the fetal heart rate electronically is that beat-to-beat variabilities can be determined readily. Obtaining the rate with a fetoscope permits only a sampling of the fetal heart rate at comparatively infrequent intervals. Options 1, 2, and 3, although they may be true, are not primary reasons for using electronic monitoring.

229. 3. The fetal heartbeat is normally between 120 and 160 beats per minute.

230. 3. The complication least likely to occur is perforation of the uterus. The most common complication is intrauterine infection due to faulty aseptic technique.

231. 2. Changing positions is not contraindicated when an internal monitor is used. Lying flat on the back during labor is usually

contraindicated as it may compress major abdominal vessels and decrease blood supply to the fetus. Telling a patient not to worry is not helpful. There is no need to have the patient lie as described in option 4.

232. 2. During a contraction, the fetal heart rate decreases. As the contraction begins nearing its end, the fetal heart rate will normally increase again.

233. 4. Pressure on the fetal head by the cervix is normal during labor and delivery. Options 1, 2, and 3 describe ominous conditions.

234. 4. If the baby is stimulated to cry before suctioning, the baby is likely to aspirate mucus. Options 1, 2, and 3 describe recommended procedure in relation to bulb suctioning of the newborn.

235. 3. Deep suctioning of the nasopharynx immediately after birth carries the danger of stimulating the vagus nerve which causes a slow heartbeat. If the suctioning is carried out carelessly, mucus membranes can be injured. Suctioning does not abolish the infant's efforts to clear mucus. Oversuctioning may remove too much oxygen which can cause respiratory distress.

236. 3. In order to provide the most room for lung expansion and to place the upper respiratory tract in the best position for receiving oxygen, the infant should be placed on his back with the neck slightly extended.

237. 1. The oxygen is being administered properly when oxygen reaches the lungs. This will be observed to occur when the chest rises with each contraction of the hand-operated bag.

238. 2. The hand should not be used to compress the sternum of an infant when CPR is used. The sternum should be compressed with two fingers. Options 1, 3, and 4 describe proper procedure.

239. 2. There is no need to cover the infant's eyes when administering oxygen via the hood. Options 1, 3, and 4 describe proper procedure.

240. 2. The percentage of oxygen in normal room air is approximately 20.

241. 3. The infant with retrolental fibroplasia is most likely to be blind. The cause of this condition is believed to be excessive use of oxygen therapy in the newborn.

242. 4. The parents should be told of the baby's actual condition. It would be unfair to withhold information that indicates the negative aspects. Options 1, 2, and 3 are recommended procedures.

243. 4. When the catheter is in the trachea, air bubbles will appear when the end of the catheter is placed under water. One or two air bubbles may also escape from the end of the catheter when it is in the stomach, but if the catheter is in the trachea, the air bubbles will be at intervals with each exhalation.

244. 4. Respiratory problems for the premature infant may be grave. Observations for evidence of respiratory distress should receive highest priority when caring for a premature infant.

245. 2. Giving birth to a premature infant is most often associated with feelings of guilt by the parents. They tend to ask questions in relation to what they might have done to cause it—or had not done that could have prevented it.

MARILYN O'BRIEN

246. 1. In the ABO system, of the blood types given here, the combination that is most likely to produce hemolytic disease of the newborn is O− mother and A+ father. Incompatabilities due to the Rh factor occur when the mother is Rh− and the father, Rh+. The fetus must be Rh+ for the incompatability to occur.

247. 4. The problem with Rh sensitivity arises when the mother's blood has developed antibodies when fetal red blood cells enter the maternal circulation. In cases of Rh sensitivity, this usually does not occur until the first pregnancy and, hence, hemolytic disease of the newborn is rare when a mother is having her first baby. A mismatched blood transfusion in the past could result in hemolytic disease also since the transfusion would have had the same effects on the mother.

248. 2. Although transfusion with improperly matched blood types can cause Rh sensitization, the usual or most common cause is delivery of an Rh+ baby. Factors described in options 1 and 4 are not related to Rh sensitization.

249. 3. Jaundice is not present at birth because the liver of the mother breaks down the bilirubin and excretes it. As the severity of hemolytic disease of the newborn increases, anemia due to the destruction of red cells by antibodies may occur. Heart failure occurs as the heart decompensates because of the severe anemia. The edema results from the heart failure. The severe form of this condition is hydrops fetalis.

250. 4. The antibodies appear in the mother's blood. Hence, the specimen required for antibody titer is maternal blood.

251. 2. The indirect Coombs' test is done to determine the presence of antibodies in the mother's blood. If the Coombs' test is positive, the infant will be observed for increases in bilirubin levels and anemia.

252. 4. A direct Coombs' test is done on cord blood to detect antibodies coating the baby's red blood cells. Indirect Coombs' test on cord blood may be positive because of "free" immune antibody.

253. 2. The fetus severely affected by hemolytic disease is transfused because the severe anemia can produce grave results. The transfusion is one to replace destroyed red blood cells.

254. 2. Cross-matching blood and getting the consent form signed are not legal responsibilities of the nurse although she might assist with both. However, preparing the equipment necessary for the procedure is a nursing responsibility.

255. 4. The vein most commonly used for an exchange transfusion is the umbilical vein. The catheter is placed in the vein and enters the body. The umbilical vein is a large and easily accessible vein.

256. 3. A premature infant (this baby was delivered at 32 weeks of gestation) has an unstable temperature regulating mechanism. Hence, an elevated temperature is not necessarily a good guide for determining the presence of infection. In fact, the temperature is frequently subnormal in a premature with an infection. Signs described in options 1, 2, and 4 are better guides.

257. 2. The albumin provides binding sites for the bilirubin. This is important because it is the free or unbound bilirubin which causes problems, such as kernicterus, in the infant. Options 1, 3, and 4 are inaccurate statements.

258. 3. The aim of care for this infant is to reduce the blood's concentration of bilirubin, in addition to relieving the infant's anemia.

259. 1. The organ most subject to damage when uncontrolled hemolytic disease is present is the brain. The bilirubin forms a coating over the brain cells which oxygen cannot penetrate.

260. 1. Phototherapy is often used in the presence of jaundice. The infant's eyes should be patched while the infant is under the light in order to prevent eye damage.

261. 4. Tenets of the Roman Catholic Church hold that it would be acceptable for anyone to baptize an infant regardless of his religious beliefs. Local practice may vary.

262. 3. If the mother wishes to view the body, it is her right to be able to do so. Viewing the body has been found to help complete the grieving process.

263. 2. Only the parents of an infant may legally give permission for an autopsy to be done.

264. 1. Option 1 gives the mother an opportunity to explore. A course

of action is more likely to be effective once this information is known. Options 2, 3, and 4 offer advice which the mother is not necessarily seeking. She is asking for help and the final decision concerning a course of action will be hers. Also, options 2 and 3 may serve to make the child afraid that God will take him too, or afraid to go to sleep at night.

265. 4. An antibody is best defined as a protein substance that reacts with specific other proteins to maintain homeostasis. Options 1, 2, and 3 are inaccurate statements.

266. 1. An antigen is best defined as a substance that acts to produce an immune reaction in the body. Options 2, 3, and 4 are inaccurate statements.

BECKY ANDREW

267. 4. Although pregnancy may occur in relationships described in options 1, 2, and 3, observations have shown that the most typical characteristic of the father of a baby whose mother is an unmarried adolescent is that he is a member of the mother's peer group and she has had a relationship with him over a period of time.

268. 4. Pregnant adolescents have been observed to have iron deficiency anemia more frequently than other pregnant women.

269. 4. The fetus needs iron, protein, and calcium for proper growth and the mother should have increased amounts of these nutrients in her diet to supply the fetus. It has not been demonstrated that increased amounts of vitamin D are indicated since the amount the mother normally ingests is adequate for her needs and that of the fetus.

270. 1. The patient's marital status is unimportant in relation to this patient's nutritional needs. Factors given in options 2, 3, and 4 are important to take into consideration.

271. 1. The daily requirements from the basic four foods for an adolescent are approximately as follows:
Milk—four or more cups
Meat—two or more servings
Vegetables and fruit—four or more servings
Bread and cereal—four or more servings
This patient's diet had no milk, two servings of meat, one serving of vegetables, and five servings of bread. Therefore, she needs four cups of milk and three servings of fruit and vegetables. Option 1 most nearly meets these requirements.

272. 2. Preeclampsia is characterized by weight gain in excess of what

would be expected when caloric intake is considered. The gain is due to water retention with resulting symptoms of edema. The patient is most likely to note swelling of her fingers.

273. 3. The three most common signs/symptoms of preeclampsia are elevated blood pressure, edema, and albuminuria.

274. 4. Although the cause of preeclampsia is unknown, it has been found that vasospasm and vasoconstriction occur which results in an elevated blood pressure and decreased glomerular filtration in the kidneys. The circulating blood volume is increased in pregnancy. An increase in aldosterone would increase sodium retention and fluid retention, but this is not associated with preeclampsia.

275. 3. Congenital anomalies are not associated with toxemias of pregnancy. Conditions given in the other options are commonly associated with toxemias of pregnancy.

276. 2. Option 2 is the best action for the nurse to take because the patient's symptoms are severe enough to warrant her being seen by the physician.

277. 3. The patient with preeclampsia may develop eclampsia which is characterized by convulsions. To decrease the likelihood of convulsions and attending dangers, it would be best to place this patient in a quiet room in order to decrease stimuli that could trigger a convulsion and in a room convenient for frequent observations by nursing personnel.

278. 3. In view of impaired kidney functioning, the patient with a toxemia tends to produce scanty amounts of urine. When the hourly output is less than approximately 20 to 30 ml., therapy may need to be instigated. Hence, in this situation, the nurse should notify the physician of her observation.

279. 4. Most foods that are good sources of protein contain substantial amounts of sodium. Thus, to reduce sodium intake, it is necessary to reduce protein intake. A pregnant woman needs an increase in her protein intake. This may be difficult when a low sodium diet is prescribed.

280. 3. After the infusion was started, a desired result would be the increase in urinary output. Headaches often occur prior to an eclamptic convulsion and should be reported. Options 2 and 4 are signs that the patient may be experiencing a fluid overload and it is most likely that the physician will wish to adjust the order in relation to the infusion.

281. 1. Urinary estriol levels are used primarily to help assess fetal well-being. Estriol levels rise during pregnancy and from this knowledge, the physician can make certain judgments in

relation to fetal maturity. Also, a study of the estriol levels helps judge the placental functioning and the fetoplacental unit which allows certain deductions concerning fetal well-being.

282. 1. A vaginal speculum is of least importance. The equipment described in options 2, 3, and 4 are essential for protecting the patient should a convulsion occur and for administering intravenous medications should the patient's condition deteriorate.

283. 3. A typical symptom of impending convulsion is epigastric pain. Symptoms described in the other options are not typical of impending convulsions.

284. 3. Magnesium sulfate is an excellent central nervous system depressant and, therefore, is often used as an anticonvulsant. However, the agent tends to depress respirations and, hence, the patient should be observed carefully for respiratory abnormalities.

285. 1. The antidote for magnesium sulfate is calcium which is commonly administered as calcium gluconate. It should be readily available when magnesium sulfate is being used.

286. 2. Highest priority during this patient's labor is to prevent convulsions and to deliver the baby safely. Goals described in options 1, 3, and 4 are desirable but do not have the same high priority that option 2 has.

287. 4. Option 4 best describes the prognosis for this patient. It takes about 10 to 14 days usually for the blood pressure to return to normal.

288. 1. It can be expected that the height of the patient's uterus will be felt slightly above the umbilicus. This is normal approximately 12 hours after delivery. Unless complications occur, this mother, despite having eclampsia, could expect normal progress of involution. Immediately after delivery, the top of the uterus will normally be midway between the umbilicus and the symphysis pubis. It descends at the rate of approximately 1 fingerbreadth each day. It will have reached the level described in option 3 approximately 7 to 10 days after delivery. Although there is individual variation, common normal ranges have been defined, as described above.

289. 3. A full bladder is likely to push the uterus to the right of the midline. When the bladder is empty, the uterus normally lies approximately in the midline. Other causes when the uterus is observed to be on one side is that the mother is lying or sleeping on the side or there is relaxation of the uterus due to bleeding.

290. 2. Of the positions given, it has been found that lying on the abdomen several times a day tends to promote involution. The position helps to firm up the uterus.
291. 4. The symptoms suggest that the airway is not open. Hence, the nurse should first clear the airway with gravity (lower the infant's head) and/or suction. Option 3 is contraindicated. Other measures may be necessary if clearing the airway proves to be insufficient.
292. 1. In the past, many persons believed that it was best for the mother not to see an infant she was giving up for adoption. However, it is now general procedure to allow the mother to see the baby if she wishes since authorities agree the mother has the right.

ANDREA NICOL

293. 4. The nurse should first check the fetal heart tones and the mother's blood pressure. A vaginal examination is contraindicated, as is an enema, at this time since these procedures may increase placental separation and bleeding. There is no need to prepare the patient for delivery since she is not in labor.
294. 2. The most typical sign when the placenta separates prematurely is a rigid abdomen. Pain is common. The amnion does not ordinarily rupture nor are uterine contractions likely to be present.
295. 2. Hypofibrinogenemia is a coagulation defect. Fibrinogen is destroyed and the patient then has a tendency to bleed. Conditions described in options 1, 3, and 4 are not associated with this condition.
296. 1. Placenta previa is present when the placenta has attached itself in the lower segment of the uterus. It may partially or completely cover the cervical os. The most characteristic sign of placenta previa is painless bleeding during the last trimester of pregnancy.
297. 2. Option 2 is an accurate description of the sonogram. Telling a patient not to worry is of little help. Option 1 and 3 offer the patient neither information nor help and they tend to put the patient down. Option 4 is an inaccurate account of a sonogram.
298. 1. The best guide is described in option 1. The patient needs guidance but is not asking for advice, as described in options 2 and 3. The advice may also be inappropriate. The patient needs to remain in bed; option 4 is contraindicated.

299. 1. The anesthesia for a pudendal block is injected through the sacrospinous ligament into the posterior areolar tissue where the pudendal nerve is located. Entry is either through the perineal skin or through the vaginal mucosa.

300. 4. The best description of the purpose for using pudendal block is offered in option 4. This type of anesthesia will not accomplish goals in options 1, 2, or 3. It has no effect on uterine contractions.

301. 4. First-degree lacerations involve the fourcet, the perineal skin, and the vaginal mucosa. No muscles are involved. Second-degree lacerations involve the muscles of the perineal body but not the rectal sphincter. Third-degree lacerations extend completely through the skin, the mucous membrane, the perineal body, and the rectal sphincter.

302. 3. An Apgar score of 1 to 3 denotes very poor condition. A score of 4 to 6 means the baby is in fair condition. A score of 7 to 10 indicates the infant's condition is good. These scores are obtained by assessing the infant's heart rate, respiratory effort, muscle tone, reflex irritability, and color.

303. 2. The first temperature of a newborn is taken to determine patency of the infant's rectum. The temperature reading itself is of less importance since it will usually reflect the temperature of the infant's immediate environment. In the newborn, axillary temperatures are as accurate as rectal temperatures.

304. 2. The newborn's temperature-regulating mechanism is not fully developed at birth. It has been found that it usually takes about 8 hours before the temperature stabilizes. It will ordinarily be lower than normal during this period. The temperature of a newborn may drop 1 to 2 degrees in the delivery room if care is not taken to protect the infant from heat loss.

305. 1. Research has shown that the axillary and rectal temperatures will be approximately the same immediately after delivery. Because an infant has little subcutaneous tissue and does not perspire, his axillary temperature is accurate and within about .5° F. of a rectal reading.

306. 2. Ergonovine maleate is an alkaloid ergot. It is used to check bleeding after the delivery of the placenta which occurs as a result of uterine contractions. The nurse should continue to monitor the vital signs every 15 minutes since the drug acts to raise blood pressure. Note that the patient's diastolic blood pressure is close to normal. The patient had one dose of the medication in the delivery room which explains her present blood pressure. No more is ordered and the nurse can

expect the blood pressure to return to normal as the medication wears off.

307. 3. The most frequent cause of a "boggy" fundus shortly after delivery is a relaxed uterus. The nurse's first course of action would be to massage the fundus. If the fundus does not firm up with this action, it may then be necessary to call the physician. Options 2 and 4 will not help firm up a relaxed uterus.

308. 4. The catheter may have caused a temporary spasm at the internal orifice. Best action would be as described in option 4. Option 1 is not indicated and would mean having to introduce the catheter a second time. Options 2 and 3 are contraindicated because of the danger of introducing organisms which could cause urinary tract infections.

309. 2. No special treatment is indicated when the ecchymotic area is observed. Ice is effective immediately to reduce bleeding or swelling but not on the second postpartal day. Heat would be more appropriate but the number of sitz baths would appear adequate; the nurse would need a physician's order to increase the number to six a day.

310. 3. When ambulating for the first time, patients will sometimes feel faint due to the sudden change in the blood distribution in the body. It is for this reason primarily that the nurse should accompany the patient when she takes her first shower after delivery.

311. 1. The mother's behavior is typical of the "taking in" phase of childbearing and usually indicates sleep hunger. The patient tends to be passive and dependent. The "taking hold" phase is characterized by a readiness to assume active care of the infant. "Postpartal blues" are characterized by irritability and generally occur later in the puerperium. Psychological counseling is rarely necessary. The "let down" phase is sometimes used to describe the "postpartal blues."

312. 1. Excessive perspiration is common during the puerperium as the skin works to rid the body of wastes. It is temporary and does not ordinarily require any treatment other than to keep the patient comfortable. Options 2, 3, and 4 are inaccurate statements.

313. 4. Breast feeding stimulates the secretion of oxytocin which causes the uterine muscles to contract. These contractions account for the discomfort associated with afterpains. They are not related to blood loss. Afterpains tend to be more common when there is retention of small placental tags, when there has been excessive stretching of the uterus, and with increasing parity. Primiparas seldom have afterpains.

314. 3. The most appropriate guideline is to suggest that the mother give the 2-year-old some undivided time each day. Option 1 may not be feasible. The youngster will not be helped to meet her needs if behavior typical of jealousy is ignored. Option 4 suggests a course of action which does not meet the problem and is ill-advised.

315. 3. Options 1, 2, and 4 describe unlikely behavior on the part of a 2-year-old. Usually while in search of attention, a 2-year-old will display regressive behavior, such as wanting a bottle, even though she had no longer been using one.

316. 4. For the first few days after delivery, the recommended exercise is perineal contractions. The exercise stimulates muscle tone in the area of the perineum and around the urinary meatus and vaginal orifice. The exercises described in options 1, 2, and 3 are too strenuous for the first few days postpartum.

317. 3. Option 3 illustrates the knee-chest position.

LAURIE BECKER

318. 3. It is most important, first of all, that the physician be told of the patient's heroin addiction since this knowledge will influence the care of the mother and her baby. The information is used only in relation to the patient's care. With the patient's consent, the information may be shared with other community health agencies that become involved with patient's long-term needs.

319. 3. Usual symptoms of withdrawal include nervousness and wakefulness. Symptoms given in the other options are not likely.

320. 1. The newborn can be expected to demonstrate symptoms of heroin withdrawal relatively promptly after birth, within the first day.

321. 4. The mother should be taught that symptoms of heroin addiction may be present in her infant for as long as 4 months and even longer.

322. 3. The characteristic cry of an infant suffering from heroin withdrawal is a shrill cry.

323. 4. Chlorpromazine hydrochloride is the drug of choice. It acts as a tranquilizer and helps control agitation and tension. Options 1 and 2 are narcotic antagonists but do not help control the symptoms of withdrawal. Meperidine hydrochloride is a narcotic and depressant that would be inappropriate for this infant.

324. 3. A spontaneous abortion is one that occurs without provocation. An induced abortion is brought on for personal or therapeutic reasons.

325. 2. It has been found that patients with an incompetent cervical os will almost always abort during the second trimester of pregnancy, as the fetus enlarges enough to cause spontaneous abortion.

326. 1. When an abortion is incomplete, the treatment of choice is to remove the contents of the uterus by dilatation and curettage. Procedures given in options 2, 3, and 4 are contraindicated and may tend to aggravate the condition of retained tissues.

327. 3. The cerclage procedure is done by encircling the cervical os with suture-type material in order to give extra strength to the relaxed and dilated cervix.

328. 4. If the mother is in labor, steps will most likely have to be taken either to attempt to halt labor or to empty the uterus. Hence, it is especially important for the physician to know the quality and frequency of contractions. Since the cervix cannot dilate with the cerclage intact, uterine rupture is a danger if contractions are strong.

BABY GIRL HARRIS

329. 1. In order to avoid examining the infant immediately before a feeding, when the baby may be irritable and hungry, and immediately after a feeding when the manipulation may cause regurgitation or vomiting, it would be best to examine her approximately midway between feedings.

330. 3. This baby's weight falls within average normal range in relation to gestation. The average weight of girls at birth is 7 pounds; the average weight of boys at birth is 7½ pounds.

331. 1. The normal head circumference of an infant at birth is approximately 33 to 34 cm., 12 to 13 inches. Normal chest circumference is about 34 to 35 cm., 13 to 14 inches. Beginning at about age 2, the chest circumference will exceed the head circumference.

332. 2. During normal vaginal delivery, the cranial bones tend to override as the head accommodates the size of the birth canal. This overriding is called "molding."

333. 3. The anterior fontanel is normally diamond-shaped. The posterior fontanel, the smaller of the two, is triangle-shaped.

334. 4. The best way is to occlude one nostril at a time and observe respirations while doing so. An infant breathes through his

nose and must learn to breathe through his mouth. Therefore, it is not necessary to cover the mouth while occluding a nostril.

335. 2. It is abnormal for a newborn to have an expiratory grunt. A heart murmur is sometimes heard but is not necessarily abnormal at this time. The heartbeat is within normal range, which is between approximately 120 and 160 beats per minute. The respiratory rate is within normal range which is between 35 and 50 per minute.

336. 4. Option 4 best describes the normal tonic neck reflex. This is also described as the fencing position.

337. 1. Bruises from the use of forceps ordinarily require no treatment, and, hence, options 2, 3, and 4 are not recommended.

338. 2. Oculomotor coordination is poor in the newborn and, hence, it is normal that the eyes will appear crossed. It is believed that a newborn has vision although it is not as acute as an adult's.

339. 1. All babies have blue or slate grey eyes at birth. By about 3 months of age, the baby's eyes will have their permanent color.

340. 4. The substance described in this stem is vernix caseosa. Milia are small white nodules on the skin and generally appear on the nose and forehead. Lanugo is fine hair generally observed on all parts of the body except for the soles and palms. Smegma is a thick cheesey substance found under the prepuce and in the region of the clitoris and labia minora.

341 3. It has been observed that a single crease across the palm is most often associated with chromosomal abnormalities, notably Down's syndrome.

342. 4. The liver, spleen, and kidneys are palpable but the thyroid gland is normally not palpable.

343. 3. The most accurate statement is that creases are normally found spread over the entire bottom of the feet in a full-term infant.

344. 2. The physician should be notified if moisture is present since this is often a sign of infection. The findings described in option 1 and 3 are normal.

345. 3. Normally, the anterior fontanel closes between about 12 and 18 months. Premature closure (craniostenosis or premature synostosis) prevents proper growth and expansion of the brain with consequent mental retardation. If signs of premature closure are present, it is ordinarily treated surgically.

346. 2. Normally, the posterior fontanel closes between about 2 and 3 months.

347. 1. Changing color of the hands and feet described here is not abnormal. The feet and hands are probably cold and the nurse's first course of action should be to wrap the baby warmly.

348. 2. It is believed that the sense of touch is most highly developed at birth.
349. 4. All babies normally cry about the same amount at birth but learn to cry more or less as their needs are responded to in some way. Investigations have shown that there is a close relationship between the amount of crying an infant does and the kind and amount of comforting he receives. Factors given in the other options have not been found to be associated with crying.
350. 3. The normal range of hemoglobin in the normal newborn is between about 15 and 20 Gm. per 100 ml. of blood. This is higher than for older children and adults. The fetus has a higher hemoglobin in order to obtain proper oxygenation. After birth, a gradual decrease takes place.

BARBARA HENDERSON

351. 1. The size of the breasts depends on the amount of adipose tissue which does not influence the production of milk. Options 2, 3, and 4 are inaccurate statements.
352. 3. The best preparation is to brush the nipples and roll them each day in order to stimulate them enough to protrude and to toughen them to prepare for the nursing of the baby. Options 2 and 4 are not recommended.
353. 1. The fluid from the nipples is colostrum. It may leak as early as the third or fourth month of pregnancy—or not at all. Options 2, 3, and 4 are contraindicated.
354. 3. Medications can be picked up by the milk and then influence the baby. Hence, except for prescribed drugs, medications are not recommended. Options 1, 2, and 4 may or may not be true but these statements do not explain the primary reason why using drugs without prescriptions is contraindicated.
355. 2. Of the food constituents given, protein in larger-than-average amounts is recommended by the Food and Nutrition Board of the National Research Council. Other constituents that are recommended in larger-than-average amounts include calcium, iron, vitamin A, thiamine, riboflavin, niacin, vitamin B6, vitamin B12, and ascorbic acid.
356. 1. An increased fluid intake is recommended during lactation in order to foster milk production and to replace the fluids which the baby consumes with nursing.
357. 3. The rooting reflex will cause the baby to turn to an object brushed across his lips and cause him to grasp the nipple for nursing. Options 1, 2, and 4 have not been found to be effective for helping the newborn become oriented to nursing.

358. 4. While it is true that breast-fed babies do not swallow as much air as bottle-fed babies, the breast-fed babies still should be bubbled. Options 1, 2, and 3 are inaccurate statements.

359. 3. On the average, a baby accustomed to breast feeding will spend about 20 minutes nursing. The breast is emptied in about 5 to 7 minutes; the baby then continues to nurse to satisfy his need to suck.

360. 1. Options 2, 3, and 4 are indicated procedure when the nipples become sore. Applying a breast binder will do nothing to alleviate the condition and may aggravate it.

361. 1. It is important to empty the breasts regularly. If this is not done, the ducts become occluded by congested tissues and the secretions become thick and tenacious. Other measures, as described in options 2, 3, and 4, may become necessary but of first importance is emptying the breasts regularly.

362. 1. Oxytocin is believed to be responsible for bringing on the "let-down" sensation when milk is carried to the nipples. Prolactin stimulates milk production. Thyrotropin promotes growth and secretion in the thyroid gland. Parathormone acts principally to regulate calcium concentration in body fluids.

363. 2. Option 2 describes the best procedure. Manipulating the nipples may cause injury to the tissues. The position also causes pressure at the area of the collecting sinuses and will result in milk being forced out of the nipples.

364. 2. The most effective way to stimulate the production of milk is to empty the breasts at each feeding. Option 1 is not necessary, nor is option 4. Occasional substitution of formula for a breast feeding is not contraindicated.

365. 1. The milk supply diminishes normally as the baby nurses less. Actions described in options 2 and 3 are not indicated. Option 4 is not an accurate statement—some mothers nurse well beyond 4 to 6 months.

366. 1. The LeLeche League was formed to assist mothers who wish to learn the art of breast feeding. The other organizations given here may give advice but teaching and helping nursing mothers is not their primary function.

367. 3. The incidence of breast cancer and thrombophlebitis is lower in women who breast feed. Since nursing releases oxytocin which stimulates the uterus to contract, postpartal hemorrhage is less likely. Option 3 is not related to breast feeding.

DISCUSSION OF FORMULA PREPARATION

368. 1. It is the fat in cow's milk that infants tolerate poorly. When

cow's milk is diluted, the carbohydrate content is also decreased. Hence, carbohydrate then must be added to formula so that the amount approximates mother's milk.

369. 2. The number of calories in mother's milk normally is about 20 per ounce.

370. 4. When evaporated milk is diluted to approximate mother's milk in other respects, the carbohydrate level is too low. Hence, the physician ordinarily prescribes adding carbohydrate to the diluted evaporated milk.

371. 4. The vitamins most commonly found in preparations for infants contain vitamins A, C, and D, the three most essential for the infant's health.

372. 4. Commercially premodified milk formula contains supplemental vitamins and, hence, it is unnecessary to prescribe additional supplemental amounts. Breast milk, cow's milk formula, and evaporated milk formula do not contain certain vitamins so that prescribing supplemental amounts becomes necessary.

373. 3. The more active a baby is, the more calories he will require. Factors given in options 1, 2, and 4 do not influence caloric intake.

374. 4. It has been demonstrated that as a general rule, most newborns will require about 50 to 55 calories each day per pound of body weight.

375. 2. The recommended procedure for enlarging the holes in a feeding nipple is to pierce the hole with a hot needle. Option 1 describes unsatisfactory procedure since the rubber will return to original position once the toothpick is removed. Options 3 and 4 are dangerous for the person attempting to enlarge the nipple holes. Also, the size of the holes are very likely to be too big since it is difficult to control a scissors or knife for this procedure.

376. 4. The procedure described in the stem will help prevent the formation of film on top of the formula. It will not influence options 1, 2, and 3.

377. 3. Because the atmospheric pressure is less at higher altitudes, the boiling point of water is lower. Factors given in options 1 and 4 have nothing to do with the time needed to sterilize at various altitudes.

378. 2. Most authorities recommend that in order to be sure of sterilization, the bottles of formula should be boiled for a minimum of 25 minutes.

379. 1. It is recommended that the nipples be washed as soon after use as possible. This prevents remaining formula from

coagulating and drying in the nipples. Then they should be boiled. Boiling unclean equipment makes it less easy to sterilize since organisms can lodge in waste materials on the article. Rinsing nipples under hot water will tend to coagulate remaining milk and, hence, make sterilization more difficult. A disinfectant is not considered necessary.

JANET BROWN

380. 2. The most important preparation for saline solution injection is to have the bladder empty to prevent possible perforation of the bladder with the instrument used to inject saline. The other options describe preparation that is contraindicated, as in option 1, or not necessary, as in options 3 and 4.

381. 4. Spinal and general anesthetics and pain relieving medications are rarely indicated when an abortion with saline injection is used. Also, it is best to have an alert patient who can report adverse symptoms; see item 382. The most accurate description of what will occur is described in option 4.

382. 3. The symptoms given in option 3 are typical when intravascular injection of hypertonic saline has occurred. Signs/symptoms given in options 1, 2, and 4 are not related to the situation described in the stem.

383. 2. The movements which the patient felt are normal and will stop when the fetus dies. Feelings of guilt are not known to be related to movement of the fetus.

384. 1. The contractions are likely to be uncomfortable and an analgesic may be given. Option 1 describes how the nurse is best able to offer the patient physical and emotional support. Vaginal examinations are contraindicated since they are not necessary and are likely to result in infection. Neither option 3 or 4 gives the patient emotional or physical support which the patient needs at this time.

385. 2. The best course of action is to stay with the patient until the fetus is expelled. The delivery room is ordinarily not used for this. The physician does not ordinarily need to be present for the procedure. Rectal pressure is a symptom indicating that expulsion of the fetus is imminent.

386. 1. The best course of action is for the nurse to clamp the cord and remove the fetus. The placenta will ordinarily be delivered in due time so that surgical intervention is unnecessary. Kneading the abdomen will not help with the delivery of the placenta and exerting pull on the cord is contraindicated.

387. 2. These drugs act to inhibit the release of the lactogenic hormone from the pituitary, thereby preventing lactation and

breast engorgement. They play no part in factors described in options 1, 3, and 4.

388. 4. It is best that the patient be examined by the physician rather than having her follow instructions described in options 1 and 2. It is unlikely that she is about to hemorrhage. The symptoms are more indicative of infection.

389. 3. Abortion became a legal act in 1973 by a ruling made by the Supreme Court of the United States.

390. 1. The longer the pregnancy lasts, the greater is the danger of performing an abortion. Hence, the abortion carries the least danger when it can be carried out during the first 4 weeks of gestation.

HELEN OLSON

391. 2. The best course of action in this situation is to stand by quietly as the patient is allowed to express her feelings. There is little help offered by telling her that she will adjust to pregnancy nor is there emotional support described in option 4. To press the patient for explanations (option 3) is usually futile and may make the patient feel antagonistic when asked to explain her feelings.

392. 2. It is most important to observe this patient for signs of hemorrhage. Massaging the fundus following an abortion at this stage of gestation is not indicated. It is better to wait for a period of time after the patient awakens before discontinuing the infusion because, if complications occur, an open intravenous makes therapy easier. There is no need to be prepared to catheterize this patient as soon as 1 hour after awakening.

393. 3. Methylergonovine maleate is a semisynthetic form of ergot. It acts to cause uterine contractions and, hence, abdominal cramping is to be expected after it is administered. The best course of action for the nurse to follow is to give the patient the prescribed analgesic. The cramping is not an adverse effect, ambulating the patient will be of no avail, and there is no need to call the physician at this time when the drug is acting in the desired manner.

394. 2. The ability to prevent Rh sensitization is now possible with the use of human anti-D globulin. This agent can bring about clearance from the maternal circulation of Rh positive fetal cells and thereby prevent sensitization.

395. 2. The legally accepted procedure is for the nurse to draw a line through the error and add the correction. It is not legally acceptable to erase an error or to destroy original records on which the error occurred.

396. 1. According to statistics, most women who seek abortions are in their teens and early twenties; requests are less frequent among older women.

JANET ADAMER

397. 1. It has been determined that it takes only 1 to 5 minutes for the sperm to reach the ovum under ideal conditions.

398. 3. Oral contraceptives prevent conception by inhibiting ovulation. They play no role in accomplishing results described in options 1, 2, and 4.

399. 1. The most commonly observed side effects of oral contraceptives include those described in option 1. Those given in options 2, 3, and 4 are infrequently observed.

400. 3. The recommended procedure when a contraceptive pill has been inadvertently omitted is to take it as soon as the person remembers and also take the next pill at the regular time.

401. 3. Ordinarily, it is unnecessary to use a lubricant when a condom is used and when sexual foreplay has been used. When a lubricant is necessary, petrolatum is least often recommended because it destroys rubber. For this same reason, it is recommended that petrolatum not be used when inserting a diaphragm.

402. 3. It is generally advised that a douche be delayed for 8 hours after using a contraceptive cream. Flushing the cream from the vagina earlier may allow some of the sperm to survive and possibly fertilize the ovum.

403. 4. It is believed that the IUD prevents conception by preventing the implantation of the fertilized ovum. Most oral contraceptives act to suppress ovulation and IUDs play no role in depressing progesterone production or in preventing the sperm from entering the fallopian tube.

404. 1. During menstruation, the cervix is ordinarily more relaxed and open, making it easier to insert the IUD. Also, it can be assumed that the IUD is not being inserted into a pregnant uterus.

405. 2. The recommended minimum time to leave a diaphragm in place after intercourse is 6 hours. If it is removed earlier, sperm may continue to be alive and could then cause conception.

406. 3. The patient was most likely ovulating between August 24 and 26 when her basal temperature was lowest. It is during that time that she is likely to be most fertile.

407. 4. It is recommended that the patient take her temperature every morning upon awakening and before arising. At this time in

the day, her temperature is least likely to be influenced by other factors.

408. 3. Of the conditions given here, the only one that will result in infertility is occluded fallopian tubes. This condition prevents sperm from making contact with the ovum.

MISCELLANEOUS ITEMS

409. 2. A man with undescended testicles is sterile. Conditions described in options 2, 3, and 4 result in infertility but not sterility.

410. 2. It is recommended that the pregnant woman increase her daily protein intake to 65 Gm. The extra protein is necessary for the proper growth and development of the fetus.

411. 4. Although a cesarean operation may not be ordered for any of these women, the one who is least likely to require one is the patient whose engagement occurred one week before admission. The other conditions present the possibility of a cesarean operation.

412. 3. The most important guide when caring for a pregnant woman with heart disease is to consider how well her heart is able to function. Factors given in options 1, 2, and 3 are of lesser significance.

413. 2. A convulsion confirms the presence of eclampsia. When toxemia is present, until a convulsion occurs, the patient is said to have preeclampsia.

414. 3. The cause of toxemias of pregnancy is not known. However, it has been observed that diabetes, vascular diseases, and multiple pregnancies predispose to the condition. Eclampsia is most often seen during the last trimester of pregnancy. Young primigravidae are prone to toxemias of pregnancy.

415. 2. *Neiserria gonorrhoeae* cause gonorrhea and this condition has serious implications. It can cause blindness in the baby if the eyes are infected during birth and not properly treated. The disease causes scar tissue in the mother's fallopian tubes and can then ultimately cause sterility. *Candida albicans* is a yeast and may invade the genital tract. The symptoms may be annoying but the infection does not have serious consequences. Trichomonas vaginalis is relatively easy to treat and does not have serious implications. Streptococcal infections can be serious, especially for the baby, but they re ordinarily effectively handled with various antibiotics.

416. 2. When an amniotomy is performed while the head is still high in the pelvis, the cord is likely to prolapse since it can easily pass by the fetal head as amniotic fluid travels through the

birth canal. The head causing pressure on the cord cuts off circulation to the fetus which is a grave complication. The fetal heart rate will drop when in circulatory distress.

417. 1. Small fibrin clots in the capillaries consume fibrinogen, leaving the patient with nonclotting blood. However, to prevent fibrin clots, heparin is the drug of choice. The patient must be observed for symptoms of bleeding. Substances that help to promote blood coagulation are made in the liver and require vitamin K for certain biochemical reactions. Hence, vitamin K acts to increase ability of the blood to coagulate. Folic acid is vitamin B_{12} which is used primarily for the treatment of pernicious anemia. Estriol is a hormone and during pregnancy, stimulates the growth and development of the uterus, among other things.

418. 3. A patient who has bright red vaginal bleeding should not be given an enema. Whatever the cause, the enema may aggravate the condition. Enemas are not contraindicated for patients described in options 1, 2, and 4.

419. 4. Nalorphine hydrochloride is a specific antidote for the depressing effects of narcotics. Drugs described in options 2 and 3 are stimulants but do not counteract the effects of a narcotic.

420. 4. A tonic contracted uterus should be reported to the physician promptly. The condition may lead to fetal distress rather quickly. Options 1 and 3 describe common occurrences during the first stage of labor. A patient should be taught not to bear down during the first stage of labor since it may delay rather than hasten birth. See item 95 also. Bearing down is used effectively during late labor and delivery.

421. 3. The instrument used for a breech delivery is the Piper forceps. The overall length of the forceps is longer than that of forceps used when the head will be delivered first.

422. 2. Of the patients described here, the diabetic multipara is least likely to require the use of forceps. Forceps may be used to conserve the strength of a mother with heart disease. Many mothers having their first babies are assisted during delivery with the use of forceps. This instrument is frequently used when the fetus is in the breech position.

423. 4. In order to release pressure of the presenting part on the prolapsed cord, it would be best to push upward on the head, or presenting part, with a sterile-gloved hand. It would be futile to try to replace the cord. After relieving pressure, the physician should be called. Turning the mother will not alleviate the problem. See item 416 also.

424. 4. Uterine atony is more common when the uterus has been

distended during pregnancy by fetal twins. Hence, the patient should be observed closely for postpartal hemorrhage.

425. 1. A mother who has delivered ten babies is more likely to have uterine atony following delivery than the woman who had delivered only one or two babies. The conditions described in the other options are not associated with multiple pregnancies and deliveries.

426. 4. Afterpains while nursing the baby are due to the uterus being stimulated to contract by oxytocin. The other options do not relate to afterpains.

427. 2. It has been found that the major cause of genetic malformation syndromes appears to be mutation of a single gene.

428. 1. Down's syndrome is believed to be due to a chromosome abnormality. It is not related to conditions described in the other options.

429. 2. Options 1, 3, and 4 are true statements concerning Down's syndrome. It is a condition that is relatively easy to diagnose at the time of birth.

430. 3. Postterm babies may suffer due to placental deterioration. Conditions described in options 1 and 4 are unlikely and option 2 is inaccurate.

431. 4. A postmature baby is most likely to have a larger-than-average head size. Molding is resisted because of advanced bone formation. Conditions described in options 1, 2, and 3 are commonly observed on a postmature infant.

432. 4. Although all of the factors given here *may* influence the fetus, the most important determiner is the stage of embryonic development when the drug was taken.

433. 1. A score of 3 or less indicates that the baby is in poor condition and emergency measures are indicated. See also item 302.

434. 2. Caput succedaneum is caused by pressure on the head during labor. It is an edematous area that occurs over the place where the scalp was encircled by the cervix. Cephalhematoma is caused by blood between the bone and the periostem. Since the bleeding is under the periostem, it cannot cross a suture line while a caput can. Hence, the area of involvement best differentiates the two.

435. 3. The symptoms described in the stem are typical of hypoglycemia. Hypothermia results in a low body temperature. Hypocalcemia is characterized by irritability, twitching, and convulsions, although hand tremors may also be present. Apnea and an expiratory grunt are the prime manifestations of respiratory distress.

436. 4. Impetigo neonatorum should be reported promptly. It is a

very infectious skin disease and can have grave consequences, especially if the umbilicus becomes infected. See item 434 in relation to options 1 and 3. Erythema toxicum is a red, blotchy rash that is often seen on newborns. It is not infectious, clears of its own accord, and requires no special treatment.

437. 1. The condition described here is normal. The mother need not consider bottle feeding at this time.

438. 4. It has been observed that when there are less than the normal number of umbilical cord vessels, the baby is most likely to have congenital anomalies, especially of the gastrointestinal or urinary tract. The cause for the relationship is unknown.

439. 3. The persistent and shrill cry is not typical of a newborn. A shrill cry is typical of an infant suffering from heroin withdrawal or experiencing increased intracranial pressure.

440. 2. When surfactant is not present, the aveoli do not extend properly and respiratory distress occurs.

441. 1. Bacteria that inhabit the large intestine synthesize vitamin K which is then absorbed. Vitamin K is often given to newborns because they are unable to synthesize the vitamin due to lack of bacteria in the intestines.

442. 1. Meconium can cause an inflammatory reaction. Thus, it should be flushed out with lavage. The actions described in options 2, 3, and 4 are not indicated unless the infant's condition deteriorates.

443. 3. Meconium provides good nutrition for bacterial growth in the respiratory passages. Options 1, 2, and 4 are inaccurate statements in relation to meconium.

444. 1. The indiscriminate use of oxygen causes retrolental fibroplasia. Blindness is likely to result.

445. 1. It is the patient who may legally give permission for a copy of the record to be sent to a physician.

446. 1. Vital statistics are considered public information. Therefore, the patient's age can be given without legal implications. Giving out any other information may lead to legal problems.

447. 4. In this case, the nurse must obtain permission to use hospital records for research purposes from a hospital representative.

448. 4. First, the nurse should check the patient's condition. Then she should notify the physician who may wish to order an antidote, depending on the patient's condition. The error should be recorded but this is not as urgent as checking the patient when the error is noted.

449. 1. The best course of action is described in option 1. Options 2, 3, and 4 do not describe satisfactory courses of action since the

patient's care may be jeopardized because of the nurse's attitude about abortions.

450. 4. Maternal death rates are reported as the number of deaths per 100,000 live births.
451. 4. Although all conditions given here may lead to death, the most frequent cause of maternal deaths is hemorrhage.
452. 1. Although all factors given here may influence decreasing maternal death rates, the greatest single factor is improved antenatal care.
453. 2. Infant mortality rates are reported as the number of deaths per 1000 live births.
454. 4. Infant mortality rates include deaths up to the age of 1 year.
455. 1. Most infant deaths occur between the ages of birth and 7 days.
456. 1. The cause of most neonatal deaths in the United States is prematurity.

nursing of children

Tommy Taylor was born with a cleft palate and lip. He is transferred from the hospital's newborn nursery to a pediatric unit for care.

Items 1 through 14 relate to this situation.

1. Tommy's parents are shocked when they see Tommy for the first time. Which one of the following nursing actions would be *most beneficial* to help the parents accept Tommy's anomaly?
   1. Bring Tommy to them more often.
   2. Tell them that surgery will correct the defect.
   3. Show them pictures of babies prior to and after surgery.
   4. Allow them to adjust and complete their grieving process prior to seeing Tommy again.

2. Which one of the following factors is of *primary* concern while caring for Tommy preoperatively?
   1. Preventing an infection in his mouth.
   2. Altering usual methods for feeding him.
   3. Using techniques to minimize his crying.
   4. Preventing him from placing his fingers in his mouth.

3. Which one of the following nursing measures is *most likely* to help Tommy retain his feedings?
   1. Bubble him at frequent intervals.
   2. Feed him small amounts at a time.
   3. Place the nipple on the back of his tongue.
   4. Hold him in a lying position while feeding him.

4. Tommy has surgery for the repair of his cleft lip. If the nurse observes that Tommy is having difficulty breathing postoperatively, which one of the following nursing actions would be *most helpful* to bring relief?

1. Turn Tommy on his abdomen.
2. Hold Tommy's nose momentarily.
3. Insert an airway into Tommy's mouth.
4. Place downward pressure on Tommy's chin.

5. The nurse should assess Tommy as having an *early* sign of respiratory distress when she notes an increase in his
   1. amount of crying.
   2. abdominal breathing.
   3. respiratory secretions.
   4. difficulty with eating.

6. The *most common* cause of respiratory distress following the repair of a cleft lip is that the infant
   1. has swelling of the tongue and nostrils.
   2. is less active than he normally would be.
   3. is secreting more than normal amounts of mucus.
   4. has had considerable medication and anesthesia during surgery.

7. Of the following methods, the *most common* one for feeding an infant during the first few days after the repair of a cleft lip is to use
   1. gastric gavage.
   2. intravenous fluids.
   3. a large-holed nipple.
   4. a rubber-tipped medicine dropper.

8. To keep Tommy's suture line clean and free of crusting, it would be *best* to swab the area carefully with
   1. mineral oil.
   2. distilled water.
   3. hydrogen peroxide.
   4. a mild antiseptic solution.

9. Tommy's parents ask the nurse when it is likely that the cleft palate will be repaired. The nurse should base her response on knowledge that the first repair of a cleft palate is *usually* done
   1. prior to the development of speech.
   2. prior to the eruption of teeth.
   3. after the child learns to sit alone.
   4. after the child learns to drink from a cup.

10. Which one of the following eating utensils would be *most appropriate* for Tommy after the repair of his cleft palate?
    1. A cup.
    2. A drinking tube.
    3. An Asepto syringe.
    4. A large-holed nipple.

11. When irrigating his mouth after the repair of his cleft palate, which one of the following positions would be *best* for Tommy?
    1. An upright sitting position.
    2. On his back with his head turned to the side.
    3. On his abdomen with his head over the side of the bed.
12. Which one of the following types of restraints would be *best* to use for Tommy immediately postoperatively after the repair of his cleft palate?
    1. A safety jacket.
    2. Elbow restraints.
    3. Arm and leg restraints.
    4. Arm and body restraints.
13. For the first few days after the repair of Tommy's cleft palate, Ms. Taylor is encouraged to stay with him as much as possible. Which one of the following activities should the nurse encourage the mother to perform?
    1. Hold and cuddle Tommy.
    2. Help Tommy to play with some of his toys.
    3. Read some of Tommy's favorite stories to him.
    4. Stay at Tommy's bedside and hold his hand in hers.
14. Of the following problems, which one is *most common* among children who have had cleft palate repairs?
    1. A speech defect.
    2. Nutritional inadequacies.
    3. Difficulty in developing a healthy self-image.
    4. Difficulty in developing an independent personality.

Several hours after Michael Stephens was born, it was noted that he had an esophageal atresia.
Items 15 through 28 relate to Michael's care.

15. Mr. and Mrs. Stephens express feelings of guilt about Michael's anomaly. Which one of the following approaches would be *best* for the nurse to use to help the parents?
    1. Encourage them to discuss long-term plans for Michael.
    2. Explain that they did nothing to cause Michael's birth defect.
    3. Help them to accept their feelings as being a normal reaction.
    4. Have them visit Michael as often as they possibly can during his hospitalization.
16. Michael displays one of the *most classic* signs of esophageal atresia which is having
    1. large frothy stools.
    2. diaphragmatic breathing.

3. bluish discoloration of his mouth.

4. excessive amounts of mucus in his mouth.

17. If an attempt is made to feed Michael, which one of the following signs would further indicate the presence of esophageal atresia?

1. His refusal to eat.

2. His inability to suck.

3. Projectile vomiting.

4. Continuous drooling.

18. Michael was diagnosed as having a blind upper pouch and a fistula into the trachea from the lower pouch of the esophagus. In his case, aspiration of material into his lungs occurs *primarily* from the

1. inability to expectorate mucus.

2. overflow of secretions from the upper pouch.

3. reflux of gastric secretions into the bronchi.

4. obstruction of the fistula leading into the trachea.

19. While suctioning the upper pouch, of the following positions, it would be *best* to place Michael

1. flat on his back.

2. on his abdomen with his head turned to either side.

3. on either side.

4. on his back with his head higher than the rest of his body.

20. Which one of the following signs should indicate to the nurse that Michael is in need of tracheal suctioning?

1. A brassy cough.

2. Decrease in activity.

3. Substernal retractions.

4. Increased respiratory rate.

21. Michael is placed in a heated isolette with high humidity. The *major* reason for maintaining high humidity is to help

1. lower his metabolic rate.

2. replace some of his fluid losses.

3. decrease the likelihood of infection.

4. decrease the viscosity of his respiratory secretions.

22. Michael has surgery for the repair of his anomaly. He has a chest tube in place, the end of which is in a bottle under water. Michael's mother accidently trips and the tube comes out of the bottle. What action should the nurse take *immediately?*

1. Clamp the tubing with a hemostat.

2. Put the tubing back into the bottle.

3. Leave the tubing out and note the respiratory rate.

4. Remove the tubing and cover the incision with a sterile dressing.

23. Michael has a gastrostomy tube in place for feeding. The physician orders a pressure clamp on the tube and a syringe barrel is used for introducing feedings into the tube. While feeding Michael, which one of the following techniques will help *most* to prevent air from entering the stomach after the syringe barrel has been attached to the tube?
1. Open the clamp after pouring all of his formula into the syringe barrel.
2. Open the clamp before pouring all of his formula into the syringe barrel.
3. Open the clamp and continuously pour his formula down the side of the syringe barrel.
4. Open the clamp and allow a small portion of his formula to enter the stomach before pouring additional formula into the syringe barrel.

24. Which one of the following nursing measures will *best* help to meet Michael's psychological needs while giving him his formula through the gastrostomy tube?
1. Hold him.
2. Talk or sing to him.
3. Give him a pacifier.
4. Lightly stroke his abdomen.

25. After feeding Michael through the gastrostomy tube, the nurse rocks him for a while, the *primary* purpose being to help
1. promote relaxation and rest.
2. prevent regurgitation of his formula.
3. associate eating with a pleasurable experience.
4. relieve pressure on his surgical repair and gastrostomy.

26. When beginning oral feedings, Michael's nursing care plan should be based on the principle that
1. a well-followed feeding schedule helps the infant accept oral feedings more readily.
2. an infant adjusts to oral feedings better when small, frequent feedings are offered.
3. oral feedings following intubation are best accepted when offered by the same nurse or by the infant's mother.
4. oral feedings following intubation are best planned in conjunction with observations of the infant's behavior.

27. Which one of the following signs, if observed in Michael, would strongly suggest that he is developing a stricture?
1. Constipation.
2. Watery stools.
3. Increased thirst.
4. Pronounced coughing.

28. Which one of the following conditions, if it had been observed during Ms. Stephens' pregnancy for Michael, would have provided a clue that Michael might have had an anomaly of the gastrointestinal tract?
   1. Low implantation of the placenta.
   2. Increased amount of amniotic fluid.
   3. Premature separation of the placenta.
   4. Presence of meconium in the amniotic fluid.

   A nurse has been assigned to care for four toddlers, all of whom have had surgery.
   Items 29 through 42 relate to the care of these children.

29. Twenty-two-month old Johnny Brown was hospitalized for the repair of a right inguinal hernia. His hernia was visible only when he cried and he had no signs of discomfort. Which one of the following statements offers the *best* explanation concerning why Johnny's hernia repair was done at this time?
   1. From a physiological viewpoint, Johnny has reached an ideal age for tolerating surgery.
   2. The experience of surgery is less frightening at Johnny's age than it would be at any later age.
   3. There is less danger of complications when surgery is an elective procedure rather than an emergency procedure.
   4. There is a preference for doing surgery near the genital organs at an age before the child becomes conscious of his sexual identity.
30. If Johnny were to develop a complication, the one that would *most likely* occur is
   1. sterility.
   2. wound infection.
   3. rupture of the wound.
   4. excessive scar formation.
31. The term which *best* describes the complication when part of the intestine becomes lodged in the hernial sac is
   1. rupture.
   2. dehiscence.
   3. intussusception.
   4. incarceration.
32. Eighteen-month-old Jane Green had an appendectomy. When compared with older children and adults, young children have a higher incidence of perforation of the appendix and peritonitis because they
   1. have a greater pain tolerance.

2. describe their symptoms poorly.

3. have a weaker appendiceal wall.

4. have less resistance to infection.

33. Jane's appendix was not perforated. Since there was no loss of bowel integrity, how soon after surgery would the physician *most likely* order a diet for her?

1. For the following evening's meal.

2. As soon as she retains fluids.

3. After her intravenous infusion is discontinued.

34. Which one of the following dietary items would *not* ordinarily be recorded as fluid on Jane's fluid intake record?

1. Gelatin.

2. Ice cream.

3. A popsicle.

4. Baked custard.

35. Tommy Black, who is 24 months old, was hospitalized for a tonsillectomy and an adenoidectomy. Which one of the following signs, if observed in Tommy, should alert the nurse to the possibility that he is having a postoperative hemorrhage?

1. A slow pulse rate.

2. Frequent swallowing.

3. Labored respirations.

4. Expectoration of reddish-brown saliva.

36. Which one of the following liquids is *most likely* to be tolerated *poorly* by Tommy during the first few hours postoperatively?

1. Milk.

2. Apple juice.

3. A carbonated beverage.

4. A fruit-flavored drink.

37. Tommy's mother tells the nurse that she is having problems toilet training Tommy. The *most common* reason for failing when toilet training toddlers is that

1. the rewards for the desired behavior are too limited.

2. the child is not ready to be trained.

3. the training equipment is of an inappropriate size for the child.

4. the child is trying to demonstrate his own individuality.

38. Suzy Blue, who is 28 months old, was hospitalized for a bilateral myringotomy. Otitis media occurs more frequently in infants and young children than in older children and adults because of the different anatomical position of the younger person's

1. esophagus.

2. eustachian tubes.

3. tympanic membranes.

4. external ear canals.

39. Suzy is ordered to have eardrops instilled after discharge from the hospital and the nurse should teach the procedure to the parents. The drops are instilled by pulling Suzy's earlobe in a direction that is
    1. up and forward.
    2. up and backward.
    3. down and forward.
    4. down and backward.
40. A practice that is often recommended to help prevent recurrence of otitis media in a child, such as Suzy, is to
    1. eliminate a bedtime bottle given when the child is in bed.
    2. cleanse the ears thoroughly and often.
    3. use continuous small-dose antibiotic therapy.
    4. have the child blow the nose well and regularly.
41. Which one of the following techniques for assessing pain would be *least effective* for the nurse to use when caring for toddlers postoperatively?
    1. Ask them about their pain.
    2. Observe them for restlessness.
    3. Watch their faces for grimaces.
    4. Listen for pain clues in their cries.
42. When performing a procedure on an uncooperative small child, if all of the following courses of action are possible for the nurse to use, which one would be *best* to try *first?*
    1. Use restraints.
    2. Sedate the child.
    3. Allow a parent to assist.
    4. Obtain another nurse to assist.

> Five-year-old Sally Horner was brought to the emergency room by her parents. She had fallen from a tree and broken her humerus.
> Items 43 through 47 relate to this situation.

43. Sally demonstrates fear and cries, "Mommy, I want to go home. Is the doctor going to cut off my arm? Will it hurt? I hate the nurse and want to go home!" Of the following actions, which one is the *most appropriate* for the nurse to take in this situation?
    1. Have another nurse care for Sally because of Sally's dislike for the present arrangement.
    2. Ask Sally's parents to leave the room for a while until the nurse has had a chance to calm the child.
    3. Suggest to Sally that she will be acting like a big girl if she is quiet while the doctor fixes her arm.

4. Explain to Sally what the doctor will be doing during the procedure in language she can readily understand.

44. Sally is to be sent home after her fracture is reduced and her arm is casted. Her parents should be instructed to bring Sally back to the emergency room promptly if
   1. Sally refuses to eat dinner.
   2. Sally is irritable and insistent that the cast is too heavy.
   3. Sally's cast feels damp as long as 6 hours after being applied.
   4. Sally's fingers below the cast feel cool and appear bluish.

45. The nurse teaches Sally's parents the importance of a good diet to help the bone to heal. *All* of the following food substances help promote bone healing *except*
   1. iron.
   2. sodium.
   3. calcium.
   4. vitamin D.

46. When the nurse explains that healing can be expected in about 4 to 6 weeks, Mr. Horner expresses surprise and says, "My father broke his arm and it took much longer than that to heal!" The nurse's response to this comment should be based on knowledge that a youngster's fracture normally heals more rapidly than an adult's because a child's bones
   1. are more pliable than an adult's bones.
   2. have a more abundant blood supply than an adult's bones.
   3. Have epiphyseal plates while, in an adult, these plates have closed.
   4. rarely sustain a comminuted fracture while an adult's bones will almost always comminute.

47. Below are three physiological stages of bone healing:
   1. osteoid formation.
   2. granulation tissue formation.
   3. callus formation.
   Indicate the order in which these three stages of bone healing normally occur.
   1. 1, 2, 3.
   2. 2, 3, 1.
   3. 3, 1, 2.
   4. 3, 2, 1.

Five-year-old Cindy Kare was admitted to the hospital for diagnostic studies and heart surgery for repair of tetralogy of Fallot. She was cyanotic at the time of admission.
Items 48 through 64 relate to this situation.

48. What is the underlying cause of Cindy's cyanosis?

1. The aorta is constricted.
2. There is stenosis of the mitral valve.
3. There is stenosis of the pulmonic valve.
4. The aorta receives blood directly from the vena cava.

49. Cindy is ordered to have a low sodium diet. Which one of the following foods would be *inappropriate* for her diet?
    1. Eggs.
    2. Fruited yogurt.
    3. Cottage cheese.
    4. Cheddar cheese.

50. The nurse observes clubbing of Cindy's fingers. The *most likely* cause is that Cindy has
    1. peripheral hypoxia.
    2. low blood pressure.
    3. electrolyte imbalances.
    4. red bone marrow destruction.

51. Cindy's blood studies reveal that her hemoglobin and hematocrit levels are above average values. The *primary* reason for these above average findings is that her body is attempting to compensate for Cindy's having
    1. an enlarged heart.
    2. poorly oxygenated blood.
    3. a below normal blood pressure.
    4. a below normal quantity of blood.

52. Of the following positions, which one is likely to give Cindy the *most* relief when she experiences dyspnea?
    1. Knee-chest.
    2. Semisitting.
    3. Trendelenburg's.
    4. Right side-lying.

53. A cardiac catheterization is ordered for Cindy. Cindy asks the nurse if the procedure will hurt. Which one of the following statements offers the nurse the best guide for responding to Cindy's query?
    1. Some pain may be felt when the catheter is introduced into the vein.
    2. Momentary sharp pain will usually occur when the catheter enters the heart.
    3. It is unusual for a 5-year-old to be aware of discomfort or pain during the procedure.
    4. It is a painless procedure although there is often a tingling sensation noted in the extremities.

54. Cindy has an electrocardiogram (EKG). The *primary* reason for the procedure is to determine

1. pressure of the blood in the heart.
2. electrical activity in heart muscle.
3. various sounds made by each heartbeat.
4. amount of blood supplying heart muscles.

55. Cindy is taught coughing and deep-breathing exercises preoperatively. All of the following teaching-learning principles are important for the nurse to consider when planning teaching activities for Cindy. Which one should assume the *first* priority?
   1. Place information in a logical sequence.
   2. Present material from simple to complex.
   3. Build on the child's level of knowledge.
   4. Use actual equipment for the demonstrations.

56. Hypothermia was used for Cindy during surgery *primarily* because it helps to decrease
   1. blood loss.
   2. pain perception.
   3. the body's metabolic rate.
   4. the heart's contractability.

57. Postoperatively, Cindy has a chest tube in place. Which one of the following actions should the nurse take *first* if Cindy's chest tube becomes clogged?
   1. Irrigate the tubing with normal saline.
   2. Milk the tubing toward the drainage bottles.
   3. Apply suction with a bulb-type syringe to remove debris.
   4. Assemble the necessary supplies for the physician to change the tubing.

58. Most authorities recommend that, in order to help avoid complications, Cindy's hourly postoperative urinary output should be a *minimum* of approximately
   1. 10 to 15 ml.
   2. 25 to 30 ml.
   3. 40 to 45 ml.
   4. 55 to 60 ml.

59. Cindy stops breathing on her second postoperative day. Which one of the following measures should the nurse take *first* when the patient stops breathing?
   1. Clear her airway.
   2. Start administering oxygen.
   3. Begin external cardiac massage.
   4. Give her mouth-to-mouth resuscitation.

60. Which one of the following techniques should the nurse use for applying pressure to the heart when she is performing cardiopulmonary resuscitation on a small child, such as Cindy?
   1. Apply pressure to the sternum with the heel of one hand.

2. Apply pressure to the sternum with the tips of two fingers.
3. Apply pressure over the apex of the heart with the heel of one hand.
4. Apply pressure over the apex of the heart with the tips of two fingers.

61. It is generally recommended that, for a child Cindy's age, the number of compressions delivered each minute when using cardiopulmonary resuscitation should be approximately
1. 60 to 80.
2. 80 to 110.
3. 100 to 110.
4. 110 to 120.

62. When all of the following arteries are equally available, which one is *most often* recommended for checking the pulse during cardiopulmonary resuscitation?
1. Radial.
2. Femoral.
3. Carotid.
4. Dorsalis pedis.

63. Cindy's parents express concern when they note that Cindy wants to be held more frequently than usual, postoperatively. The term that *best* describes this behavioral response to stress is
1. regression.
2. depression.
3. repression.
4. rationalization.

64. The nurse should anticipate that the *most likely* fear Cindy's parents will have when they plan to take Cindy home is fear of
1. allowing Cindy to lead a normal active life.
2. persuading Cindy of the need for extra rest.
3. Cindy's developing a postoperative complication.
4. having Cindy's siblings compete for equal attention.

One-year-old Billy Wright was admitted to the hospital with a fracture of the left femur. He was accompanied by his parents, both of whom appeared well developed and in good health. Mr. and Ms. Wright gave different descriptions of the accident that caused Billy's fracture. Child abuse was suspected.

Items 65 through 71 relate to this situation.

65. The physician orders Billy's legs placed in traction. Which one of the following statements is an *unlikely* reason for the physician's order?
1. Traction will help to reduce the fracture.

2. Traction will help decrease muscle contractions.
3. Traction will help prevent infection at the fracture site.
4. Traction will help keep the broken bone in proper alignment.
66. Skin traction, using moleskin, is applied to Billy's legs. Billy is placed in bed on his back and his legs are extended upwardly with his hips flexed at a 90° angle. Weights are used to obtain traction. Countertraction in Billy's case will be obtained by
1. the weight of his body.
2. the weight of his legs.
3. elevating the foot of the bed.
4. elevating the head of the bed.
67. If a nurse is observed carrying out all of the following actions in relation to Billy's traction, which one would be considered an *appropriate* nursing measure?
1. Allow the weights on his traction to hang freely.
2. Decrease the amount of weight on his traction slightly each day.
3. Change the moleskin used on his legs for obtaining traction each day.
4. Remove the weights while inspecting his legs for evidence of friction over bony prominences.
68. If the nurse notes that Billy displays the following behaviors while being cared for, which one *most strongly* suggests that possibly he has been experiencing child abuse?
1. He sucks his thumb.
2. He eats his lunch without urging.
3. He is underdeveloped for his age.
3. He appears happy when personnel work with him.
69. If all of the following findings are noted when Billy's parents are interviewed by the nurse, which one should the nurse judge as being *least typical* of parents who are potential child abusers?
1. The parents speak more about themselves than about their children.
2. The parents indicate that they participate in many school activities.
3. The parents describe Billy as being different from other children his age.
4. The parents reveal that they have financial problems since both have lost their jobs recently.
70. When the nurse suspects that Billy has been abused by his parents, it would be *best* for her to
1. inform the parents that she suspects that Billy has been abused.

2. see to it that her findings are reported to the designated authorities in the state in which she practices.
3. keep the findings confidential since they are considered legal privileged communication between a nurse and her patient.
4. report her findings to the physician since, legally, reporting evidence of child abuse falls within the province of medical practice.

71. Statement A, below, is a correct statement. What is the relationship between statements A and B?
Statement A: The art of parenting is learned behavior.
Statement B: A person who has a history of being abused by his parents rarely abuses his own children.
1. Statement B is true; statement A explains or confirms statement B.
2. Statement B is true; statement A neither helps explain nor confirm statement B.
3. Statement B is false; statement A contradicts or indicates the falsity of statement B.
4. Statement B is false; statement A neither contradicts nor indicates the falsity of statement B.

The team leader in a hospital's emergency room scheduled a conference on common accidents involving children.
Items 72 through 90 relate to information discussed in the conference.

72. While all of the following factors influence a preschooler's tendency to ingest substances that are poisonous to him, recent findings indicate that the *most influential* factor is the child's
1. immature understanding of danger.
2. curiosity with the world around him.
3. desire to imitate adults around him.
4. growing freedom for independent activity.
73. If a youngster has ingested an undetermined amount of drain cleaner, with which of the following measures should the nurse be prepared to assist during the child's initial care?
1. Tracheostomy.
2. Gastric lavage.
3. External cardiac massage.
4. Administration of an emetic.
74. After the acute stage following the ingestion of drain cleaner, the *most common* complication is the development of esophageal

1. ulcers.
2. varices.
3. strictures.
4. diverticuli.
75. The reason a physician orders methylprednisolone sodium succinate (Solu-Medrol) for a child who has ingested drain cleaner is that the drug helps to
    1. sedate the child.
    2. reduce the inflammatory process.
    3. regulate the child's fluid balance.
    4. mobilize the child's resources to fight infection.
76. Which of the following signs/symptoms is *most often* the *earliest* to occur after taking an overdose of aspirin?
    1. Convulsions.
    2. A nosebleed.
    4. Nausea and vomiting.
    4. Deep and rapid respirations.
77. When a child arrives in an emergency room with aspirin poisoning, the nurse should be prepared to assist with the administration of
    1. oxygen.
    2. an emetic.
    3. a diuretic.
    4. a sedative.
78. The *most common* complication following the ingestion of a hydrocarbon, such as gasoline, is
    1. uremia.
    2. pneumonia.
    3. hepatitis.
    4. meningitis.
79. A mother calls the emergency room of the hospital after her 3-year-old child has eaten some poisonous wild mushrooms. In addition to telling the mother to bring the child to the emergency room, it would be *best* for the nurse to tell her to
    1. induce the child to vomit.
    2. have the child drink milk.
    3. have the child eat some burnt toast.
    4. keep the child quiet while bringing him to the hospital.
80. Which one of the following nursing actions should be taken *first* when administering emergency care to the affected areas of a burn victim?
    1. Expose the burned areas to air.
    2. Apply cool water to the burned areas.

3. Apply an oil-base ointment to the burned areas.

4. Cover the burned areas with dry sterile dressings.

81. Which one of the following treatments is *most often* used for children with lead poisoning?

1. Detoxification with chelating agents.

2. Exchange transfusions with whole blood.

3. Radiation therapy with low voltage x-rays.

4. Gastric lavages with fluids high in electrolyte content.

82. The nurse can anticipate that the effectiveness of deleading therapy is determined by examinations of the child's

1. blood.

2. feces.

3. spinal fluid.

4. stomach contents.

83. Which one of the following complications is *most commonly* noted in children with long-standing, untreated lead poisoning?

1. Retarded growth rate.

2. Neurological changes.

3. Pathological fractures.

4. Cirrhosis of the liver.

84. Most children with lead poisoning today have acquired the lead accidently by

1. eating paint that contains lead.

2. inhaling fumes of leaded gasoline.

3. drinking water delivered through lead pipes.

4. sucking on clothing colored with dyes that contain lead.

85. Of the following measures, the one that has been found to be the *most effective* in relation to preventing lead poisoning is to

1. condemn old housing developments.

2. educate the public concerning common sources of lead.

3. educate the public concerning the importance of good nutrition.

4. inoculate children who live in areas where lead poisoning is common.

86. A youngster being cared for in the emergency room following an accident demonstrates fear of being exposed for the physical examination. In which of the following age groups is this fear *most typical?*

1. Toddlerhood (ages 1 to 3 years).

2. Preschool (ages 4 to 5 years).

3. School age (ages 6 to 12 years).

4. Adolescence (ages 13 to 15 years).

87. Which one of the following diagrams illustrates how *best* to apply an automobile's seat belt to protect an infant while traveling?

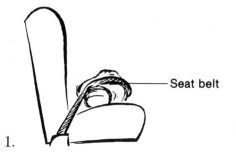 Baby should be lying on car seat with seat belt around it. Better to have infant facing driver.

1.

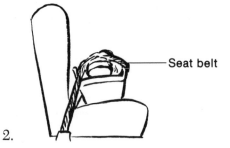 Infant seat is sitting flat on car seat with infant facing driver. Seat belt around infant seat.

2.

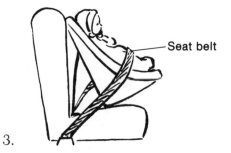 Infant seat facing forward with seat belt around infant and seat.

3.

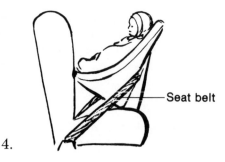 Infant seat facing backwards with face of infant toward back of car with seat belt in place.

4.

88. Which of the following accidents occurring in the home account(s) for the largest number of deaths each year?
1. Falls.
2. Poisoning.
3. Asphyxiation.
4. Scalds and burns.

89. Fatal accidents during the first year of life are *most often* caused by
1. drowning.
2. suffocation.
3. choking with aspiration.
4. motor vehicle collisions.

90. In the United States, *most* deaths in persons between the ages of one and 14 years of age are due to accidents associated with
1. swimming.
2. electricity.
3. toxic poisons.
4. motor vehicles.

A nurse was asked to participate in a screening program for musculoskeletal disorders.
Items 91 through 104 relate to musculoskeletal disorders.

91. If the physician wishes to determine the physiological age of a child, he would *most likely* order
1. hormonal studies.
2. bone marrow biopsy.
3. creatinine blood levels.
4. an x-ray examination of the left hand and wrist.

92. While assessing some of the children, the nurse measures the length of their legs. Which skeletal landmarks should she use when taking the measurements?
1. The ischial tuberosity and the calcaneus.
2. The middle of the acetabulum and the patella.
3. The anterior superior iliac crest and the medial malleolus of the tibia.
4. The top of the greater trochanter of the femur and the bottom of the foot.

93. Torticollis ("wry neck") is an abnormality affecting the
1. clavicle.
2. trapezius muscle.
3. cervical vertebrae.
4. sternocleidomastoid muscle.

94. The *primary purpose* for prescribing corrective shoes for a child

with flat feet is to help
1. strengthen the arches of the feet.
2. keep the legs in proper alignment.
3. prevent the development of pigeon toes.
4. maintain proper weight-bearing balance on the feet.

95. Osgood-Schlatter disease ("growing pains") is characterized by discomfort in the area of the tuberosity on the
1. tibia.
2. femur.
3. fibula.
4. calcaneus.

96. The medical term that describes having an excess number of fingers and toes is
1. zygoma.
2. polypodia.
3. polydactyly.
4. zygodactyly.

97. Current opinion holds that the *most probable* cause of muscular dystrophy is
1. trauma.
2. infection.
3. a hereditary factor.
4. a hormonal imbalance.

98. The nurse plans to screen only the high-risk children for scoliosis. Therefore, of the following groups of children, she should screen only the
1. last-born children.
2. first-born children.
3. children 4 to 7 years of age.
4. children 8 to 14 years of age.

99. The nurse should suspect scoliosis of she notes that a youngster has a skeletal change that results in his
1. walking in a waddling manner.
2. having a hump of the shoulder blade.
3. walking while thrusting the body forward.
4. having a longer than average trunk.

100. Which position taken by the children will help *most* in detecting scoliosis among those children the nurse has screened?
1. Lying flat on the floor while extending the legs straight from the trunk.
2. Bending forward at the waist while allowing the head and arms to fall freely.
3. Standing against a wall while pressing the length of the back against the wall.

4. Sitting in a chair while lifting the feet and legs to a right angle with the trunk.

101. Mary Anne Long was found to have scoliosis. Which of the following statements should the nurse use as a rationale for her response when Mary Anne is fitted for and asks about the purpose of the Milwaukee brace which was prescribed for her?
1. It stretches soft tissue and muscle.
2. It applies countertraction to the pelvis.
3. It facilitates separation of the cervical vertebrae.
4. It provides longitudinal traction and lateral pressure.

102. Mary Anne asks the nurse how long each day she has to wear the brace. The nurse should base her response on knowledge that common therapeutic regimens indicate that Mary Anne's brace may be removed only while she
1. sleeps—about 10 hours a day.
2. is at school—about 7 hours a day.
3. eats—about 3 hours a day.
4. carries out personal hygiene measures—about 1 hour a day.

103. Mary Anne is ordered to do certain exercises each day *primarily* in order to help
1. prevent contractures of her spine.
2. decrease spasms in her back muscles.
3. improve the traction effect of her brace.
4. increase the strength of the muscles in her trunk.

104. Mary Anne says she has difficulty shampooing her hair. Of the following courses of action, it would be *best* for the nurse to recommend that Mary Anne
1. use a form of dry shampoo.
2. plan to shampoo her hair while she takes a shower.
3. have her mother shampoo her hair while Mary Anne bends over a sink.
4. have her mother shampoo her hair while Mary Anne lies over the edge of her bed.

Five-year-old Bobby White was admitted to the hospital with burns received while playing with matches. His legs, hands, and lower abdomen were burned. Some smoke inhalation occurred also. The physician's orders for Bobby include the following:

5% dextrose in Ringer's lactate intravenously; 3 ml./Kg./% of burn to be received in first 24 hours.
Tetanus prophylaxis.
Nothing by mouth.

Indwelling Foley catheter.

Ampicillin (Amcill), 250 mg. by IV push q.8h.

Items 105 through 137 relate to this situation.

105. Bobby weighs 44 pounds (20 Kg.) and it is estimated that approximately 44 percent of his body surface was burned. How much intravenous fluid should he receive in the first 24 hours?
   1. 1760 ml.
   2. 2640 ml.
   3. 3520 ml.
   4. 4400 ml.

106. Of the 24-hour amount of intravenous fluid ordered for Bobby, how much will the physician *most likely* allocate to be infused in the first 8-hour period?
   1. ⅓ of the total mount.
   2. ½ of the total amount.
   3. ⅔ of the total amount.
   4. ¾ of the total amount.

107. Which one of the following laboratory determinations will the physician *most likely* use to help estimate the amount of fluid replacement Bobby requires?
   1. The hematocrit level.
   2. The blood creatinine level.
   3. The blood oxygen tension (pO_2).
   4. The leukocyte differential count.

108. Six hours after Bobby's intravenous infusion was begun, the nurse notes that the rate of infusion is less than that prescribed and is approximately 2 hours behind the ordered schedule. Which of the following courses of action would be *best* for the nurse to take?
   1. Consult the physician concerning a new schedule for the intravenous infusion.
   2. Calculate a new drip rate so that within a 24-hour period, the total amount of ordered solution will be infused.
   3. Increase the drip rate enough so that the total amount of ordered solution will be infused within the 8-hour period.
   4. Correct the drip rate to the prescribed rate even though less than the total ordered amount of solution for the 8-hour period will be infused.

109. Which one of the following statements explains *best* why water intoxication may occur if Bobby receives *excessive* amounts of fluids?
   1. The heart rate and cardiac output are decreased.
   2. The hormonal responses are sluggish and depressed.

3. The kidneys are conserving fluids and electrolytes.

4. There is vasodilatation and increased blood flow to cell tissue.

110. Two common signs/symptoms when the body is suffering with water intoxication are

1. cyanosis and dyspnea.

2. muscular tremors and twitching.

3. a slow pulse rate and chest pain.

4. a sore throat and hoarseness.

111. Tetanus prophylaxis is ordered for Bobby because necrotic tissue in burn areas supports *Clostridium tetani* well. A characteristic of these organisms is their ability to

1. acidify body fluids.

2. agglutinate red blood cells.

3. live without access to oxygen.

4. take up sodium ions from body tissues.

112. When the nurse learns that Bobby's tentaus immunization is up-to-date, she should anticipate that the biological product that will be used to offer Bobby further protection will be

1. a toxoid.

2. a vaccine.

3. an antitoxin.

4. immune globulin.

113. The physician's *primary* reason for withholding oral fluids and food initially from Bobby is to help prevent

1. hiccoughs.

2. paralytic ileus.

3. aspiration pneumonia.

4. irritation to his smoke-sensitive throat.

114. The physician orders an indwelling Foley catheter for Bobby *primarily* in order to help

1. prevent urinary retention.

2. decrease the workload of the kidneys.

3. facilitate accurate output measurements.

4. obtain urine specimens with ease as necessary.

115. The nurse notes that Bobby may be having an allergic reaction while she is administering ampicillin 36 hours after Bobby's admission. Of the following courses of action, which one should the nurse take *first?*

1. Administer oxygen.

2. Stop administering the drug.

3. Decrease the rate of infusing intravenous fluids.

4. Place Bobby in bed with his head lower than his body.

116. Which one of the following signs/symptoms is *most typical* of an allergic reaction to ampicillin?

1. A skin rash.
2. Joint pains.
3. Mental confusion.
4. An unusually rapid pulse.
117. The physician orders that Bobby lie flat in bed for the first 48 hours after admission *primarily* in order to help prevent
1. postural shock.
2. respiratory infection.
3. contracture of joints.
4. unnecessary expenditure of energy.
118. After initial debridement of burned areas, the physician orders mafenide acetate (Sulfamylon) applied topically to burned areas every 8 hours. Because topical mafenide acetate therapy may have an effect on certain normal blood values, the nurse should anticipate that Bobby will require monitoring of his blood's
1. pH level.
2. platelet level.
3. leukocyte level.
4. hemoglobin level.
119. In addition to its possible effects on Bobby's blood, another disadvantage of mafenide acetate therapy is that the drug
1. stains linen permanently.
2. tends to disintegrate easily.
3. has a disagreeable, strong odor.
4. causes a burning sensation when applied.
120. When a child feels that he has control of what is happening to him, he is more likely to cooperate. Which one of the following nursing measures would allow Bobby to feel *most* in control during his mafenide acetate treatments?
1. Allow him to help apply the cream.
2. Delay the treatment if he seems unwilling to cooperate.
3. Arrange to have a parent to support him during the treatments.
4. Tell him it is all right for him to cry during the treatments.
121. The staphylococcus organism often invades and infects burn areas. Under the microscope, these organisms look like
1. rods.
2. chains.
3. spheres.
4. spirals.
122. Shortly after admission, Bobby receives a xenograft on his left thigh which means that the grafting material came from
1. an animal.
2. Bobby's body.

3. another person's body.

4. synthetic ingredients.

123. The *primary* purpose of a xenograft is to
1. decrease the patient's pain.
2. stimulate the growth of granulation tissue.
3. facilitate the patient's range of body motion.
4. cover the burned areas until other grafts are available.

124. After Bobby has received split-thickness skin grafts to the worst burned areas, the physician orders that Bobby's legs be splinted. The *primary* purpose for splinting is to help prevent
1. edema.
2. phlebitis.
3. contractures.
4. pathological fractures.

125. What recommendations do most persons of authority give concerning the use of gloves when caring for victims with severe burns?
1. Gloves are a desirable precautionary measure, but wearing them is optional.
2. Gloves should be worn whenever any kind of care is being given to the burn victim.
3. Gloves should be worn whenever giving direct care to burn areas; one pair is recommended for removing soiled dressings and applying new dressings.
4. Gloves should be worn whenever giving direct care to burn areas; one pair is used for removing soiled dressings and one pair is used for applying new dressings.

126. Which one of the following signs should suggest to the nurse that Bobby may be hemolyzing red blood cells?
1. His feet are reddish.
2. His stools are black.
3. His eyes are bloodshot.
4. His urine is dark brown.

127. When Bobby starts eating after being burned, it is *particularly* important that his diet have a high content of
1. fats.
2. minerals.
3. proteins.
4. carbohydrates.

128. If a potassium deficit occurs in Bobby following his burns, which one of these liquids would provide him with the *most* potassium when he begins taking fluids orally?
1. Ginger ale.
2. Grape juice.

3. Orange juice.
4. Cranberry juice.
129. Which one of the following measures is *least likely* to interest Bobby in eating?
1. Serve small amounts of food at one time.
2. Allow his mother to help feed him.
3. Offer foods that he can eat with his fingers.
4. Explain that dessert will be served when other foods have been eaten.
130. Hydrotherapy with exercising, which is ordered for Bobby during his recovery period, is *least effective* in helping to prevent
1. contractures.
2. muscle atrophy.
3. calcium deposits in his joints.
4. infection at the site of his skin grafts.
131. Bobby is fitted with elastic pantyhose before discharge. The *primary* purpose of the hose is to help
1. support Bobby's weakened leg muscles.
2. prevent infection in the grafted areas.
3. improve circulation to the grafted areas.
4. keep Bobby's trousers from adhering to his grafted areas.
132. For a child under teen age, the percentage of body surface allocated to the different body parts following the "Rule of Nines" differs from that of a teenager or adult. The usual modification made for young children is that a larger percentage of total body surface is given to the child's head and a lower percentage is given to the child's
1. anterior trunk.
2. posterior trunk.
3. upper extremities.
4. lower extremities.
133. Silver nitrate solution is sometimes used for treating burns. If it is used carelessly, there is danger of upsetting the body's ability to maintain
1. water balance.
2. nitrogen balance.
3. temperature control.
4. electrolyte balance.
134. When a serious burn has occurred, the *primary* shift in the location of body fluids is from
1. interstitial to intravascular spaces.
2. intracellular to interstitial space.
3. insterstitial to intracellular spaces.
4. intravascular to interstitial spaces.

135. Which one of the following electrolytes is lost in the *largest* amounts during the first 48 hours following a severe burn?
    1. Sodium.
    2. Potassium.
    3. Magnesium.
    4. Phosphorus.
136. Metabolic acidosis, which may occur following serious burns, is characterized by respirations that are
    1. deep and rapid.
    2. slow and difficult.
    3. labored and stridulous.
    4. interspersed with periods of no breathing.
137. A complication commonly associated with extensive and infected burns is
    1. Curling's ulcers.
    2. Cushing's disease.
    3. diabetes insipidus.
    4. chronic hypertension.

> Eight-year-old Gary Ray was hospitalized. His diagnosis is nephrotic syndrome.
> Items 138 through 148 relate to this situation.

138. Which one of the following orders would Gary's physician be *least likely* to prescribe for Gary at the time of his admission?
    1. Weigh daily.
    2. Observe bed rest.
    3. Restrict oral fluids to 1000 ml. each day.
    4. Obtain blood pressure readings every 4 hours.
139. At the time of admission, the nurse can anticipate that Gary's vital signs will *most probably* reveal
    1. a slow pulse rate.
    2. a rapid respiratory rate.
    3. a low grade temperature.
    4. an elevated blood pressure.
140. The nurse can expect that Gary's laboratory reports will indicate that he has
    1. an elevated blood pH.
    2. a decreased blood platelet count.
    3. a decreased blood creatinine level.
    4. an elevated blood urea nitrogen (BUN).
141. Gary is edematous. When edema is present, in which of the following body spaces do fluids accumulate?
    1. Interstitial spaces.

2. Intracellular spaces.
3. Intravascular spaces.

142. Of the following nursing measures, in order to help reduce edema in Gary's eyelids, it would be *best* for the nurse to
1. elevate the head of Gary's bed.
2. irrigate Gary's eyes with warm normal saline.
3. limit Gary's reading to short periods of time.
4. apply cool compresses to Gary's eyes several times a day.

143. Which one of the following signs will the nurse *most likely* observe when Gary begins to develop renal failure?
1. Lethargy.
2. Insomnia.
3. Hypotension.
4. Excessive perspiration.

144. Which one of the following vitamins is *most likely* to be prescribed in supplemental doses when Gary starts dialysis therapy after his kidneys fail?
1. Vitamin A.
2. Vitamin B.
3. Vitamin C.
4. Vitamin D.

145. Of the following minerals, the one that will *most likely* be prescribed in supplemental doses while Gary receives dialysis therapy is
1. sodium.
2. calcium.
3. magnesium.
4. phosphorus.

146. Of the following medications, the one that has been *most effective* for reducing the mortality rate of children with nephrotic syndrome is
1. streptomycin.
2. prednisone (Deltra).
3. epinephrine (adrenaline).
4. ascorbic acid (vitamin C).

147. Cyclophosphamide (Cytoxin), another drug sometimes used to treat nephrotic syndrome, has the disadvantage of having undesirable side effects. A *common* side effect is that it causes
1. sodium retention.
2. loss of muscular coordination.
3. a decreased white blood cell count.
4. an interference with the normal growth rate.

148. A characteristic sign of nephrotic syndrome that reflects its pathology is that the body

1. excretes protein in the urine.
2. retains red blood cells in the bloodstream.
3. excretes urine of an abnormally low specific gravity.
4. retains unusually large amounts of albumin in the bloodstream.

Nine-month-old Sara Holt was hospitalized with a skin rash. Her diagnosis is atopic dermatitis (eczema). The physician's orders include the following:

Differential blood count.
Specimen for urinalysis.

Items 149 through 154 relate to this situation.

149. The nurse can anticipate that Sara's blood findings will *most likely* reveal
    1. a lowered hemoglobin level.
    2. an elevated neutrophil count.
    3. an elevated eosinophil count.
    4. a lowered blood urea nitrogen (BUN) level.
150. The laboratory report indicates that the specific gravity of Sara's urine is 1.015. Specific gravity is *best* defined as the weight of a substance compared with the weight of an equal amount of
    1. water.
    2. blood.
    3. plasma.
    4. normal saline.
151. Because infection is present, the physician orders a penicillin preparation for Sara which is given intramuscularly. Which one of the following measures has been found to meet an infant's emotional needs *best* when the infant experiences an uncomfortable procedure, such as an intramuscular injection?
    1. Allow the infant's mother to be present during the procedure.
    2. Rock the infant for a few minutes before beginning the procedure.
    3. Allow the infant to become familiar with the equipment to be used.
    4. Provide the infant with his nursing bottle of formula during the procedure.
152. The *most* characteristic sign/symptom of Sara's eczematous rash can be expected to be
    1, pain.
    2. edema.
    3. burning.
    4. itching.

153. Which one of the following types of night wear would be *best* for Sara?
1. Nylon night-sack.
2. One-piece cotton pajamas.
3. Two-piece flannel pajamas.
4. Woolen sleeper with feet and mittens.

154. If only the following agents were available, it would be *best* for the nurse to cleanse Sara's skin with
1. lanolin.
2. normal saline solution.
3. a mild, antiseptic soap.
4. a nonoily, cleansing lotion.

Six-year-old Billy Casper, who has asthma, was brought to the hospital's emergency room when he was having an acute asthmatic attack.
Items 155 through 159 relate to this situation.

155. During Billy's acute attack, his breathing is *most likely* to be characterized by
1. crowing on inspiration.
2. wheezing on expiration.
3. frequent periods of apnea.
4. stertorous abdominal breathing

156. Unless complications occur, the color of Billy's expectorations will *most likely* be
1. green.
2. brown.
3. white.
4. yellow.

157. Cromolyn sodium (Aarane) is prescribed for Billy. This drug acts to
1. dilate the bronchioles.
2. decrease an inflammatory process.
3. inhibit the release of histamine.
4. reduce the viscosity of respiratory secretions.

158. After Billy's attack subsides and he is ready to go home, his mother tells the nurse that Billy wishes to have a pet. Of the following pets, the one that would be *most appropriate* for Billy is a
1. cat.
2. dog.
3. fish.
4. parakeet.

159. During an acute asthma attack, *all* of the following conditions occur in the body *except*
1. collapse of the alveoli.
2. spasms of the bronchioles.
3. an increase in the production of mucus.
4. an edema of the mucosa in the respiratory passages.

Jennifer Stone, who is 1 year old, was admitted to the hospital with a diagnosis of sickle cell anemia in crisis.
Items 160 through 168 relate to this situation.

160. Which one of the following treatments should the nurse anticipate the physician will *most likely* order for Jennifer upon her admission?
1. A low fat diet.
2. Gavage feedings.
3. A transfusion with packed cells.
4. Administration of intravenous fluids.

161. The local tissue damage Jennifer is likely to show at admission is due to
1. a general inflammatory response due to an autoimmune reaction complicated by hypoxia.
2. air hunger and resultant respiratory alkalosis due to deoxygenated red blood cells.
3. local tissue damage with ischemia and necrosis due to the obstruction of circulation.
4. hypersensitivity of the central nervous system due to high serum bilirubin levels and adrenocortical imbalance.

162. Which one of the following pathological developments is responsible for the jaundice Jennifer displays upon admission?
1. Enlarged spleen.
2. Red blood cell destruction.
3. Renal infarction and necrosis.
4. Hyperplasia of the bone marrow.

162. Jennifer's crisis subsides in about 3 days and she is to be discharged. Mr. and Ms. Stone should be taught to bring Jennifer to her physician for immediate care in the future when she shows signs of
1. infection and fever.
2. headache and nausea.
3. fatigue and lassitude.
4. excessive hunger and thirst.

164. Mr. and Ms. Stone are planning a vacation. Which one of the following geographic areas would be *contraindicated* for Jennifer?

1. Desert areas.
2. Ocean-side areas.
3. Large urban areas.
4. Mountainous areas.

165. Of the following statements, which one offers the *best* explanation of why Jennifer had been symptom-free since birth until the present time?
    1. Jennifer had not had an elevated temperature until now.
    2. The placenta barred the passage of sickle hemoglobin from the mother to Jennifer in utero.
    3. Antibodies transmitted from her mother in utero provided Jennifer with temporary immunity against the disease.
    4. Fetal hemoglobin was rich in oxygen content at the time of Jennifer's birth and for a period of time thereafter.

166. As Jennifer grows older, which one of the following conditions is *least likely* to result from her having sickle cell anemia?
    1. Hepatitis.
    2. Gallstones.
    3. Osteomyelitis.
    4. Kidney disease.

167. Sickle cell anemia is an autosomal recessive disease. What percent of Mr. and Ms. Stone's children can be predicted to be carriers of the sickle cell trait?
    1. 25 percent.
    2. 50 percent.
    3. 75 percent.
    4. 100 percent.

168. Sickle cell anemia has a high incidence among blacks. In which other ethnic group is there also a significant incidence of the disease?
    1. Greeks.
    2. Germans.
    3. Japanese.
    4. Spanish-Americans.

Three-year-old Patty Young was admitted to the hospital with a diagnosis of bronchopneumonia. She has cystic fibrosis. The physician's orders include the following:

Sputum specimen for culture.
Isoproterenol hydrochloride (Isuprel) in saline, 1 ml. per inhalation every 4 hours for 10 minutes.
Postural drainage and percussion to chest wall every 4 hours following inhalation therapy.

Items 169 through 186 relate to this situation.

169. What is the *primary* reason for ordering a sputum culture for Patty?
1. To ascertain the organism responsible for the pneumonia.
2. To ascertain if Patty's cystic fibrosis is under control.
3. To ascertain if there is blood present in the tracheobronchial tree.
4. To ascertain the proportion of Patty's lungs affected by the pneumonia.

170. Isoproterenol hydrochloride is ordered for Patty because the drug acts to
1. relax and dilate the bronchial tree.
2. constrict enlarged pulmonary vessels.
3. coat and protect the mucous membrane of the bronchial tree.
4. stimulate the respiratory center in the medulla of the brain.

171. At which of the following times in the day is it *best* to carry out the procedures of postural drainage and percussion?
1. Shortly after meals.
2. Shortly before meals.
3. Halfway between meals.

172. The *primary* reason for postural drainage for Patty is that it helps to
1. dilate the bronchioles.
2. clear the lungs of debris.
3. force better use of the diaphragm.
4. provide more room for lung expansion.

173. The organism causing Patty's bronchopneumonia is found to be Diplococcus pneumoniae. A characteristic of the organism is that it does not ordinarily survive in a host body without its
1. spores.
2. capsule.
3. fibrils.
4. flagella.

174. Patty was placed in a cool, high humidity tent, operated with compressed air. The *primary* reason for using this tent for Patty is that it helps to
1. provide oxygen.
2. lower her temperature.
3. reduce the viscosity of her secretions.
4. provide a means for administering inhalant drugs.

175. Statement A below is a correct statement. What is the relationship between statements A and B?
Statement A: When several unmet needs are present, the body

will direct intense energies toward those needs that are most essential for sustaining life.

Statement B: The increased respiratory rate often observed while caring for children with respiratory diseases, such as bronchopneumonia, is the result of the body's efforts to obtain sufficient oxygen for its needs.

1. Statement B is true; statement A explains or confirms statement B.
2. Statement B is true; statement A contradicts or indicates the falsity of statement B.
3. Statement B is false; statement A contradicts or indicates the falsity of statement B.
4. Statement B is false; statement A neither contradicts nor indicates the falsity of statement B.

176. The type of diet ordered for Patty would *most likely* be high in *all* of the following content *except*
1. fat.
2. protein.
3. calories.
4. carbohydrate.

177. Which one of the following statements describes the stool Patty is *most likely* to have?
1. It will be bulky and foul in odor.
2. It will be watery and sweet in odor.
3. It will be dry and have the odor of ammonia.
4. It will be dark in color with almost no odor.

178. Which of the following toys would be *best* for Patty while she is hospitalized?
1. A tricycle.
2. Her favorite doll.
3. A fuzzy, stuffed animal.
4. Scissors, paper and paste.

179. Which of the following instructions should the nurse include when she teaches Patty's parents how to care for her at home?
1. Restrict her activities so as not to overtire her.
2. Give her a cough suppressant at bedtime to allow restful sleep.
3. Continue inhalation treatments, percussion, and postural drainage at home.
4. Regulate her medication dosage according to daily urine tests for bilirubin.

180. Patty's parents should be taught that the National Cystic Fibrosis Foundation is available to assist them with
1. financial help for medical care.

2. obtaining necessary dietary supplements.

3. educational materials concerning Patty's care.

4. Patty's education by home tutoring.

181. The reason that hot weather is hazardous for Patty is that characteristically, a person with cystic fibrosis

    1. has no sweat glands.

    2. lacks skin pigments to prevent sunburn.

    3. has a poorly developed temperature control center.

    4. loses excessive amounts of salt through perspiration.

182. Patty's parents ask for genetic counseling. Following the principles of Mendelian recessive inheritance, what percentage chance does each of their children have for developing cystic fibrosis?

    1. 10 percent.

    2. 25 percent.

    3. 50 percent.

    4. 75 percent.

183. Patty's long-term prognosis can *best* be described as

    1. good; she is likely to outgrow the disease during her teen years.

    2. fair; she can look forward to a full life as an adult provided she has excellent medical and nursing care during childhood.

    3. unfavorable; she is unlikely to survive past early adulthood.

184. Of the following statements, which one *best* describes cystic fibrosis?

    1. It is a disease of the glands of the body that secrete mucus.

    2. It is a disease in which fibrous cysts form in various body organs.

    3. It is a disease due to an interaction between antigens and antibodies.

    4. It is a disease resulting from the faulty development of the bile ducts.

185. Which of the following organs is *least likely* to be affected by cystic fibrosis?

    1. The lungs.

    2. The kidneys.

    3. The pancreas.

    4. The salivary glands.

186. Which of the following conditions is often the result of the heart's trying to adapt to the pathology of cystic fibrosis?

    1. Mitral stenosis.

    2. Atrial fibrillations.

    3. Ventricular tachycardia.

    4. Right ventricular hypertrophy.

Eight-year-old Stevie Field was admitted to the hospital in an unconscious state. His diagnosis is diabetic coma.

Items 187 through 209 relate to this situation.

187. The nurse judges that Stevie's blood sugar level upon admission is about what can be expected in his case. Of the following findings, which one would be *most typical* when diabetic coma is present?
    1. 10 mg. per 100 ml. of blood.
    2. 110 mg. per 100 ml. of blood.
    3. 150 mg. per 100 ml. of blood.
    4. 350 mg. per 100 ml. of blood.
188. Which of the following laboratory findings can the nurse expect will be found when Stevie's blood CO_2 tension (pCO_2) and pH are calculated?
    1. A low pCO_2 and low pH.
    2. A low pCO_2 and high pH.
    3. A high pCO_2 and low pH.
    4. A high pCO_2 and high pH.
189. The physician orders intravenous therapy with normal saline for Stevie. The physician's rationale for ordering the therapy is that it will help to
    1. bring up the blood glucose level.
    2. stimulate the production of urine.
    3. correct fluid and electrolyte imbalances.
    4. improve circulation to vital brain centers.
190. The physician states that he will order insulin for Stevie, to be administered by "intravenous push." The nurse can anticipate that the type of insulin the physician will order is
    1. insulin zinc suspension (Lente).
    2. insulin injection (regular insulin).
    3. isophane insulin suspension (NPH Iletin).
    4. protamine zinc insulin suspension (Protamine zinc).
191. The physician orders 10 units of insulin for Stevie. There are 100 units of insulin per ml. in the bottle the nurse obtains from the refrigerator. How many ml. of insulin will the nurse use for Stevie?
    1. 0.1 ml.
    2. 0.2 ml.
    3. 1.0 ml.
    4. 2.0 ml.

192. Which of the following substances, when found in excess in the bloodstream, would account for the sweet, fruity odor that the nurse notes on Stevie's breath?
   1. Urea.
   2. Glycogen.
   3. Amino acids.
   4. Ketone bodies.
193. Which of the following signs/symptoms is *least likely* to appear in Stevie's nursing history?
   1. Having had a recent rapid weight gain.
   2. Feeling more hungry and thirsty than usual.
   3. Feeling more tired after exercise than usual.
   4. Having involuntary urination in bed almost nightly.
194. When Stevie begins to recover, which one of the following examinations is *most likely* to be used in ascertaining the amount of insulin he should receive?
   1. Urine sample to determine the level of pH and specific gravity.
   2. Urine sample to determine the amount of glucose and acetone present.
   3. Blood sample to determine the amount of glucose and acetone present.
   4. Blood sample to determine the amount of albumin and globulin present.
195. At what times in the day should tests be done to determine the amount of insulin Stevie needs?
   1. Shortly before meals and at bedtime.
   2. Approximately halfway between meals.
   3. Immediately after meals and at bedtime.
   4. Upon awakening in the morning and at bedtime.
196. Stevie and his parents should be taught that *all* of the following factors increase the body's requirements for insulin *except*
   1. overeating.
   2. acute infections.
   3. increased emotional strain.
   4. increased physical exercise.
197. Stevie's parents ask the nurse why Stevie cannot take insulin by mouth. The nurse explains that insulin is not given by mouth because it is
   1. excreted before being absorbed.
   2. absorbed too slowly to be effective.
   3. too irritating to stomach mucous membranes.
   4. rendered inactive by gastrointestinal secretions.

198. The nurse teaches Stevie and his parents to rotate the site for injecting insulin. Which sites in the diagram below are the *least appropriate* to use?
   1. The sites labeled A.
   2. The sites labeled B.
   3. The sites labeled C.
   4. The sites labeled D.

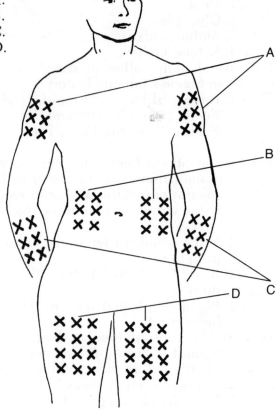

199. Before preparing to remove insulin from its vial, what step should the nurse teach Stevie and his parents to take *first?*
   1. Inject at least two times more air into the vial than the amount of insulin to be removed.
   2. Inject about the same amount of air into the vial as the amount of insulin to be withdrawn.
   3. Inject approximately half as much air into the vial as the amount of insulin to be withdrawn.
   4. Be sure the plunger is completely into the barrel of the syringe so that no air can be injected into the vial.

200. An exchange diet is to be used for Stevie. Which one of the following foods can be substituted in his diet for one piece of bread?
   1. One cup of whole milk.

2. One small baked potato.

3. One-half of a small banana.

4. One-fourth cup of cottage cheese.

201. It is important that Stevie and his parents know that a *typical* sign/symptom of diabetic acidosis is

1. dilated pupils.

2. slow pulse rate.

3. excessive perspiration.

4. deep, rapid respirations.

202. Which of the following actions should Stevie and his parents be taught to take *first* when it appears that Stevie may be going into diabetic acidosis?

1. Stevie should drink a cup of hot, well-sugared tea.

2. Stevie's insulin should be withheld until he sees his physician.

3. Stevie should go to the nearest emergency room for intravenous therapy to prevent coma.

4. Stevie's urine should be checked to determine the sugar and acetone levels.

203. If after discharge Stevie presents early signs/symptoms of insulin shock, the *first best* course of action would be to

1. have him increase his activity.

2. have him eat several cubes of sugar.

3. call his physician for instructions.

4. have him rest in bed until his symptoms subside.

204. Which one of the following admonitions in relation to activities of daily living would be *inappropriate* for the nurse to make to Stevie's parents?

1. Stevie should be particularly careful to wear properly fitting shoes.

2. Stevie should be treated in a manner similar to other 8-year-old boys.

3. Stevie should avoid especially strenuous physical activities, such as contact sports.

4. Stevie should be prepared to make insulin and dietary adjustments when he develops an infection.

205. Stevie's parents ask the nurse why Stevie has diabetes mellitus. Which one of the following statements *most accurately* describes current opinion concerning the etiology of diabetes mellitus?

1. Diabetes mellitus is a disease with no known cause.

2. Diabetes mellitus is most probably a hereditary disease.

3. Diabetes mellitus is most probably due to Stevie's pancreas being damaged during a difficult birth.

4. Diabetes mellitus is most probably due to Stevie's mother having a streptococcal infection early in her pregnancy.

206. Stevie's parents ask how insulin works in the body. The nurse should base her response on knowledge that insulin affects carbohydrate metabolism by
1. increasing the rate of sugar metabolism.
2. increasing the blood sugar concentration.
3. decreasing the rate of metabolism in the body
4. decreasing the amount of sugar stored in body tissues.

207. Stevie and his parents should be taught that when he is an adult, his need for insulin will
1. decrease provided he keeps his diabetes under good control.
2. decrease so that eventually he can switch to an oral hypoglycemic agent.
3. continue in a manner similar to his need for insulin during his childhood.
4. continue until old age when dietary discretion will most likely be sufficient to control his disease.

208. Consider the following two statements:
Statement A: The liver plays a role in changing blood sugar levels.
Statement B: When the blood glucose level is above normal, the liver is failing to function properly.
1. Statement A is true but statement B is false.
2. Statement A is false but statement B is true.
3. Both statements A and B are true and statement A explains or confirms statement B.
4. Both statements A and B are true but statement A neither explains nor confirms statement B.

209. Which of the following injection methods is safe to use for *all* types of insulin?
1. Intradermal.
2. Intravenous.
3. Subcutaneous.
4. Intramuscular.

Mike Lane, an acutely ill 10-year-old, was hospitalized with an upper respiratory infection and right otitis media. He was pale and lethargic. Mike was diagnosed 3 years earlier as having acute lymphoblastic leukemia. After a long initial regimen of care at that time, Mike had a remission when he was free of symptoms and when his parents became optimistic.

Items 210 through 237 relate to this situation.

210. Which one of the following statements *best* describes Mike's leukemia?
    1. His disease is infectious in nature and characterized by increased white blood cell production.
    2. His disease is inflammatory in nature and characterized by solid tumor formation in the lymph nodes.
    3. His disease is neoplastic in nature and characterized by a proliferation of immature white blood cells.
    4. His disease is allergic in nature and characterized by an increased number of circulating antibodies in his bloodstream.

211. Mike's pallor and lethargy were *most likely* the result of
    1. excessive needs for energy due to Mike's respiratory and ear infections.
    2. an accumulation of toxic wastes in body tissues due to poor kidney functioning.
    3. a slower than normal blood flow to the body tissues due to a decreased heart rate.
    4. body tissue being starved of oxygen due to a decrease in the number of red blood cells.

212. Laboratory findings show that Mike is anemic which in his case, *most probably* has resulted from blood loss and
    1. inadequate intake of iron in the diet.
    2. failure in the formation of red blood cells.
    3. destruction of red blood cells by the lymphocytes.
    4. progressive replacement of bone marrow with scar tissue.

213. The nurse can assess the extent of Mike's anemia with knowledge that the normal hemoglobin level for a 10-year-old youngster is approximately
    1. 4 to 6 Gm. per 100 ml. of blood.
    2. 8 to 10 Gm. per 100 ml. of blood.
    3. 12 to 14 Gm. per 100 ml. of blood.
    4. 16 to 18 Gm. per 100 ml. of blood.

214. Which one of the following statements *best* describes why Mike is especially prone to infections?
    1. His white blood cells are incapable of handling an infectious process.
    2. His play activities have no doubt been too strenuous in view of his illness.
    3. His vitamin C intake has no doubt been inadequate over an extended period of time.
    4. His red blood cells are inadequate for carrying sufficient oxygen for tissue nourishment.

215. The nurse notes that Mike has developed petechiae, his gums, lips, and nose bleed easily, and there are bruises on various parts of his body. Which one of the following laboratory findings would be *typical* when these symptoms appear?
    1. Low serum calcium level.
    2. Faulty thrombin production.
    3. Insufficient platelet level.
    4. Insufficient fibrinogen concentration.
216. Mike complains of having a sore mouth. To help him maintain adequate nourishment, the nurse should offer him a diet consisting of *all* of the following foods *except*
    1. cooked fruits.
    2. warm, sugared foods.
    3. cool, soft, bland foods.
    4. high protein malted milk shakes.
217. Which one of the following interventions would be *contraindicated* for Mike's mouth care?
    1. Swab the mouth with moistened cotton swabs.
    2. Cleanse between the teeth with dental floss.
    3. Apply petrolatum jelly to the lips as indicated.
    4. Rinse the mouth frequently with nonirritating mouthwash or water.
218. Which of the following eating or drinking utensils would be *contraindicated* for Mike?
    1. A fork.
    2. A spoon.
    3. A plastic cup.
    4. A ceramic mug.
219. Which of the following sets of vital signs would be a good indication of probable increased bleeding (internal or external) in a child Mike's age?
    1. Pulse, 90 beats per minute; blood pressure, 106/76 mm. Hg.
    2. Pulse, 82 beats per minute; blood pressure, 98/70 mm. Hg.
    3. Pulse, 120 beats per minute; blood pressure, 80/56 mm. Hg.
    4. Pulse, 68 beats per minute; blood pressure, 140/90 mm. Hg.
220. Since Mike is prone to bleed easily, *all* of the following nursing measures are indicated for him *except*
    1. gentle turning and handling during his care.
    2. protection from injury when he is out of bed.
    3. giving him as many medications intramuscularly as possible.
    4. monitoring his stools and using stool softeners as indicated.
221. The physician orders a bone marrow biopsy. Which of the following bone sites is *most commonly* entered to obtain a tissue sample?

1. The femur.
2. The radius.
3. The cervical vertebrae.
4. The posterior iliac crest.

222. The physician also performs a lumbar puncture. The rationale for the procedure is that he wishes to
1. relieve undue pressure in the central nervous system.
2. determine whether the central nervous system has been invaded by the disease.
3. inject drugs that will help control an infection in the central nervous system.
4. identify organisms that may be causing an infection in the central nervous system.

223. The physician orders that Mike be transfused with two units of packed cells. Which one of the following solutions can the nurse anticipate will be used in conjunction with the administration of packed cells?
1. 5% dextrose in water.
2. Isotonic saline solution.
3. Lactated Ringer's solution.
4. 5% dextrose in half-strength saline.

224. Which one of the following statements offers the *best* reason for giving Mike packed cells rather than whole blood?
1. Mike needs red cells but no plasma.
2. Mike may have a hypersensitivity reaction to whole blood.
3. Whole blood may cause an overload on Mike's circulatory system.
4. Mike's veins may be too fragile to tolerate the time it takes to infuse whole blood.

225. The physician prescribes mercaptopurine (Purinethol), 75 mg. daily. Mercaptopurine is marketed in 50 mg. tablets for oral administration. How many tablets will be given to Mike each day?
1. One and a half tablets.
2. One and three-quarters tablets.
3. Two tablets.
4. Three tablets.

226. Which of the following signs/symptoms, if present in Mike, should suggest to the nurse that toxicity to mercaptopurine is occurring?
1. Nausea, vomiting and diarrhea.
2. Skin rash, constipation and polyuria.
3. Dry mouth, blurred vision and headache.
4. Drowsiness, malaise and low blood pressure.

227. The drug methotrexate (Amethopterin) is given to Mike by injecting it into his spinal column. This type of drug administration is called
   1. subdural.
   2. intrathecal.
   3. intradermal.
   4. intra-articular.
228. Which one of the following signs/symptoms should suggest to the nurse that toxicity to methotrexate is *most probably* occurring?
   1. Anuria.
   2. Tinnitus.
   3. Tarry stools.
   4. Blurred vision.
229. When Mike develops signs of toxicity to methotrexate therapy, the nurse should anticipate that the physician will order that Mike receive
   1. vitamin A.
   2. folinic acid.
   3. ascorbic acid.
   4. vitamin B complex.
230. Mercaptopurine and methotrexate are ordinarily classified as antimetabolites which function to
   1. selectively destroy malignant cells, thereby slowing tumor growth.
   2. create a hormonal imbalance within the body which acts to suppress tumor growth.
   3. damage deoxyribonucleic acid (DNA) within cell nuclei which in turn disrupts cell growth and division.
   4. imitate nutrients that are essential for malignant cell growth, thus preventing those cells from using natural nutrients.
231. One common side effect of antimetabolite therapy is
   1. buildup of serum calcium level.
   2. excretion of iron in the urine.
   3. release of bilirubin from destroyed body cells.
   4. formation of uric acid crystals in renal tubules.
232. When Mike develops toxicity to the antimetabolites, the physician prescribes allopurinol (Zyloprim) for him. Which one of the following nursing measures should be observed while Mike takes allopurinol?
   1. Omit fluids that are carbonated.
   2. Encourage fluids to at least 1500 ml. daily.
   3. Give foods that are high in potassium content.
   4. Limit foods that are high in natural sugar content.

233. When Mike fails to respond to therapy, as he did in the past, his parents are told of his imminent death. Which of the following statements offers the nurse the *best* guide as she makes plans to assist Mike's parents?
1. Their knowing for years that the prognosis was poor helps prepare relatives for the death of children.
2. Relatives are especially grievous when a remission in a disease process was thought to be a good sign of cure.
3. Trust in health personnel who wish to help relatives in grief is most often destroyed by a death that is considered untimely.
4. It is more difficult for relatives to accept the death of a 10-year-old than the death of a younger child whose family membership has been short.

234. Which one of the following courses of action would be *most appropriate* for the nurse while planning to meet Mike's emotional needs during his last days of living?
1. Restrict Mike's visitors to his parents so as not to overtax him.
2. Answer Mike's questions about his illness and imminent death honestly.
3. Concentrate nursing efforts on meeting his physical needs in order to help him think of things other than himself.
4. Encourage Mike to play quietly with his roommate in order to replace thoughts of sadness with thoughts of pleasurable things.

235. After Mike's death, his mother asks the nurse, "What if we had brought Mike in when he first complained of an earache? Would he have lived if we had brought him to the hospital sooner?" Which of the following statements offers the nurse the *best* guide when she responds to Ms. Lane's questions?
1. Explain that everything possible was done for Mike.
2. Suggest that Mike is better off now that he is not suffering.
3. Suggest that Mike's physician is in the best position to explain what happened.
4. Explain that infections are often the result of leukemia rather than a cause of its reappearance.

236. Authorities generally agree that in order to help others deal with death, the nurse *first* must have
1. experienced the death of a loved one herself.
2. worked out her own personal philosophy concerning life and death.
3. taken a course of study that considered how to deal with death and grieving.
4. developed a belief of her own that accepts a supreme being and a life hereafter.

237. Which of the following statements is *most accurate* concerning the incidence of leukemia?
    1. It appears that the occurrence of leukemia is gradually decreasing.
    2. Leukemia occurs more often among persons of low socioeconomic status.
    3. Leukemia, along with the lymphomas, accounts for about 20 percent of all individuals suffering with a malignancy.
    4. Leukemia is the leading cause of death from malignancy in children between the ages of 4 and 14.

      Kelly Walter appeared normal at the time of her birth. Six weeks later, she began to eat poorly, her skin was dry and scaly, and her tongue began to protrude. She was being breast fed. Her physician diagnosed her as having cretinism.
      Items 238 through 246 relate to this situation.

238. Hypothyroidism which causes cretinism is often impossible to detect in an infant at birth because the infant has
    1. little need for the deficient hormone until he is approximately 2 to 3 months old.
    2. received sufficient hormone through his mother's milk for the first few weeks of life.
    3. a gland that functioned well during fetal life but has failed to function since birth.
    4. received sufficient hormone during fetal life from its mother to prevent appearance of signs at birth.

239. Kelly is ordered to receive desiccated thyroid which acts in the body to help
    1. increase the metabolic rate.
    2. stimulate the thyroid to secrete thyroxin.
    3. limit excessive growth of the skeletal system.
    4. promote reabsorption of thyroxin in the kidney tubules.

240. Which route of administration should the nurse anticipate will be used for administering desiccated thyroid to Kelly?
    1. Oral.
    2. Intravenous.
    3. Subcutaneous.
    4. Intramusuclar.

241. Which one of the following food constituents should Kelly receive in above average amounts?
    1. Fats.
    2. Minerals.
    3. Proteins.
    4. Carbohydrates.

Items 242 through 244 relate to the following graphs, both of which illustrate by a dotted line, Kelly's weight and length from birth to 3 months of age.

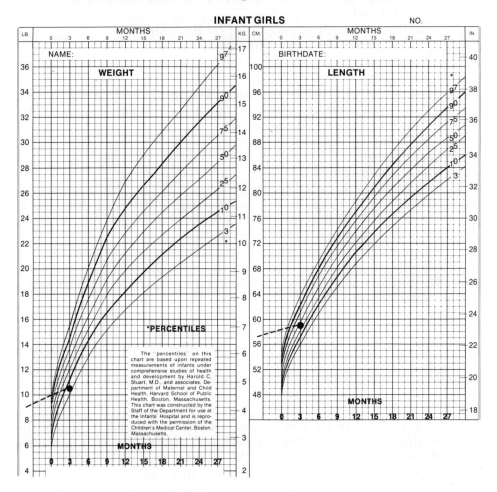

242. Kelly's weight in relationship to her length can be considered to fall within normal range.
  1. This statement is supported by the graphs.
  2. This statement is not supported by the graphs.
  3. This statement is neither supported nor contradicted by the graphs.

243. Kelly is average in length and weight when compared with other 3-month-old infant girls.
  1. This statement is supported by the graphs.
  2. This statement is not supported by the graphs.

3. This statement is neither supported nor contradicted by the graphs.

244. The weight gain for infant boys is usually more rapid than for infant girls.
1. This statement is supported by the graphs.
2. This statement is not supported by the graphs.
3. This statement is neither supported nor contradicted by the graphs.

245. When cretinism is not properly diagnosed and treated, in addition to changes in physical appearance, it can be anticipated that the child will also be
1. blind.
2. epileptic.
3. mentally retarded.
4. emotionally unstable.

246. Dwarfism that results from an endocrine disorder differs from cretinism in that, of the following glands, the one which is malfunctioning in dwarfism is the
1. pineal gland.
2. adrenal gland.
3. pituitary gland.
4. parathyroid gland.

Two-year-old Chris Little has phenylketonuria (PKU). Ms. Little has brought Chris to the physician's office for a routine checkup.
Items 247 through 254 relate to this situation.

247. Ms. Little has been taught on previous occasions about phenylketonuria and Chris's care but asks again what causes the illness. Of the following explanations, the one that describes the *least likely* reason for Ms. Little's question is that she
1. is denying that her child has the disease.
2. is hostile toward health care personnel.
3. has inadequately retained previous teaching.
4. has received ineffective reassurances from previous explanations.

248. Ms. Little asks the nurse to explain how phenylketonuria is transmitted. The nurse should base her response on knowledge that the disease is transmitted by
1. a translocation of a gene.
2. a nondisjunction of a gene.
3. an autosomal recessive gene.
4. a homozygous dominant gene.

249. Diet therapy for Chris includes keeping low blood levels of
    1. tyrosine.
    2. tryptophan.
    3. phenylalanine.
    4. phenylpyruvic acid.
250. Which one of the following foods should be omitted from Chris's diet?
    1. Cheese.
    2. Squash.
    3. Tapioca.
    4. Bananas.
251. When a 10 percent ferric chloride solution is placed on an infant's diaper that is wet with urine, the test is assessed as positive for phenylketonuria if the nurse notes that the ferric chloride and urine combine to produce
    1. a foul odor.
    2. a green color.
    3. a foaming effect.
    4. precipitate matter.
252. When testing for the presence of phenylketonuria in a newborn during his first 12 hours of life, a false negative result is *most frequently* due to his
    1. inadequate fluid intake.
    2. decreased vitamin K level.
    3. insufficient protein intake.
    4. increased bilirubin blood level.
253. When comparing the physical characteristics of a well child with those of a child with phenylketonuria, it is found that the child with PKU has
    1. a larger abdomen.
    2. a shorter stature.
    3. a larger head size.
    4. lighter skin pigmentation.
254. The enzyme in short supply or absent in the child with phenylketonuria is normally manufactured by the
    1. liver.
    2. thymus.
    3. spleen.
    4. pancreas.

Julie Ritter, who is 5 years old, was diagnosed as having measles (rubeola) by the family's physician. She has a sister who is 3 years old and a brother who is 7 years old. The nurse in the physician's office discussed various aspects of Julie's care with Ms. Ritter.

Items 255 through 263 relate to this situation.

255. For how long should Ms. Ritter be taught to keep Julie in bed?
1. For a minimum of 5 days.
2. Until Julie's rash disappears.
3. Until Julie is eating normally.
4. Until Julie's temperature returns to normal.

256. Ms. Ritter says her other two children have not received the measles vaccine and asks what might be done for them. The nurse's response should be guided by knowledge that, in order to modify the severity of the disease, the family physician would *most likely* recommend that they be given
1. a toxoid.
2. a vaccine.
3. an antibiotic.
4. an immunoglobulin.

257. The nurse explains to Ms. Ritter that rubeola is *most often* spread by
1. fecal material.
2. insects and rodents.
3. respiratory secretions.
4. contaminated water and milk.

258. Ms. Ritter is taught that rubeola spreads during its incubation period which lasts approximately
1. 1 to 2 days.
2. 6 to 8 days.
3. 10 to 21 days.
4. 24 to 30 days.

259. Julie's 3-year-old sister has become quiet and shy and demonstrates more than the usual amount of sexual curiosity, according to her mother. According to Erik Erikson's description of the central psychosocial problem of the preschooler, Julie's sister is demonstrating an attempt to resolve a conflict between
1. trust and mistrust.
2. initiative and guilt.
3. industry and inferiority.
4. autonomy and shame or doubt.

260. Which one of the following signs is *most characteristic* of rubeola and helps differentiate it from other childhood diseases?
1. Enlarged lymph nodes in the neck.
2. Inflammation of the mucous membranes of the eyes.

3. Dry, hacking cough that is not relieved with medication.

4. Reddish spots with light centers on the mucosa of the mouth.

261. Although the vaccine can be given at later ages, most physicians recommend that the measles vaccine be given when the child is approximately
1. 2 months of age.
2. 1 year of age.
3. 2 years of age.
4. 4 years of age.

262. The type of organism that causes rubeola is a
1. virus.
2. pneumococcus.
3. streptococcus.
4. staphylococcus.

263. The rubeola/rubella vaccine is usually given in combination. *All* of the following conditions are *contraindications* for receiving the vaccine *except*
1. being pregnant.
2. having active tuberculosis.
3. having a history of rubella.
4. being sensitive to neomycin sulfate.

Two-year-old Brian Jones is admitted to the hospital with gastroenteritis. His mother states that he vomited 7 or 8 times in the past 24 hours and had large, green, liquid stools.

Items 264 through 287 relate to this situation.

264. Ms. Jones states that she cannot stay with Brian because she has two other young children at home. It would be *best* for the nurse to respond to Ms. Jones by saying.
1. "You really should stay. Brian is a very sick child."
2. "I understand. You may visit any time or call to see how he is doing."
3. "It really isn't necessary to stay with Brian since we are here to care for him."
4. "Is it possible to obtain help to stay with your children? Brian needs you since he seems very afraid of us."

265. Brian is placed on enteric precautions. The purpose of this procedure is to help prevent the spread of pathogenic organisms by
1. airborne routes.
2. droplets expelled by sneezing and coughing.
3. animals, insects, and such vehicles as contaminated water and blood.

    4. contact with contaminated feces and such vehicles as linens and clothing.

266. If Brian's cloth teddy bear becomes contaminated while Brian is hospitalized, of the following methods, it would be *best* to render it safe to play with again by using
1. sunlight.
2. hot-air oven.
3. free-flowing steam.
4. a germicidal solution.

267. Which one of the following precautionary measures is *unnecessary* when caring for Brian?
1. A mask should be worn while caring for Brian.
2. A gown should be worn while caring for Brian.
3. Gloves should be worn while caring for Brian.
4. Dishes and leftover food should be handled as contaminated items.

268. A culture shows that Brian's diarrhea is due to Salmonella bacillus. Which one of the following statements *best* describes the course of Salmonella enteritis?
1. Some persons become chronic carriers of the causative organism and remain infectious for long periods of time.
2. Once the acute stage of the disease is past, it is rare that the causative organism continues to be shed from the body.
3. The causative organism may live in the body indefinitely but it becomes so attenuated in time that it is of no danger to anyone.
4. For persons excreting the causative organism as long as 2 to 3 months after contracting Salmonella, an antitoxin has been found helpful to destroy the organism.

269. The *most unlikely* source of Salmonella in the home is
1. fresh eggs.
2. kitty litter.
3. a pet turtle.
4. tropical fish.

270. Brian is suffering from moderate (10 percent) dehydration. Which one of the following signs is characteristic of this degree of dehydration?
1. Vomiting.
2. Increased perspiration.
3. Absence of tear formation.
4. A decrease in the specific gravity of urine.

271. The physician orders that Brian is to receive 500 ml. of intravenous fluid every 8 hours. The drip factor for the equipment being used for the intravenous therapy is 60 drops per ml. How many drops of fluid should be infused each minute?

1. 10 drops.
2. 25 drops.
3. 42 drops.
4. 62 drops.

272. Since the physician ordered that 500 ml. of fluid be infused every 8 hours, how many ml. of intravenous fluid will Brian receive every 24 hours?
    1. 1000 ml.
    2. 1500 ml.
    3. 2000 ml.
    4. 2500 ml.

273. If Brian's renal functioning is normal, which one of the following electrolytes should the nurse anticipate Brian's physician is *most likely* to order added to the intravenous fluid?
    1. Sodium.
    2. Calcium.
    3, Magnesium.
    4. Potassium.

274. Which one of the following methods to restrain Brian is recommended *most often* to help assure that the intravenous needle is not dislodged from his left hand?
    1. Support left wrist and elbow on an armboard; restrain left arm to bed rail.
    2. Support left wrist on an armboard; restrain left arm and left leg loosely to the bed frame.
    3. Support left wrist on an armboard; restrain the four extremities loosely so they may move but do not meet at the midline.
    4. Support the left wrist on an armboard; restrain both arms loosely so that they may move but do not meet at the midline.

275. Which one of the following factors has the *least amount* of influence on Brian's intravenous flow rate?
    1. The height of the solution bottle.
    2. The size of the intravenous needle.
    3. The amount of solution in the bottle.
    4. The position of the needle in the vein.

276. The nurse can anticipate a change in the intravenous flow rate when Brian
    1. eats.
    2. cries.
    3. dreams.
    4. urinates.

277. One of the dangers of infusing Brian's intravenous fluid too rapidly is that he is likely to develop
    1. renal shutdown.

2. liver necrosis.

3. pulmonary edema.

4. insulin insufficiency.

278. Heart failure, another complication when intravenous solutions are allowed to infuse too rapidly, is usually *first* noted when the child has

1. a slow pulse rate.

2. an enlarged abdomen.

3. distention of neck veins.

4. scanty production of urine.

279. Pain with swelling in the region where the intravenous needle was inserted *usually* means that the

1. patient has a low pain tolerance.

2. needle has come out of the vein.

3. intravenous site has been used too long.

4. patient is allergic to the metal in the needle.

280. Which one of the following statements *best* explains why young children require more fluid in proportion to body weight than older children, teenagers, and adults?

1. The younger the person, the lower is the osmolarity of his blood.

2. The younger the person, the less extracellular water his body contains.

3. The younger the person, the less ability his body has to secrete the antidiuretic hormone (ADH).

4. The younger the person, the greater the surface area of the body in relation to his body weight.

281. The physician advises Ms. Jones to serve Brian yogurt during his convalescence. The *primary* reason for this measure is that yogurt

1. helps to promote water absorption in the colon.

2. will form a protective coating on his gastrointestinal tract.

3. helps destroy pathogenic organisms in the gastrointestinal tract.

4. will help reestablish the normal flora in his gastrointestinal tract.

282. A public health nurse calls to see Brian at home after he is discharged from the hospital. Ms. Jones reports seeing what looked like blood in Brain's last stool. If Brian has had the following foods in his diet, which one is likely to color his stool red?

1. An apple.

2. Rare meat.

3. Cherry-flavored gelatin.

4. Strawberry yogurt.

283. Ms. Jones tells the nurse that Brian answers "No!" to everything and is difficult to manage. The *most probable* explanation for his behavior is that Brian is
1. exhibiting beginning leadership qualities.
2. demonstrating an inherited personality trait.
3. beginning to assert himself as an individual.
3. showing typical 2-year-old disinterest in everything.

284. Ms. Jones should be taught that when Brian has a temper tantrum, it would be best to
1. ignore the outburst of anger.
2. let him have his way occasionally.
3. help him find other ways to expend his energy.
4. give him part of what he is demanding to have.

285. Which one of the following behaviors, all of which Brian has exhibited since hospitalization, is *least typical* of regressive behavior?
1. He refuses to drink from his cup.
2. He sleeps 10 to 12 hours each day.
3. He cries when a stranger approaches him.
4. He wets and soils diapers more often than he did.

286. Of the following courses of action, which is the *best* for Brian's parents to take when Brian demonstrates regressive behavior?
1. Punish Brian's unacceptable behavior.
2. Explain to Brian that he is a good boy.
3. Accept Brian's behavior as a coping mechanism.
4. Compare Brian's behavior with that of his sister.

287. At home, Brian is beginning to play with his older sister. The play of a normal 2 year old is described as
1. parallel.
2. associative.
3. cooperative.
4. distributive.

Seven-year-old Karen Sardin visited the family physician's office with her mother. Her health history and signs of being ill led the physician to have Karen admitted to the hospital with a diagnosis of rheumatic fever. The physician's orders include the following:

Complete bed rest.
Procaine penicillin (Crysticillin), 300,000 units IM every 12 hours.
Acetylsalycetic acid (ASA), 5 grains every 4 hours, PO.

Complete blood study (details included in the order).

Items 288 through 309 relate to this situation.

288. Activity is restricted during the acute phase of Karen's illness *primarily* in order to help
   1. reduce the work of the heart.
   2. promote full benefit of drug therapy.
   3. prevent additional pressure on tender joints.
   4. allow the inflammatory process to run its course.

289. Pencillin acts on the causative organism by
   1. destroying it.
   2. inhibiting its growth.
   3. neutralizing its toxins.
   4. decreasing its pathogenicity.

290. Which one of the following signs/symptoms should lead the nurse to suspect that Karen is experiencing early salicylate toxicity?
   1. Pain in the chest.
   2. Pink-colored urine.
   3. Ringing in the ears.
   4. Increased blood pressure.

291. Of the following laboratory blood findings, which one would help the physician *most* to confirm his diagnosis of rheumatic fever?
   1. A high leukocyte count.
   2. A low hemoglobin count.
   3. Sensitivity of the causative organism to penicillin.
   4. The presence of antibodies of the causative organism.

292. The health-illness continuum can be used to assist the nurse in evaluating Karen's needs for care. The continuum helps to illustrate that
   1. the human body has the ability to adapt within a rather wide range.
   2. there is an exact point at which a patient should be considered terminally ill.
   3. there are certain well-defined points at which a patient should be considered well or ill.
   4. the human body handles illness in a direct relationship to its ability to regenerate diseased tissues.

293. Maslow's theory concerning a hierarchy of needs can be used to plan Karen's nursing care. The theory holds that before humans can satisfy other of their own needs, they must *first* meet their
   1. love needs.

2. esteem needs.

3. physiological needs.

4. self-actualization needs.

294. Which one of the following findings is *most likely* to be present if Karen develops carditis?
    1. Heart murmur.
    2. Irregular pulse rate.
    3. Elevated blood pressure.
    4. Decreased vital lung capacity.

295. Karen is diagnosed as having carditis and a digitalis preparation is prescribed for her. The *primary* reason for giving the drug is it helps to
    1. relax the walls of heart capillaries.
    2. improve the strength of the heartbeat.
    3. decrease the likelihood of thrombus formation.
    4. prevent irregularities in ventricular contractions.

296. The physician prescribes digoxin (Lanoxin), 0.15 mg. PO daily. The digoxin is available in liquid form with 0.05 mg. in each ml. How much of the medication should the nurse administer with each dose?
    1. 0.2 ml.
    2. 0.5 ml.
    3. 3.0 ml.
    4. 5.0 ml.

297. The nurse elvates the head of Karen's bed slightly and supports her arms on pillows. The *primary* purpose of this nursing care was to help
    1. prevent skin irritation on her elbows.
    2. limit the possibility of joint contractions.
    3. allow for maximum respiratory functioning.
    4. promote circulation in her upper extremities.

298. The nurse noted that Karen had a bruise on her left leg when she was admitted. The term commonly used to describe the purplish color of skin due to blood in subcutaneous tissue is
    1. cyanosis.
    2. jaundice.
    3. ecchymosis.
    4. diaphoresis.

299. Karen complains of abdominal pain. The cause of her pain is *most probably* due to
    1. pain referred to the area from her joints.
    2. poor circulation of the blood in the area.
    3. pressure from enlarged mesenteric lymph nodes.
    4. a decrease in the normal mobility of the gastrointestinal tract.

300. Which one of the following measures is likely to be *most effective* in *minimizing* the joint pain Karen is experiencing?
1. Massage the affected joints.
2. Immobilize the affected joints.
3. Apply ice to the affected joints.
4. Put the affected joints through range of motion.
301. Of the following nursing measures, which one is also likely to help prevent Karen's joint pains?
1. Change Karen's position in bed frequently.
2. Apply gentle traction to the affected joints.
3. Support Karen's body in proper alignment with rolled pillows.
4. Use a bed cradle to remove the weight of bed linens on the joints.
302. During the acute phase of Karen's illness, of the following diversional activities, it would be *least desirable* to have Karen
1. read a book.
2. play with dolls.
3. watch television.
4. listen to the radio.
303. Karen has developed subcutaneous nodules on the surface of her joints. A characteristic of these nodules is that they are *usually*
1. soft.
2. painless.
3. immovable.
4. symmetrical.
304. Which of the following eating utensils would be *contraindicated* if Karen develops chorealike movements?
1. A fork.
2. A spoon.
3. A plastic cup.
4. A drinking tube.
305. Which one of the following illnesses is *most likely* to have appeared in Karen's health history?
1. Measles.
2. Chickenpox.
3. Otitis media.
4. A sore throat.
306. Which one of the following agencies would offer the best source of help for Karen and her family following Karen's discharge from the hospital?
1. The Cerebral Palsy Foundation.
2. The Christmas Seal Foundation.
3. The County Health Department.

4. The American Heart Association.

307. Congestive heart failure that often accompanies rheumatic fever is due to pathology involving the
1. aorta.
2. heart valves.
3. sinoatrial node.
4. coronary arteries.

308. Which one of the following statements *best* describes research findings in relation to predisposing factors for rheumatic fever?
1. Rheumatic fever is most common among children in their teens.
2. Rheumatic fever is most common among persons of the Caucasian race.
3. Rheumatic fever is most common in families of a low socioeconomic status.
4. Rheumatic fever strikes without regard for socioeconomic status, race, or age.

309. Rheumatic fever is frequently classified as one of the collagen diseases. In which body tissue is pathology observed when a collagen disease is present?
1. Nerve tissue.
2. Muscular tissue.
3. Connective tissue.
4. Epithelial tissue.

Four-year-old Mindy Titus was brought to the hospital by her parents. She has a stiff neck and a severe headache. Her parents state that she has vomited several times. Her temperature is 39° C. The physician's orders include the following:

500 ml. of 5% dextrose in water—to run 12 hours.
Spinal tap.
Complete bed rest.

Items 310 through 322 relate to this situation.

310. When measured on the Fahrenheit scale, Mindy's temperature of 39° C. is equivalent to
1. 101.3° F.
2. 102.2° F.
3. 103.1° F.
4. 104.0° F.

311. Approximately how many drops per minute of the dextrose in water should Mindy receive if 500 ml. of intravenous solution

is to infuse over a 12-hour period when the drop factor is 60 drops per ml.?

1. 32 drops.
2. 42 drops.
3. 52 drops.
4. 62 drops.

312. While doing the spinal tap (lumbar puncture) to obtain the cerebrospinal fluid pressure, a falsely low reading may be obtained if, just prior to reading the manometer,
    1. the child cries.
    2. the child coughs.
    3. specimens of fluid are obtained.
    4. a medication is injected into the fluid.

313. While maintaining complete bed rest for Mindy, which of the following measures will help *least* to prevent Mindy from developing decubitus ulcers over bony prominences?
    1. Keep the skin dry.
    2. Massage pressure areas.
    3. Place Mindy on a firm mattress.
    4. Change Mindy's position frequently.

314. Mindy is weighed upon admission. Her parents ask why this has to be done in view of Mindy's acute illness. The nurse explains that the weight is important to obtain in this instance because it is used to
    1. evaluate Mindy's nutritional status.
    2. determine Mindy's developmental stage.
    3. determine how much edema is present.
    4. permit accurate calculation of drug dosages.

315. The physician diagnoses Mindy as having pneumococcal meningitis which is a likely complication of
    1. diarrhea.
    2. nephritis.
    3. septic arthritis.
    4. middle ear infection.

316. During the neurological examination, the nurse notes that Mindy's Kernig's sign is positive. Which one of the following responses to stimuli indicates a positive Kernig's sign?
    1. A loud noise causes extension followed by flexion of the arms.
    2. Passive flexion of the neck causes bending of the hips and kness.
    3. The large toe extends and the other toes fan outward when the bottom of the foot is stroked.
    4. Straightening of the legs at the knees is met with resistance when the thigh is flexed at a right angle to the body.

317. During the acute stage of illness, Mindy is irritable and restless. Which one of the following nursing measures should assume top priority?
1. Omit bathing her.
2. Avoid talking to her.
3. Perform treatments as quickly as possible.
4. Keep extraneous noise in her room to a minimum.
318. In addition to a change in level of consciousness, a sign of increased intracranial pressure is
1. dyspnea.
2. deafness.
3. seizure activity.
4. unusually rapid pulse rate.
319. When discontinuing Mindy's intravenous therapy, the nurse allows Mindy to apply a dressing to the area where the needle was removed. The nurse bases her action on knowledge that Mindy needs to
1. find more diversional activities.
2. protect her image of an intact body.
3. relieve the anxiety of separation from her home.
4. enhance her confidence in personnel caring for her.
320. Which of the following signs observed by the nurse would help the physician *most* to diagnose that Mindy had developed disseminated intravascular coagulation (DIC)?
1. Cyanosis.
2. Swollen glands.
3. Dyspnea on exertion.
4. Hemorrhagic skin rash.
321. Which one of the following body postures do children characteristically assume when they are seriously ill with meningitis?
1. The patient will lie on his back with his legs crossed.
2. The patient will lie on his abdomen with his legs drawn up under him.
3. The patient will lie on his side with his legs and head drawn backwards.
4. The patient will lie in a fetal position with his legs and head drawn forward.
322. Which one of the following diseases *most commonly* predisposes to viral meningitis?
1. Mumps.
2. Hepatitis.
3. Chickenpox.
4. Whooping cough.

Items 323 through 337 relate to chronic diarrhea in infants and children.

323. Diarrhea is *best* defined on the basis of the stool's
    1. color.
    2. amount.
    3. frequency.
    4. consistency.

324. Which one of the following enzymes is *least likely* to be involved when carbohydrate malabsorption is present?
    1. Lactase.
    2. Sucrase.
    3. Maltase.
    4. Amylase.

325. The skin of an infant with diarrhea that is caused by carbohydrate malabsorption is especially susceptible to breakdown because the stool contains more than average amounts of
    1. bile.
    2. acids.
    3. bacteria.
    4. potassium.

326. After thorough study, an infant is diagnosed as having diarrhea due to an irritable colon. Which one of the following statements describes the *most typical* course of this disorder?
    1. The presence of diarrhea is likely to be a lifelong problem despite treatment.
    2. The diarrhea tends to terminate of its own accord without any special treatment.
    3. The diarrhea tends to worsen until excision of the diseased colon is performed.
    4. Remission of the diarrhea most often occurs when a constipating diet is maintained.

327. An infant suffering with chronic diarrhea needs special care to prevent skin irritation. In addition to the effects of the stool on the skin, which one of the following practices is believed to contribute *most* to the breakdown of the infant's skin?
    1. Cleansing the area with soap that is inadequately rinsed away.
    2. Using disposable diapers to which the infant eventually develops a sensitivity.
    3. Dusting the area with powder so often that the skin becomes dry and subject to easy breakdown.
    4. Lubricating the area so generously with oil that the skin becomes soft and subject to easy breakdown.

328. A baby with chronic diarrhea often is irritable and cranky.

Which one of the following measures is likely to be *most comforting* for the baby?
1. Offer the baby a pacifier.
2. Sit at the baby's bedside and talk to him.
3. Hold the baby and rock him in a rocking chair.
4. Have soft, soothing music playing in the baby's room.

329. Heat lamp treatments are often used when caring for infants with diarrhea. Which of the following explanations *best* describes why the application of dry heat is effective for skin irritation?
1. Heat acts as a local anesthetic to damaged tissues.
2. Heat relaxes the baby which helps him to remain on his abdomen.
3. Heat increases the blood supply to damaged tissues to help in healing.
4. Heat constricts blood vessels in damaged tissues to decrease the swelling.

330. The minimum number of inches a heat lamp should be placed away from the child's skin is
1. 6 inches.
2. 12 inches.
3. 18 inches.
4. 24 inches.

331. Which one of the following situations is *most likely* to lead to an acute attack of ulcerative colitis?
1. Emotional stress.
2. A poorly balanced diet.
3. An inadequate fluid intake.
4. Poor habits of elimination.

332. With which one of the following conditions is a youngster with chronic ulcerative colitis often afflicted?
1. Anemia.
2. Anorexia.
3. Heartburn.
4. Dehydration.

333. Celiac disease is characterized by a disturbance in the absorption of
1. fats.
2. proteins.
3. vitamins.
4. minerals.

334. In addition to diarrhea, a characteristic sign of celiac disease is
1. enlarged liver.
2. rapid weight gain.
3. protuberant abdomen.

4. tender inguinal lymph nodes.

335. Which of the following foodstuffs is *contraindicated* in the diet of a child with celiac disease?
    1. Grains, such as wheat.
    2. Tubers, such as potatoes.
    3. Leavening agents, such as yeast.
    4. Fermented foods, such as yogurt.
336. For how long is it likely that a child with celiac disease will need to remain on a special diet?
    1. For the rest of his life.
    2. Until the disease is well controlled.
    3. Until approximately the age of puberty.
    4. For the period required to desensitize him to the offending foods.
337. A mother whose infant is diagnosed as having celiac disease asks the nurse what safety precautions she should take with the infant's reusable diapers. Which one of the following statements should guide the nurse when she responds to the mother's question?
    1. The diapers should be boiled after they are washed.
    2. The diapers should be soaked in an antiseptic solution before they are washed.
    3. It would be best to use disposable diapers until the diarrhea is under control.
    4. There are no special precautions necessary in the care of this infant's diapers.

The parent of children attending an elementary and junior high school invited the school nurse to attend some of their meetings to discuss common childhood problems related to health.
Items 338 through 386 relate to this situation.

338. Which one of the following symptoms is *most common* when a person has been infected with pediculosis capitis (head lice)?
    1. Itching of the skin.
    2. Scaling of the skin.
    3. Serous weeping on the skin surface.
    4. Pinpoint hemorrhagic spots on the skin surface.
339. Which one of the following statements *best* explains why infestation with pediculosis is more common among school children than among adults?
    1. An immunity to pediculosis usually is not established until adulthood.

2. Children of school age tend to be more neglectful of frequent handwashing than are adults.
3. Pediculosis is most often spread by close contact with infected children in the classroom.
4. The skin of adults is more capable of resisting the invasion of lice than the skin of children.

340. One mother comments, "My children had head lice and I thought we were rid of them. I was so careful but in about a week's time, they were back!" The *most probable* reason for this recurrence was that
1. the nits had not been destroyed.
2. immature lice had withstood treatment.
3. the lice developed resistance to the treatment.
4. infestation had occurred with another type of lice.

341. The organism responsible for causing tinea capitis (ringworm of the scalp) is classified as a
1. virus.
2. fungus.
3. bacillus.
4. protozoan.

342. Which one of the following techniques is *most often* recommended to prevent the spread of scalp ringworm?
1. Wearing mittens.
2. Shaving infected areas.
3. Having a daily shampoo.
4. Wearing a stocking cap.

343. One mother comments, "The doctor prescribed griseofulvin (Grisactin) to treat my son's ringworm of the scalp. He said it was essential to take the medication exactly as ordered for several weeks. Why was this so important?" The response by the nurse should be based on knowledge that
1. a sensitivity to the drug may occur if not taken as ordered.
2. fewer side effects occur as the body adjusts to the new substance.
3. fewer allergic reactions occur if the drug is maintained at the same level.
4. the antiinfective agent should be maintained at a therapeutic level in the bloodstream.

344. It is believed that the pinworm is spread *most commonly* by contaminated
1. food.
2. hands.
3. toilet seats.
4. drinking water.

345. When one of the parents asks what disease is spread by under-cooked pork, the nurse should respond by saying
1. tularemia.
2. trichinosis.
3. paratyphoid fever.
4. bacillary dysentery.

346. When a parent says that his family will be traveling abroad where drinking water must be boiled, he asks what disease will be prevented. In addition to various types of dysentery, contaminated drinking water is *most often* responsible for the transmission of
1. typhus.
2. brucellosis.
3. typhoid fever.
4. poliomyelitis.

347. What type of immunity does a person have when he has had rubella (German measles)?
1. Natural immunity.
2. Passive immunity.
3. Active acquired immunity.
4. Artifically acquired immunity.

348. The *most common* reason why females after the age of puberty are *rarely* given rubella vaccine is that
1. risks to the fetus are high if the female is pregnant.
2. chances of contracting the disease are much lower after puberty than before.
3. changes occurring within the immunological system may affect the rhythm of the menstrual cycle.
4. dangers associated with a strong reaction to the vaccine are increased after puberty.

349. Parents are concerned about problems that acne creates in their children and they ask the nurse how a teenager should cleanse the affected areas. Of the following courses of action, it would be *best* for the nurse to recommend that teenagers use
1. witch hazel.
2. soap and water.
3. hydrogen peroxide.
4. lotions and creams.

350. Which of the following pharmaceutical preparations are used by many physicians today to help decrease the severity of mumps?
1. Antibiotics.
2. Corticosteroid agents.

3. Antiinflammatory drugs.

4. Immunological products.

351. A mother asks if her teenage son who has not had mumps is likely to become sterile if he acquires the disease. The nurse should base her response on knowledge that the occurrence of sterility in males who acquire mumps after the age of puberty is

1. rare.

2. frequent.

3. likely in about half of the cases.

352. If a male does become sterile because of complications following mumps, tissue damage has *most likely* occurred in his

1. testes.

2. prostate.

3. seminal vesicles.

4. ejaculatory duct.

353. The organism responsible for causing chickenpox is a

1. virus.

2. fungus.

3. bacterium.

4. rickettsia.

354. Which one of the following types of lesions *best* describes a mature chickenpox lesion?

1. Macule with smooth edges.

2. Vesicle with a red areola.

3. Pustule with irregular edges.

4. Macule with depressed center.

355. The care of a child with chickenpox is directed *primarily* toward the prevention of

1. anemia and dehydration.

2. anorexia and malnutrition.

3. infection at the site of lesions.

4. infection in the respiratory system.

356. Of the following symptoms, the one that is most typical of mononucleosis is

1. liver tenderness.

2. enlarged lymph nodes.

3. persistent nonproductive cough.

4. generalizing blushing-type skin rash.

357. A parent in the group says that his neighbor's youngster has mononucleosis and asks the nurse what type of precautions should be used to prevent its spread. Which one of the following responses would *most accurately* reflect present opinion concerning the spread of mononucleosis?

1. No particular precautionary measures are advised.
2. The youngster's eating utensils should be boiled before being reused.
3. A mask should be used when giving the youngster direct personal care.
4. The youngster's linens should be washed separately in hot, soapy water.

358. A positive tuberculin skin test in a child who has not previously been vaccinated with BCG is *most often* interpreted to mean that the child
1. is presently infectious.
2. is immune to tuberculosis.
3. has an active case of tuberculosis.
4. has been infected with tubercle bacilli.

359. How is tuberculosis *most commonly* spread?
1. By vectors.
2. By droplet nuclei.
3. By contaminated milk.
4. By contaminated water.

360. Which one of the following drugs is *commonly* used for the treatment of tuberculosis?
1. Colchicine.
2. Isoniazid (INH).
3. Propantheline (Pro-Banthine).
4. Quinidine sulfate (Quinidex).

361. Public health measures to help control the spread of tuberculosis are *most often* directed toward
1. case finding.
2. health teaching.
3. isolation of active cases.
4. maintenance of patients on chemotherapy.

362. Which one of the following statements is *least accurate* concerning the venereal disease syphilis?
1. It is difficult to treat.
2. It is a reportable disease.
3. It is often associated with promiscuity.
4. It has reached epidemic proportions in parts of this country.

363. The causative organism for syphilis is the
1. Plasmodium vivax.
2. Trypanosoma cruzi.
3. Treponema pallidum.
4. Trichomonas vaginalis.

364. Which one of the following venereal diseases is *commonly* referred to as "clap" by lay persons?

1. Syphilis.
2. Chancroid.
3. Gonorrhea.
4. Genital herpes.
365. Public health measures geared to control the incidence of venereal diseases are *most often* directed toward
   1. mass screening for venereal diseases.
   2. locating the sources of venereal diseases.
   3. treating persons who have or are suspected of having venereal diseases.
   4. isolating persons who have or are suspected of having venereal diseases.
366. Of the following practices, the one which is *most* responsible for the marked decrease in the incidence of diphtheria in the past 50 years is the widespread use of
   1. water purification.
   2. milk pasteurization.
   3. early disease detection methods.
   4. immunization against the disease.
367. Hemophilia is transmitted by a sex-linked
   1. nondisjunction of the X chromosome.
   2. recessive gene from each parent carried to males.
   3. recessive gene carried by the female X chromosome to males.
   4. dominant gene from the female which joins with an affected gene from the male.
368. If a child with hemophilia has a wound on his leg, after it has been cleansed, the parents should be taught to care for the area by applying
   1. an ice bag.
   2. gentle pressure.
   3. warm moist compresses.
   4. a tourniquet above the wound.
369. Which one of the following drugs should be avoided by a child with hemophilia?
   1. Acetaminophen (Tylenol).
   2. Phenylbutazone (Butazolidin).
   3. Aspirin (acetylsalicylic acid).
   4. Tetracycline hydrochloride (Achromycin).
370. A mother says that a physician described her youngster as having vision that is 20/60. She asks the nurse what 20/60 means. The nurse should base her response on knowledge that the child
   1. has lost approximately one-third of his visual acuity.
   2. is seeing at 60 feet what he should be seeing at 20 feet.

3. is seeing at 20 feet what he should be seeing at 60 feet.

4. has visual acuity approximately three times better than the average child.

371. A parent asks, "Why should vomiting be discouraged when a child drinks kerosene?" The nurse should base her response on knowledge that vomiting after kerosene has been ingested is dangerous because of the likelihood of its resulting in

1. aspiration of the kerosene.

2. a perforation of the esophagus.

3. swelling of the mouth and pharynx.

4. the formation of scar tissue in the esophagus.

372. When compared with the food requirements of preschoolers and adolescents, the food requirements of children between about 6 and 12 years of age are less because they have a lower

1. growth rate.

2. metabolic rate.

3. level of activity.

4. hormonal secretion rate.

373. When the eating habits of children in middle childhood (ages 6 through 12) are discussed, the nurse is guided by knowledge that eating habits of children during this period are *most* influenced by

1. food preferences of their peers.

2. the smell and appearance of food offered them.

3. the atmosphere and examples provided by parents at meal-times.

4. parents encouraging their children to eat foods that are good for them.

374. Which one of the following vitamins must be included in the diet regularly because it cannot be stored by the body in any appreciable amount?

1. Vitamin A.

2. Vitamin B.

3. Vitamin D.

4. Vitamin E.

375. The most common disorder of speech in children over 4 years of age is

1. lisping.

2. stuttering.

3. baby talking.

4. being nonfluent.

376. Which one of the following factors has been *least often* found to be a cause of enuresis (bed wetting)?

1. Organic diseases.

2. Emotional stress.

3. Premature toilet training.

4. Permissive home environments.

377. One parent says, "No matter how careful I am about trying to keep my 2-year-old child away from dangerous things, she is constantly into everything! Why is this?" The nurse should explain that, at age 2, such behavior is

1. normal; the child is striving to gain independence.

2. normal; the child is exploring to satisfy curiosity.

3. abnormal; this type of behavior is typical of children who are 3 to 5 years of age.

4. abnormal; a 2-year-old child should be checked by a physician when behavior is as mischievous as the mother describes.

378. The parents ask the school nurse how they can best prepare their children for entering school. Of the following courses of action, it would be *best* for the nurse to recommend that the parents

1. have an older sibling tell their children about school.

2. orient their children to the school's physical environment.

3. offer to stay with their children for the first few days of school.

4. discuss school with their children if they ask questions about school.

379. It has been found that the *most common* cause for the unhappiness some children experience when first entering school is their

1. feeling of insecurity.

2. emotional maladjustment.

3. poor language development.

4. inability to pay attention.

380. Children between 6 and 11 years of age often develop feelings of inferiority and inadequacy when they have not had sufficient experience to

1. finish tasks.

2. develop skills.

3. think subjectively.

4. work cooperatively.

381. Which of the following tasks is likely to help a 9-year-old girl *most* to acquire a sense of industry and success?

1. Assign her to bake a premixed cake.

2. Assign her to pick up her baby brother's toys.

3. Assign her with an older sister to do the family laundry.

4. Assign her to repair the on-off switch on her record player.

382. One mother asks the nurse what to do in a situation she describes: Her 12-year-old son wants to use television after 10

P.M. to watch a half-hour mystery show. "Rule of the house" is that there is to be no television after 10 P.M. Based on the knowledge that the nurse has of growth and development, her guide for this mother should be that the son's request is

1. all right but only for this one time.
2. all right but only for the first 15 minutes.
3. not all right until the policy has been modified.
4. not all right and there can be no exceptions made.

383. According to Erik Erikson, of the following developmental tasks, the central problem of early adolescence is the establishment of a sense of
   1. intimacy.
   2. industry.
   3. identity.
   4. initiative.

384. Which one of the following statements *most accurately* describes findings in relation to the onset of adolescence in boys and girls?
   1. Girls and boys experience the onset of adolescence at approximately the same age.
   2. Boys experience the onset of adolescence approximately 1 to 2 years earlier than girls.
   3. Girls experience the onset of adolescence approximately 1 to 2 years earlier than boys.
   4. Findings do not support a sexual relationship concerning the onset of adolescence.

385. Which one of the following statements would be *most typical* of a normal adolescent in the United States?
   1. "I can hardly wait to grow up."
   2. "I know who I am and where I wish to go in life."
   3. "I usually prefer being with my parents rather than being alone in my room."
   4. "I like my friends and I don't mind their choice of clothes and hair-do. But I want to be different."

386. Which one of the following proverbs reflects an attitude toward child-rearing that *most often* leads to conflicts between parents and teenagers?
   1. Do as I say, not as I do.
   2. A stitch in time saves nine.
   3. Spare the rod and spoil the child.
   4. Nature is more important than nurture.

Shawn Baxter was delivered prematurely. He weighed 4 pounds and 8 ounces at birth. After initial emergency care was given in the delivery room, he was transferred to the intensive care nursery in the pediatric department.

Items 387 through 401 relate this situation.

387. Upon admission to the intensive care nursery, the nurse can expect that Shawn will normally display *all* of the following physical findings *except*
1. a Moro response.
2. pliable earlobes.
3. fine hair over much of his body.
4. numerous creases on the soles of his feet.

388. Shawn is ordered to receive sodium bicarbonate through an umbilical catheter. The rationale for the physician's order is to help alleviate
1. edema.
2. acidosis.
3. alkalosis.
4. dehydration.

389. Which one of the following effects will the sodium bicarbonate have on Shawn's blood chemistry?
1. It will increase the blood's pH value.
2. It will decrease the blood's osmolarity.
3. It will decrease the blood's chloride level.
4. It will decrease the blood's potassium level.

390. Shawn is ordered to be fed by gavage. Which one of the following statements describes how the nurse may *best* judge whether after the catheter is inserted, it is in Shawn's stomach?
1. The catheter is introduced the desired length without resistance.
2. There is an absence of periodic bubbling when the end of the catheter is placed under water.
3. After inserting water into the catheter with a syringe, the water returns easily with aspiration.
4. While inserting air into the catheter with a syringe, auscultation over the lungs reveals air sounds.

391. The nurse wishes to determine whether Shawn is developing abdominal distention. Which one of the following techniques, performed before and after a feeding, would be *best* to determine distention?
1. Weighing him.
2. Palpating his abdomen for degree of firmness.
3. Measuring the circumference of his abdomen with a tape measure.

4. When he is placed on his abdomen, observing for abdominal spread on each side of his body.

392. Which one of the following conditions is Shawn *very likely* to develop if he is given oxygen at too high a concentration?
   1. Glaucoma.
   2. Cataracts.
   3. Ophthalmia neonatorum.
   4. Retrolental fibroplasia.

393. Which one of the following measures would be of *least* importance when caring for Shawn?
   1. Providing him with sensory stimulation.
   2. Maintaining his fluid and electrolyte balance.
   3. Minimizing the workload on his cardiovascular system.
   4. Preventing him from experiencing discomfort when administering treatments.

394. Shawn develops a pneumothorax. A chest tube, kept under water in a drainage bottle is used. Which one of the following observations will help the physician *most* to make the decision that the tube be removed?
   1. Shawn no longer has a respiratory grunt.
   2. X-ray films reveal a reexpansion of Shawn's lung.
   3. The water in Shawn's drainage bottle is no longer bubbling.
   4. Shawn's blood oxygen tension (pO_2) is within normal limits.

395. Shawn's parents are frightened about his condition. Which one of the following measures is likely to be of *most help* in relieving the parents' fears?
   1. Allowing them to see and touch him.
   2. Arranging a visit with another couple with a premature baby.
   3. Excouraging them to participate in feeding and caring for him.
   4. Explaining to them that their fear is needless since he is doing well.

396. During a feeding, Shawn aspirates some of his formula. Which one of the following observations is an *early* sign of aspiration?
   1. Choking.
   2. Cyanosis.
   3. Lethargy.
   4. Abdominal breathing.

397. Although all of the following techniques are beneficial, authorities generally agree that the *single most effective* way to control infection in a premature nursery is to
   1. require personnel to wear gowns and masks.
   2. have personnel use frequent hand and arm washing techniques.
   3. keep each infant in an isolette that is opened as infrequently as possible.

4. maintain a ventilation system in the nursery that provides for continuous clean air exchange.

398. Of the following criteria, the one *most appropriate* for classifying an infant as being premature is the infant's
1. birth weight.
2. gestation age.
3. central nervous system development.
4. musculoskeletal system development.

399. Idiopathic respiratory distress syndrome (hyaline membrane disease) is a common complication of prematurity. It is generally believed that this disease is caused *primarily* by a lack of
1. bilirubin.
2. vitamin K.
3. surfactant.
4. phenylalanine.

400. Shawn is unable to walk or stand when he is 18 months old. His physician diagnoses him as having cerebral palsy. Cerebral palsy is a neurological condition that results from damage to the
1. brain.
2. meninges.
3. spinal cord.
4. peripheral nerves.

401. When it is learned that Shawn has cerebral palsy, the public health nurse working with Shawn and his parents sets up an objective of care. The *best* objective for this family is one that
1. sets behavior goals for Shawn that are consistent with his capabilities.
2. helps the parents seek financial assistance for Shawn's extensive medical care needs.
3. prepares Shawn and his parents for a series of corrective surgical and medical procedures.
4. provides an environment that helps keep emotional and physical stress for Shawn at a minimum.

Four-month-old Timmy Lee is brought to the well child clinic by his mother. He appears to be in good health.
Items 402 through 410 relate to this situation.

402. Ms. Lee asks the nurse when she should wean Timmy from breast feedings and have him use a cup. The nurse should explain that Timmy will show readiness to be weaned when he is
1. taking solid foods well.
2. sleeping through the night.

3. shortening his nursing time.

4. eating on a regular schedule.

403. Ms. Lee says that Timmy's physician recommended solid foods but Timmy is refusing to eat them after his breast feedings. The nurse should suggest that Ms. Lee feed Timmy by

1. offering him dessert followed by his vegetables and meat.

2. giving him breast milk as long as Timmy refuses solid food.

3. mixing puréed food with cow's milk and feeding it through a large-holed nipple.

4. giving him a small amount of milk and then feeding him his solid foods.

404. Which one of the following abilities would be considered *un-usual* for an infant Timmy's age?

1. Sitting up without support.

2. Responding to pleasure with smiles.

3. Grasping a rattle when it is offered to him.

4. Turning himself from his back to either side.

405. The nurse discusses immunization with Ms. Lee. In addition to immunizing for diphtheria, pertussis, and tetanus (DPT), most physicians recommend that during the first 6 months of life, children also be immunized against

1. mumps.

2. measles.

3. tuberculosis.

4. poliomyelitis.

406. Ms. Lee states, "The soft spot near the front of Timmy's head is still big. When will it close?" The nurse's response should be guided by knowledge that the anterior fontanel normally closes between the ages of

1. 4 and 8 months.

2. 8 and 12 months.

3. 12 and 18 months.

4. 24 and 30 months.

407. Ms. Lee asks about "cradle cap." What structure in the skin is involved when an infant is diagnosed as having "cradle cap"?

1. The sweat glands.

2. The hair follicles.

3. The sebaceous glands.

4. The ceruminous glands.

408. It is *most often* recommended to remove "cradle cap" by

1. using dry powdered shampoos until the infant outgrows it.

2. rubbing it gently but firmly with terry cloth while giving a shampoo.

3. softening it with a lotion or ointment and follow this with a shampoo.

4. applying alcohol or witch hazel and follow this with a brushing of the scalp.

409. The nurse plans to administer the Denver Developmental Screening Test (DDST) to Timmy. The nurse should explain to Ms. Lee that the test measures a child's
1. intelligence quotient.
2. emotional development.
3. social and physical abilities.
4. predisposition to genetic and allergic illnesses.

410. An early supplement to the diet of most infants is orange juice. Which one of the following diseases does orange juice help to prevent?
1. Scurvy.
2. Rickets.
3. Beriberi.
4. Pellagra.

Items 411 through 422 relate to developmental tasks at various ages of childhood and youth.

411. It has been observed that most normally developed infants begin play activities with their
1. food.
2. rattle.
3. clothing.
4. own body.

412. Of the following developmental achievements, the one that is normal for a 1-month-old infant is that he will be able to
1. smile and laugh aloud.
2. roll from his back to his side.
3. hold a rattle for a brief period of time.
4. turn his head from side to side when lying on his abdomen.

413. Michelle is observed by the nurse to be competent in the following developmental skills: she holds her head erect when in a sitting position; she stares at an object placed in her hand and takes it to her mouth; she coos and gurgles when talked to; and she sustains part of her own weight when held in a standing position. The nurse is correct when she assesses Michell's age to be approximately
1. 2 months.
2. 4 months.
3. 6 months.
4. 8 months.

414. *All* of the following developmental tasks are typical of a normal 9-month-old child *except*

1. creeping and crawling.
2. holding his bottle with good hand-mouth coordination.
3. putting his arm through a sleeve while being dressed.
4. beginning to use specific imitative verbal expressions.

415. Which of the following tasks is *most typical* of a normally developed 18-month-old child?
1. Copying a circle.
2. Pulling toys behind him.
3. Playing tag with other children.
4. Building a tower of eight or more blocks.

416. Tommy is normally developed 3-year-old. He is to start nursery school. For which of the following tasks can the teacher expect Tommy to be *least* skilled?
1. Riding a tricycle.
2. Tying his shoelaces.
3. Stringing large beads.
4. Letting her know when he must go to the bathroom.

417. Of the following therapeutic play activities, which one will help the hospitalized 4-year-old child *most* to relieve pent-up hostilities?
1. Stacking blocks.
2. Pounding a peg board.
3. Painting with watercolors.
4. Having a story about the hospital read to him.

418. A normally developing 4-year-old child requires sutures for a deep forehead gash. Which of the following fears is *most typical* for a child his age in this situation?
1. Fear of bodily harm or disfigurement.
2. Fear of being separated from his mother.
3. Fear of having no control over what will happen to him.
4. Fear of the pain associated with the suturing procedure.

419. Which of the following activities is *least therapeutic* for a hospitalized 4-year-old child?
1. Finger painting.
2. Watching television.
3. Cutting and pasting.
4. Playing with puppets.

420. Of the following play materials, which can a school-age child use *best* to communicate fears and feelings to the nurse?
1. A deck of cards.
2. Drawing paper and pencil.
3. A paint-by-number set and paints.
4. A game that challenges players to tell the truth.

421. Of the following diversional items, which is likely to appeal to

most teenagers who must observe strict bed rest?
1. A book to read.
2. Modeling clay.
3. Letter-writing equipment
4. A record player and records.

422. Which of the following tasks is typical of late adolescence and young adulthood?
1. Exploring and collecting things.
2. Beginning separation from family.
3. Establishing relationships with own-sex friends.
4. Establishing a lasting relationship with a member of the opposite sex.

Items 423 through 456 are miscellaneous items.

423. A well, normally developed newborn has aspirated some of his formula. Which one of the following emergency nursing actions should the nurse use?
1. Begin oxygen therapy.
2. Stimulate the infant to cry.
3. Insert an endotracheal tube.
4. Suspend the infant by his feet.

424. Recent research indicates that pica (compulsive eating, usually of nonfood items) is *most probably* caused by
1. an iron deficiency.
2. a magnesium excess.
3. a potassium excess.
4. a sodium deficiency.

425. It is believed that secretions of the thymus gland are related to the body's
1. rate of sexual maturation.
2. ability to develop immunity.
3. distribution of adipose tissue.
4. competency to maintain electrolyte balance.

426. A physician writes an order for a drug for a child, the dosage of which is 1 grain. The metric equivalent for 1 grain is
1. 0.06 Gm.
2. 0.60 mg.
3. 1.00 mg.
4. 0.10 Gm.

427. Which one of the following types of behavior is characteristic of a child with autism?
1. Being unusually combative.
2. Repeating what is said to him.

3. Being unable to pronounce words.

4. Withdrawing from social contacts.

428. Which one of the following statements *best* describes current opinion concerning the cause of Sudden Infant Death Syndrome (SIDS)?

1. It is an immunological abnormality.

2. It is due to an overwhelming viral infection.

3. It is due to a lack in respiratory secretions.

4. No single etiological factor has been confirmed.

429. In order to help the parents *most*, it is generally agreed that when sudden, unexplained death of an infant occurs, it is *best* for the nurse to

1. remain in control of her own feelings.

2. reinforce the physician's words to the parents.

3. help the parents express their feelings about the death.

4. encourage the parents to view the infant for private grieving.

430. The parents refuse a blood transfusion for their child because of their religious beliefs. Of the following courses of action, it would be *best* for the nurse to

1. consult with the parents' clergyman for assistance in seeking a solution to the problem.

2. give the transfusion since the physician indicated it was important for the child's survival.

3. allow the parents to make the decision without seeking further assistance since the child is a minor.

4. begin an intensive teaching program so that the parents will understand the importance of the transfusion.

431. Among children, which one of the following neoplasms remains *most ominous* in relation to cure rates?

1. Lymphoma.

2. Wilms' tumor.

3. Neuroblastoma.

4. Soft tissue sarcoma.

432. It is generally recommended that a comatose child is *best* positioned on

1. his back.

2. either side.

3. his abdomen.

433. A public health nurse is suspicious when she sees a child in his home with an illness that she thinks could possibly be diphtheria. In order to assist the physician with the diagnosis, the nurse should obtain a specimen for a

1. blood culture.

2. urine culture.

3. stool culture.

4. throat culture.

434. When in Bryant's traction, a child should be positioned on his back and his legs should be
   1. straight in line with his body resting flat on the bed.
   2. flexed at a 90° angle at his hips and his hips should be slightly off the bed.
   3. flexed at a 45° angle at his hips and his hips should be resting flat on the bed.
   4. separated with the affected leg at a right angle to his body and the unaffected leg in any position of comfort.

435. If a public health nurse plans to include all the following points when teaching an adolescent girl about syphilis, which one is in *error?*
   1. Syphilis can be spread to a fetus.
   2. A douche after sexual intercourse prevents acquiring syphilis.
   3. Treatment for syphilis would not provide her immunity to the disease.
   4. She should have her partner wear a condom during sexual intercourse to prevent acquiring syphilis.

436. In most instances, the diet for children who have kidney diseases will be ordered low in its content of
   1. sodium.
   2. calcium.
   3. magnesium.
   4. phosphorus.

437. Which one of the following descriptions *best* defines a meningomyelocele?
   1. It is an inflammation of the meninges.
   2. It is an absence of a portion of the meninges.
   3. It is a cystlike growth derived from embryonic cells.
   4. It is a saclike mass that protrudes through a defect in the spine.

438. Of the following objectives, the one that should receive *highest* priority when caring for a child with hydrocephalus is one that will help prevent
   1. decubitus ulcers on the head.
   2. infection in the urinary tract.
   3. infection in the central nervous system.
   4. herniation of the cerebrum into the ventricles of the brain.

439. To date, the *most successful* treatment for hydrocephalus has been therapy using
   1. drugs.
   2. surgery.
   3. radiation.

4. electrocautery.

440. Hirschsprung's disease has many signs/symptoms similar to those of
1. inguinal hernia.
2. pyloric stenosis.
3. esophageal atresia.
4. intestinal obstruction.

441. A characteristic of Hirschsprung's disease which must be considered when administering an enema or colonic irrigation to a child with the disease is that the
1. anus is relaxed.
2. anus is stenosed.
3. colon is spastic.
4. colon is enlarged.

442. The incidence of intussusception occurs more frequently in infants than in adults *primarily* because infants
1. eat at frequent intervals.
2. lack roughage in their diets.
3. tend to swallow air during their feedings.
4. have a hyperactive lower intestinal tract.

443. Which one of the following signs is *most typical* of pyloric stenosis?
1. Diarrhea.
2. Constipation.
3. Projectile vomiting.
4. Abdominal distention.

444. An infant suffering with pylorospasms is often given thickened feedings *primarily* because, in contrast to regular formula, the thickened formula
1. is vomited less readily.
2. tends to be taken with greater ease.
3. provides the infant with more calories.
4. moves through the gastrointestinal tract more slowly.

445. Of the following conditions, the one which *most often* accounts for the death of a leukemic child is
1. infection.
2. hemorrhage.
3. heart failure.
4. liver failure.

446. Which one of the following statements best describes the *most widely* recommended way to begin an infant on new foods?
1. Mix new foods with formula.
2. Mix new foods with more familiar ones.
3. Offer new foods on a one-at-a-time basis.

4. Offer new foods after formula is taken.

447. Which one of the body's systems is particularly dependent on adequate amounts of vitamin D for proper growth and development?
   1. The nervous system.
   2. The skeletal system.
   3. The muscular system.
   4. The endocrine system.

448. Which one of the following secretions initiates the digestion of carbohydrates?
   1. Ptylin.
   2. Pepsin.
   3. Trypsin.
   4. Steapsin.

449. The mineral magnesium is important to the body because it functions to help
   1. coagulate blood.
   2. activate enzymes.
   3. regulate metabolism.
   4. initiate cellular oxidation.

450. When compared with a 14-year-old youngster, the percentage of water a 2-year-old's body normally contains is
   1. less.
   2. more.
   3. approximately the same.

451. Which of the following persons are the "significant others" to the child during toddlerhood (ages 1 to 3 years)?
   1. Peers.
   2. Parents.
   3. Siblings.
   4. Neighbors.

452. During the last decade, which one of the following trends has *most* influenced the increased support for preparing nurses to meet the primary health needs of children?
   1. The increased demand for health care by the consumer.
   2. The increased number of health maintenance organizations.
   3. The increased number of associate degree programs preparing nurses.
   4. The increased emphasis on prevention rather than on the cure of disease.

453. Of the following health services, the one receiving *most* emphasis in well-child care within the past decade has been
   1. rehabilitation.
   2. health promotion.

3. disease detection.

4. disease prevention.

454. Many authorities believe that we become less judgmental of other people's behavior as we attempt to
   1. give up our values and learn to accept people as they are.
   2. recognize the origins of our own values and understand why we hold them.
   3. work purposefully to overlook other people's values that are contrary to our own.
   4. gradually work to change other's values when we consider them detrimental to their well-being.

455. A public health nurse works in an area where many of the children are from families whose cultural backgrounds are different from hers. Anthropologists generally agree that an undesirable aspect of ethnocentricism (preoccupation with one's own culture) is that it tends to
   1. produce cultural changes too rapidly.
   2. ignore hereditary influences on behavior.
   3. stand in the way of understanding people of other cultures.
   4. place too much emphasis on studying groups of people rather than on studying individuals.

456. The nuclear family is defined as consisting of
   1. mother and father.
   2. mother, father, and their children.
   3. the children of one set of parents.
   4. mother, father, their children, and the children's four grandparents.

answer sheet for nursing of children

Read each question in the examination carefully and select which one of the options is the *best* or *correct* answer. If the answer you would prefer is not given, select the one which seems *most appropriate*.

Locate on the answer sheet the number of the item you are answering. With a pencil, blacken the circle corresponding to the answer you have selected. Be sure you are recording your answer in the proper space.

	1 2 3 4		1 2 3 4		1 2 3 4		1 2 3 4
1	○○○○	18	○○○○	35	○○○○	52	○○○○
2	○○○○	19	○○○○	36	○○○○	53	○○○○
3	○○○○	20	○○○○	37	○○○○	54	○○○○
4	○○○○	21	○○○○	38	○○○○	55	○○○○
5	○○○○	22	○○○○	39	○○○○	56	○○○○
6	○○○○	23	○○○○	40	○○○○	57	○○○○
7	○○○○	24	○○○○	41	○○○○	58	○○○○
8	○○○○	25	○○○○	42	○○○○	59	○○○○
9	○○○○	26	○○○○	43	○○○○	60	○○○○
10	○○○○	27	○○○○	44	○○○○	61	○○○○
11	○○○○	28	○○○○	45	○○○○	62	○○○○
12	○○○○	29	○○○○	46	○○○○	63	○○○○
13	○○○○	30	○○○○	47	○○○○	64	○○○○
14	○○○○	31	○○○○	48	○○○○	65	○○○○
15	○○○○	32	○○○○	49	○○○○	66	○○○○
16	○○○○	33	○○○○	50	○○○○	67	○○○○
17	○○○○	34	○○○○	51	○○○○	68	○○○○

	1 2 3 4		1 2 3 4		1 2 3 4		1 2 3 4
69	○○○○	91	○○○○	113	○○○○	135	○○○○
70	○○○○	92	○○○○	114	○○○○	136	○○○○
71	○○○○	93	○○○○	115	○○○○	137	○○○○
72	○○○○	94	○○○○	116	○○○○	138	○○○○
73	○○○○	95	○○○○	117	○○○○	139	○○○○
74	○○○○	96	○○○○	118	○○○○	140	○○○○
75	○○○○	97	○○○○	119	○○○○	141	○○○○
76	○○○○	98	○○○○	120	○○○○	142	○○○○
77	○○○○	99	○○○○	121	○○○○	143	○○○○
78	○○○○	100	○○○○	122	○○○○	144	○○○○
79	○○○○	101	○○○○	123	○○○○	145	○○○○
80	○○○○	102	○○○○	124	○○○○	146	○○○○
81	○○○○	103	○○○○	125	○○○○	147	○○○○
82	○○○○	104	○○○○	126	○○○○	148	○○○○
83	○○○○	105	○○○○	127	○○○○	149	○○○○
84	○○○○	106	○○○○	128	○○○○	150	○○○○
85	○○○○	107	○○○○	129	○○○○	151	○○○○
86	○○○○	108	○○○○	130	○○○○	152	○○○○
87	○○○○	109	○○○○	131	○○○○	153	○○○○
88	○○○○	110	○○○○	132	○○○○	154	○○○○
89	○○○○	111	○○○○	133	○○○○	155	○○○○
90	○○○○	112	○○○○	134	○○○○	156	○○○○

2   nursing of children answer sheet

	1 2 3 4		1 2 3 4		1 2 3 4		1 2 3 4
157	○○○○	179	○○○○	201	○○○○	223	○○○○
158	○○○○	180	○○○○	202	○○○○	224	○○○○
159	○○○○	181	○○○○	203	○○○○	225	○○○○
160	○○○○	182	○○○○	204	○○○○	226	○○○○
161	○○○○	183	○○○○	205	○○○○	227	○○○○
162	○○○○	184	○○○○	206	○○○○	228	○○○○
163	○○○○	185	○○○○	207	○○○○	229	○○○○
164	○○○○	186	○○○○	208	○○○○	230	○○○○
165	○○○○	187	○○○○	209	○○○○	231	○○○○
166	○○○○	188	○○○○	210	○○○○	232	○○○○
167	○○○○	189	○○○○	211	○○○○	233	○○○○
168	○○○○	190	○○○○	212	○○○○	234	○○○○
169	○○○○	191	○○○○	213	○○○○	235	○○○○
170	○○○○	192	○○○○	214	○○○○	236	○○○○
171	○○○○	193	○○○○	215	○○○○	237	○○○○
172	○○○○	194	○○○○	216	○○○○	238	○○○○
173	○○○○	195	○○○○	217	○○○○	239	○○○○
174	○○○○	196	○○○○	218	○○○○	240	○○○○
175	○○○○	197	○○○○	219	○○○○	241	○○○○
176	○○○○	198	○○○○	220	○○○○	242	○○○○
177	○○○○	199	○○○○	221	○○○○	243	○○○○
178	○○○○	200	○○○○	222	○○○○	244	○○○○

	1 2 3 4		1 2 3 4		1 2 3 4		1 2 3 4
245	○○○○	267	○○○○	289	○○○○	311	○○○○
246	○○○○	268	○○○○	290	○○○○	312	○○○○
247	○○○○	269	○○○○	291	○○○○	313	○○○○
248	○○○○	270	○○○○	292	○○○○	314	○○○○
249	○○○○	271	○○○○	293	○○○○	315	○○○○
250	○○○○	272	○○○○	294	○○○○	316	○○○○
251	○○○○	273	○○○○	295	○○○○	317	○○○○
252	○○○○	274	○○○○	296	○○○○	318	○○○○
253	○○○○	275	○○○○	297	○○○○	319	○○○○
254	○○○○	276	○○○○	298	○○○○	320	○○○○
255	○○○○	277	○○○○	299	○○○○	321	○○○○
256	○○○○	278	○○○○	300	○○○○	322	○○○○
257	○○○○	279	○○○○	301	○○○○	323	○○○○
258	○○○○	280	○○○○	302	○○○○	324	○○○○
259	○○○○	281	○○○○	303	○○○○	325	○○○○
260	○○○○	282	○○○○	304	○○○○	326	○○○○
261	○○○○	283	○○○○	305	○○○○	327	○○○○
262	○○○○	284	○○○○	306	○○○○	328	○○○○
263	○○○○	285	○○○○	307	○○○○	329	○○○○
264	○○○○	286	○○○○	308	○○○○	330	○○○○
265	○○○○	287	○○○○	309	○○○○	331	○○○○
266	○○○○	288	○○○○	310	○○○○	332	○○○○

	1 2 3 4		1 2 3 4		1 2 3 4		1 2 3 4
333	○○○○	355	○○○○	377	○○○○	399	○○○○
334	○○○○	356	○○○○	378	○○○○	400	○○○○
335	○○○○	357	○○○○	379	○○○○	401	○○○○
336	○○○○	358	○○○○	480	○○○○	402	○○○○
337	○○○○	359	○○○○	381	○○○○	403	○○○○
338	○○○○	360	○○○○	382	○○○○	404	○○○○
339	○○○○	361	○○○○	383	○○○○	405	○○○○
340	○○○○	362	○○○○	384	○○○○	406	○○○○
341	○○○○	363	○○○○	385	○○○○	407	○○○○
342	○○○○	364	○○○○	386	○○○○	408	○○○○
343	○○○○	365	○○○○	387	○○○○	409	○○○○
344	○○○○	366	○○○○	388	○○○○	410	○○○○
345	○○○○	367	○○○○	389	○○○○	411	○○○○
346	○○○○	368	○○○○	390	○○○○	412	○○○○
347	○○○○	369	○○○○	391	○○○○	413	○○○○
348	○○○○	370	○○○○	392	○○○○	414	○○○○
349	○○○○	371	○○○○	393	○○○○	415	○○○○
350	○○○○	372	○○○○	394	○○○○	416	○○○○
351	○○○○	373	○○○○	395	○○○○	417	○○○○
352	○○○○	374	○○○○	396	○○○○	418	○○○○
353	○○○○	375	○○○○	397	○○○○	419	○○○○
354	○○○○	376	○○○○	398	○○○○	420	○○○○

	1 2 3 4		1 2 3 4		1 2 3 4		1 2 3 4
421	○○○○	430	○○○○	439	○○○○	448	○○○○
422	○○○○	431	○○○○	440	○○○○	449	○○○○
423	○○○○	432	○○○○	441	○○○○	450	○○○○
424	○○○○	433	○○○○	442	○○○○	451	○○○○
425	○○○○	434	○○○○	443	○○○○	452	○○○○
426	○○○○	435	○○○○	444	○○○○	453	○○○○
427	○○○○	436	○○○○	445	○○○○	454	○○○○
428	○○○○	437	○○○○	446	○○○○	455	○○○○
429	○○○○	438	○○○○	447	○○○○	456	○○○○

answer sheet for nursing of children

Read each question in the examination carefully and select which one of the options is the *best* or *correct* answer. If the answer you would prefer is not given, select the one which seems *most appropriate*.

Locate on the answer sheet the number of the item you are answering. With a pencil, blacken the circle corresponding to the answer you have selected. Be sure you are recording your answer in the proper space.

	1 2 3 4		1 2 3 4		1 2 3 4		1 2 3 4
1	○○○○	18	○○○○	35	○○○○	52	○○○○
2	○○○○	19	○○○○	36	○○○○	53	○○○○
3	○○○○	20	○○○○	37	○○○○	54	○○○○
4	○○○○	21	○○○○	38	○○○○	55	○○○○
5	○○○○	22	○○○○	39	○○○○	56	○○○○
6	○○○○	23	○○○○	40	○○○○	57	○○○○
7	○○○○	24	○○○○	41	○○○○	58	○○○○
8	○○○○	25	○○○○	42	○○○○	59	○○○○
9	○○○○	26	○○○○	43	○○○○	60	○○○○
10	○○○○	27	○○○○	44	○○○○	61	○○○○
11	○○○○	28	○○○○	45	○○○○	62	○○○○
12	○○○○	29	○○○○	46	○○○○	63	○○○○
13	○○○○	30	○○○○	47	○○○○	64	○○○○
14	○○○○	31	○○○○	48	○○○○	65	○○○○
15	○○○○	32	○○○○	49	○○○○	66	○○○○
16	○○○○	33	○○○○	50	○○○○	67	○○○○
17	○○○○	34	○○○○	51	○○○○	68	○○○○

	1 2 3 4		1 2 3 4		1 2 3 4		1 2 3 4
69	○○○○	91	○○○○	113	○○○○	135	○○○○
70	○○○○	92	○○○○	114	○○○○	136	○○○○
71	○○○○	93	○○○○	115	○○○○	137	○○○○
72	○○○○	94	○○○○	116	○○○○	138	○○○○
73	○○○○	95	○○○○	117	○○○○	139	○○○○
74	○○○○	96	○○○○	118	○○○○	140	○○○○
75	○○○○	97	○○○○	119	○○○○	141	○○○○
76	○○○○	98	○○○○	120	○○○○	142	○○○○
77	○○○○	99	○○○○	121	○○○○	143	○○○○
78	○○○○	100	○○○○	122	○○○○	144	○○○○
79	○○○○	101	○○○○	123	○○○○	145	○○○○
80	○○○○	102	○○○○	124	○○○○	146	○○○○
81	○○○○	103	○○○○	125	○○○○	147	○○○○
82	○○○○	104	○○○○	126	○○○○	148	○○○○
83	○○○○	105	○○○○	127	○○○○	149	○○○○
84	○○○○	106	○○○○	128	○○○○	150	○○○○
85	○○○○	107	○○○○	129	○○○○	151	○○○○
86	○○○○	108	○○○○	130	○○○○	152	○○○○
87	○○○○	109	○○○○	131	○○○○	153	○○○○
88	○○○○	110	○○○○	132	○○○○	154	○○○○
89	○○○○	111	○○○○	133	○○○○	155	○○○○
90	○○○○	112	○○○○	134	○○○○	156	○○○○

	1 2 3 4		1 2 3 4		1 2 3 4		1 2 3 4
157	○○○○	179	○○○○	201	○○○○	223	○○○○
158	○○○○	180	○○○○	202	○○○○	224	○○○○
159	○○○○	181	○○○○	203	○○○○	225	○○○○
160	○○○○	182	○○○○	204	○○○○	226	○○○○
161	○○○○	183	○○○○	205	○○○○	227	○○○○
162	○○○○	184	○○○○	206	○○○○	228	○○○○
163	○○○○	185	○○○○	207	○○○○	229	○○○○
164	○○○○	186	○○○○	208	○○○○	230	○○○○
165	○○○○	187	○○○○	209	○○○○	231	○○○○
166	○○○○	188	○○○○	210	○○○○	232	○○○○
167	○○○○	189	○○○○	211	○○○○	233	○○○○
168	○○○○	190	○○○○	212	○○○○	234	○○○○
169	○○○○	191	○○○○	213	○○○○	235	○○○○
170	○○○○	192	○○○○	214	○○○○	236	○○○○
171	○○○○	193	○○○○	215	○○○○	237	○○○○
172	○○○○	194	○○○○	216	○○○○	238	○○○○
173	○○○○	195	○○○○	217	○○○○	239	○○○○
174	○○○○	196	○○○○	218	○○○○	240	○○○○
175	○○○○	197	○○○○	219	○○○○	241	○○○○
176	○○○○	198	○○○○	220	○○○○	242	○○○○
177	○○○○	199	○○○○	221	○○○○	243	○○○○
178	○○○○	200	○○○○	222	○○○○	244	○○○○

	1 2 3 4		1 2 3 4		1 2 3 4		1 2 3 4
245	○○○○	267	○○○○	289	○○○○	311	○○○○
246	○○○○	268	○○○○	290	○○○○	312	○○○○
247	○○○○	269	○○○○	291	○○○○	313	○○○○
248	○○○○	270	○○○○	292	○○○○	314	○○○○
249	○○○○	271	○○○○	293	○○○○	315	○○○○
250	○○○○	272	○○○○	294	○○○○	316	○○○○
251	○○○○	273	○○○○	295	○○○○	317	○○○○
252	○○○○	274	○○○○	296	○○○○	318	○○○○
253	○○○○	275	○○○○	297	○○○○	319	○○○○
254	○○○○	276	○○○○	298	○○○○	320	○○○○
255	○○○○	277	○○○○	299	○○○○	321	○○○○
256	○○○○	278	○○○○	300	○○○○	322	○○○○
257	○○○○	279	○○○○	301	○○○○	323	○○○○
258	○○○○	280	○○○○	302	○○○○	324	○○○○
259	○○○○	281	○○○○	303	○○○○	325	○○○○
260	○○○○	282	○○○○	304	○○○○	326	○○○○
261	○○○○	283	○○○○	305	○○○○	327	○○○○
262	○○○○	284	○○○○	306	○○○○	328	○○○○
263	○○○○	285	○○○○	307	○○○○	329	○○○○
264	○○○○	286	○○○○	308	○○○○	330	○○○○
265	○○○○	287	○○○○	309	○○○○	331	○○○○
266	○○○○	288	○○○○	310	○○○○	332	○○○○

	1 2 3 4		1 2 3 4		1 2 3 4		1 2 3 4
333	○○○○	355	○○○○	377	○○○○	399	○○○○
334	○○○○	356	○○○○	378	○○○○	400	○○○○
335	○○○○	357	○○○○	379	○○○○	401	○○○○
336	○○○○	358	○○○○	480	○○○○	402	○○○○
337	○○○○	359	○○○○	381	○○○○	403	○○○○
338	○○○○	360	○○○○	382	○○○○	404	○○○○
339	○○○○	361	○○○○	383	○○○○	405	○○○○
340	○○○○	362	○○○○	384	○○○○	406	○○○○
341	○○○○	363	○○○○	385	○○○○	407	○○○○
342	○○○○	364	○○○○	386	○○○○	408	○○○○
343	○○○○	365	○○○○	387	○○○○	409	○○○○
344	○○○○	366	○○○○	388	○○○○	410	○○○○
345	○○○○	367	○○○○	389	○○○○	411	○○○○
346	○○○○	368	○○○○	390	○○○○	412	○○○○
347	○○○○	369	○○○○	391	○○○○	413	○○○○
348	○○○○	370	○○○○	392	○○○○	414	○○○○
349	○○○○	371	○○○○	393	○○○○	415	○○○○
350	○○○○	372	○○○○	394	○○○○	416	○○○○
351	○○○○	373	○○○○	395	○○○○	417	○○○○
352	○○○○	374	○○○○	396	○○○○	418	○○○○
353	○○○○	375	○○○○	397	○○○○	419	○○○○
354	○○○○	376	○○○○	398	○○○○	420	○○○○

	1 2 3 4		1 2 3 4		1 2 3 4		1 2 3 4
421	○○○○	430	○○○○	439	○○○○	448	○○○○
422	○○○○	431	○○○○	440	○○○○	449	○○○○
423	○○○○	432	○○○○	441	○○○○	450	○○○○
424	○○○○	433	○○○○	442	○○○○	451	○○○○
425	○○○○	434	○○○○	443	○○○○	452	○○○○
426	○○○○	435	○○○○	444	○○○○	453	○○○○
427	○○○○	436	○○○○	445	○○○○	454	○○○○
428	○○○○	437	○○○○	446	○○○○	455	○○○○
429	○○○○	438	○○○○	447	○○○○	456	○○○○

nursing of children examination

correct answers and rationales

TOMMY TAYLOR

1. 3. Of the options given, it would be best to show the parents pictures of children prior to and after corrective surgery. It is simply not enough to say that surgery will help when the parents are emotionally disturbed. Options 1 and 4 are not recommended as satisfactory since they offer the parents little if any support.

2. 2. It is important that this newborn have food and fluids. In order to feed him, methods for feeding will need to be adjusted to fit his needs. Infection in the mouth is uncommon and minimizing crying is of no particular help. There is no special need at this point to keep his fingers out of his mouth since this may upset him even further.

3. 1. With whatever method is used to feed an infant with a cleft palate and lip, the baby is likely to swallow large amounts of air. Hence, it is particularly important to bubble the infant frequently to help minimize regurgitation. Feeding him small amounts at a time is of no particular help. Actions described in options 3 and 4 are likely to cause the child to choke and aspirate.

4. 4. This infant must become accustomed to nasal breathing postoperatively. If he is having difficulty breathing, it would be best to open his mouth by placing downward pressure on his chin. In some instances, an airway is used routinely post-

operatively but when it is not in place, it is best to try pressure on the chin first. Options 1 and 2 describe actions that are likely to aggravate the situation.

5. 4. An early sign of respiratory distress in this infant is most likely to be difficulty with eating as he tires and has trouble breathing. Amount of crying and respiratory secretions are not good guides to assess that the child has respiratory problems. Abdominal breathing is a later sign.

6. 1. The most common cause of respiratory distress is the swelling of the tongue and nostrils, which is common after surgery has been performed in this area. Options 2, 3, and 4 do not describe common causes of respiratory distress.

7. 4. Of the methods given, a rubber-tipped medicine dropper has been found to be the most satisfactory method for feeding an infant that has had surgical repair of a cleft palate and lip. Gastric gavage and intravenous feedings are ordinarily not used. A large-holed nipple may cause the child to aspirate since feedings may enter the mouth too rapidly.

8. 3. Of the agents given, hydrogen peroxide is the agent of choice because of the effectiveness with which it bubbles and cleans the area.

9. 1. Optimal time for the surgical repair of the palate depends on many factors, but it is best when it can be done before speech development. Factors given in the other options are not ordinarily used to determine time of surgery.

10. 1. A cup is the preferred utensil for eating after the repair of a cleft palate. At the age when repair is done, the child is ordinarily able to drink from a cup and its use avoids having to place a utensil in the mouth where surgery has just been completed.

11. 1. The upright position is best since other positions are likely to cause the child to choke and aspirate fluid.

12. 2. In order to keep restraints at a minimum and still prevent the child from injuring the repair with his fingers and hands, the recommended type of restraint is elbow restraint.

13. 1. In order to offer this child the most emotional support, the mother should be encouraged to hold and cuddle the child. Options 2, 3, and 4 are not contraindicated but do not offer as much support.

14. 1. Of the conditions given, a speech defect is the most common problem following surgical repair of a cleft palate. Conditions given in options 2, 3, and 4 are uncommon if adequate care and support are given.

15. 3. The parents of children born with defects often have feelings of guilt and ask what they might have done (or should not have done) to have caused the condition. It is important to allow parents to express their feelings as being normal reactions. Actions described in options 1, 2, and 4 are generally of little help when offering emotional support in situations such as this.

16. 4. A characteristic sign of esophageal atresia is that the infant has excessive amounts of mucus in his mouth since the atresia does not allow mucus to enter the stomach. The other signs given here are not characteristic.

17. 3. Since the food has no way of entering the stomach, the infant with esophageal atresia will have projectile vomiting after eating. The other options do not describe typical signs.

18. 3. Gastric secretions enter the tracheobronchial tree by way of the defect and will cause aspiration into the lung. Options 1, 2, and 4 are not related to this phenomenon.

19. 4. In order to suction the upper pouch of the defect, the child should be on his back but with his head higher than the rest of the body. This position minimizes the chances of aspiration of pouch contents into the lungs.

20. 3. Substernal retractions are the most characteristic sign that suctioning the trachea is indicated.

21. 4. The humidity in the air helps decrease the viscosity of respiratory secretions. Low humidity air tends to cause drying of the membranes and secretions. Adding humidity to the air plays no role in factors described in other options.

22. 1. In order to prevent air from entering the chest cavity and causing collapse of the lung, it is most important to clamp the tubing with a hemostat immediately.

23. 1. The best way to prevent air from entering the stomach is to open the clamp after the formula has been placed in the syringe barrel. The other three options describe methods that will allow air to enter the stomach via the tubing.

24. 3. Giving the child a pacifier while feeding him by gavage allows normal sucking activity. Talking or singing would not be contraindicated. It is difficult to feed an infant by tube while holding him. It would be better to hold him before and/or after feeding. Stroking his abdomen may not be contraindicated but does not meet the child's need to suck.

25. 3. Helping meet this infant's psychological needs can be accomplished when the child is rocked after feeding him and he will

soon learn to associate eating with a pleasurable experience. Holding and rocking the child may accomplish goals described in other options but they are not primary goals in this instance.

26. 4. It is best to follow a care plan based on the principle that oral feedings following intubation are best planned in conjunction with observations of the child's behavior. Statements made in options 1, 2, and 3 have not been found to be of any particular help since they tend not to focus on the infant and his needs.

27. 4. The stricture decreases the passageway and the child coughs in an attempt to allow more air to enter the lungs. The mucus also increases and further blocks the passage and coughing occurs in an attempt to expectorate mucus. Other conditions may occur but they are not necessarily related to the stricture.

28. 2. Maternal polyhydramnios occurs in about 40 percent of children born with gastrointestinal tract anomalies, according to statistics.

POSTOPERATIVE CARE OF FOUR TODDLERS

29. 3. There tend to be fewer complications when surgery can be done on an elective basis since emergency situations are more likely to require some compromises in treatment and care. Explanations described in options 1, 2, and 4 have not been found to be significant.

30. 2. The most likely complication, if one develops, would be a wound infection. The complications in options 3 and 4 are rare, and sterility (option 1) has not been associated with hernia repair.

31. 4. The term described in this stem is incarceration. A rupture is a break opening an organ to its environment. Dehiscence refers to a splitting open and is often used to describe an opening of a surgical wound. Intussusception refers to a telescoping of the intestines.

32. 2. An 18-month old child will have difficulty describing symptoms and, hence, complications when appendicitis is present are more frequent than when older children or adults have the illness. Factors described in options 1, 3, and 4 have not been found to be accurate.

33. 2. For youngsters who have had an uncomplicated appendectomy, it is customary to start offering a diet as soon as the youngsters are retaining fluids.

34. 4. Baked custard is not considered a fluid. For purposes of

keeping intake records, the foods listed in options 1, 2, and 3 are considered liquids.

35. 2. When a child is bleeding following a tonsillectomy and adenoidectomy, he will swallow the blood. Hence, observing that a child is swallowing frequently is a typical sign of hemorrhage. The pulse rate will increase. Labored respirations are not associated with this complication. Reddish-brown saliva can be expected later since it is tinged with old blood.

36. 1. Most children tolerate milk poorly following anesthesia and surgery. The liquids described in options 2, 3, and 4 are much more likely to be tolerated than milk.

37. 2. The most common reason for failing when toilet training toddlers is that they are not ready for the training. Even with rewards and proper equipment, the child who is not ready for training will not learn voluntary control. Option 4 is possible but it is not the most common reason for problems.

38. 2. The eustachian tubes in a child are short and lie in a relatively horizontal position. This anatomical position favors the development of otitis media since it is easy for materials from the nasopharynx to enter the tubes. Also, a child's eustachian tubes are lined with cartilage that has not reached maturity so that the tubes are incapable of distending and opening appropriately. This too contributes to the incidence of otitis media.

39. 4. In a child, the auditory canals are almost straight. The recommended procedure for holding the earlobe is to pull it downward and backward to facilitate entry of the drops. In an adult, since the auditory canals are directed inward, forward, and down, the earlobe is pulled upward and backward.

40. 1. It has been found that a child subject to otitis media does better when a bedtime bottle is eliminated. This helps prevent material from entering the eustachian tubes. Options 2 and 3 are not recommended. Options 4 predisposes to otitis media since the blowing may cause material to enter the tubes.

41. 1. It is not particularly valuable to ask a small child about pain. He may not understand nor be able to describe what he feels. It is best to assess pain using methods described in options 2, 3, and 4.

42. 3. Most authorities recommend that a parent be allowed to assist. Poor cooperation is due to fright and the child will feel more secure with a parent present. Other methods may be necessary but trying to use the parent as an assistant is recommended as a first course of action.

SALLY HORNER

43. 4. A 5-year-old child often responds to explanations when given in language she understands. This child is demonstrating fear and expressing it as anger; calling another nurse is not likely to help. See item 42 concerning the role of a parent. Reprimanding a child who is fearful is unlikely to produce satisfactory results.

44. 4. If the child's fingers below the cast feel cool and appear bluish, the child should be seen by the physician promptly. These signs indicate poor circulation and if it continues, damage to tissue, including gangrene, can occur. The signs described in options 1, 2, and 3 are not grave in nature and the signs in option 4 are.

45. 2. This child's bones are still growing and a diet including sufficient amounts of iron, calcium, and vitamin D is important. Salt intake is not related to bone development.

46. 2. The reason healing occurs more quickly is that the bones of a child have a richer blood supply than that of an adult. Options 1, 3, and 4 are accurate statements about a child's bones but do not state the reason why bones heal relatively quickly.

47. 2. The stages of bone healing have been well described and they normally occur in a particular order. The order is described in option 2.

CINDY KARE

48. 3. Tetralogy of Fallot has four underlying pathological conditions: pulmonary stenosis, ventricular septal defect, dextroposition of the aorta, and right ventricular hypertrophy. The cause for cyanosis is the pulmonic valve stenosis. This part of the defect prevents blood from leaving the heart normally which results in poor blood oxygenation and underlies the cause of cyanosis.

49. 4. Of the foods given here, cheddar cheese has a high level of salt content. The other foods do not.

50. 1. As explained in item 48, the child with tetralogy of Fallot suffers from poorly oxygenated blood. This causes peripheral hypoxia which is believed responsible for the clubbing of fingers. The other three conditions are not related either to clubbing of the fingers or necessarily to tetralogy of Fallot.

51. 2. Chronic hypoxia causes the stimulation of red blood cell production and, hence, this child's hemoglobin and hematocrit levels may be expected to be above average values. None of the conditions described in options 1, 3, and 4 is likely to

contribute to this typical finding of the child with poor blood oxygenation.

52. 1. Children with tetralogy of Fallot soon learn that when they experience dyspnea, they will have relief by assuming the knee-chest position. The reason why this position affords relief is not understood.

53. 1. The best guide for the nurse to follow is to explain that the child will experience some pain when the catheter is introduced. It is a truthful statement and the child's trust will be quickly lost if the nurse's words prove to be wrong. Statements made in options 2, 3, and 4 are inaccurate statements concerning heart catheterization.

54. 2. An EKG records electrical activity in heart muscle. It does not determine information as described in options 1, 3, and 4.

55. 3. Before beginning teaching, the nurse should first learn what the child already knows. The child's interest will soon be lost if material with which she is well familiar is repeated. Options 1, 2, and 4 are still recommended but should be used after baseline information is obtained, as described in option 3.

56. 3. Hypothermia is frequently used when surgery on the heart is performed in order to decrease the body's metabolic rate. Hypothermia does not help accomplish goals described in options 1, 2, and 4.

57. 2. The first course of action when a chest tube becomes clogged is to attempt to dislodge debris by milking the tubing toward the drainage bottle—away from the chest. Irrigating the tubing may force debris into the chest cavity. Applying suction with a syringe is not likely to clear the debris from the tubing. Option 4 may become necessary as a last resort if the tube cannot be cleared.

58. 2. It is recommended that the child's urinary output should reach approximately 25 to 30 ml. per hour. Less than that amount suggests a complication that may require prompt therapy.

59. 1. Although techniques described in options 2, 3, and 4 may be necessary when cardiac arrest occurs, the first course of action should be to clear the patient's airway. If the airway is not clear, other measures will most likely prove to be futile.

60. 1. When pressure is applied to massage the heart during CPR, the sternum should be compressed. It, in turn, will cause pressure (massage) on the heart. For a child of 5 years, the pressure should be applied with the heel of one hand. The tips of the fingers are used for an infant.

61. 2. For a child of 5 years, 80 to 100 compressions per minute are recommended when CPR is being administered. For adults,

the recommended number of compressions per minute is 60.

62. 3. The carotid artery is recommended because it is nearest the operator, it is ordinarily easily accessible, and it will usually have a pulse when smaller, less central arteries may be pulseless.

63. 1. Regression is defined as the act of moving backward. In psychology, the term is used to describe a person who reverts to an earlier stage of acting or feeling. Depression is characterized by feelings of sadness, gloom, and "low spirits." Repression is a defense mechanism by which an unacceptable or painful experience is put out of the conscious mind. Rationalization is characterized by the person's making explanations and excuses for behavior.

64. 1. After being with a child that has not been well for 5 years and whose activities have had to be restricted, most parents will find it especially difficult to allow the child to lead a normal active life. Fears as described in options 2, 3, and 4 are least likely to be present.

BILLY WRIGHT

65. 3. Traction plays no role in helping to prevent infection in this child but is used for reasons given in options 1, 2, and 4.

66. 1. Countertraction when traction is applied in the manner described in the stem is obtained by the weight of the child's body. The other three factors will not serve to counteract the traction being applied through the use of weights.

67. 1. The weights used when traction is applied should be allowed to hang free. Actions described in options 2, 3, and 4 are contraindicated unless specific reason exists for doing so.

68. 3. Any number of symptoms have been observed in children suffering from child abuse, including those described in these four options. However, the most frequent finding is that the abused child will be underdeveloped for his age either from lack of an adequate diet or from lack of supportive parenting, or both.

69. 2. When researchers studied the parents of abused children, it was found that these parents frequently behave in ways described in options 1, 3, and 4. Participation in school activities has not been found to be related to child abuse.

70. 2. Evidence of child abuse is a reportable condition and hence, the nurse should report her findings to the designated authorities. Reporting such findings is a nursing responsibility.

71. 3. Statement B is false and statement A explains why: parents

learn their roles from their parents and, hence, a person with a history of being abused is also likely to abuse his children.

COMMON ACCIDENTS INVOLVING CHILDREN

72. 3. Although all factors described here may well play a role when a child ingests poisons, research has indicated that the most influential factor is the child's desire to imitate adults whom he has seen "pill popping" frequently and with apparent casualness.

73. 1. Drain cleaner usually contains lye. Hence, the mouth, pharynx, and esophagus may well be burned from the caustic effects of the lye. The nurse should be prepared to assist with a tracheostomy. Gastric lavage and emetics are contraindicated since they will tend to aggravate the situation and cause still more tissue injury. External cardiac massage is not indicated since lye does not poison by interfering with heart functioning.

74. 3. As the burn areas heal in the esophagus, scar tissue is most likely to cause strictures. Ulcers, varices, and diverticuli following ingestion of lye are not ordinarily seen.

75. 2. Methylprednisolone sodium succinate is an adrenocorticosteroid drug. It has been observed that drugs of this type are effective for relieving an inflammatory process which can be expected to be present at the site of this child's injury to mucous membranes.

76. 4. The salicylate ion in aspirin stimulates the respiratory center. The most frequently observed early sign of aspirin poisoning is deep, rapid respirations. Other signs may occur later, convulsions being one when the overdose is large.

77. 2. Emergency treatment of the child who has taken an overdose of aspirin is to induce vomiting and hence, an emetic is almost always given. Vomiting will stop absorption of drug removed from the stomach and it is not contraindicated since there has been no damage to tissues in the mouth, pharynx, and esophagus when aspirin is ingested. Other measures may need to be prescribed later.

78. 2. Of the complications given, pneumonia is the most common following ingestion of hydrocarbons. This is due to irritation from the hydrocarbon which has been aspirated or is being excreted via the lungs.

79. 1. Mushrooms do not irritate the mouth, pharynx, and esophagus and, hence, the mother should be told to induce vomiting in order to avoid continued absorption of mushrooms. Courses

of action given in the other options will not eliminate the danger of further absorption of a poison.

80. 2. The suggested course of action when a burn is present is to apply cool water to the area. This acts to reduce the temperature of the area and, hence, stops further tissue damage. Applying dressings or agents to the burn area is contraindicated and usually acts to aggravate the injury caused by the burn.

81. 1. Treatment of a child with lead poisoning is aimed toward getting lead out of tissues and especially brain tissues. The metal ions damage nervous system cells. Chelating agents are used which tie up the metal ions in the blood and tissues before they enter cells. The lead is then excreted from the body via the kidneys. Treatments described in options 2, 3, and 4 are ineffective for accomplishing the goal described above.

82. 1. The blood is examined to determine effectiveness of therapy. As the metal leaves the body via the kidneys, the blood will no longer distribute the metal to tissues and cells. Residual particles are removed from the bowel during therapy but blood examination is the best way to determine effectiveness of therapy.

83. 2. Neurological changes can be expected when lead poisoning goes untreated. Complications given in the other options are less likely to occur.

84. 1. There are many sources of lead in the environment, such as lead paint, ore smelters, contaminated dust, pottery, and lead found in paint used in printing. Lead is present in fumes of gasoline and in battery casings. However, most children who suffer with lead poisoning ingested it from eating paint containing lead. The paint may be on furniture or on walls.

85. 2. Education of the public concerning sources of lead that could cause poisoning has been found to be the most effective preventive measures. Condemning old housing developments has been insufficient—lead paint still exists in other dwellings. Education concerning good nutrition will not be an effective preventive measure. There is no agent for inoculating children against lead poisoning.

86. 3. It has been observed that children of school age are most fearful of being exposed due to increasing body awareness. This may occur at about 11 years of age. Other ages have concerns about body image but not to the extent of being unduly modest about exposure.

87. 4. In the event of a front end impact, the infant seat will be held securely by the seat belt and the child's head will be protected

by the back of the infant seat and the back of the car seat. The other positions offer less satisfactory positioning of an infant seat in the car. The infant seat may be tipped forward and the child's head and neck will be unprotected. If the infant seat is flat on the car seat, the seat belt is in an awkward position and the infant can slip out of both the seat and the belt.

88. 1. Falls account for nearly half of the accidental deaths that occur in the home. Scalds and burns rank second. Poisoning and asphyxiation occur less frequently than falls and burns.

89. 3. During the first year of life, deaths from choking with aspiration occur most frequently. Drowning and suffocation are rare with this age group as are motor vehicle accidents.

90. 4. Under 15 years of age, about 43 percent of all deaths are caused by accidents and about half of the deaths are caused by motor vehicle accidents.

SCREENING AND CARING FOR MUSCULOSKELETAL DISORDERS

91. 4. The left hand and the wrist are most often used to determine the physiological age of a child. There is a small bone near the left thumb which appears at preadolescence. Options 1 and 2 may be used but are costly and take more time.

92. 3. Extremity lengths should be made for objective comparison of the two legs. The measurement is taken between two bony prominences with the legs extended. The lower extremity landmarks are the crests of the anterior superior iliac spines and the medial malleoli of the ankles.

93. 4. The sternocleidomastoid muscle appears to be contracted when torticollis is present. The condition is often called "wry neck." It causes lateral inclination and a rotation of the head away from the midline of the body.

94. 2. There is no treatment for flat feet. However, corrective shoes are often prescribed in order to help keep the legs in proper alignment. Being pigeon-toed is not associated necessarily with flat feet and the shoes will not change weight bearing.

95. 1. The osteochondroses are a group of diseases affecting various parts of the body, the most common one of this group being Osgood-Schlatter disease. This disease involves the tibial tubercle.

96. 3. Supernumerary digits is called polydactyly. Zygoma is the name of the bone which bridges the temperal fossa. Polypodia refers to supernumerary feet. Zygodactyly is used to describe webbing between the fingers and toes.

97. 3. Muscular dystrophy is a genetically determined, sex-linked condition. The cause has not been associated with other

factors. It is a progressive degenerative disease of the skeletal muscles.

98. 4. Scoliosis, a hereditary condition, occurs about six times more often among girls than among boys and usually between approximately 8 and 15 years of age. Order of birth has not been demonstrated to influence the condition.

99. 2. The characteristic sign of scoliosis is having a hump of the shoulder blade which is due to the spinal curvature.

100. 2. The recommended position of the child while screening for scoliosis is to have the youngster bend forward at the waist while allowing the head and arms to fall freely. The hump then becomes noticeable. The child should be observed by the examiner from the anterior and posterior views.

101. 4. The Milwaukee brace extends from the pelvis to the occiput. It provides longitudinal traction and lateral pressure which helps to decrease the curvature. Children who for one reason or another cannot use the brace often require surgical procedures for correction of the curvature.

102. 4. Common procedure is to have the patient wear the brace at all times except while carrying out personal hygiene measures.

103. 4. Exercises are prescribed primarily in order to strengthen muscles that will help prevent curvature. Exercises are only effective for children with very minor scoliosis for reasons given in the other options.

104. 2. Recommended procedure is to have the child shampoo the hair while the brace is off and the youngster is showering. Dry shampoo is satisfactory as a short-time measure but ineffective for cleaning for long-term use. Procedures described in options 3 and 4 are awkward and unnecessary.

BOBBY WHITE

105. 2. The formula used to determine this child's requirements for fluids was 3 ml./Kg. of body weight times percent of burn, that is, 3 X 20 X 44 = 2640. Various formulas have been used to determine fluid needs; they serve as good guides but additional observations, especially blood volume estimates, should also be used in conjunction with the formula.

106. 2. It is generally recommended that half of the total amount of intravenous fluid prescribed for the burn victim be given in the first 8 hours. The remainder should be given over the next 16 hours. These amounts may vary, depending on the child's condition, but they serve as guides to health practitioners.

107. 1. Of the examinations given, the physician is most likely to study the child's hematocrit levels to estimate fluid replace-

ment requirements. If the hematocrit level decreases, the speed of giving intravenous fluids may be decreased. Hemoglobin examination may also be used and in the same manner as described above.

108. 1. The physician should be consulted in the situation described in this stem. If options 2 or 3 are used, the patient may receive the fluids too quickly and suffer with overload and water intoxication. If option 4 is followed, the patient may suffer for having had an insufficient amount of fluid.

109. 3. Water intoxication occurs when the kidneys are not excreting fluids and electrolytes properly, or, are conserving fluids and electrolytes. Water intoxication is not related to factors given in options 1, 2, and 4.

110. 2. Signs of water intoxication include muscular twitchings and tremors, apathy, loss of visual acuity, headaches, diarrhea, scanty urine production, and finally generalized seizures.

111. 3. Clostridium tetani have the unique property of surviving without the presence of air. They are gram positive, motile rods which produce extremely resistant endospores. They release an exotoxin which is potent and can be lethal.

112. 1. Since this child had been immunized previously, the nurse can anticipate that a toxoid will be used. Had he not been immunized, he would most probably receive immune globulin.

113. 2. Paralytic ileus occurs frequently following burns. Conditions described in options 1, 3, and 4 are unlikely to be prevented by withholding fluids and food.

114. 3. Accurate determination of the patient's intake and output can be a crucial factor in the care of a burn victim. Hence, to assure accuracy concerning output, it is common procedure to use an indwelling catheter. Keeping the bladder empty does not decrease the workload of the kidneys. An indwelling catheter prevents urinary retention and its use may make it easier to obtain specimens but these are not primary purposes for using the catheter.

115. 2. When a patient demonstrates an allergy to a drug, the nurse's first course of action should be to stop administering the drug. An allergic reaction can be serious! In some instances, patients must receive other drugs to relieve symptoms, histamine being one frequently used, but measures described in options 1, 3, and 4 are not indicated at this time. Oxygen should be readily available for emergency use if the patient's condition deteriorates.

116. 1. A skin rash is the most common sign when an allergic reaction

occurs following the use of ampicillin. A serum sickness type of reaction may also occur, often with arthritic joint pains, but this type of reaction is much less common than a skin rash.

117. 1. The reason for keeping this child flat in bed is to help avoid postural shock. Because of fluid losses, peripheral circulation and circulation to the head may become inadequate if the patient's head is elevated or the patient sits up. Nursing care should take into account conditions described in options 2, 3, and 4 and take measures to help avoid them. However, a flat position in bed will not necessarily help to avoid them.

118. 1. Mafenide acetate is a strong carbonic anhydrase inhibitor. It may adversely affect the blood's pH level. The condition that will result with the indiscriminate use of this agent is metabolic acidosis.

119. 4. Mafenide acetate therapy causes a burning sensation when applied. The discomfort can last as long as an hour in some patients. Silver nitrate, which is also used on burns, has the disadvantage of staining.

120. 1. Allowing the patient to participate by having him apply some of the ointment increases the child's self-esteem and helps him feel that he is in control. Option 2 is contraindicated since the therapy is important for his well-being. It may be advantageous to have a parent nearby to offer the child support and he should know it is all right for him to cry if he wishes. But these two measures will not accomplish the desired goal of helping him to feel in control.

121. 3. Staphylococcus organisms are spherical cells. They may occur singly or in pairs but most often, they appear in irregular clumps.

122. 1. Tissues taken from animal sources are called xenografts. Tissues taken from the same person are called autografts. Tissue taken from another person is called an allograft.

123. 4. The primary purpose for a xenograft is to cover the burn areas until other grafts are available. It will help to minimize the growth of granulation tissue. It may also help decrease discomfort and thus even promote movement but these are not primary reasons for using a xenograft.

124. 3. When splints are used, their primary purpose is to prevent contracture. They play no role in preventing conditions described in options 1, 2, and 4.

125. 4. Gloves are recommended to be used when any care is given. However, their effectiveness will be limited unless the gloves are changed after removing soiled dressings and before handling and applying new dressings.

126. 4. A sign of hemolysis is hemoglobinuria. The presence of hemolyzed red blood cells in the urine will cause the urine to appear dark brown.

127. 3. Hypoproteinemia is not uncommon following severe burns. Hence, the patient's diet should be high in protein content. The child will also almost always require a high caloric diet and one rich in iron to help prevent anemia.

128. 3. Of the fluids given, orange juice contains the highest amount of potassium.

129. 4. Measures described in options 1, 2, and 3 are recommended when a child loses interest in eating. Option 4 is a type of punishment and rarely meets with success.

130. 3. Hydrotherapy is frequently used in order to help prevent contractures, muscle atrophy, and infection. However, it plays no role in preventing calcium deposits.

131. 3. Elastic pantyhose help prevent venous stasis in the legs. Hence, their use will improve circulation to the legs and to grafted areas. Options 1, 2, and 4 are not related to the use of pantyhose.

132. 4. The percentage of body surface allocated to the head of a 5-year-old is 13; for an adult, it is 7. The percentage of body surface allocated to the lower extremities, including feet, for a 5-year-old is 33; for an adult, it is 30. The anterior and posterior trunks and the upper extremities, including the hands, are allocated the same percentage of body surface in adults and children.

133. 4. A disadvantage of using moist silver nitrate dressings is that there is a loss of electrolytes into the wet dressings which may cause an electrolyte imbalance if care is not taken.

134. 4. The first effect of a burn is to produce dilatation of capillaries and small vessels in the area, and capillary permeability increases. Plasma (fluid) seeps into the surrounding tissues to produce blisters and edema. The primary fluid shift, then, is from the vascular spaces to interstitial spaces.

135. 1. Persons severely burned are predisposed to many electrolyte imbalances, the most common ones during the first 48 hours being these: sodium deficit, potassium excess, and calcium deficit.

136. 1. When metabolic acidosis is present, the body attempts to rid itself of carbon dioxide. It can be noted by the nature of the patient's respirations which are characteristically deep and rapid.

137. 1. Stomach and duodenal ulcers occur relatively often when severe burns are present. These ulcers are called Curling's ulcers.

138. 2. Admission orders are most likely to include those described in options 1, 3, and 4. Ambulation for this patient can be expected to be encouraged to help prevent the complications associated with prolonged bed rest, such as skin breakdown and venous thrombosis.

139. 4. Of the signs given here, the nurse can anticipate that the patient's blood pressure will be elevated. This may be minimal if the disease is in early stages.

140. 4. Typical laboratory findings include an increased creatinine and BUN level. Both indicate destructive renal changes in progress. The BUN may be used as a guide for determining whether protein intake should be decreased in order to lower the amount of protein catabolic end products.

141. 1. When edema is present, plasma accumulates in interstitial spaces.

142. 1. In order to reduce edema in this patient's eyelids, it would be best to elevate the head of his bed. The force of gravity will tend to reduce the edema. Other measures described here will not influence this edema.

143. 1. Characteristically, as renal failure occurs, the patient will become lethargic and drowsy. Hypertension is almost always present. Options 2 and 4 are not likely. The cause for the lethargy is not clear but is believed related to uremic toxins.

144. 4. Vitamin D, along with increased intake of calcium, are pre-
145. 2. scribed for patients receiving dialysis therapy to minimize the risk of bone disease. The patient may become anemic due to inevitable blood loss associated with the procedure of dialysis; blood transfusions are most often prescribed for this.

146. 2. It has been found that the use of prednisone has been effective for treating many children with nephrotic syndrome. The reason for its effectiveness is not known but it is credited for reducing the mortality rate markedly.

147. 3. Because of its side effects which can be severe, cyclophosphamide will probably never replace prednisone. These are some of the most common side effects: decrease in white blood cell count and increased susceptability to infection; hair loss; cystitis from bladder irritation when the drug accumulates in the bladder prior to excretion; and sterility.

148. 1. There is altered glomerular permeability in the presence of nephrotic syndrome which results in the excretion of protein in the urine. The other symptoms are not characteristic of this syndrome.

SARA HOLT

149. 3. The most characteristic laboratory finding in a child with eczema is an elevated eosinophil count. Eosinophils engulf the bacteria (phagocytize) and contribute to body defense.

150. 1. Specific gravity is defined as the weight of a substance when compared with water. A specific gravity of 1.000 means the substance has the same weight as water. Amounts above 1.000 indicate the substance weighs more than water.

151. 1. See item 42. An infant of 9 months will not be comforted by action described in option 3. The child is not likely to be distracted by giving him formula and such action may cause the child to associate eating with an unpleasant experience.

152. 4. The most characteristic sign of eczema is itching. The skin is basically dry. Scratching often predisposes to skin breakdown and skin infections.

153. 2. Itching is intensified when the patient is warm and perspiring and when in contact with itchy clothing, such as wool. The best night garment would be a one-piece cotton garment; there is no elastic at the waist to irritate the skin and cotton is unlikely to be irritating and is cool. Nylon tends to be hot.

154. 4. Although the skin is dry, heavy oils, such as lanolin, are not recommended. Nor is an antiseptic soap. Normal saline does not have good cleansing ability. The best agent, of those given here, is the nonoily cleansing lotion.

BILLY CASPER

155. 2. During an acute attack of asthma, there is a narrowing and obstruction of the bronchi and bronchioles making breathing difficult. Since the obstruction for the flow of air is more marked during expiration, air tends to be trapped in the lungs and the child must use great effort to rid the lungs of air. This produces a characteristic wheeze on expiration.

156. 3. The characteristic color of expectorations of the patient with asthma is white. Complications are likely to be present if the expectorations are of a different color. Greenish and yellowish colors are common when infection is present.

157. 3. Cromolyn sodium plays no role in accomplishing options 1, 2, and 4. The drug is used to prevent attacks of asthma because it is believed it interferes with the release of histamine.

158. 3. Exposure to inhaled antigens are likely to bring on asthma attacks. Pets, such as those mentioned in options 1, 2, and 4, are common offenders. However, a fish would be appropriate for this child.

159. 1. Characteristic processes that occur during an acute attack of asthma are described in options 2, 3, and 4. The alveoli do not collapse but fill with trapped air.

JENNIFER STONE

160. 4. A child with sickle cell anemia in crisis almost always is in need of additional fluids for good hydration and, hence, it can be expected that intravenous fluids will be ordered.

161. 3. The characteristic sickle cell tends to "log jam" in the capillaries. This results in poor circulation to local tissue because of ischemia and necrosis. Options 1, 2, and 4 are inaccurate statements in relation to this disease.

162. 2. Jaundice is due to an accumulation of bilirubin in the blood. When sickle cell anemia is present, the bilirubin is elevated due to the release of hemoglobin when red blood cells destruct. Options 1, 3, and 4 do not play a role in this patient's jaundice.

163. 1. Children with sickle cell anemia are prone to infection which often will bring on a crisis. Hence, the parents should be taught to take extra precautions should an infection develop and do whatever is possible to prevent one.

164. 4. Sickling is more likely to occur where atmospheric pressure is low. Hence, mountainous areas and flying in nonpressurized planes are contraindicated. The areas described in options 1, 2, and 3 are not in themselves contraindicated unless they are in mountainous areas (options 1 and 3).

165. 4. The best explanation concerning freedom from symptoms for the first year of life for this child with sickle cell anemia is given in option 4. Some people are free until a crisis occurs, one precipitating factor being an infection. However, option 1 is less likely than option 4. Statements given in options 2 and 3 are not accurate in relation to this disease.

166. 1. Of those given here, the least likely condition a child with sickle cell anemia is likely to develop is hepatitis. Gallstones are likely to form because of the high bilirubin content in the blood. Local cell damage in the bones and kidneys accounts for a high incidence of osteomyelitis and kidney disease.

167. 2. A child with sickle cell anemia must receive a defective gene from both parents. If only one parent is a carrier, the child may be a carrier but will not have the disease. Fifty percent of the children of parents, both of whom are carriers, can be expected to have the disease.

168. 4. Sickle cell anemia is found almost entirely among blacks and Spanish-Americans.

169. 1. When sputum is ordered for culturing, the primary purpose is to determine what organism is causing an infection in the respiratory system. This patient has pneumonia and, hence, it becomes important to determine the causitive organism. Blood may be found in the sputum but this will be determined using methods other than cultures. Sputum cultures will not assist in accomplishing goals described in options 2 and 4.

170. 1. Isoproterenol hydrochloride is an adrenergic drug; it acts to relax and dilate the bronchial tree but plays no role in actions described in the other options.

171. 3. In order to avoid interfering with eating and in order to avoid the possibility of vomiting or regurgitating food, it is generally recommended that postural drainage be used about halfway between meals.

172. 2. Postural drainage uses the force of gravity to accomplish its goal. The position of the patient is such that debris will leave the respiratory passages with the assist of gravity. Postural drainage plays no role in accomplishing goals described in the other options.

173. 2. Diplococcus pneumoniae organisms can survive and produce disease only when their capsules are intact. Once the capsule is absent, the organism can be readily phagocytosed and destroyed. The organism is lancet shaped and is without spores, fibrils, and flagella.

174. 3. The primary reason for using the type of tent described here is to offer the patient humid air. This, in turn, will reduce the viscosity of her secretions.

175. 1. Oxygen is an essential of life. Hence, when a respiratory disease is present, the body will place first priority on obtaining oxygen by increasing the respiratory rate.

176. 1. Pancreatic enzymes are blocked when cystic fibrosis is present. These enzymes can then not enter the duodenum and are not available to break down ingested fat. Thus, the diet most frequently ordered for a patient with cystic fibrosis is one low in fat content.

177. 1. Poor digestion and absorption of fats result in stools that are frequent, bulky, greasy, and very foul smelling. Microscopic study often reveals excess fat droplets in the stool.

178. 2. For a 3-year-old, her favorite doll would be the best choice of toy among those given here. The doll provides support and is a familiar toy. A tricycle provides exercise that is too strenuous for this child. In view of lung pathology, a fuzzy stuffed

animal is not advised. Scissors, paper, and paste are not appropriate for a 3-year-old unless there is supervision present when used.

179. 3. The best course of action for this child's home care is to continue inhalations, percussion, and postural drainage. While the child should not exert herself to the point of fatigue, in general, children are encouraged to do as much as they can to improve ventilation. A cough suppressant is contraindicated since it is important to expectorate debris from the respiratory passages. Her medication dosage will not be altered according to the test given in option 4.

180. 3. The National Cystic Fibrosis Foundation assists parents of children with cystic fibrosis with educational materials. It is not organized to help with factors discussed in options 1, 2, and 4.

181. 4. A characteristic of cystic fibrosis is that excess amounts of salt are lost during perspiration. During warm weather or whenever the child perspires more than usual, salt supplements are almost always necessary. Options 1, 2, and 3 do not describe conditions related to cystic fibrosis.

182. 2. Twenty-five percent of the children of these parents are likely to develop cystic fibrosis. The disease is an autosomal recessive trait.

183. 3. Although some people with cystic fibrosis have survived beyond early adulthood, most do not. The prognosis for this disease remains unfavorable.

184. 1. The best definition of cystic fibrosis, among those given here, is that it is a disease of the glands of the body that secrete mucus. Statements in options 2, 3, and 4 do not accurately reflect the nature of this disease.

185. 2. The organs most often attacked by cystic fibrosis are the pancreas, lungs, liver, and salivary glands. The kidneys are not involved.

186. 4. Because of lung pathology, the right ventricle of the heart has extra work in order to produce sufficient pressure to carry blood from the heart to the lungs. This results in hypertrophy of the right ventricle.

STEVIE FIELD

187. 4. Normal blood sugar is approximately 80 to 120 mg. per 100 ml. of blood. In diabetic coma, the blood sugar level is elevated. Hence, of the blood sugar levels given, the one that would be most typical of diabetic coma is 350 mg. per 100 ml. of blood.

188. 1. When diabetic coma is present, glucose cannot be brought to cells because of lack of insulin. The body then draws upon fat

supplies for energy. The liver, to which fat supplies move, produces ketone bodies for catabolism by tissue cells. However, the liver may produce too many ketone bodies for the cells to catabolize and ketonosis results. Metabolic acidosis results when the rate of ketogenesis is so great that the pH of the blood falls below normal and the pCO_2 falls below normal.

189. 3. Therapy is ordered to help correct fluid and electrolyte imbalances. The blood glucose level for this patient is too high and stimulating the production of urine will not correct the underlying problem. Circulation is not at fault when diabetic acidosis is present.

190. 2. To produce prompt results, the insulin the physician is most likely to order is regular insulin. The other types of insulin given here are slower acting.

191. 1. Using ratios, the number of ml. is determined as follows:
10 units : X ml. :: 100 units : 1 ml.
$$100 X = 10, \text{ or } X = \frac{10}{100}, \text{ or } X = 1/10$$
0.1 ml. of 100 unit insulin will provide 10 units of insulin.

192. 4. The characteristic odor of the breath of a patient in diabetic coma is sweet which is due to acetone that is being excreted by the lungs. When fatty acids are converted to ketones, they accumulate in the blood (ketonemia) and are carried to the kidneys and to the lungs, as acetone, for excretion.

193. 1. The classic signs/symptoms of diabetes mellitus include weight loss, polyuria (in children, often resulting in bedwetting), polydipsia, polyphagia, and hyperglycemia.

194. 3. The best way to determine this patient's insulin needs following diabetic coma is to use blood samples which will be used to measure the amount of glucose and acetone present. Once the child is on his way to recovery, and insulin doses are more stabilized, urine samples will help to regulate insulin dosages.

195. 1. Tests to determine dosages of insulin are best done before meals and at bedtime when blood sugar levels should normally be lower than at other times in the day.

196. 4. Increased exercise stimulates the body to produce more insulin. Hence, exercise tends to reduce the body's needs for insulin. Factors given in options 1, 2, and 3 tend to increase the body's need for insulin.

197. 4. Insulin is rendered inactive by gastrointestinal juices and, hence, cannot be given by mouth.

198. 3. The least appropriate site is the forearm. Subcutaneous tissue in the forearms is sparse and, hence, areas of the body where subcutaneous tissue is more abundant are advised for the injection of insulin.

199. 2. A vial has a cap which makes the vial air tight. It is recommended that one should inject about the same amount of air into the vial as the amount of insulin to be withdrawn. If less or no air is injected, the vial will develop a partial vacuum, making removal of insulin difficult. If more air is injected than insulin is removed, the vial will have positive pressure. When a needle is then inserted, the pressure is likely to blow out the plunger or make it difficult to measure the amount of insulin desired.

200. 2. One piece of bread has been determined to be equivalent to one small baked potato. Exchange lists for foods for diabetic diets have been prepared by the American Diabetic Association (ADA). These exchange lists are widely used throughout the country.

201. 4. When acidosis is present, the body tries to compensate by taking extra efforts to rid itself of carbon dioxide. The patient will take deep, rapid respirations and breathe as though he is experiencing air hunger. This type of breathing is often referred to as Kussmaul's breathing.

202. 4. To establish the possibility of impending diabetic acidosis, the first course of action is to check the urine for sugar and acetone levels. If they are elevated, the patient should be prepared to take insulin. Taking sugar and withholding insulin are contraindicated and will aggravate the situation. It may be necessary to take a patient with impending diabetic acidosis to the emergency room of a hospital for care but the first course of action should be as described in option 4.

203. 2. Insulin shock is the result of hypoglycemia which often occurs if the patient has had too much insulin or insufficient food. It is best to relieve the symptoms by taking sugar, such as eating several cubes of sugar or drinking a glass of orange juice. Eating a piece of hard candy will accomplish the same thing. Increasing activity will aggravate the situation. Resting in bed will not alleviate the signs. The physician may need to be consulted if conservative care does not help.

204. 3. It would be inappropriate to suggest that this child should refrain from strenuous sports. Many diabetics lead completely normal lives and often do participate in strenuous sports. Suggestions offered in options 1, 2, and 4 are indicated.

205. 2. Diabetes mellitus is a disorder of carbohydrate metabolism. The cause is unknown. It is believed to be an inherited disease, although somewhat unpredictably. It is not related to the process of birth or to intrauterine influences.

206. 1. Insulin affects carbohydrate metabolism. It helps to decrease blood sugar levels but does not influence the rate of metabolism directly nor does it decrease the amount of stored sugar in the body.
207. 3. Diabetes mellitus cannot be cured and, hence, this child can be expected to need insulin and dietary adjustments throughout life. The severity of the disease cannot be decreased. Maturity-onset diabetes can often be controlled with oral hypoglycemics but diabetes that began during childhood will amost always require the use of insulin throughout life.
208. 1. The liver plays an important part in changing blood sugar levels. When the level falls, glycogen which is stored in the liver, is converted to glucose to enter the bloodstream. When the blood glucose level is above normal, it is not the liver that is at fault. The pancreas is the organ at fault when diabetes mellitus is present since insulin is not being produced in the pancreas in a normal manner.
209. 3. Insulin is more quickly absorbed and utilized when injected into subcutaneous tissue. Subcutaneous sites allow for more smooth, consistent rates of absorption and these tissues also lack sensitivity so the injections will not be unduly painful.

MIKE LANE

210. 3. Leukemia is a malignant type of disease characterized by a proliferation in immature white blood cells. It is not an infectious, inflammatory, or allergic disease.
211. 4. A typical manifestation of leukemia is the presence of anemia. Red blood cell precursors are decreased. The anemia starves body cells of needed oxygen with the resulting pallor and lethargy. Statements in options 1, 2, and 3 do not accurately describe this child's condition.
212. 2. See item 211.
213. 3. Twelve to 14 Gm. per 100 ml. of blood is a normal hemoglobin level for a 10-year-old. As an adult, it can be expected that values would be somewhat higher, normally about 14 to 18 Gm. per 100 ml. of blood.
214. 1. Normal white blood cells are markedly decreased and hence, a child with leukemia is subject to infections. Options 2, 3, and 4 do not accurately explain the cause for repeated infections.
215. 3. Megakaryocytes from which platelets derive are decreased when leukemia is present. Hence, platelet counts are low and the patient is subject to easy bruising. The other options do not play a role in this sign of leukemia.

216. 2. The only food that would not be recommended, among those given here, is food that is sugared. The sugar offers bacteria an excellent medium in which to grow. Since the patient's mouth is already sore, excessive sugar may only compound mouth problems.

217. 2. The mucous membranes of the mouth are easily damaged and may be ulcerated. Hence, it would be better to avoid using dental floss at this time to prevent the possibility of injury to gum tissues. Options 1, 3, and 4 are indicated care.

218. 1. A fork is contraindicated because of the danger of injuring mouth tissues. See item 217.

219. 3. Just as for an adult, this child's pulse rate can be expected to increase and his blood pressure will fall when bleeding is present. Option 3 describes these findings most accurately.

220. 3. The trauma of the needle and the drug when giving medications intramuscularly may be sufficient to cause bleeding in the area and injury to the tissues. Hence, option 3 is contraindicated. Options 1, 2, and 4 are indicated procedures.

221. 4. Although bone marrow specimens may be obtained from various sites, of the sites given here, the most commonly used one is the posterior iliac crest. The area is close to the body's surface and removed from vital organs. Also, the area is large in terms of being able to obtain a specimen easily.

222. 2. A lumbar puncture is performed to determine whether the central nervous system has been invaded by the disease. Reasons given in options 1, 3, and 4 are unlikely for this patient.

223. 2. Packed red cells are most often administered with isotonic saline solution because the packed cells are thick and the saline solution helps clear the tubes. Saline is closest to normal body fluid and may be used more safely if more packed cells are required.

224. 3. Packed cells are preferred over whole blood to avoid fluid overload.

225. 1. Using ratios, the number of tablets can be determined as follows:

1 tablet : 50 mg. :: X tablets : 75 mg.

$50X = 75$

$X = \dfrac{75}{50} = 1\frac{1}{2}$ tablets

226. 1. Toxic doses of mercaptopurine are most likely to produce nausea, vomiting, and diarrhea. The drug also tends to cause

bone marrow depression and, hence, observations of the blood count are important.

227. 2. The drug was administered intrathecally. This route is also called the intraspinal route. The drug is placed immediately under the skin when the intradermal route is used. It is placed directly into a joint when the intra-articular route is used.

228. 4. Toxicity affects the central nervous system. Blurred vision is one of the first toxic symptoms noted and usually the patient can readily help identify this early sign. Other symptoms may occur later.

229. 2. Folinic acid is the antidote used when patients display signs/symptoms of toxicity to methotrexate therapy.

230. 4. Antimetabolites have a chemical structure resembling various dietary substances that malignant cells need to grow. The drugs keep cancer cells from using natural nutrients in metabolic processes and hence, they interfere with the cellular growth and development of cancer cells.

231. 4. Antimetabolites are largely excreted via the kidneys and may damage kidney tissues when uric acid crystals are formed. In order to help avoid this complication, adequate fluid intake and alkalinization of the urine with sodium bicarbonate is essential.

232. 2. Allopurinol reduces the production of uric acid which lowers its level in the urine and blood. This helps prevent kidney damage from uric acid crystals. When administered, the patient should be encouraged to increase his fluid intake in order to promote good urinary output.

233. 2. The patient's parents are reported as being optimistic when the child is in remission. It has been found that parents are more grievous when optimism is followed by defeat and, hence, option 2 offers the nurse the best guide. Options 1, 3, and 4 have not necessarily been found to be true.

234. 2. Most patients are aware when their death appears imminent. The best policy is to answer the patient's questions honestly. When this is not done, patients tend to feel isolated and alone during their decline to death. Actions described in options 1, 3, and 4 are not recommended.

235. 4. Just as with the patient, it is best to answer relatives honestly. Suggestions offered in options 1, 2, and 3 avoid the issue and offer the parents no support.

236. 2. The nurse caring for terminally ill patients is better equipped to do so when she has worked out her own philosophy concerning death. Although experiences as described in the

other options may be helpful to assist the nurse in her thinking about death, of prime importance are her own feelings about life and death.

237. 4. Option 4 is the only accurate statement made here in relation to leukemia.

KELLY WALTER

238. 4. Thyroxin can cross the placental barrier and, hence, if the fetus has received an adequate supply, signs of hypothyroidism may not be present at the time of birth. Options 1, 2, and 3 are not accurate statements in relation to hypothyroidism.

239. 1. Dessicated thyroid acts as the hormone does and stimulates metabolism so that normal growth and development may be possible.

240. 1. Dessicated thyroid is administered orally. It can be crushed and offered with food, such as fruit.

241. 3. This child needs a high protein intake to foster the best possible growth and development.

242. 2. This infant's weight in relation to its length does not fall within normal average ranges.

243. 2. This infant's weight and length do not fall within normal average ranges.

244. 3. This statement is neither supported nor contradicted by the graph.

245. 3. The hallmark signs of cretinism that have not been effectively treated are mental retardation and poor physical development. The other conditions given here are not associated with hypothyroidism.

246. 3. Dwarfism is due to the hypofunction of the anterior lobe of the pituitary gland.

CHRIS LITTLE

247. 2. It is unlikely that this mother is expressing hostility toward health personnel but it is likely that factors given in options 1, 3, and 4 are present, any one or all of which often stand in the way of learning.

248. 3. It has been found that PKU is transmitted by an autosomal recessive gene.

249. 3. PKU involves abnormal amino acid metabolism. The liver fails to convert the amino acid phenylalanine to tyrosine by addition of a hydroxyl group. Hence, the diet should be directed toward keeping the phenylalanine at low levels.

250. 1. Milk has a good supply of phenylalanine and hence, the contraindicated food is cheese which is made from milk. The other foods given here are low in this substance.

251. 2. The ferric chloride solution combined with urine containing phenylpyruvic acid will produce a green color. Children with PKU have been observed to have a peculiar body odor but the urine has no distinguishing odor.

252. 3. The result of testing for PKU is likely to be negative unless the infant is receiving either formula or breast milk. A 12-hour-old infant is unlikely to be receiving either. This insufficiency of protein intake causes the false negative.

253. 4. The characteristic skin coloring of a child with PKU is light. The other options are not particularly characteristic of a child with PKU.

254. 1. The liver is the organ at fault. See item 249.

JULIE RITTER

255. 4. It is generally recommended that children with rubeola be kept in bed until the temperature returns to normal. In the past, longer bed rest was often used but this no longer is common practice.

256. 4. Immunoglobulin is ordinarily used for children who have been exposed to rubeola and have not had the disease. Vaccine is in wide use today and is given to children to protect them from the disease before they have already been exposed.

257. 3. The virus which causes rubeola is spread by respiratory secretions. The organism lives in the nose, mouth, and throat and their discharges. The virus also can be found in the eyes and their secretions.

258. 3. The incubation period for rubeola is between about 10 and 21 days. Rubeola is a highly communicable disease.

259. 2. The central task for the preschool child is to develop a sense of initiative versus guilt. Any environmental change may have a difficult effect on a child. Here, the sister is feeling less attention from her mother and is attempting to resolve the conflict.

260. 4. The characteristic that differentiates rubeola from other childhood diseases is the reddish spots with light centers on the mucosa of the mouth. They are called Koplik's spots.

261. 2. Most physicians recommend immunization against measles at about one year of age. Antibodies transmitted across the placenta from the mother are ordinarily still present until about that age.

262. 1. The causative organism for rubeola is a virus.

263. 3. If an individual has had rubella, there is no need to give the vaccine although it would not be harmful if given. Rubella usually is acquired once in a lifetime. If any acute infection is present or if pregnancy is suspected, vaccine should not be given.

BRIAN JONES

264. 2. The mother's decision was that she could not stay with the child because of her other responsibilities. In this situation, the nurse's best course of action is to support the mother and this can be done effectively with the comment described in option 2. Option 1 is critical of the mother and seems insensitive. Option 3 suggests the mother is not necessary, which is not true. The nurse seems to be telling the mother how to solve her dilemma without sufficient knowledge to warrant it in option 4.

265. 4. Gastroenteritis is spread from fecal matter. Hence, the precautions for this child are aimed at preventing contact with contaminated feces.

266. 2. An oven is recommended for an item such as a teddy bear. Steam and solutions are likely to ruin the toy. Sunlight will probably not be sufficiently effective.

267. 1. It is unnecessary to use a mask while caring for a child with gastroenteritis. The organisms are not spread by droplet infection.

268. 1. A difficulty in the control of an infection due to the Salmonella bacillus is that some persons become chronic carriers. Options 2, 3, and 4 are inaccurate statements in relation to the disease caused by the Salmonella bacillus.

269. 4. Of the possible sources given here, the only one which has not been found to spread Salmonella bacillus is tropical fish.

270. 3. In this state of dehydration, absence of tears is typical. The specific gravity of the urine is most likely to be elevated. Options 1 and 2 are not considered to be signs of dehydration.

271. 4. The number of drops the patient should receive each minute is determined as follows:

$$\frac{500 \text{ ml.}}{8 \text{ hrs.}} = 63 \text{ ml. approximately is to be infused each hour}$$

$$\frac{63 \text{ ml.} \times 60 \text{ (drop factor)}}{60 \text{ (minutes)}} = \frac{3780}{60} = 63$$

The number of drops to be infused each minute is about 62 to 63 drops.

272. 2. If the patient is to receive 500 ml. of fluid every eight hours, in every 24 hours, he should receive 1,500 ml.

$\frac{24}{8} = 3.$ $3 \times 500 = 1500$ ml.

273. 4. The loss of potassium is likely to be high since it is excreted in the stools in large quantities when the child has gastroenteritis. Hence, it is most likely that potassium will be added to the intravenous fluid. This procedure would be contraindicated if the child's renal functioning is poor because it would produce additional burden on the kidneys.

274. 4. The suggested restraint described in option 4 is the only safe procedure. It allows for movement, prevents the child from touching the tubing and needle, and prevents him from rolling over upon himself.

275. 3. The amount of solution in the bottle has least amount of influence on the rate of flow. Solution enters the body by force of gravity and, hence, the height of the solution bottle will influence rate. So also will the size of intravenous needle and the position of the needle in the vein. If the needle is resting near or on the wall of the vein, the flow will be slow or might stop entirely, even though the needle is in the vein.

276. 2. Crying indicates the child is upset and probably moves more quickly. Eating, dreaming, and urinating are usually associated with pleasurable feelings and the child is more relaxed and moves less.

277. 3. If fluids are introduced too rapidly, pulmonary congestion and edema are most likely to occur. The other conditions given here are not associated with rapid infusion of intravenous fluids.

278. 3. There is usually pulmonary congestion and venous engorgement. There is a backup or reflux engorgement of the upper trunk, and the neck veins will be engorged and distended as a result. The other signs appear later.

279. 2. When swelling occurs at the site of injection, the needle has very likely come out of the vein. The swelling occurs as the fluid goes into subcutaneous tissues. Signs described in options 1, 3, and 4 are not related to swelling at the site of injection.

280. 4. Option 4 describes why infants need more fluids in proportion to body weight than do older persons. Options 1, 2, and 3 are inaccurate statements.

281. 4. Yogurt is made with cultured organisms. The yogurt helps to establish normal flora in the gastrointestinal tract and is often

used for children who have diarrhea. It is easily tolerated and digested. For infants, it may be diluted with plain water.

282. 3. Cherry-flavored gelatin has been observed to appear red in the stool, due apparently to food coloring added to the gelatin which passes through the gastrointestinal tract unchanged. Rare meat is likely to result in a dark stool since the blood is digested before it leaves the body as waste. The strawberry and apple should be expected to digest normally, leaving the stool normal in color.

283. 3. This child's behavior is typical for his age and he is attempting to assert himself as an individual. The behavior does not illustrate disinterest nor is it inherited. This age (2 years) is too early to assess leadership qualities.

284. 3. Toddlers have difficulty coping with frustration but once their anger has been released, they usually quickly return to composure. To help conquer the tantrums, it is usually recommended that other ways be found for the child to expend his energy. Options 2 and 4 are likely to aggravate tantrums and to ignore the outbursts has avoided the problem without solving it.

285. 2. Regressive behavior is behavior that reverts to actions typical of an earlier age. Regressive behavior for a two-year-old is described in options 1, 3, and 4. Option 2 is normal behavior.

286. 3. It is best to accept regressive behavior for what it is—a coping mechanism being used by the child. Actions described in options 1, 2, and 4 are unlikely to help and may aggravate the behavior.

287. 1. A two year old is egocentric, self-loving, and deeply absorbed in his own self. Hence, when he plays in the company of others, the play is characteristically parallel play, that is, the child is in the company of others without actually participating in cooperative play.

KAREN SARDIN

288. 1. During the acute phase of rheumatic fever, every effort should be taken to reduce the work of the heart. Bed rest with limited activities is recommended to help attain that goal.

289. 1. Penicillin acts to kill—or destroy—organisms.

290. 3. Antiinflammatory therapy with salicylic acid (aspirin) is usually prescribed for the patient with rheumatic fever. An early sign of toxicity is ringing in the ears. The other signs/symptoms given here are not associated with aspirin toxicity.

291. 4. Antibodies that form to counteract enzymes produced by the causitive organism are usually present in high titers within

several weeks of an infection and are elevated when rheumatic fever is present.

292. 1. The health-illness continuum is based on the concept that there is no one point at which health or illness occurs. Both are relative and there is considerable range and latitude in what might be called illness or wellness. The continuum can be used for planning all patients' care plans, including this acutely ill child.

293. 3. Dr. Maslow built his theory on knowledge that needs motivate behavior. These needs fall into a characteristic order. Basic first is that the human being meet physiological needs. The remaining needs, according to this theory, are safety needs, belongingness and love needs, esteem needs, and self-actualization needs, in that order of highest to lowest.

294. 1. Of the signs given here, a heart murmur is most characteristic of carditis. The valves most often involved are the mitral and aortic.

295. 2. Digitalis preparations act to improve and strengthen the heartbeat. The drugs also act to slow the heart rate. Digitalis is not prescribed for reasons given in options 1, 3, and 4.

296. 3. The following method describes how the correct amount of medication is determined:

0.15 mg. : Xml. :: 0.05 mg. : 1 ml.

$0.05X = 0.15$

$X = \dfrac{0.15}{0.05} = 3$

The correct dosage will be contained in 3 ml. of the drug in solution.

297. 3. The position described helps relieve dyspnea. When arms are supported, they are less likely to rest on the abdomen and further restrict breathing capacity. The child's position should be changed at regular intervals to prevent joint stiffness and skin breakdown.

298. 3. Ecchymosis is defined in the stem. Cyanosis is a bluish coloring of the skin, most frequently due to poor blood oxygenation. Jaundice is a yellowing of the skin, most often due to an accumulation of bilirubin in the blood. Diaphoresis is excessive perspiration.

299. 3. The lymph nodes are characteristically enlarged when rheumatic fever is present. Enlargement of the mesenteric lymph nodes is likely to produce abdominal pain. The cause of the pain is unlikely to result from conditions described in options 1, 2, and 4.

300. 2. Pain will be best minimized by immobilizing the affected

joints. The other measures described here are likely to cause more pain.

301. 4. To help minimize the weight of bed clothing on painful joints, using a bed cradle is recommended. Supporting the body in good alignment and changing the patient's position are recommended but these nursing measures are not likely to relieve pain. Placing traction on the joints is not recommended.

302. 2. During the acute stage of illness, obtaining rest is of utmost importance. Therefore, playing with dolls and the activity such play involves would be the least desirable type of recreational diversion for this child. It is generally recommended that when bed rest is essential, programs of a violent or frightening nature on radio or television should also be avoided.

303. 2. The characteristic subcutaneous nodules associated with rheumatic fever are small, hard, painless, and moveable.

304. 1. In the presence of chorealike movements, this child should avoid trying to use a fork which may cause injury to the mouth and face with the tines of the fork.

305. 4. Rheumatic fever follows an infection, most often in the throat, caused by a beta-hemolytic streptococcus. It has been said that if every case of streptococcal sore throat was adequately cared for, rheumatic fever could probably be eliminated.

306. 4. The heart is the organ most often damaged following rheumatic fever. The American Heart Association is the agency of choice, of those given here, to help this child following hospitalization.

307. 2. The heart valves are functioning poorly when congestive heart failure accompanies rheumatic fever. See item 294 also.

308. 3. It has been observed that rheumatic fever occurs most often among older children and young adolescents who are of the lower socioeconomic group.

309. 3. Collagen is an albuminoid constituent of fibers of connective tissues. Rheumatic fever is a collagen disease because it is destructive of connective tissues.

MINDY TITUS

310. 2. To convert centigrade to Fahrenheit, multiply the centigrade temperature by 9/5 and add 32. Using this formula, the conversion is determined as follows:
$39 \times 9/5 = 70.2$
$70.2 + 32 = 102.2$

311. 2. The number of drops the patient should receive each minute is determined as follows:

$$\frac{500 \text{ ml.}}{12 \text{ hrs.}} = 41\text{-}42 \text{ ml. approximately to be infused each hour}$$

$$\frac{42 \text{ ml.} \times 60 \text{ (drop factor)}}{60 \text{ minutes}} = \frac{2520}{60} = 42 \text{ drops to be infused every minute}$$

312. 3. If specimens are obtained prior to reading the manometer when obtaining cerebrospinal fluid pressure, the reading is likely to be falsely low since the fluid removed for the specimens will reduce the pressure. Injecting a medication prior to the reading is likely to increase the pressure falsely. Options 1 and 2 would not ordinarily influence the pressure.

313. 3. Placing a patient on a firm mattress to help prevent decubitus ulcers is false reasoning since the firmness of the mattress may produce pressure and predispose to decubitus ulcers. Measures described in options 1, 2, and 4 are indicated.

314. 4. The most important reason for weighing an acutely ill child is to permit accurate calculation of drug dosages. Especially for children, weight serves to help determine dosages. Weighing is often used when edema is present; comparing weights indicates whether fluid is being lost or more is being retained. However, this was not a likely factor for this patient.

315. 4. Of the illnesses given here, pneumococcal meningitis is a likely complication of a middle ear infection. The other illnesses are not associated with the pneumococcal organism.

316. 4. Kernig's sign is positive when the response described in option 4 occurs. Option 1 describes the Moro response. Option 2 describes Brudzenski's sign; it is often seen when meningitis is present. Option 3 describes the Babinski response.

317. 4. During the time when the child is acutely ill and irritable, the patient is hypersensitive to loud noises and prefers to remain undisturbed. Extraneous noises should be kept at a minimum. The child should be bathed and spoken to and treatments must be carried out. However, they should be done with an air of calmness and with gentleness while avoiding unnecessary noise and sudden movements.

318. 3. One cause of seizure activity in a child with meningitis is increased intracranial pressure. The pulse rate tends to decrease. Dypsnea and deafness are not associated with seizure activity.

319. 2. Children of this patient's age (4 years) are concerned about an intact body and become fearful when there is a threat to the

body's integrity.   Allowing the child to participate as possible with some of the care helps to protect the child's image of an intact body.   Reasons for allowing participation with care as described in options 1, 3, and 4 are invalid.

320. 4. The typical sign of DIC is hemorrhagic skin rash.   When the condition occurs, it is important to report it; usual therapy includes an anticoagulant, such as heparin.

321. 3. Muscle rigidity may progress to spasms of the paraspinal muscles.   This causes the legs and head to draw backward and the child will ordinarily lie on his side to accommodate.   The position is referred to as the opisthotonic position.

322. 1. Mumps is the disease which most commonly predisposes to viral meningitis.

INFANTS AND CHILDREN WITH CHRONIC DIARRHEA

323. 4. Diarrhea is best defined on the basis of the stool's consistency which is usually liquid in nature.   Frequency of stool itself is not sufficient although patients with diarrhea commonly do have frequent stools.   The amount and color of stools do not differentiate.

324. 4. Carbohydrates are normally digested by salivary and pancreatic amylase and become disaccharides.   Malabsorption does not occur with the absence of amylase but does occur when the specific enzyme that splits disaccharides into components, such as fructose, glucose, and galactose, is absent.

325. 2. The stools contain both acid and sugar; it is the acid which tends to irritate the skin and cause it to break down.

326. 2. An infant with diarrhea due to an irritable colon rarely requires treatment.   The condition is self-limiting and tends to disappear spontaneously.   Options 1, 3, and 4 are inaccurate in relation to irritable colon in infants.

327. 1. Many authorities believe that of the practices given here, the one that contributes the most to skin breakdown is cleansing the area with soap that is inadequately rinsed away.   This same theory holds for adults whose skin breaks down in the presence of diarrhea.

328. 3. A baby with chronic diarrhea needs comforting and support. Experience has shown that the best way to offer the child comfort and support is to hold the infant and rock him.   An infant is very sensitive to touch.   Options 1, 2, and 4 do not provide for touch and the soothing influence of rocking.

329. 3. The heat lamp provides heat.   Heat increases the blood supply to damaged tissue and enhances healing.   Cold tends to act as a local anesthetic and initially causes vasoconstriction

(option 1). Heat may be relaxing but this is not the primary reason for using the heat lamp. Heat brings blood to the area because the heat causes vasodilatation (option 4).

330. 2. It is recommended that a heat lamp should be placed at least 12 inches from the skin surface. A 25-watt bulb is recommended. The bulb should be protected with a wire cage to help prevent burns when handling this piece of equipment.

331. 1. Although ulcerative colitis is a physical disorder, it is associated with emotional stress. Psychotherapy is often required in chronic cases. Factors given in options 2, 3, and 4 have not been found to bring on acute attacks of colitis— emotional stress is very likely to bring on an attack.

332. 1. Bleeding in the colon usually occurs during acute attacks. The child then is likely to develop anemia and may require iron supplements or, in more severe instances, blood transfusions. Dehydration is not often associated with the disease although if fluid intake is poor and the colitis severe, the youngster needs observation for signs of dehydration. Anorexia and heartburn do not ordinarily occur.

333. 1. Celiac disease is due to fat malabsorption.

334. 3. The malabsorption of fat in celiac disease typically leads to abdominal distention to the extent that it is common to note a protuberant abdomen. The signs described in options 1, 2, and 4 are not associated with celiac disease.

335. 1. Gluten is involved in the pathology of celiac disease. Grains, such as wheat, oats, and rye, are contraindicated in the diet. The offending gluten causes poor fat absorption in the intestinal tract.

336. 1. It is believed that celiac disease is inherited and it is a lifelong disease. When care is good, the severity of the disease can be limited.

337. 4. There is no reason why special precautions, such as boiling or soaking diapers in an antiseptic, should be necessary. The disease is not infectious. If reusable diapers are used, they should be well rinsed following washing in soap since soap remaining in the diapers is irritating to the skin.

COMMON CHILDHOOD PROBLEMS RELATED TO HEALTH

338. 1. The most characteristic symptom of head lice is severe itching. Itching is also present when lice infect other parts of the body. Scratch marks can almost always be found when lice are present.

339. 3. Lice are spread by personal contact or by infested articles of clothing. Head lice are more common among school children

because of their close contact with each other. The statements in options 1, 2, and 4 are inaccurate.

340. 1. The nits of lice have a sticky coating which eventually dries. They are resistant to treatment and, hence, although the lice may have been destroyed, the nits may survive. Nits hatch in about one week's time. Preparations that are advertised as being capable of destroying nits are now on the market.

341. 2. Ringworm of the scalp is caused by a fungus. The fungus is grouped under the name of dermatophytes.

342. 4. Sterilized stocking caps are worn to prevent the spread of infected hair follicles. Measures described in options 1, 2, and 3 are not as effective for preventing spread.

343. 4. Griseofulvin is an antifungal antibiotic. The medication should be taken as prescribed since the agent will be ineffective unless a therapeutic level is maintained in the bloodstream. This same principle applies to the use of other drugs as well. Options 1, 2, and 3 do not offer satisfactory explanations concerning why it is important to take the drug exactly as prescribed.

344. 2. Pinworms live in and about the anus. Although pinworms can be spread by food and water contaminated with pinworm, the most frequent manner in which it is spread is with hands that become infested during toileting.

345. 2. Trichinosis is one of the roundworms. Embryo of the parasite, Trichinella spiralis, become encysted in the muscle fibers of infected pigs. Thorough cooking of pork destroys the parasite. Tularemia is spread to man from rodents through the bite of a fly. Paratyphoid is caused by a bacillus. Bacillary dysentery is caused by the Shigella organism.

346. 3. Water is usually the culprit for spreading typhoid fever. Typhus is spread through insect bites. Brucellosis (undulant fever) is spread by cow's milk. Poliomyelitis is most probably spread through respiratory secretions.

347. 3. There are two types of immunity: natural and acquired. A natural immunity is inherited. An acquired immunity is developed either actively or passively. An active acquired immunity results when an individual has immunity because he has had the disease. An artificially acquired immunity results from an injection of antibodies or vaccines.

348. 1. When a vaccine is used, the person develops a mild form of the disease which stimulates his body to develop an immunity. It has been found that when pregnant women have rubella early in pregnancy, the fetus may be deformed. Hence, after puberty, vaccine is rarely used because if the girl is pregnant, (she

may not know that she is), the danger for the fetus is serious. Options 2, 3, and 4 are inaccurate statements in relation to rubella vaccine.

349. 2. The lesions of acne are caused by plugging of the pores which eventually become infected. During adolescence, the skin produces more oil than usual. The best suggestion to give parents concerning the care of a child with acne is to recommend that the affected areas be washed frequently with soap and water. Lotions and creams tend to aggravate an already oily skin. Hydrogen peroxide has not been found to be an effective skin cleanser. Astringents, which tend to close pores, may be used after cleaning with soap and water.

350. 4. Many physicians are recommending the use of immunological products to help decrease the severity of mumps. Agents given in options 1, 2, and 3 are not used except in situations when a complication may have occurred. Mumps can be a serious disease—it predisposes to meningitis.

351. 1. The male may develop orchitis following mumps. Despite common opinion, sterility occurs rarely following orchitis.

352. 1. If sterility does develop following orchitis, the tissue damage will be in the testes where sperm are produced.

353. 1. Chickenpox is caused by a virus. It is a highly contagious disease spread through the respiratory tract.

354. 2. The lesion of chickenpox first appears as a macule but the mature pox is a vesicle with a red areola. Pustules may develop when the pox becomes infected; this occurs most commonly when the vesicle has been scratched. Itching is a common annoying symptom of the disease.

355. 3. See item 354.

356. 2. Infectious mononucleosis is characterized by swollen lymph nodes. Other typical signs/symptoms include a sore throat and fever.

357. 1. Although various procedures have been used in the past when a person had mononucleosis, at the present time, most authorities agree that no particular precautionary measures are necessary.

358. 4. A positive tuberculin test signifies only that the person has been infected with tubercle bacilli. However, the person may not have clinical evidence of the disease even though he may have been infected with the organism.

359. 2. Although other vectors are capable of spreading tuberculosis, it is most commonly spread by droplet nuclei and inhaled into the respiratory tract.

360. 2. Of the drugs given, the one used specifically for the treatment

of tuberculosis is isoniazid. It is commonly administered with aminosalicylic acid or streptomycin.

361. 1. Although measures described in options 2, 3, and 4 are important in controlling the incidence of tuberculosis, public health measures are most often directed toward case finding. The disease is infectious but with the use of drugs, it can be controlled and "cured" with relative ease.

362. 1. Syphilis is a relatively easy disease to treat. The drug of choice is penicillin. Options 2, 3, and 4 are true statements in relation to syphilis.

363. 3. The causitive organism for syphilis is Treponema pallidum. It is a spirochete.

364. 3. Gonorrhea is often referred to by lay persons as "clap." It is also called "whites," "drips," "strain," and "dose."

365. 2. Public health measures are most often directed toward locating sources. When a person is diagnosed as having a venereal disease, an important responsibility is to learn of all of the person's sexual contacts and urge contacts to have treatment. Although venereal diseases are prevalent, mass screening is impractical. Isolating persons, once they have therapy, is unnecessary. Treatment is important but for effective control, all contacts should also be treated.

366. 4. Although other measures have helped decrease the incidence of diphtheria, the measure which is credited as being most responsible for the marked decrease in the disease is immunization.

367. 3. Hemophilia is transmitted by a sex-linked recessive gene and carried by the female chromosome to males.

368. 2. Hemophilia is a bleeding disorder due to faulty coagulation of blood. Breaks in the skin can lead to serious bleeding. Hence, once a wound is cleansed, pressure should be applied to help stop the bleeding. Other measures are less effective (option 1) or contraindicated (options 3 and 4).

369. 3. Aspirin affects platelet formation and prolongs the bleeding time and, hence, is contraindicated.

370. 3. A child with 20/60 vision is seeing at 20 feet what he should be seeing at 60 feet. 20/200 is considered the boundary of legal blindness.

371. 1. When vomiting is induced after the ingestion of kerosene, there is danger of aspirating the kerosene and the local irritating effects predispose to pneumonia. Complications described in options 2, 3, and 4 are not likely to occur.

372. 1. Children between 6 and 12 years of age have a slower growth rate than either younger children or adolescents. Hence,

their food requirements are comparatively smaller.

373. 3. Children are most likely to be influenced by examples and the atmosphere provided by parents, although at times, they may be influenced some by their peers. It has been found that coaxing and badgering children to eat is most likely to aggravate the situation when eating habits are poor.

374. 2. Water soluble vitamins are not stored by the body. They include vitamins B and C. Fat soluble vitamins (A, D, E, and K) can be stored by the body.

375. 2. Stuttering has been found to be the most common speech disorder in children over four years of age. The problem usually requires some type of therapy because of the psychological tension the condition causes.

376. 4. Enuresis can be related to conditions described in options 1, 2, and 3 but is not associated with a permissive home environment.

377. 2. At the age of 2, the child becomes more mobile and is beginning to assert his independence. By this time, he has acquired some sense of independence and hence, option 1 is not entirely correct. The child is curious and begins to explore and this is normal behavior.

378. 2. It is generally recommended that the child be taken to the school so that he may become oriented to the school's physical environment. Older siblings are likely to put the younger child down and option 3 is generally ill-advised. The child may not ask questions because of his fears and so preparation as described in option 4 cannot be accomplished effectively.

379. 1. The child about to enter school has experienced great security in his home environment. He now must enter an entirely new world and hence, unhappiness results most commonly from feelings of insecurity. Options 2, 3, and 4 do not describe typical conditions for the child about to enter school.

380. 2. When the child enters school, he also enters a wider social world. Skills must be sufficiently well developed in order to free the child to interact with other children and to begin to acquire new knowledges and skills. Other options are important but are not specifically related to feelings of inadequacy.

381. 1. Giving a child increasing amounts of responsibility and opportunities to accept the consequences are most likely to develop a sense of industry and success. Of the tasks described here, having the youngster bake a premixed cake could best accomplish these goals. Picking up after baby brother is likely to be interpreted as a put-down and does not offer a good experience for self-esteem. Repairing a record player is likely to be too

complicated for a 9-year-old girl and could end in frustration and a feeling of defeat. Having an older sibling act as the supervisor will not usually foster a sense of success and independent action.

382. 3. Democratic guidance protects self-esteem and adaptive capacity. Hence, it would be best to deny the privilege of watching television until the policy has been modified. Options 1 and 2 do not foster decision-making on a cooperative basis. Option 4 offers no relief and could cause friction and hard feelings between the 12 year old and parents.

383. 3. According to Erikson's theory, the central problem confronting adolescents is establishing a sense of identity. The core problem of young adulthood is concerned with intimacy. School age children (6 to 13 years of age) are concerned with industry and preschool children, with initiative.

384. 3. Girls experience the onset of adolescence approximately one to two years earlier than boys. The reason for this phenomenon is not understood. Options 1, 2, and 4 are inaccurate.

385. 1. The typical statement of a normal adolescent in the United States is expressed in option 1. Most children of this age are in the process of discovering themselves and do not know where they wish to go in life. Teenagers prefer peers to parents or being alone. These youngsters do not want to be different and strive to be like their peers.

386. 1. Of the proverbs given here, the one that is likely to cause the most problems between teenagers and parents is the proverb quoted in option 1. Teenagers are generally quick to note when parents "preach" one thing but do another. The other proverbs are less likely to cause conflicts.

SHAWN BAXTER

387. 4. This premature infant is likely to display all signs except numerous creases on the soles of the feet. Prior to 36 weeks of gestation, there is likely to be only one sole crease but by 39 weeks of gestation, the soles of the feet are normally covered with creases.

388. 2. Acidosis in premature infants is common due to pulmonary vasoconstriction which increases the degree of hypoxia. Due to immaturity of the respiratory system, the oxygen and carbon dioxide exchange may be hampered and periods of apnea occur.

389. 1. Administering bicarbonate increases the level of the blood's pH. It will have no effect on factors described in options 2, 3, and 4.

390. 2. Of the procedures given here, the best one is to observe the

catheter after it is in place to see whether air bubbles occur. If they do, the catheter is most likely not in the stomach but in the trachea. The catheter can be introduced the desired length and still not be in the stomach (option 1). The water will return if the catheter is in the stomach but if it does not, the water would be introduced into respiratory passages (option 3). Action described in option 4 is not a recommended procedure for determining where the catheter has been placed.

391. 3. The best method for determining distention is to measure the circumference of the abdomen. Obtaining weight will not help to determine distention. Palpating the abdomen is not dependable. Observing for abdominal spread is also not accurate nor a dependable method.

392. 4. The indiscriminate use of oxygen for this premature infant is likely to cause retrolental fibroplasia. The condition often results in blindness.

393. 4. While comfort is of concern when administering treatments, it is of less significance than measures described in options 1, 2, and 3, all of which are highly recommended when caring for a premature infant.

394. 2. The best way to determine whether the lung has reexpanded is by x-ray examination. The other methods are less accurate when making this type of assessment.

395. 1. The best procedure is to allow the parents to see and touch their premature infant. Option 2 is not likely to give support to the same degree. If parents are fearful, their fears may be aggravated by action described in option 3. Also, their skills may not make it advisable to have them assist with the infant's care. Explaining that fear is needless ignores the problem at hand and offers no support.

396. 1. An early sign of aspiration is choking. Cyanosis is likely to occur later. Lethargy is unusual; the choking infant tends to become restless. Abdominal breathing is not associated with choking.

397. 2. Authorities hold to the opinion that the single most effective way to control the spread of infections is to have personnel use frequent hand and arm washing techniques, even though no one would deny that practices mentioned in options 1, 3, and 4 are important too.

398. 2. The most recent definition of a premature infant is one born at less than 39 weeks of gestation. Birth weight and stage of development have been found to be unsatisfactory guides in determining prematurity since many factors can influence growth in utero.

399. 3. Hyaline membrane disease is also called surfactant deficiency

or progressive neonatal atelectasis. Surfactant which lines the alveoli is deficient and the alveoli tend to collapse or become atelectic. Factors given in the other options do not appear involved in the presence of hyaline membrane disease.

400. 1. When cerebral palsy is present, the damage has occurred in the brain. It is a nonprogressive neurological disorder characterized by lack of uniformity in terms of signs and severity. About one-third of children with cerebral palsy are mentally retarded.

401. 1. The best objective is to set goals for the child with cerebral palsy that are consistent with his capabilities. Capabilities vary widely among children so afflicted and, hence, each child requires individual evaluation. Options 2, 3, and 4 are not necessarily required, desirable, or practical.

TIMMY LEE

402. 3. Readiness for weaning is usually present when the child begins to shorten his feeding time. He will be showing independence and will be ready to take a cup and learn a new skill. The child ready for weaning may also demonstrate behavior described in options 1, 2, and 4 but these behaviors in themselves are not necessarily evidence of readiness for weaning.

403. 4. Starting an infant on solid foods is a new experience and requires new skills. It is typical for the infant to spit out foods because he has not learned how to swallow them. Also, he is hungry and is used to having milk to satisfy his hunger. It is generally recommended that the infant be given at least some milk first and then offered solids. If his hunger has been satisfied by taking all of the milk, he will be less interested in learning to accept solid foods. Options 1, 2, and 3 have not been found to be satisfactory when helping an infant learn to eat solid foods.

404. 1. A 4-month-old infant is not normally able to sit without support, but will normally display behavior described in options 2, 3, and 4. It is normal to expect a child of 7 or 8 months to be able to sit without support.

405. 4. Most physicians recommend that during the first 6 months of life the child should be immunized for DPT and for poliomyelitis. Protection from measles and mumps is recommended at about 1 year of age and a tuberculin test is also recommended then.

406. 3. The anterior fontanel normally closes at about 12 to 18 months of age. The posterior fontanel normally closes when the infant is between approximately 6 and 8 weeks of age.

407. 3. "Cradle cap" is a mild form of seborrheic dermatitis. The sebacious glands are involved and there are greasy scales on the scalp. The condition usually clears spontaneously by about one year of age.

408. 3. The treatment for "cradle cap" consists of softening it and then removing it with a shampoo. Methods described in options 1, 2, and 4 are not ordinarily recommended.

409. 3. The DDST measures a child's social and physical abilities. It is not designed to measure intelligence and emotional development nor does it measure predisposition to illnesses.

410. 1. Orange juice which is rich in vitamin C helps prevent scurvy. Rickets results when a child has an inadequate intake of vitamin D. Vitamin B_1 (thiamine chloride) is the antiberiberi vitamin. Pellagra is likely to develop when the intake of niacin (nicotinic acid) is inadequate.

DEVELOPMENTAL TASKS OF CHILDREN AND YOUTH

411. 4. The infant receives cues from the environment which stimulate a deep body sensitivity and he responds in terms of internal needs. The infant is generally uninterested in the external world through his own body. During the creeping stage, he is likely to begin play with toes and genitals.

412. 4. Normally, a baby 1 month old will turn his head from side to side when lying on his abdomen. A 2- to 3-month-old baby will smile and laugh aloud. A 4-month-old baby can be expected to roll from his back to his side. A 5- to 6-month-old baby will hold a rattle for a brief period of time.

413. 2. According to behaviors described, this baby can be expected to be about 4 months old.

414. 3. Normally, a 9-month-old infant will not be able to put his arm through a sleeve while being dressed but will be able to carry out activity described in options 1, 2, and 4. He will be between approximately 2 and 3 years old before being able to put an arm through a sleeve.

415. 2. Of the activities given here, the most typical of an 18-month-old child is being able to pull toys behind him. Activities described in options 1, 3, and 4 occur later.

416. 2. A 3-year-old child can be expected to carry out activity described in options 1, 3, and 4 but he will not be able to tie his own shoelaces until about age 4 or 5 years.

417. 2. An emotionally tense child with pent-up hostilities needs a physical activity that will release energy and frustrations. Having him pound on a peg board offers him this opportunity. Options 1, and 3 suggest play activity that requires

concentration and fine movements. This is likely to aggravate the situation. Having a story read to him allows no opportunity to express emotions and has the child playing a passive role.

418. 1. The major fear of a preschooler is fear of bodily mutilation or harm. Infants and toddlers fear most being separated from mother. School age children fear most for their loss of self-control.

419. 2. Of the activities given here, television would be considered least therapeutic. It requires no imagination and does not provide opportunities for self-expression nor interaction with people, objects, and environment.

420. 2. Drawing, writing, and even doodling are expressive and the nurse could use the products of a school age child's drawings best as a communication vehicle. Option 1 and 3 do not offer the child opportunities for free expression. Option 4 is likely to be challenging and a fearful experience.

421. 4. While teenagers may enjoy all activities listed here, most are at that time in age when a record player and records are most appealing.

422. 4. Late adolescence and young adulthood persons are normally concerned with establishing lasting relationships with members of the opposite sex. Activity described in option 1 normally occurs earlier in childhood, as does establishing relationships with own-sex friends. Separation from family begins early in adolescence and continues but it is not the central concern of the age.

MISCELLANEOUS ITEMS

423. 4. Suspending the newborn by the feet allows the aspirated formula to drain from the lungs. After feeding, the newborn should be placed on his right side or on his abdomen so that if he vomits, the material will drain from the mouth. The airway should be cleared first prior to initiating further treatment.

424. 1. Investigations have illustrated that children with pica almost always have an iron deficiency.

425. 2. The thymus gland has been found to play an important role in the development of immunological competence. Its function is not related to factors described in the other three options.

426. 1. One grain is a measure of weight in the apothecary system. It is equivalent to 0.064 Gm. or 0.06 Gm. A milligram is one-thousandth of a gram and equivalent to about 1/65 of a grain.

427. 4. The autistic child withdraws, even to the point of failing to respond to his mother. It has been said that autism is charac-

terized by the "desire for the preservation of sameness."

428. 4. Although many theories have been advanced concerning the cause of SIDS, no single etiological factor has been confirmed to date.

429. 3. The stricken parents should be given opportunities to express their feelings about the death. A nurse has feelings too; option 1 does not necessarily help the parents and if the nurse shows no feelings when they are there, the parents may interpret her as cold and heartless. The physician should be reinforced as indicated but someone else's word is not particularly helpful at this point. It is up to the parents to decide whether they wish to view the body.

430. 1. In a situation such as this, it is best to consult with the family's clergyman. Giving the transfusion without parenteral consent may have legal implications for the nurse, even though the measure may be considered life-saving. Option 3 has not opened other avenues for the parents to consider. Option 4 may be too late and also may not be appropriate, especially if the parents are uninterested in medical reasons for the transfusion.

431. 3. Neuroblastoma presents the gravest prognosis. Metastasis usually occurs even before a diagnosis is made and this type of neoplasm has not responded well to any type of therapy. Lymphomas have been contained with current forms of therapy. Wilms' tumor carries a high recovery rate. Many soft tissue sarcomas have been well contained and even cured with continued aggressive therapy.

432. 2. A comatose child should be placed on either side with a pillow propped at his back. This position allows best drainage from the mouth to prevent aspiration. A comatose person should not be placed flat on his back in bed. Placing the person on the abdomen may become dangerous due to the possibility of suffocating.

433. 4. Diphtheria is caused by Corynebacterium diphtheriae. It is noninvasive and grows best on the mucous membranes of the throat. The organism produces a toxin which causes most of the symptoms of the disease. A throat culture should be taken when diphtheria is suspected. Blood, urine, and stool cultures will be of no value to assist in diagnosing this disease.

434. 2. When in Bryant's traction, the child should be on his back and his legs should be flexed at a 90° angle at his hips; his hips should be slightly off the bed. This positioning provides for the best body alignment and traction.

435. 2. Options 1, 3, and 4 are true statements in relation to the spread

of syphilis. It may be desirable to douche after intercourse for personal hygiene reasons, but a douche will not help to prevent the spread of syphilis.

436. 1. Edema accompanies most kidney diseases and hence, in order to help limit edema, the diet is restricted in its sodium content.

437. 4. Option 4 offers the best definition of a meningomyelocele. An inflammation of the meninges is called meningitis.

438. 1. The child with hydrocephalus has an enlarged head due to a defect in cerebrospinal fluid dynamics. Nursing care should be directed toward preventing pressure sores from developing on the head and toward keeping the child well nourished. Complications described in options 2, 3, and 4 are not ordinarily associated with hydrocephalus.

439. 2. To date, the only successful treatment for hydrocephalus has been surgery. The surgical procedure involves providing a shunt from the lateral ventricle of the brain to the peritoneum or to the heart. The shunt helps drain the ventricle of excessive fluid.

440. 4. Hischsprung's disease often presents signs/symptoms similar to those of bowel obstruction. Obstruction is caused by lack of peristalsis in the enlarged colon.

441. 4. Since the colon is enlarged in the child with Hirschsprung's disease, the nurse should anticipate that she will need to make adjustments in the procedures of enemas and colonic irrigations in relation to the amount of solution to use. The colon is not spastic nor is the anus involved when a child has this disease.

442. 4. Intussusception is a telescoping of the bowel within itself. It is believed that it occurs in infants more often than in older children and adults since the infant's intestinal tract is comparatively hyperactive. Factors described in the other three options are not associated with intussusception.

443. 3. When pyloric stenosis is present, there is an obstructing lesion at the pylorus and food cannot move freely into the intestines from the stomach. The classical sign of pyloric stenosis is projectile vomiting.

444. 1. The primary reason for giving an infant with pyloric stenosis thickened formula is that it is less easily vomited.

445. 1. Because of the disease process and the therapy, persons with leukemia almost always succumb to an infection. Reverse isolation is often used for patients with leukemia to help prevent the risk of infections.

446. 3. It is recommended that infants be offered new foods on a one-at-a-time basis in order to be able to recognize any aller-

gies to specific foods. If foods are mixed, this assessment is not possible.

447. 2. Vitamin D is essential for the proper growth and development of the skeletal system. Inadequate intake of vitamin D leads to a bone condition known as rickets.

448. 1. Carbohydrate digestion is initiated by ptylin which is found in saliva. The digestion is completed in the intestines by various intestinal secretions. Pepsin and trypsin are concerned with protein digestion and steapsin is a fat splitting enzyme.

449. 2. Magnesium functions in the body to activate enzymes. It is also important in neuromuscular activity, the synthesis of protein, and the formation of bones and teeth. Calcium is important for the proper coagulation of blood. Iodine helps in the regulation of body metabolism and is required for normal growth.

450. 2. A newborn's body is approximately 80 percent water. By adulthood, this has changed to 55 to 65 percent. The child does not approach adulthood levels until sometime after the age of two.

451. 2. During toddlerhood, the most significant persons in the child's life are his parents. Siblings usually appear next most important. When children begin school, peers and others become more important.

452. 1. During the last one or two decades, the consumer's demands for health services have increased markedly. This trend greatly influenced preparing nurses to meet primary health needs of children. Health maintenance organizations were set up to help meet demands and to help place more emphasis on the prevention of disease. Associate degree programs have helped meet general demands for more nursing services.

453. 2. Health promotion has been receiving the most emphasis in well-child care within the past decade, although health services described in options 1, 3, and 4 continue to play important roles in total health care.

454. 2. Behavior is caused. Once we know why we behave as we do, we can then learn to become less judgmental about the behavior of others. Options 1 and 3 are not effective ways to become less judgmental of others. We may wish to work toward changing values that have been determined to be detrimental to well-being but an ethical and moral concept is at stake. Anthropologists generally agree that if change seems indicated, it is better to present the person with alternatives and consequences and let the person decide whether he wishes to give up or retain a cultural value.

455. 3. Preoccupation with one's culture stands in the way of understanding others. Ethnocentricism has positive values and can
help the survival of a society. But it is defeating if used to
stand in the way of understanding persons of different cultures.
456. 2. The nuclear family is defined as consisting of mother, father,
and their children. Option 4 describes the extended family.

psychiatric nursing

Forty-two-year-old Mr. John South was an unemployed laborer who was picked up by the police for disturbing the peace. He was brought voluntarily to the county hospital for admission to the psychiatric unit after it was discovered that his language was incoherent and that he was hallucinating. His admitting diagnosis was chronic undifferentiated schizophrenia.

Items 1 through 22 relate to this situation.

1. Upon admission, Mr. South docilely goes with the admitting nurse to his room, where he cocks his head to one side and says, "What? Oh yeah, that's right!" and then laughs uproariously to himself. Which one of these possible responses by the nurse would be *best* to make at this time?
   1. "Why are you laughing, Mr. South?"
   2. "Are you hearing voices, Mr. South?"
   3. "You're laughing, Mr. South. I wonder what's so funny."
   4. "I'm glad you find this hospital so amusing, Mr. South."
2. When Mr. South verbalizes thoughts related to his fantasy world and unrelated to reality, the nurse can *best* intervene by
   1. quickly interrupting his reveries.
   2. maintaining a discreet silence with him.
   3. talking to him in abstract terms about his past life.
   4. speaking to him in simple, concrete sentences about present happenings.
3. Since Mr. South is a shy, aloof patient, it is *especially* important that the nature of his initial hospital environment be
   1. hygienic.
   2. exciting.
   3. restrictive.
   4. nonstressful.

4. At dinner, Mr. South is seated in the dining room with his tray placed in front of him but he appears preoccupied and makes no attempt to eat. When helping the patient to maintain an adequate intake, which one of the following actions by the nurse would be *best* to take *first?*
   1. Spoon-feed him.
   2. Promise him an extra dessert if he cleans his plate.
   3. Put a fork full of food in his hand and guide it to his mouth.
   4. Remind him that he is not a child and that he is expected to do as much as he can for himself.
5. Mr. South invests most of his emotional energy in himself. Which one of the following terms is used to describe this attachment of significance and feelings to the self?
   1. Cathexis.
   2. Blocking.
   3. Imprinting.
   4. Narcissism.
6. The patient who withdraws from reason and reality is *most likely* to have a defect in his personality structure that is called a
   1. dominant id.
   2. lax superego.
   3. fragmented ego.
   4. punishing superego.
7. Mr. South expresses the feeling that he has seen the room to which he was admitted before although he is new to the city. This feeling of reliving an entirely new experience is called
   1. autism.
   2. déjà vu.
   3. depersonalization.
   4. hypnagogic imagery.
8. During the early stages of a one-to one relationship with a withdrawn patient like Mr. South, many authorities recommend that the nurse focus *most* of her attention on helping the patient to develop a sense of
   1. trust.
   2. autonomy.
   3. independence.
   4. decisiveness.
9. One afternoon, the nurse finds Mr. South sitting in the lounge fondling his genitals. Of the following actions the nurse could take with the patient who is masturbating, which one would be *best* for the patient?
   1. Ignoring the patient's behavior.
   2. Telling the patient his behavior is not acceptable.

3. Covering the patient with a blanket to hide his behavior.
4. Allowing the patient to continue the behavior in his room.

10. Of the following statements about the causes and effects of masturbation, which one expresses the belief held by the majority of psychiatric practitioners today?
   1. It might lead to impotency.
   2. It can cause mental deterioration.
   3. It is engaged in by those who are immoral and lack will power.
   4. It is a harmless and normal sexual outlet for unmarried young adults.

11. Mr. South is a member of a minority racial group. For which one of the following reasons do many progressive mental health centers try to hire workers of the same background and race as their clientele?
   1. To save money on interpreters for the institution.
   2. To meet affirmative action and federal funding requirements.
   3. To lessen the possibility of the workers' misjudging the patient's behavior.
   4. To take advantage of the workers' abilities to better understand the needs of the patients.

12. Mr. South views his physician, a member of the same minority race as he is, as "okay, but not as good as a white doctor." Which one of the following phenomena of stigmatization is the patient illustrating?
   1. The tendency to isolate negatively valued individuals.
   2. The tendency to punish willfully deviant members of one's group.
   3. The tendency to view one's own devalued group members as inferior.
   4. The tendency to attribute all one's difficulties to one's differentness.

13. Mr. South receives an antipsychotic medication four times a day. *All* of the following drugs are classified as major tranquilizers or antipsychotic agents *except*
   1. haloperidol (Haldol).
   2. trifluoperazine (Stelazine).
   3. thioridazine hydrochloride (Melleril).
   4. nortriptyline hydrochloride (Aventyl).

14. Of the following adverse effects Mr. South might experience as a result of using a major tranquilizer, which ones have the *gravest* implications for his physical health and well-being?
   1. Agranulocytosis and jaundice.
   2. Photosensitivity and dermatitis.
   3. Gynecomastia and corneal opacities.

4. Sedation and orthostatic hypotension.

15. Mr. South attends a remotivational group session daily with three other patients who manifest regression and withdrawal. Which one of the following themes would constitute a suitable topic for this remotivational group session?
1. Concepts of love.
2. Marital relations.
3. Religious beliefs.
4. Types of occupations.

16. According to remotivational therapy concepts, which one of the following qualities is the patient with a chronic psychiatric disorder assumed to have?
1. A creative instinct.
2. An intact intelligence.
3. A potential for improvement.
4. An obliviousness to surroundings.

17. Which one of the following changes in patient behavior would indicate to the nurse that the remotivational group is making progress and fulfilling its main purpose?
1. There is increased eye contact among the patients.
2. There is decreased absenteeism among the patients.
3. The patients spend less of the group time socializing.
4. The patients spend more of the group time bumming cigarettes.

18. The *most common* effect on staff members when remotivational techniques are used effectively with chronically disturbed patients is that it increases the staff members'
1. workload.
2. career goals.
3. anxiety levels.
4. job satisfaction.

19. Music and dance therapy are also available for the patients on Mr. South's unit. Such therapy has been observed to help withdrawn patients *most* by
1. stimulating interest in the arts.
2. increasing physical activity levels.
3. permitting open expression of feelings.
4. earning tokens for desired weekend passes.

20. After being hospitalized for 3 weeks, Mr. South shows little behavioral change. The staff decides that he likes the hospital too well and needs to be "pushed" more. When directed by the nursing aide to pick up his clothes and make his bed, Mr. South asks, "Why are you so mean to a soul brother? Just let me rest." Which one of the following possible responses by

the aide would be *best* in this situation?
1. "It's for your own good."
2. "The doctor ordered it; he wants you to do more for yourself."
3. "The object is to make you more independent. You have to admit, you have had it pretty easy here so far."
4. "By taking care of yourself here, you will be better able to manage later when it's time to leave the hospital."

21. If Mr. South continues with appropriate treatment, which one of the following statements *best* describes his prognosis?
    1. He will probably spend the remainder of his life in an institution.
    2. He will probably return to his previous level of adjustment in the community.
    3. He will probably be more economically and socially successful than he was before on the outside.
    4. He will probably have to stay in a halfway house or supervised boarding home for an indefinite period.

22. In the United States, approximately what percentage of the total mental hospital population do schizophrenic patients presently comprise?
    1. 25 percent.
    2. 50 percent.
    3. 75 percent.
    4. 90 percent.

Mr. Jerry Rand, a slender man in his early 40s, glanced disdainfully around the adult inpatient unit on his arrival at the hospital. He was neatly and attractively dressed and clutched a leather briefcase tightly in his arms.
Items 23 through 41 relate to this situation.

23. Mr. Rand refuses to let the psychiatric technician who admitted him touch his briefcase or check it for valuables or contraband. Which one of the following approaches would be *best* for the technician to use in determining the contents of the briefcase at this time?
    1. Obtain help to take the briefcase away from the patient.
    2. Ask the patient for a description of the items in his briefcase.
    3. Inspect the briefcase when the patient is temporarily out of his room.
    4. Tell the patient it is necessary to observe hospital policy if he wishes care.

24. The psychiatric technician stands near the window while explaining to Mr. Rand how his bed operates. The patient

shouts, "Come away from the window! They'll see you!"
Which one of the following responses by the technician would
be *best* to make?

1. "Who are 'they,' Mr. Rand?"
2. "No one will see me, Mr. Rand."
3. "You have no reason to be afraid, Mr. Rand."
4. "What will happen if they do see me, Mr. Rand."

25. The technician should refrain from moving away from the window quickly as the patient requested because moving away would

1. reveal a lack of poise in the technician.
2. make the patient feel the technician is only humoring him.
3. indicate nonverbal agreement with the patient's false ideas.
4. let the patient think he will have his way whenever he wishes it.

26. Mr. Rand thinks he is being followed by foreign agents who are after the secret papers in his briefcase. The thought disorder from which he is suffering is called

1. an idea of reference.
2. an idea of influence.
3. a delusion of grandeur.
4. a delusion of persecution.

27. Mr. Rand has not eaten anything since his admission because he says, "I know you people have put something in the food to make me sleep." Which one of the following actions would be best for the nursing staff to take in order to get the patient to eat?

1. Have his wife bring food from home for him to eat.
2. Keep food in sealed containers from which he can help himself.
3. Arrange with the diet kitchen for him to supervise cooking for himself.
4. Point out to him that other patients are not afraid to eat the food.

28. The team leader overhears a nursing assistant respond to Mr. Rand's statement that he is the only person alive who has the answer to the world food shortage with, "How can that be? Tell me more, Mr. Rand." On which one of the following facts about the effects of questioning a patient closely about his false ideas should the team leader base her subsequent comments to the nursing assistant?

1. It leads the patient to defend his thinking.
2. It leads the patient to reverse his thinking.
3. It leads the patient to share more of his thinking.

4. It leads the patient to clarify some of his thinking.

29. Which one of the following characteristics of a suspicious patient makes it *especially* difficult for the nurse to establish and maintain a therapeutic relationship with him?
    1. The patient's tendency to question the motives of others.
    2. The patient's tendency to ridicule and belittle other persons.
    3. The patient's tendency to believe he is always right and others are wrong.
    4. The patient's tendency to see others as part of the conspiracy against him.

30. Mr. Rand is ordered to receive chlorpromazine (Thorazine). To avoid problems with Mr. Rand possibly "cheeking" the medication, in which one of the following forms would it initially be *best* to give the patient the medication?
    1. Liquid.
    2. Capsule.
    3. Suppository.
    4. Intramuscular injection.

31. After 3 days of taking chlorpromazine, Mr. Rand shows an inability to sit still, motor restlessness, fidgeting, and a tendency to pace around the unit. Of the following extrapyramidal side effects, the patient is showing signs of
    1. dystonia.
    2. akathisia.
    3. parkinsonism.
    4. tardive dyskinesia.

32. Which one of the following medications can the nurse anticipate the physician will order to treat Mr. Rand's extrapyramidal side effects?
    1. Chlordiazepoxide (Librium).
    2. Benztropine mesylate (Cogentin).
    3. Imipramine hydrochloride (Tofranil).
    4. Thioridazine hydrochloride (Melleril).

33. Which one of the following observations about Mr. Rand warrants the *most prompt* reporting and the nurse's use of safety precautions for him?
    1. He cries when he talks about his divorce.
    2. He starts a petition to end the curfew hour.
    3. He declines to attend a daily group therapy session.
    4. He names another patient who he says is his adversary.

34. Beneath Mr. Rand's air of arrogance and superiority lie deep-seated feelings of inferiority and inadequacy. Which one of the following defense mechanisms is Mr. Rand using to protect his self-esteem?

1. Denial.
2. Projection
3. Idealization.
4. Introjection.

35. The nursing assistant who is assigned to care for Mr. Rand comments to the nurse, "That Mr. Rand! He surely gets on my nerves. Just who does he think he is?" Which one of the following replies would be *best* for the nurse to make?
1. "He cannot help being the way he is."
2. "It sounds like you are angry with him."
3. "You should not talk that way about a patient."
4. "I wonder if you might try to consider his feelings."

36. Which one of these hospital regulations should the staff be *especially* tactful in enforcing with Mr. Rand?
1. Patients may not leave the unit without an escort.
2. Patients may not have alcoholic beverages on the unit.
3. Patients must keep sums over $7 in the business office safe.
4. Patients can only smoke in designated areas, such as in the lounge.

37. Which one of the following phrases is *most likely* to describe the personality of Mr. Rand prior to his illness?
1. A man-about-town.
2. Inclined to be sentimental.
3. A self-sacrificing individual.
4. Secretive in his dealings with others.

38. During which of the following age periods do the characteristic signs of a paranoid reaction *commonly first* appear in a patient?
1. In early childhood.
2. During adolescence.
3. At young adulthood.
4. Past the age of 30.

39. The nurse tries to provide support for Mr. Rand by using touch. For example, she puts her arm around his shoulder and pats his hand. For which one of the following reasons would it be *best* for the nurse to avoid touching this patient?
1. The action may cause the patient to reject the nurse.
2. The action may arouse transference feelings in the patient.
3. The action may lead to dependency on the part of the patient.
4. The action may be interpreted by the patient as an aggressive move.

40. Which one of the following recreational activities would be the *least suitable* choice for Mr. Rand at any time during his hospitalization?
1. Playing solitaire.

2. Playing basketball.
3. Attending a concert.
4. Working a crossword puzzle.

41. The secure atmosphere of the hospital eventually helps effect a decrease in Mr. Rand's paranoid ideation. *All* of the following activities of the nurse *very likely* contributed to the patient's recovery *except*
1. acting as a role model for the patient in everyday social situations.
2. taking a passively friendly, slow approach in conversations with the patient.
3. trying to minimize making promises to the patient but keeping those that were made.
4. letting the patient see the nurse talking with other patients outside his hearing range.

Ms. Dinah Wallace, who is 43 years old, was brought to the hospital by her husband. She wore sandals, revealing dirty and swollen feet, and had on a rumpled dress with a stain down the front. She moved slowly and looked confused.
Items 42 through 56 relate to this situation.

42. The *initial* actions of the nurse who admits Ms. Wallace should be focused on
1. making the patient feel safe and accepted.
2. helping the patient get acquainted with others.
3. giving the patient information about the program.
4. providing the patient with clean, comfortable clothes.

43. When asked about herself during the admission interview, Ms. Wallace stares blankly at the nurse and mutters unintelligibly to herself. This behavior is *best* charted as
1. "uncooperative during admission procedure."
2. "not able to answer questions at this time."
3. "responded to questions with blank look and incomprehensible mumble."
4. "stared at nurse when asked questions and was disoriented and incoherent."

44. Fluphenazine decanoate (Prolixin Decanoate), an antipsychotic drug, is prescribed for Ms. Wallace. The outstanding characteristic of this drug is that it
1. is inexpensive and can be self-administered.
2. quickly relieves the patient of his symptoms.
3. has fewer side effects than the other major tranquilizers.
4. needs to be administered only once every 2 to 4 weeks.

45. While Ms. Wallace receives fluphenazine decanoate, it is recommended that *all* of the following observations should be made on a regular schedule *except*
1. weight checks.
2. white blood cell count
3. pulmonary function test.
4. blood pressure measurements.

46. Ms. Wallace is in a catatonic state for the first few days after admission. She speaks to no one and sits in one place for long periods of time. When her arm is placed over her head, it remains passively in this position. This abnormal posturing is termed
1. echolalia.
2. neurasthenia.
3. waxy flexibility.
4. reaction formation.

47. Of the following nursing actions, which one is *most likely* to help a mute patient like Ms. Wallace express herself verbally?
1. Ask questions to draw the patient out.
2. Use hand signals to entice the patient to communicate.
3. Say out loud what she thinks the patient is experiencing.
4. Make frequent remarks to the patient about neutral topics.

48. Ms. Wallace often does the opposite of what she is requested to do. For example, if asked to stand up, she sits down; if asked to dress, she undresses. In view of the patient's negativism, which of the following actions would be *best* for the nurse to take to get Ms. Wallace to the dining room for meals?
1. Ask her to eat in her room away from the other patients.
2. Wait for her to get hungry enough to come to the dining room by herself.
3. Tell her it is time for lunch and lead her firmly by the arm to the dining room.
4. Promise her a reward if she eats in the dining room and get help to take her there if she refuses.

49. Like many other schizophrenic patients, Ms. Wallace was severely traumatized emotionally in her first years of life. Which one of the following adjectives probably *best* describes the type of parenting she might have experienced to foster her subsequent withdrawal from reason?
1. Ambiguous.
2. Sheltered.
3. Authoritarian.
4. Overpermissive.

50. When upset, Ms. Wallace curls up in a fetal position in bed.

Which one of the following defense mechanisms is she using when she displays behavior reminiscent of an earlier level of emotional development?

1. Fixation.
2. Regression.
3. Substitution.
4. Symbolization.

51. The nurse pays close attention to nonverbal communications whenever conversing with Ms. Wallace. Of the following statements, which one *best* describes why the nurse's observations of nonverbal messages are important?
   1. Nonverbal communications convey feelings more accurately than do verbal communications.
   2. Nonverbal communications reveal inner defects in a person better than do verbal communications.
   3. Nonverbal communications allow for a healthier expression of negative emotions than do verbal communications.
   4. Nonverbal communications provide better concealment for the true feelings of a person than do verbal communcations.

52. It is known that catatonic patients may suddenly behave in an impulsive, hyperactive, and unpredictable manner. Which one of the following approaches would be *best* for the nurse to use *first* if Ms. Wallace becomes violent?
   1. Provide a physical outlet for her energies.
   2. Let her know her behavior is not acceptable.
   3. Get enough help to handle the situation safely.
   4. Use heavy sedation to ensure calmness of the patient.

53. The physician orders restraints for Ms. Wallace to be used according to the nurse's discretion. With which one of the following offenses could the nurse be charged in the event she uses the restraints on the patient without good cause and a legal suit develops?
   1. Fraud.
   2. Assault.
   3. False imprisonment.
   4. Invasion of privacy.

54. Although Ms. Wallace shows signs of progress daily, her husband complains to the nurse, "Why isn't she well yet? She's been here over 2 weeks already. Aren't you people doing your job?" Which one of the following replies by the nurse would be the *most* therapeutic?
   1. "You are anxious for your wife to get better. Shall we talk about it for a while?"
   2. "She is really doing a lot better than you think. It won't be

long before she will be home again."

3. "We are doing the best we can. She has deep-seated conflicts which cannot be cured overnight."

4. "I know it is difficult for you. But you wouldn't want to rush her and have her get worse again, would you?"

55. Ms. Wallace's children are being cared for by her mother-in-law. One day, after a visit with the children, Ms. Wallace becomes agitated and shaky and whispers to the nurse, "That woman has turned my children against me." Which one of the following interventions would be *best* for the nurse to make *first*?

1. Arrange for a social worker to visit the home.

2. Determine the identity of the woman to whom the patient referred.

3. Assign a staff member to watch the patient carefully the rest of the day.

4. Tell the family they cannot visit anymore if they are going to upset the patient.

56. This is Ms. Wallace's first admission to a mental hospital. With which one of the following factors would a favorable prognosis for her *most likely* be associated?

1. Low socioeconomic status.

2. Gradual onset of illness.

3. Lengthy illness prior to hospitalization.

4. Good social adjustment prior to present illness.

Six-year-old Melissa Corning is a patient at a residential treatment center for children. She is an autistic child. Her primary nurse therapist, Ms. Pratt, meets with her three times a week for an hour. For her one-to-one sessions with Melissa, Ms. Pratt keeps on hand a supply of simple games and toys, a doll family, and drawing material.

Items 57 through 78 relate to this situation.

57. During play, which one of the following possible areas of malfunctioning of the child is usually *most open* to the therapist's scrutiny?

1. The patient's moral deficiencies.

2. The patient's organic impairments.

3. The patient's intellectual deficits.

4. The patient's interpersonal difficulties.

58. For which one of the following reasons are play techniques, rather than psychoanalytic methods, often used while diagnosing and treating the emotionally disturbed child?

1. A child has stronger ego defenses than does an adult.

2. Play therapy requires less skill on the part of the therapist.

3. Play is the child's natural medium of expression and learning.

4. The child is not amenable to internal change and psychoanalytic insights.

59. Ms. Pratt notes that Melissa is sensitive to the nonverbal behaviors of others. In which one of the following manners, then, is it *especially* important for the nurse to try to convey her messages to the child during their one-to-one sessions?

1. In a covert manner.

2. In a verbal manner.

3. In a genuine manner.

4. In a nonverbal manner.

60. Although at many of her previous sessions with Ms. Pratt, Melissa had been hyperactive and silent, at one she is able to play with the toys and utter a few words. In relation to ending a productive session of this nature, which one of the following practices should be followed by the nurse?

1. The session should be terminated at the usual time.

2. The session should be cut short on a positive note.

3. The session should be extended beyond the usual hour.

4. The session should be ended as usual with the next session made longer.

61. Ms. Pratt watches Melissa take the little girl doll from the doll family grouping and set it apart from the others. Of the following comments that the nurse could make in relation to the child's manipulation of the doll, which one would be the *most appropriate and therapeutic?*

1. "Is that how you feel, separated from your family?"

2. "Why did you put the little girl doll so far away from her family?"

3. "It must be lonely for the little girl, with her family way over there."

4. "The little girl is sitting all by herself; I guess no one must care for her."

62. In general, which one of the following terms *best* sums up the kind of oral response the nurse should make initially to each of Melissa's actions and words in the one-to-one situation?

1. Agreement.

2. Exploration.

3. Interpretation.

4. Acknowledgment.

63. Melissa's growth and development has been adversely affected by her illness. Tools that a "normal" 6-year-old is expected to have at her disposal for accomplishing the tasks of childhood

that occur between about 6 and 9 years of age include *all* of the following skills *except*

1. a sense of self.
2. the ability to compete.
3. the ability to collaborate.
4. a basic command of language.

64. Ms. Pratt reports on Melissa's progress at the weekly meeting of the health team. Of the following items of information that are shared by staff members in the meeting, which one is likely to have the *most bearing* on the patient's progress?
1. The staff's knowledge of Melissa's past history.
2. The staff's personal reactions to Melissa's behavior.
3. The staff's areas of disagreement about Melissa's care.
4. The staff's ideas on suitable long-term goals for Melissa.

65. A major role of the nurse with Melissa is the mother surrogate role. Which one of the following basic needs of the psychotic child is *primarily* met through this role?
1. The child's dependency needs.
2. The child's need for prestige.
3. The child's need for adequacy.
4. The child's achievement needs.

66. Melissa is prone to strike out at the other children when she is upset. Which one of the following actions should the nurse take *first* when Melissa starts to flail her arms about in an emotional outburst?
1. Hold her arms firmly so she cannot hit anyone.
2. Encourage her to talk about what is upsetting her.
3. Remind her that the punching bag is available if she needs it.
4. Explain to her that she will not be allowed to hurt herself or anyone else.

67. One day Melissa sees her mother coming to visit her. She runs to the nurse and clings to her skirt. Which one of the following actions by the nurse is indicated in this situation?
1. Scold the child for her behavior and take her to her room.
2. Move toward the mother with the child and calmly welcome the mother.
3. Stand quietly beside the child and observe the mother's reaction.
4. Smile sympathetically at the mother and ask her to come back later.

68. On a visit to Melissa's home for a family interview, Ms. Pratt observes that the youngest child, John, who was 2 years old, looks malnourished and neglected. *All* of the following signs

and symptoms are also commonly indicative of parental abuse *except*

1. clubbing of the fingers and toes.
2. cigarette burns on the extremities.
3. apathy or fearfulness toward strangers.
4. the presence of old scars and fractures.

69. In the event of suspected child abuse, *primary* consideration and protection should be given to the rights of the
   1. parents.
   2. child victim.
   3. nurse doing the case finding.
   4. case finder's affiliated agency.

70. Once the legal issues of a child abuse have been decided, which one of the following explanations that the nurse could make to the parents about her availability as a resource person for them would *most positively* influence their utilization of her services?
   1. "It could go very badly for you if you hurt John again, so be sure to call me before you do anything you will regret."
   2. "You have the center's phone number and know where I can be reached if you need me. I do hope it won't come to that, though."
   3. "Remember, you can depend on me to help you, whatever the problem. Just give me a ring and I will come right over to save the day."
   4. "Call me anytime, day or night, when you feel yourself getting tense or upset with John and when you need to get away from him for a while."

71. Which one of the following descriptions of the parents of a neglected or battered child is *least likely* to characterize them?
   1. They demonstrate role reversal.
   2. They are perceptive of how their child feels.
   3. They are chiefly concerned about themselves.
   4. They have defects in their character structures.

72. Which of the following terms *best* describe the way in which the abuse-prone parent was himself usually treated as a child?
   1. Critically and punitively.
   2. Variably and unorthodoxly.
   3. Adequately and protectively.
   4. Permissively and overindulgently.

73. Of the following ways to intervene in the child abuse cycle, which one is *most likely* to be cited by authorities as the *earliest* and *best* form of prevention?

1. Arranging for prompt medical treatment of the battered child.
2. Educating prospective parents about normal growth and development.
3. Coordinating the work of separate diagnostic and treatment agencies.
4. Providing parental alternatives in the form of foster homes or day care.

74. Of the following forms of therapy that could be initiated for Melissa and her neglected brother to help resolve their problems, which one is likely to have the *most* beneficial effect on their future welfare and be suitable for their present needs also?
   1. Behavioral therapy.
   2. Conjoint family therapy.
   3. Individual psychotherapy.
   4. Small group psychotherapy.

75. All of the following items of information contained in the medical record are helpful when assessing Melissa's mental state and interpersonal difficulties. The observations that nurses are likely to find *most useful and applicable* to Melissa's care are the
   1. reports from school representatives.
   2. records of nurse participant observations.
   3. scores of psychological tests that were administered.
   4. summaries of social service interviews with parents and siblings.

76. Melissa spends every other weekend with her family. On returning Melissa to the center following a weekend pass, her parents complain about her disruptiveness at home. Which one of the following qualities do the parents *most likely lack* in dealing with Melissa in the home setting?
   1. Warmth.
   2. Tolerance.
   3. Consistency.
   4. Spontaneity.

77. Long-range aims of therapy for a psychotic child like Melissa should include helping her develop *all* of the following skills *except* being able to
   1. relate to other human beings.
   2. integrate her concept of herself.
   3. tolerate strict routines of daily living.
   4. identify her own body as separate from those of other people.

78. Melissa has been a patient at the center for approximately 8 months. Which one of the following behaviors offers the *best*

evidence that Melissa is beginning to accept herself as a worthwhile and important individual?
1. She refuses to eat with other children.
2. She walks around with an air of aloofness.
3. She chooses a clean, attractive outfit to wear.
4. She laughs when her finger gets shut in the door.

Ms. Stephanie Jamet, who is 56 years old, insisted on being taken to her room immediately upon admission to the hospital. She ordered one nurse to unpack her clothes, another to bring her some coffee, and a third to get her agent on the phone for her. She stated, "I am the greatest actress since Sarah Bernhardt. I will take my meals in my room; you may prepare my bath now." Mr. Jamet said his wife had not slept for 3 nights and had spent her days writing checks to charitable institutions which they can ill afford to do. Ms. Jamet is diagnosed as manic-depressive psychosis, manic phase.
Items 79 through 97 relate to this situation.

79. For which one of the following qualities would the nursing staff *most likely* look when deciding in which room to house Ms. Jamet?
1. A quiet atmosphere.
2. A cordial roommate.
3. A view of the hospital grounds.
4. A large amount of storage space.
80. Mr. Jamet apologizes to the nurse for his wife's demanding behavior. Which one of the following possible replies would be *best* for the nurse to make?
1. "I am sure she is doing the best she can."
2. "It's all right. We have been treated worse."
3. "It must be hard for you to see her like this."
4. "I understand. What happened to set her off like this?"
81. Ms. Jamet is scheduled to go to the radiology department for a routine x-ray examination of the chest. Before taking the patient for her x-ray examination, which one of the following actions should the nurse take?
1. Explain the x-ray procedure to her in simple terms.
2. Say nothing to the patient before taking her to the x-ray department.
3. Give her a detailed explanation of the x-ray procedure.
4. Bring another staff member along in case she resists going to the x-ray department.
82. The nurse notes that Ms. Jamet is too busy investigating the unit

and overseeing the activities of other patients to eat much of her dinner. In order to help Ms. Jamet obtain sufficient nourishment, which of the following plans would be *best* for the nurses to implement?

1. Serve foods that she can carry with her.
2. Allow her to send out for her favorite foods.
3. Serve food in small attractively arranged portions.
4. Allow her in the unit kitchen for extra food as she pleases.

83. Later the same evening, Ms. Jamet appears at the nurses' station with brightly rouged cheeks, ornaments in her hair, and wearing three pairs of false eyelashes. She has on a sheer nightgown, high heels, and bracelets up to her elbows. Which one of the following actions should the nurse take in relation to the patient's attire?

1. Remind her gently that she is not on the stage now.
2. Assist her matter-of-factly to put on proper apparel.
3. Show her several magazine illustrations of well-groomed women.
4. Explain to her what clothing is considered appropriate for the hospital setting.

84. While watching television in a lounge, Ms. Jamet says quickly and abruptly to the nurse, "The sun is shining. My son is in Virginia. Who's afraid of Virginia Woolf?" Which one of the following disorders is the patient displaying?

1. Concreteness.
2. Flight of ideas.
3. Depersonalization.
4. Use of neologisms.

85. The speech pattern described in item 84 is *chiefly* due to

1. feelings of anxiety.
2. loose ego boundaries.
3. distortions in the self-concept.
4. abnormalities in the hypothalamus.

86. When Ms. Jamet makes the statements described in item 84, which one of the following responses would be the *most therapeutic* for the nurse to make?

1. "Let's talk about what you did today instead."
2. "How does the sun shining relate to your son being in Virginia?"
3. "You are talking nonsense; why don't you try to stay on one subject?"
4. "I cannot follow you; it would help me if you would speak a little slower."

87. If all of the following activities are available on the unit, which

one would probably be *best* for Ms. Jamet during the *acute* stage of her illness?
1. Sewing.
2. Reading.
3. Checkers.
4. Ping-Pong.

88. Which one of the following feeling states does the behavior a patient exhibits during a manic episode reflect?
1. Guilt, projected onto others.
2. Anger, turned against the self.
3. Distrust, focused on the family.
4. Hostility, directed against the environment.

89. Ms. Jamet sometimes makes inappropriate requests. For example, she asks to have a nearby shop deliver 30 bars of expensive soap to her room. For this particular request, which one of the following plans that the staff discussed would be *best* suited to the patient's needs?
1. Ignore the request.
2. Fill the request promptly.
3. Offer to supply part of the request.
4. Allow the request to be filled with a less expensive product.

90. Which one of the following terms *best* describes the personality that Ms. James *most likely* exhibited prior to her present illness?
1. Shy.
2. Rigid.
3. Submissive.
4. Extroverted.

91. The nurse makes a daily check of Ms. Jamet's physical condition. During the patient's period of euphoria, for which of these conditions should the nurse be *especially* alert?
1. Gastritis and vertigo.
2. Exhaustion and infections.
3. Convulsions and dermatitis.
4. Bradycardia and palpitations.

92. The drug regimen for the management of Ms. Jamet's hyperactivity includes administration of lithium carbonate (Lithane). While Ms. Jamet is taking this drug, the nurse should make certain that the patient has an adequate intake of
1. salt.
2. iron.
3. iodine.
4. calcium.

93. Ms. Jamet expresses the belief that she is the illegitimate daugh-

ter of a famous family. When dealing with this delusion of grandeur the nurse should *first* try to
1. get the patient to discuss another topic.
2. involve the patient in a simple group project.
3. convince the patient that she is wrong in her belief.
4. meet the implied need of the patient to feel important.

94. One day when Ms. Jamet's charmingly delivered request for a pass is refused by the physician, she becomes angry and utters a stream of profanities. On which one of the following considerations should nursing intervention into the use of abusive language by the patient be based?
1. It is often upsetting to others.
2. It indicates serious organic pathology.
3. It is a sign of disrespect that cannot be tolerated.
4. It will decrease as the patient's condition improves.

95. Ms. Jamet improves with the help of drug and relationship therapy. She appears less often at the nurses' station and makes fewer demands. In relation to her prognosis, when this particular illness has abated, it is *most likely* that the symptoms of her mood disorder will
1. not occur again.
2. recur periodically.
3. prove ultimately fatal.
4. increase in occurrence with age.

96. Mr. Jamet asks the nurse what he can do to help his wife when she goes home from the hospital. Of the following actions, which one would probably be *least helpful* for the family members to take on behalf of the patient?
1. Try to keep the patient free from worry and anxiety.
2. Relieve the patient of some home responsibilities she had.
3. Develop effective communication techniques with the patient at home.
4. Learn to recognize when the patient is showing signs of drug toxicity.

97. Since Ms. Jamet's illness is diagnosed as manic-depressive psychosis, to which one of the following factors is her condition *most likely* related?
1. Having been molested as a preschool child.
2. Having a family history of manic-depression.
3. Building up high serotonin levels in the brain.
4. Drinking alcoholic beverages more frequently than usual.

Ms. May Bullen, age 49, was an involuntary admission to the psychiatric hosptial. Her admission is for 30 days by court order. Documents sent with her cite, among other things, that she will not eat because she feels her stomach is "missing," her bowels have "turned to jelly," and she views this as "just punishment for my past wickedness and for the evil I have brought on my family."

Items 98 through 117 relate to this situation.

98. To have been considered legally commitable, which one of the following criteria did Ms. Bullen *most likely* have to meet?
   1. She had to be psychotic.
   2. She must have tried to harm herself or others.
   3. She must have been unable to afford private treatment.
   4. She must have made threatening remarks to others.
99. Of the following rights, which one did Ms. Bullen lose by virtue of being admitted involuntarily to a mental hospital?
   1. The right to send and receive mail.
   2. The right to vote in a national election.
   3. The right to make a will or a legally binding contract.
   4. The right to sign out of the hospital against medical advice.
100. Through which one of the following legal methods could Ms. Bullen seek release from the psychiatric hospital if she believes she is being improperly detained?
   1. Through a malpractice suit.
   2. Through a guardianship hearing.
   3. Through a writ of habeus corpus.
   4. Through a lien of property petition.
101. Ms. Bullen is suffering from the grandiose delusion that she is the "worst sinner in the world." Her delusion of sinfulness *most likely* had its origin in her unconscious image of herself as a
   1. superior being.
   2. helpless child.
   3. pitiable victim.
   4. detestable failure.
102. Ms. Bullen is to receive tube feedings since she refuses food in any form. Gastric gavage is usually used as a last resort with the suspicious involutional patient because the feedings are *very likely* to
   1. be aspirated by the person.
   2. arouse fears of dying in the person.
   3. be viewed as an attack on the person.
   4. increase the irritability of the person.
103. At night Ms. Bullen becomes restless and increasingly incoherent. Besides administering prescribed antipsychotic medi-

cation, which one of the following actions by the nurse would be *most helpful* for the patient at this time?
1. Encourage her to talk about her family life.
2. Read to her with the lights turned down low.
3. Help her to take a cool shower before retiring.
4. Sit quietly with her until the medication takes effect.

104. Despite the nurse's good intentions, Ms. Bullen demands to be let alone to die. "If you try to cheat the avenger, you will suffer," Ms. Bullen tells the nurse. Which one of the following possible replies by the nurse would be *best?*
1. "Are you trying to frighten me, Ms. Bullen?"
2. "I'd like to help you, Ms. Bullen, and I'm not afraid."
3. "I'm not trying to cheat anyone, Ms. Bullen, just doing my work."
4. "Do you really expect me to let this 'avenger' get you, Ms. Bullen?"

105. In addition to her mood disorder, Ms. Bullen is prone to "hot flashes" and dizzy spells. She is started on estrogen replacement therapy for her bothersome menopausal symptoms. The use of estrogen is *contraindicated* in *all* of the following disorders *except*
1. kidney and liver disease.
2. emphysema and osteoporosis.
3. fibroids and endometriosis.
4. cancer and recurrent cysts.

106. Of the following signs/symptoms that Ms. Bullen might present, which one is *least likely* to be a side effect of estrogen therapy?
1. Nausea.
2. Weight gain.
3. Hypotension.
4. Breast tenderness.

107. Of the following factors, which one probably had the *most* bearing on the unhealthy and negative impact of the menopause on Ms. Bullen?
1. The severity of her sex steroid deficiency.
2. The psychosocial losses menopause signal for her.
3. The lack of financial security in her declining years.
4. The fluctuation in her adrenal gland production of cortisone.

108. After voicing his concern for his wife's welfare, Mr. Bullen asks the nurse if it is true that men also go through a "change of life." The nurse should base her reply on knowledge that
1. the climacteric occurs in men but years later than in women.
2. the climacteric occurs in men but years earlier than in women.
3. men do not undergo a menopausal "change of life" as women do.

4. men undergo a negligible physiological reduction of capacity quite dissimilar to the female menopause.

109. Prior to Ms. Bullen's present episode of involutional melancholia, which of the following characteristics did she *most likely* exhibit?
1. Manic-depressive behavior.
2. Lack of concern for bodily ailments.
3. Symptoms of psychomotor retardation.
4. Personality traits of conscientiousness and rigidity.

110. In view of her agitated state and rumination, Ms. Bullen is placed on suicidal precautions and scheduled for electroconvulsive therapy. When the therapy is explained to her and her family, a family member asks "Won't the shock treatment be terribly traumatic for her?" Which one of the following responses by the nurse would be the *most accurate and therapeutic?*
1. "She will be asleep during the treatment and probably won't remember it at all."
2. "The treatment is not an unpleasant procedure and it will make her feel better."
3. "She may experience a little discomfort initially but she will soon become accustomed to the sensation."
4. "The treatment has few drawbacks but exhaustive research has shown them to be outweighed by the advantages to the patient."

111. Before the series of electroconvulsive treatments is begun, which one of the following items should be obtained from Ms. Bullen?
1. A urine sample.
2. A skull and jaw x-ray.
3. A signed consent form.
4. A blood sample for an SMA_{16}.

112. One of the nurses feels very strongly that electroconvulsive therapy is a "barbarous treatment" and that "any doctor who uses it ought to be made to go through it himself." When asked about the treatment by a patient or family member, which one of the following courses of action would be *most prudent* for this nurse to take?
1. Give the questioner her honest opinion of the treatment.
2. Refer the questioner to another knowledgeable party for information on the treatment.
3. Tell the questioner she does not know enough about the treatment to be of help to him.
4. Inform the questioner that there are books available about the treatment in any public library.

113. When preparing Ms. Bullen for her electroconvulsive treatment,

the nurse should perform *all* of the following activities *except*
1. toileting the patient.
2. inserting the patient's dentures.
3. removing the patient's eyeglasses.
4. assisting the patient into loose clothing.

114. Of the following drugs often administered before electroconvulsive therapy, which one functions to block the myoneural junction, thereby relaxing the skeletal musculature?
1. Atropine sulfate.
2. Succinylcholine chloride (Anectine).
3. Thiopental sodium (Pentothal Sodium).

115. Which one of the following undesirable conditions is *least likely* to occur when electroconvulsive therapy is used?
1. Residual epilepsy.
2. Dislocation of the jaw.
3. Temporary memory loss.
4. Compression fracture of the spine.

116. In terms of time, Ms. Bullen's recovery from her illness will *most likely* be
1. rapid.
2. gradual.
3. spontaneous.
4. intermittent.

117. Which one of the following actions generally constitutes the *best* preventive measures against involutional problems in middle-aged persons?
1. Encouraging them to have yearly medical checkups.
2. Enabling them to profit from tax relief programs.
3. Providing them with adequate recreational facilities.
4. Supporting them in their efforts toward role satisfaction.

Mr. Archie Rowland was driven to the emergency department of the hospital by his brother. Mr. Rowland is 52 years old. On admission, he was perspiring profusely, breathing rapidly, and complaining of dizziness and heart palpitations. Problems of a cardiovascular nature were promptly ruled out. Mr. Rowland's diagnosis was tentatively listed as acute anxiety reaction.

Items 118 through 137 relate to this situation.

118. It is noted by the emergency department staff that Mr. Rowland is hyperventilating. Which one of the following electrolyte imbalances is *most likely* to occur when the patient hyperventilates?

1. Metabolic acidosis.
2. Respiratory acidosis.
3. Metabolic alkalosis.
4. Respiratory alkalosis.

119. To ease the symptoms caused by hyperventilation, which one of the following measures would be *best* for the nurse to try *first* with Mr. Rowland?
   1. Have him rebreathe into a paper bag.
   2. Instruct him to put his head down between his knees.
   3. Give him a low concentration of oxygen via nasal cannula.
   4. Tell him to take several deep, slow breaths and exhale normally.

120. In addition to the nursing measure selected in item 119, which one of the following nursing interventions would also be indicated during Mr. Rowland's severe anxiety reaction?
   1. Putting him in restraints until he is calmer.
   2. Staying with him until he regains his self-control.
   3. Telling him to "cool it" in a firm no-nonsense manner.
   4. Leaving him alone briefly to enable him to collect himself.

121. As opposed to Mr. Rowland's behavior at a severe level of anxiety, which one of the following descriptions *best* depicts what the patient's thought processes and behavior would be like at a *mild* level of anxiety?
   1. Attentive, emotional, sensitive, stereotyped.
   2. Selectively inattentive, adequate, slow, rigid.
   3. Attentive, alert, logical, relevant, integrated.
   4. Inattentive, automatic, illogical, disorganized.

122. Mr. Rowland's episode of severe anxiety lasted for approximately 30 minutes. He was then admitted to the inpatient psychiatric unit for further evaluation and treatment, based on his urgent plea for definitive help. Mr. Rowland is aware that his anxiety is of neurotic origin. Neurotic anxiety differs from normal anxiety in that neurotic anxiety is
   1. out of proportion to the cause.
   2. lessened with the passage of time.
   3. a rational response to an objective danger.
   4. easily traceable to a consciously recognized stimulus.

123. *All* of the following nursing measures are usually therapeutic in nature when helping to reduce a neurotic patient's anxiety level *except*
   1. responding for the patient in family-staff discussions.
   2. encouraging the patient to express his negative feelings.
   3. providing the patient with physical activity and diversion.
   4. making decisions for the patient in the form of suggestions.

124. The nursing staff learns that Mr. Rowland was recently promoted at work although he had not yet assumed his new duties and was ambivalent about doing so. To which of the following underlying feelings are the patient's present anxiety reactions to his promotion, and his chronic anxiety neurosis, *most likely* related?
1. To feelings of distrust.
2. To feelings of alienation.
3. To feelings of inadequacy.
4. To feelings of superiority.

125. The main coping method used by persons with an anxiety neurosis involves excluding from awareness unacceptable self-knowledge. The term used to describe this type of behavior is
1. projection.
2. repression.
3. regression.
4. sublimation.

126. Mr. Rowland often jumps when spoken to and complains of feeling uneasy. "It's as though something bad is going to happen," he says. *All* of the following nursing measures are likely to reassure Mr. Rowland *except* the nurse's
1. being physically present.
2. communicating a respectful attitude.
3. being technically competent.
4. conveying optimistic verbalizations.

127. Which one of the following physiological reactions should suggest to the nurse that Mr. Rowland is feeling anxious?
1. Bradycardia.
2. Cold, clammy skin.
3. Excess salivation.
4. Muscular flaccidity.

128. Mr. Rowland's anguish and distress are readily communicated to the nurse who conducts daily counseling sessions with him. When the nurse finds herself adversely affected or overwhelmed by the patient's painful feelings, which one of the following statements of intent would be *best* for her to make?
1. "I need to leave for a few minutes to deal with my feelings but I will return shortly."
2. "I wish I could stay to talk with you but I just remembered something I have to take care of."
3. "I hate to cut you off but I think we should talk about something less upsetting to both of us."
4. "I am feeling anxious about what you have told me but I will try to stay with you despite my feelings."

129. The *main* reason the activities planned for Mr. Rowland are directed toward increasing his contact with other people is to
1. relieve his boredom.
2. lessen his egocentricity.
3. keep him safely occupied.
4. prevent him from regressing.

130. Mr. Rowland is married but states that he cannot talk to his wife. He says he did not make sexual advances toward her because he was sure she would turn him down. Which one of the following tendencies of neurotic patients was Mr. Rowland displaying in this particular instance?
1. The tendency to set excessively high goals for oneself.
2. The tendency to anticipate negative reactions from others.
3. The tendency to use ineffective ways to satisfy one's basic needs.
4. The tendency to convert emotional conflicts into physical complaints.

131. Chlordiazepoxide (Librium) is prescribed for Mr. Rowland. Many therapists prefer that neurotic patients *not* receive anti-anxiety agents while in psychotherapy, the primary reason being that these agents tend to
1. be habit forming.
2. decrease muscular tension.
3. reduce motivation for change.
4. have little effect on anxiety of panic proportions.

132. Mr. Rowland attends a psychodrama session twice weekly. Two major purposes of psychodrama are to help patients to
1. decrease emotional spontaneity and obtain attention from others.
2. relive unpleasant situations and learn about the problems of others.
3. gain new self-perception and develop more adequate responses to situations.
4. confront individuals with unacceptable behaviors and increase group productivity.

133. In accord with the manner in which an anxiety neurosis usually develops, much of Mr. Rowland's childhood behavior was *most probably* directed toward unsuccessful efforts to
1. win parental approval.
2. decipher contradictory messages.
3. avoid harsh physical punishment.
4. find refuge in a world of fantasy.

134. Mr. Rowland progresses rapidly in this therapy and is soon discharged. He is referred to the outpatient clinic for follow-up. Which one of the following hospital-learned abilities is proba-

bly *most important* for the continued alleviation of Mr. Rowland's neurotic symptoms?

1. He recognizes when he is feeling anxious.
2. He understands the reasons for his anxiety.
3. He can alter his methods of handling anxiety.
4. He is able to describe the situations preceding his feelings of anxiety.

135. Of the following medications, which ones usually are classified as minor tranquilizers or antianxiety agents?

1. Oxazepam (Serax) and hydroxyzine pamoate (Vistaril).
2. Thiothixene (Navane) and thioridazine hydrochloride (Melleril).
3. Biperiden hydrochloride (Akineton) and procyclidine hydrochloride (Kemadrin).
4. Desipramine hydrochloride (Pertofran) and protriptyline hydrochoride (Vivactil).

136. The minor tranquilizers are more often prescribed by the physician to relieve mild to moderate anxiety symptoms than are the major tranquilizers or barbiturates because the minor tranquilizers tend to

1. induce sleep more readily.
2. cause fewer undesirable side effects.
3. be excreted from the body more quickly.
4. evoke a more rapid sensitization response.

137. In which one of the following ways can anxiety be an asset to a person?

1. It can slow down one's physiological functioning.
2. It can lead to one's use of ego defense mechanisms.
3. It can mobilize one's automatic behavior responses.
4. It can increase one's alertness to the environment.

Mr. Ned Packard, who is 62 years old, was admitted to the psychiatric unit of the hospital 1 month after retiring involuntarily. Ms. Frank, a registered nurse, was assigned to care for him. She has noted that he keeps his head bowed in a dejected manner and that his facial expression is sad.

Items 138 through 153 relate to this situation.

138. At their first meeting, although the patient asks to be called by his first name and there is no policy against this practice, Ms. Frank persists in calling the patient "Mr. Packard." Of the following statements, which one offers the *best* explanation for the nurse's noncomplying behavior?

1. She is showing respect for the patient's age.

2. She is being formal and professional with the patient.
3. She is indifferent to the needs and wishes of the patient.
4. She is uncomfortable with the peer role implied in the patient's request.

139. In her relationship with Mr. Packard, Ms. Frank should realize that their sessions will probably differ from the patient's sessions with his psychiatrist because in nurse-patient interactions, the participants discuss *primarily* the patient's
1. dreams and free associations.
2. childhood and past life history.
3. current feelings and experiences.
4. underlying conflicts and defense mechanisms.

140. After a few minutes of conversation, Mr. Packard warily asks the nurse, "Why pick me to talk to when there are so many other people here?" Which one of the following replies by the nurse would be *best?*
1. "I am assigned to care for you today, if you will let me."
2. "You have a lot of potential, and I would like to help you."
3. "Why shouldn't I want to talk to you, as well as the others."
4. "You're wondering why I am interested in you, and not the others?"

141. Ms. Frank meets with Mr. Packard on a daily basis. He stays mostly in his room and speaks only when addressed, answering briefly and abruptly while keeping his eyes on the floor. At this stage of their relationship, it would be *best* for the nurse to focus on the ability of the patient to
1. make decisions.
2. function independently.
3. express himself verbally.
4. relate to other patients.

142. Of the following behaviors of Mr. Packard, which one would *best* indicate to Ms. Frank that her relationship with the patient is in a *working* phase?
1. The patient attempts to familiarize himself with the nurse.
2. The patient makes an effort to describe his problems in detail.
3. The patient tries to summarize and evaluate his progress in the relationship.
4. The patient starts to challenge the boundaries or outer limits of the relationship.

143. Ms. Frank consciously works to become aware of the feelings and emotions of Mr. Packard. This practice of trying to comprehend the psychological state of another or of trying to perceive how he feels is called
1. empathy.

2. climate.

3. rapport.

4. sympathy.

144. On the day following an interview during which Mr. Packard talked at length and tearfully about feeling useless and unmanly since his retirement, he fails to keep an appointment with the nurse. Which one of the following actions would it be *best* for the nurse to take next?

1. Assume that he had a good reason for not coming and let him make the next move.

2. Confront him with his behavior and explain to him the probable reason for his avoidance.

3. Seek him out at the end of the scheduled interview time and tell him he was missed today.

4. Arrange for another session with him later the same day and say nothing about his absence.

145. Mr. Packard is concerned that the information he gave the nurse remain confidential. Ms. Frank explains that she will let him know beforehand if she plans to share any of the interview data with the staff or his physician. This is done *primarily* so that the patient will

1. not lose trust in the nurse.

2. not get angry with the nurse.

3. think he has some privacy left.

4. be encouraged to reveal more of himself to the nurse.

146. Mr. Packard speaks in an enthusiastic, seemingly sincere manner about his former employer who was responsible for suddenly replacing him in his position with a younger man. "He surely was a swell fellow. Best boss I ever had. It was a privilege to know him." Which one of the following defense mechanisms is Mr. Packard using?

1. Sublimation.

2. Suppression.

3. Rationalization.

4. Reaction formation.

147. Mr. Packard begins to attend group therapy daily. He explains to the group members how he lost his job after 20 years with the company. Which one of the following responses by the group members is the *most therapeutic?*

1. "It must have been very upsetting for you."

2. "Those people are foolish for letting you go."

3. "You should sue the company for age discrimination."

4. "With your skills, finding another job should be easy."

148. The physician orders a different type of drug when Mr. Packard

does not respond positively to a tricyclic antidepressant. While the patient is taking the newly prescribed drug, tranylcypromine sulfate (Parnate), which one of the following reactions is likely to occur if the patient's diet includes foods containing amines?

1. A heart block.
2. A grand mal seizure.
3. A respiratory arrest.
4. A hypertensive crisis.

149. *All* of the following substances contain amines or high tyramine levels *except*
    1. wine.
    2. beer.
    3. coffee.
    4. cheese.

150. One week after admission to the hospital, Mr. Packard obtains permission for a 24-hour pass to go home. Which one of the following preparations by his family for the visit indicates the *best* understanding of the patient's needs?
    1. Bringing his bed downstairs so he can rest during the day.
    2. Scheduling a day of interesting activities outside of the home.
    3. Arranging for a member of the family to watch him at all times.
    4. Planning to involve him in the usual at-home pursuits of the immediate family.

151. Mr. Packard's pass went well and a discharge date is set. When planning the task of dissolving the nurse-patient relationship, which one of the following courses of action by the nurse would be the *most helpful?*
    1. Meet more often with the patient.
    2. Hold future-oriented conversations.
    3. Engage in longer interview sessions.
    4. Discourage contact with other staff members.

152. Ms. Frank had kept a verbatim record (process recordings) of her interactions with Mr. Packard. What is *most often* the *ultimate* goal of this practice?
    1. To evaluate the progress of the patient.
    2. To determine the care plan for the patient.
    3. To improve the communication skills of the nurse.
    4. To increase the recording proficiency of the nurse.

153. Which one of the following possible reactions of Mr. Packard to the termination of his relationship with Ms. Frank would be considered the *most* healthy?
    1. A lack of response.
    2. A display of anger.

3. An attempt at humor.
4. An expression of regret.

A nurse who makes weekly rounds of area boarding homes observed a discharged mental hospital patient in one home. The patient, Ms. Rachel Cory who is 65 years old, was irritable and walked about her room slowly and morosely.

Items 154 through 171 relate to this situation.

154. After 10 minutes, since Ms. Cory seemed to have nothing to say, the nurse prepares to leave. But each time she tries to go, Ms. Cory plucks at her sleeve and quickly asks for help to rearrange her belongings or move small articles of furniture she could easily have moved herself. She also anxiously makes inconsequential remarks to keep the nurse with her. Which one of the following statements provides the *most likely* explanation for the patient's behavior?
1. The patient is lonely and looking for a way to pass the time.
2. The patient is self-centered and possessive of the nurse's time.
3. The patient needs attention paid to some as yet unknown concern.
4. The patient desires assistance to improve the appearance of her room.

155. The nurse has important business to attend to elsewhere so she tells Ms. Cory that she will spend more time with her at their next weekly meeting. When the nurse arrives as planned, Ms. Cory is taciturn and sits staring angrily at the nurse. When dealing with this situation, which one of the following actions that could be taken by the nurse would probably be the *least helpful?*
1. Commenting that the patient looks angry.
2. Remaining silent until the patient decides to talk.
3. Asking the patient what her thoughts are at the moment.
4. Apologizing for not being more available to the patient the previous week.

156. Before the nurse decides which strategy she will use with the patient, Ms. Cory blurts out, "You hate me, don't you?" Which one of the following replies that the nurse could make would be the *most therapeutic?*
1. "You are imagining things."
2. "I could never hate anyone."
3. "What did I do or say to give you that impression?"
4. "You are unhappy with me for not staying last week, aren't you?"

157. The nurse is careful not to act rushed or impatient with Ms. Cory and gradually learns that the patient is very "down" and feels worthless and unloved. In view of the fact that Ms. Cory made a suicidal gesture previously when unhappy, which one of the following interventions by the nurse is indicated at this time?
1. She should ask the patient frankly if she has thoughts of or plans for committing suicide.
2. She should avoid bringing up the subject of suicide to prevent giving the patient any ideas.
3. She should outline some alternative measures to suicide for the patient to use during periods of sadness.
4. She should mention others she has known who have felt like the patient and attempted suicide, to draw her out.

158. Ms. Cory volunteers the information that, while she would like to end her life, her religious beliefs keep her from doing anything fatal. Nevertheless, for Ms. Cory's safety, the nurse suggests that Ms. Cory have a friend come and be with her now. Ms. Cory is reluctant to do this because "My friends think people who try to take their lives are perverted and stupid. They will think I'm morally depraved and not want anything to do with me." Ms. Cory is expressing a fear of being
1. maltreated.
2. discredited.
3. unappreciated.
4. misinterpreted.

159. Ms. Cory would like to have someone comfort her; at the same time she dreads the questions it will raise and the explanations she will be required to make. Which one of the following phenomena is the patient exhibiting?
1. A conflict.
2. An impulse.
3. A regression.
4. An ego break.

160. When Ms. Cory turns her feelings (especially anger) against herself in a depressive episode, which one of the following defense mechanisms is she using?
1. Conversion.
2. Restitution.
3. Introjection.
4. Substitution.

161. Which one of the following events has *most likely* been experienced recently when people like Ms. Cory become depressed?
1. Financial upset.

2. Physical injury.

3. Real or imagined loss of a loved object.

4. Increased personal or social responsibility.

162. Of the following problems, with which one is Ms. Cory also likely to have difficulty at this time?

1. Obesity.

2. Diarrhea.

3. Reality testing.

4. Making decisions.

163. Ms. Cory finally agrees to let one of the other boarding home residents stay with her at night since that is when she feels the bluest and the most in need of companionship. Ms. Nathe is agreeable when approached and asks the nurse how she should act with Ms. Cory. In considering therapeutic ways of behaving with Ms. Cory, the nurse is *least likely* to recommend that Ms. Nathe act

1. firmly.

2. seriously.

3. cheerfully.

4. spontaneously.

164. Ms. Cory is ordered to receive amitriptyline hydrochloride (Elavil). At which one of the following times does this medication *usually* achieve the desired effect of lifting the patient's depression?

1. Within a few days.

2. Almost immediately.

3. In 2 to 4 weeks.

4. After about a 5-week period.

165. The nurse begins visiting Ms. Cory daily to evaluate her condition and progress. Of the following activities that could be included in a program for the patient, which one would be *best* for the nurse to try to involve Ms. Cory in at the present time?

1. Volunteer work.

2. A part-time job.

3. Group recreation.

4. A simple daily routine.

166. It is difficult to maintain effective relationships with depressed persons such as Ms. Cory because their

1. pessimism arouses frustration and anger in others.

2. poor personal grooming invites disgust and ridicule from others.

3. independence prevents them from asking for any kind of assistance.

4. laziness keeps them from putting forth the necessary effort to get well.

167. At which of the following times should the nurse be aware that the danger of a suicide attempt by Ms. Cory is the *greatest?*
 1. When her energy starts to return.
 2. At the time of her greatest despair.
 3. After she has resumed her former life style.
 4. After she has had a visit from a well-to-do brother.

168. After a week of taking amitriptyline hydrochloride, Ms. Cory complains that her mouth feels dry. Which one of the following measures would be *least* desirable to relieve the dryness in the patient's mouth?
 1. Chew sugarless gum.
 2. Suck on hard candies.
 3. Drink plenty of fluids.
 4. Rinse the mouth with water.

169. Of the following side effects of amitriptyline hydrochloride, which one is potentially the *most life-threatening* and should be reported immediately?
 1. Sedation.
 2. Tachycardia.
 3. Urinary retention.
 4. Loss of visual accommodation.

170. The nurse returns to a weekly schedule of visits when Ms. Cory is more able to function on her own. The patient gives the nurse an attractively wrapped package, "a small token of appreciation for helping me," the patient says. The *most detrimental* of the following effects of gift giving is that it could result in the nurse's feeling
 1. obligated to the patient.
 2. belittled by the patient.
 3. annoyed by the patient.
 4. ill-at-ease with the patient.

171. Although Ms. Cory's insomnia improves and her poverty of thought diminishes, she still stresses her faults in conversations with the nurses. When Ms. Cory starts to point out all the things she can't do, which one of the following responses by the nurse would provide the *best* intervention?
 1. "You can do anything you put your mind to."
 2. "Try to think more positively about yourself."
 3. "Let's talk about your plans for the weekend."
 4. "You were able to write a letter to your friend today."

Eighteen-year-old Jay Bonner arrived late for his appointment with the nurse at the outpatient clinic of the mental health center. During the interview, he fidgets restlessly in his chair and has trouble remembering what topic is being discussed. He asks for help "to keep from going crazy."

Items 172 through 186 relate to this situation.

172. Which one of the following courses of action would be the *most appropriate* for the nurse to take during the initial interview with Jay?
    1. Find out what he thinks would help him.
    2. Assist him to describe his difficulties more thoroughly.
    3. Assure him that he has come to the right place for help.
    4. Let him know that his anxious behavior has been observed.

173. Which one of the following statements by the nurse would *best* deal with Jay's fears about "going crazy"?
    1. "Everyone feels that way occasionally so you are not any different from anyone else."
    2. "I don't know enough about you to judge. Why don't you tell me more about yourself?"
    3. "You sound perfectly sane to me. Maybe your perception of 'crazy' is different from mine."
    4. "I appreciate that this is a concern you have, but so far I have yet to see evidence of irrationality in you."

174. Jay reveals that he was late for his appointment because of "my dumb habit." I have to take off my socks and put them back on 41 times. I can't stop until I do it just right." The nurse should understand that this behavior *most likely* represents an effort by the patient to
    1. relieve his anxiety.
    2. control his thoughts.
    3. gain attention from others.
    4. express hostility toward the nurse.

175. A decision is made not to hospitalize Jay. Which one of the following abilities of the patient probably influenced the decision *most?*
    1. His ability to hold a job.
    2. His ability to perform activities of daily living.
    3. His ability to behave in an outwardly normal manner.
    4. His ability to relate to members of the opposite sex.

176. Jay reports that before he leaves home to go anywhere, he counts the money in his wallet as many as 12 times. Which one of the following reasons *best* explains his motive for performing this particular ritual?
    1. To channel excessive sexual energy into an appropriate habit.
    2. To compensate for not having enough money to spend as a child.

3. To avoid the embarrassment of having a shortage of funds on hand.

4. To substitute emotions unacceptable to him with a relatively acceptable activity.

177. Which one of the following defense mechanisms is Jay employing when he overengages in ritualistic behavior?
1. Fixation.
2. Projection.
3. Conversion.
4. Displacement.

178. In addition to having the urge to perform repetitive acts, Jay is afflicted with the persistent, unwanted thought of doing harm to his brother. This latter disturbance is called
1. a phobia.
2. an obsession.
3. a compulsion.
4. a dissociation.

179. Jay's mother asks if her son will ever get over "those awful habits of his." Which one of the following replies that the nurse could make would be the *most therapeutic?*
1. "It is not always possible to free a person from his symptoms."
2. "That goal is certainly within his reach although it will require a lot of hard work on his part."
3. "With the use of behavior modification techniques, there is an excellent chance he will be cured."
4. "With long-term psychotherapy, an expensive and time-consuming process, he can definitely be helped."

180. Which one of the following actions would be *best* for the nurse to take when she observes Jay in a ritualistic pattern of behavior?
1. Isolate him so he will not disturb others.
2. Observe him closely for radical changes in behavior.
3. Remind him he can control his behavior if he wishes.
4. Enable him to continue so he won't become more agitated.

181. If the nurse is to work successfully with neurotic patients, such as Jay, which one of the following qualities is *most important* for her to possess?
1. Patience.
2. Compassion.
3. Friendliness.
4. Self-confidence.

182. After a few weeks of outpatient treatment, Jay has improved very little. His therapist arranges for Jay to meet with the day care center staff which has formulated a program for him with his collaboration. What is considered to be the *most important*

advantage of partial hospitalization treatment, such as that offered by day care centers?

1. It is closer to the client's home.
2. It offers the client a wider choice of therapies.
3. It is cheaper than inpatient hospitalization.
4. It helps the client maintain his family and social ties.

183. During a morning group meeting, Jay is introduced to the other day care patients who shortly begin to include him as part of their group. Which one of the following factors was probably the *most influential* in determining the group's positive behavior toward Jay?

1. His acceptance by the staff.
2. His self-effacing mannerisms.
3. His wardrobe of expensive clothes.
4. His ability to tell funny stories.

184. The staff considers it important to decrease Jay's dependence on others. To meet that goal, when Jay asks, "What time is it?" which one of the following replies would be the *most effective* for a staff member to make?

1. "My watch says ten o'clock."
2. "What time do you think it is?"
3. "Has anyone else got the time?"
4. "There is a clock behind you on the wall."

185. Jay eats slowly and is always the last to finish lunch which makes it difficult for the group to get started on its 1 P.M. outing. Which one of the following approaches constitutes the *best* solution for this problem?

1. Change the time of the outing to accommodate Jay.
2. Arrange for Jay to start eating earlier than the other patients.
3. Plan to go without Jay so that he will have ample time for his lunch.
4. Inform Jay he will have to eat faster so the group can leave on time.

186. As Jay progresses, he wants to take up a hobby and asks the day care nurse for some suggestions. From a therapeutic standpoint, which one of the following activities would be the *most desirable* for Jay?

1. Swimming.
2. Drama club.
3. Solo flying.
4. Photography.

Mr. Roger Cranst, a 27-year-old graduate student, was referred to the college counseling service by his academic adviser. He told the nurse counselor that he was unable to concentrate on his studies and that he recently failed several examinations. "I got so panicky during the tests that I couldn't even think straight," he explained.

Items 187 through 205 relate to this situation.

187. When a patient suffers from test anxiety, which one of the following actions should the counselor generally take *first?*
1. Teach the patient relaxation exercises.
2. Assist the patient to define and improve his study habits.
3. Explore with the patient the possible reasons for his anxiety and failing.
4. Help the patient determine whether or not he can still meet class requirements.

188. As a small child, Mr. Cranst became physically ill each morning when it was time for him to go to school. This apprehension about attending school was *most likely* related to his fear of being
1. separated from his mother.
2. criticized by his teacher.
3. ignored by his schoolmates.
4. compared with his older brothers.

189. The counselor learns that Mr. Cranst's wife left him following an argument about his "womanizing." "Now, little honey, do I seem like the Romeo type to you?" Mr. Cranst coaxingly asks the nurse. Which one of the following replies by the nurse would be *best?*
1. "You are trying to flirt with me, aren't you?"
2. "It all depends on your definition of 'Romeo.'"
3. "What way do you think you are coming across to me?"
4. "I can't say you impress me as being very seductive."

190. Mr. Cranst is inwardly uncertain of his masculine identification but he outwardly acts the "Don Juan" role. Which one of the following defense mechanisms is the patient using?
1. Sublimation.
2. Introjection.
3. Reaction formation.
4. Emotional insulation.

191. Mr. Cranst says his grades would improve if his wife would come back. The nurse and Mr. Cranst invite Ms. Cranst to meet with them for a joint session. On which one of the following characteristics of Mr. and Ms. Cranst will a successful outcome of marital counseling sessions *primarily* depend?
1. Their personal liking for the therapist.

2. Their motivation to change their behavior patterns.
3. Their ability to pay for an unlimited number of therapy sessions.
4. Their willingness to point out unpleasant mannerisms of each other.

192. A nurse undertaking to engage in therapy with a family or couple should be *especially* aware of and guard against the tendency to
1. view the family as a single, isolated entity.
2. take sides with a family member against other family members.
3. form opinions about the family before obtaining sufficient data.
4. become overwhelmed by the complexity of the family interactions.

193. An important trait that every family or marital counselor should ideally possess is the quality of
1. deference.
2. flexibility.
3. decisiveness.
4. unobtrusiveness.

194. Ms. Cranst states that since the nurse is unmarried, she would be a less effective counselor than would a married counselor. Which one of the following statements *most accurately* describes current opinion concerning Mr. Cranst's comment?
1. It is a likely possibility.
2. It is an unwarranted assumption.
3. It is a myth motivated by jealousy.
4. It is part of an unethical competitive campaign for patients.

195. In the initial interview session with Mr. and Ms. Cranst, the nurse obtains information about the coping methods commonly utilized by each of their own parents. Toward which one of the following ends did she collect this information?
1. To assure the couple that the problematic behavior did not begin with them.
2. To reacquaint the couple with older, more effective ways of dealing with stress.
3. To convince the couple of the necessity for persuading the families of origin to seek treatment also.
4. To assist the couple with lessening the influence of prior family habits on their currect interactions.

196. Ms. Cranst said that she married Mr. Cranst because she thought he would be "someone I could lean on, who would earn enough so I wouldn't have to work." Mr. Cranst replied, "I

thought you were the liberated kind who needed to pay her own way." Such misunderstandings in a marriage can *best* be avoided if the expectations of each of the participants are

1. accepted.
2. minimized.
3. projected.
4. verbalized.

197. When a person's expectations of his marital partner go unmet, with which one of the following reactions is he *least likely* to respond?

1. Distrust and withdrawal.
2. Frustration and aggression.
3. Compromise and cooperation.
4. Disappointment and anxiety.

198. The counselor attempts to investigate the transaction modes of the couple. When differences of opinion are present, *all* of the following methods in relation to family living are adaptive *except*

1. exploring preferences.
2. negotiating differences.
3. making decisions on the basis of power.
4. settling differences through the use of consensus.

199. While glancing at his wife, Marcy, Mr. Cranst tells the nurse, "I don't want her to hassle me any more." Of the following replies that the nurse could make, which one would be *best?*

1. "I don't blame you; it must be unpleasant to be hassled."
2. "Try explaining to Ms. Cranst what it is you want her to do."
3. "Perhaps you shouldn't give her reason to complain, in that case."
4. "You're talking to me but what you are really saying is 'Marcy, stop it.'"

200. Continuing couple therapy by the counselor with the Cransts would *most likely* deal mainly with the subject of

1. Ms. Cranst's dependency.
2. Mr. Cranst's insecurity.
3. their past transgressions and present transference reactions.
4. their present communications with each other and with the therapist.

201. After the nurse twice points out to Ms. Cranst that she did not respond to a seeming bid from her husband for support, Ms. Cranst says that she has a hearing loss and, therefore, does not always hear what Mr. Cranst says. Which one of the following experiences is Ms. Cranst *least likely* to have encountered as a hard-of-hearing person in this society?

1. Feeling isolated from other people.
2. Feeling alienated when meeting new people.
3. Being accommodated too pleasantly in social situations.
4. Being treated by others as if she were mentally incompetent.

202. In communicating with a hard-of-hearing person it would be *most helpful* for the nurse to
1. shout at the person.
2. exaggerate her lip movements.
3. keep her back to the window when talking.
4. establish direct eye contact with the person.

203. Mr. Cranst's mother was a frequent visitor at the Cranst home. She and her daughter-in-law were covertly and uncharacteristically united in their desire to push Mr. Cranst to "succeed." This alliance is *best* defined as a family
1. rule.
2. myth.
3. script.
4. coalition.

204. A useful technique sometimes used to analyze the interactions of a married couple is transactional analysis. In general, according to concepts of transactional analysis, most marital conflicts can *best* be solved by conducting discussion at the ego state levels of
1. adult to adult.
2. child to adult.
3. parent to child.
4. parent to parent.

205. At which one of the following times is termination of the couple-counselor relationship *most usually* indicated?
1. When the couple is satisfied with their marriage.
2. When the couple is no longer dependent on the therapist.
3. When the couple has wiped out their areas of disagreement.
4. When the couple can handle their dissensions constructively.

Mr. Eric Jasper, age 24, was admitted to the hospital with a diagnosis of chronic ulcerative colitis. He had frequent bouts of diarrhea in the last month, causing him to lose another 10 pounds from his already slight frame.
Items 206 through 224 relate to this situation.

206. Since this is Mr. Jasper's fourth admission to the hospital in 9 months, he is a familiar person to the nurse caring for him. Of the following remarks that the nurse could make to Mr. Jasper

when he is getting settled in his room, which one would be the *most beneficial* for the patient?
1. "It's nice to see you again, Mr. Jasper. Did you get lonesome for us on the outside?"
2. "I thought we had seen the last of you for a while, Mr. Jasper. What are you doing back?"
3. "It's been 2 months since you were last here, Mr. Jasper. What do you think about being back in the hospital?"
4. "I see you have your old room again, Mr. Jasper. No need to explain things to you is there, since you are such an old pro?"

207. Mr. Jasper tells the nurse that he would give anything to be rid of his illness. He sighs and says he often daydreams about being healthy, sometimes imagining himself as showing powers of endurance that would put others to shame. When he thinks of himself in this way, which one of the following ego defense mechanisms is Mr. Jasper using?
1. Fantasy.
2. Repression.
3. Projection.
4. Compensation.

208. The nurse feels sorry for Mr. Jasper but does not want him to know it. Regardless of any precautions she might take to hide her feelings, in which one of the following ways would Mr. Jasper *best* be able to detect the nurse's true feelings toward him?
1. By listening carefully to what she says to him.
2. By asking her for a description of her feelings toward him.
3. By observing her facial expressions and nonverbal behavior toward him.
4. By reading, with permission, what she has written about him on his chart.

209. When the nurse feels pity for Mr. Jasper, a trait that will *most likely* characterize her behavior is
1. attentiveness.
2. seductiveness.
3. permissiveness.
4. condescendence.

210. Mr. Jasper becomes tense and nauseated when he hears the cart containing meal trays approaching. He knows that eating increases his loose stools and discomfort. To prevent the premeal buildup of tension, which one of the following practices would be *best* for the nursing staff to institute?
1. Reroute the dietary cart so the patient will not be disturbed by it.

2. Order a special early tray for the patient to let him finish eating before the cart comes.

3. Turn the patient's television or radio on before meals to mask the noise of the approaching meal cart.

4. Arrange for someone to keep the patient engaged in a relaxing activity or conversation before the meal time.

211. Mr. Jasper should be involved in suitable activities in his room while his diarrhea is being treated. For which one of the following attributes *in particular* should the activities be chosen?

1. They should be conducive to rest and relaxation.

2. They should teach new recreational and social skills.

3. They should require attention to detail and deep concentration.

4. They should involve manual dexterity rather than intellectual processes.

212. A certain personality pattern is often attributed to persons with ulcerative colitis. Based on this pattern, which three of the following traits would the nurse expect Mr. Jasper to have?

1. Shyness, flexibility, modesty.

2. Hostility, perfectionism, dependency.

3. Perseverance, ambition, ruthlessness.

4. Irritability, suspiciousness, self-reliance.

213. Mr. Jasper had regular weekly meetings with a psychotherapist in a private agency during the periods when he was not hospitalized. For a patient with ulcerative colitis, what is the goal of psychotherapy *most likely* to be?

1. To support the defenses and endeavors of the patient.

2. To rid the patient of his anxiety and physical symptoms.

3. To draw out the hidden feelings and conflicts of the patient.

4. To bring the patient a measure of self-confidence and social ease.

214. The physical symptoms of a person with overconcern for the body often center around the gastrointestinal tract for *all* of the following reasons *except*

1. cultural rituals are related to the alimentary tract throughout life.

2. there is a strong emphasis during early childhood on eating and toileting behaviors.

3. the gastrointestinal tract is the most fragile of body parts and the most susceptible to damage.

4. the functioning of the digestive and intestinal tracts is readily noted and subject to some amount of manipulation.

215. The organs of the body involved in psychophysiological dis-

eases, such as ulcerative colitis, are ordinarily under the control of the
1. central nervous system.
2. autonomic nervous system.
3. peripheral nervous system.
4. reticular activating system.

216. An important distinction for the nurse to make between a psychophysiological disorder, such as ulcerative colitis, and a neurotic disorder, such as conversion reaction, is that in a psychophysiological disorder
1. the physical symptoms may be fatal to the person if left untreated.
2. the set of physical symptoms are consciously selected by the person.
3. the physical symptoms of the person are relieved when the mental conflict is arrested.
4. the person characteristically has an attitude of indifference toward his physical symptoms.

217. In addition to ulcerative colitis, which one of the following illnesses is considered to be partly or completely due to psychobiological factors?
1. Asthma.
2. Epilepsy.
3. Nephrosis.
4. Hepatitis.

218. A week after Mr. Jasper's admission, the physician recommends that Mr. Jasper have part of his bowel resected and an ileostomy constructed. Later Mr. Jasper says to the nurse, "That doctor of mine surely likes to play big. I'll bet the more he can cut, the better he likes it." Which one of the following replies that the nurse could make would be *most therapeutic?*
1. "You sound upset. We could talk about it, if you'd like."
2. "It's too nice a day to be talking about such a morbid subject."
3. "Aren't you being a bit hard on him? He is only trying to help you."
4. "Does that remark have something to do with the operation he wants you to have, by any chance?"

219. Mr. Jasper becomes increasingly morose and irritable after thinking more about his physician's recommendation. He is rude to his visitors and pushes nurses away when they attempt to give him his medications and treatments. Which one of the following nursing interventions would be *best* when the patient has a hostile outburst?
1. Try to prevent him from expressing anger.

2. Show disapproval of his ill-mannered behavior.
3. Encourage him to discuss his immediate concerns and feelings.
4. Continue with the assigned tasks as though nothing has happened.

220. One evening, Mr. Jasper uses a stream of profanities directed at the nurse, then abruptly hangs his head and pleads, "Please forgive me. Something just came over me. Why do I say those things?" The name for this type of behavior is
1. punning.
2. confabulation.
3. flight of ideas.
4. emotional lability.

221. The nursing staff begins teaching Mr. Jasper what to expect following surgery but finds that he does not retain the information and seems indifferent to these efforts. The *most likely* reason Mr. Jasper is not learning is because he lacks
1. an acceptance of the idea of having surgery.
2. an interest in obtaining information about his impending surgery.
3. the intelligence to grasp what he was being taught about the surgery.
4. confidence in the members of the nursing staff who are teaching him about his surgery.

222. Arrangements are made for a member of the ileostomy club to meet with Mr. Jasper. Of the following aims, which one illustrates the *chief purpose* for having a representative from the club visit Mr. Jasper preoperatively?
1. To provide support for the physician's plans for the patient.
2. To let the patient know he has resources in the community to help him.
3. To show the patient that he can still live a full life with an ileostomy.
4. To allow the patient plenty of time to consider becoming a member of the club.

223. Mr. Jasper's family saw him through many exacerbations and remissions of his illness. Of the following possible effects of chronic invalidism on the patient's family, the most detrimental to their interrelationships would *most probably* be that the illness may make family members feel
1. dominated and guilty.
2. put-upon and overworked.
3. sympathetic and concerned.
4. superior and self-sufficient.

224. If Mr. Jasper's immediate physical problems are eventually solved by successful surgical intervention, to stay healthy he will *especially* need to
1. see his physician regularly for checkups.
2. adhere faithfully to a rigid dietary regimen.
3. utilize other defenses to disguise his shortcomings.
4. find an emotionally satisfying substitute for his physical symptoms.

A nurse and a nutritionist are co-leaders of a therapy group for overweight women. The group meets once a week and is directed toward helping the eight members help themselves to lose weight. The members decided to address each other by first names.
Items 225 through 245 are related to this situation.

225. Of the following advantages for using a co-leadership approach in a group, which one usually has the *most immediate and the most directly beneficial* effect on the group members?
1. It contributes to the professional growth of the leaders through peer interaction.
2. It enables the leaders to help more clients and to cover more areas of discussion.
3. It allows the leaders to demonstrate model patterns of relating to each other and to the clients.
4. It permits the co-leaders to validate their individual perceptions and to gain support for their interventions.

226. The nurse accepts obese people but realizes that she does not always feel positively toward them. To aid in improving her attitude toward her obese patients, which one of the following actions should the nurse take *first?*
1. Talk out her feelings about obesity in a staff meeting.
2. Ask the unit psychiatrist for a referral to a good analyst.
3. Give herself time to learn to like the obese group members.
4. Share her initial reaction to the group members with them in a matter-of-fact way.

227. The women are weighed prior to each meeting. To which one of the following factors is a consistent, maintained loss of weight *most likely* related?
1. To the individual commitment of a person to lose weight.
2. To the threat of illness if a person does not lose weight.
3. To the promise of a new wardrobe if a person loses weight.
4. To the joyful responses of others when a person loses weight.

228. Many of the women in the group, ranging in age from 23 to 60

years, have contracted one or more of the physical disorders
commonly associated with obesity. Of the following conditions that a person might develop, which two are *not* closely
related to the state of obesity?
1. Atherosclerosis and gout.
2. Joint pains and hypertension.
3. Hypervitaminosis and hypotension.
4. Diabetes mellitus and malnutrition.

229. Which one of the following statements *best* explains the relationship between obesity in women and social class membership?
1. More upper-class women than lower-class women are overweight.
2. Fewer upper-class women than lower-class women are overweight.
3. Approximately the same number of upper-class and lower-
class women are overweight.
4. There is no correlation between social class membership and
obesity.

230. The nurse and the nutritionist make efforts to avoid the
authoritarian type of leadership that occurs when leaders direct but remain apart from the members in general. They try
to be democratic because authoritarianism tends to produce
group behavior that is
1. independent and disorganized.
2. apathetic or indirectly aggressive.
3. nonproductive in solving problems.
4. less demanding of attention from the leaders.

231. During the first two meetings, the co-leaders were seen as
superiors and experts and were asked many questions by
group members. To encourage the members to seek solutions
among themselves, which one of the following tactics would
be *best* for the therapists to use?
1. Ask for the opinion of other members on questions directed to
leaders.
2. Inform the members that it is up to them to provide answers to
their questions.
3. Explain that the leaders will only answer questions if the
members are stumped.
4. Use silence to force the members to find a different authority
within the group.

232. Lucille continually sighs and laments to the group, "I will never
to able to lose weight, never." Which one of the following
comments by a group member would be the *most helpful* to
Lucille?

1. "What prevents you from losing weight?"
2. "If you feel that way, why did you join the group?"
3. "I guess your situation is pretty hopeless, at that."
4. "Sure you can, once you stop feeling sorry for yourself."

233. By the fourth meeting, the members are able to start sessions by themselves and are relating to each other in a warm, considerate manner. They are proud of each others' successful dieting attempts and able to cope supportively with an occasional member's feelings of discouragement. This unity and spirit illustrates a group quality known as
1. mutuality.
2. dependency.
3. genuineness.
4. cohesiveness.

234. For members to obtain the most benefit from a group, it is desirable for them to use functional group roles. In which one of the following instances is a group maintenance or building role (versus an individual role) being utilized by a group member?
1. Jill shows the group the latest pictures of her child.
2. Grace insists that everyone try her favorite reducing product.
3. Lucille makes quiet comments to the person sitting next to her.
4. Molly proposes an alternate way to keep from thinking about food.

235. The most successful person in the group is Thelma who lost 25 pounds during the past 3 months. The others, especially Molly, have patterned their eating habits after Thelma and have unconsciously adopted her attitudes toward food. Which one of the following mental mechanisms are they using?
1. Imitation.
2. Sublimation.
3. Incorporation.
4. Identification.

236. After 6 weeks, several members of the group have reached a stage when their weight has stabilized although they say they continue to follow the diet plan faithfully. Plateaus such as these are caused *most often* by
1. a slowdown in metabolism as body size decreases.
2. the accumulation of water in the body as fat is lost.
3. a temporary shortage of the glycogen-releasing substance.
4. an unconscious underestimation of the amount of food eaten.

237. Grace asks the nutritionist, "What's wrong with fad diets?"

Which one of the following explanations by the nutritionist is likely to be the *least threatening* and the *most acceptable* to the food faddist?

1. "Fad diets are nothing more than quick moneymakers for their originators."
2. "Fad diets usually lack one or more of the essential nutrients necessary for good health."
3. "Fad diets often are boring and tempt one to cheat because of the restrictions placed on what one may eat."
4. "Fad diets are for the emotionally insecure and the gullible looking for a magical solution to their problems."

238. Most of the group members are responsible for food preparation for others at home. While these women are trying to lose weight, which one of the following practices would be *best* for them to use in their homes in relation to food preparation?

1. Prepare two different meals, one as usual and one low caloric.
2. Serve the same menu to the whole family in different-sized portions.
3. Turn over the responsibility for food preparation to another member of the family.
4. Arrange for someone else to do the grocery shopping and the cleaning up after meals.

239. Jill, the youngest member of the group, asks what she can do to discourage her mother-in-law from trying to "fatten up" her 6-month-old daughter. Which one of the following responses by group members is likely to be the *most helpful* to Jill?

1. "Tell her your child's weight is no concern of hers."
2. "Tell her it upsets you when she gives the baby more to eat than you want her to have."
3. "Tell her she cannot come to visit anymore if she persists in pushing the baby to eat."
4. "Tell her that times have changed and her ways are no longer considered good for the baby."

240. Obesity is *most often* due to

1. the intake of more calories than are expended.
2. a disturbance in the functioning of the glands.
3. a long-standing and deep-seated emotional difficulty.
4. the resistance of the body to metabolizing the thyroid hormone.

241. Obesity is a social as well as a physical phenomenon. According to many knowledgeable observers, which one of the following feelings do grossly overweight people in the American culture *more often* experience in their interactions with others?

1. A sense of invulnerability, due to their size.

2. A sense of isolation, due to their rejection by others.
3. A sense of importance, due to the deference shown them.
4. A sense of anger, due to thoughtless remarks made by others.

242. Many people of the American culture have difficulty with weight control because they unconsciously equate food with
1. power and control.
2. love and affection.
3. status and prestige.
4. survivial and growth.

243. The relatively new field in medicine and nursing which deals specifically with the problem and treatment of obesity is called
1. podiatry.
2. lithology.
3. cryogenics.
4. bariatrics.

244. Discrimination should be used when using appetite-depressant drugs, such as the amphetamines, for overweight persons. Possible adverse effects of using the amphetamines on a long-term basis include *all* of the following signs/symptoms *except*
1. insomnia.
2. gastritis.
3. depression between doses.
4. behavior of toxic psychosis.

245. The *best* approach to the future control of obesity as a public health problem is
1. screening and treating overweight school children.
2. educating young mothers to prevent obesity in their children.
3. informing the adult population of the risks of being overweight.
4. making nutrition information available at senior citizen centers.

Nineteen-year-old Gary Ord was admitted to a psychiatric unit with a nonspecific diagnosis of personality disorder. He was accompanied by his mother and by a lawyer who told the nurse he hoped his client would "stay out of mischief until we get this crank phone call business straightened out."
Items 246 through 263 relate to this situation.

246. According to Gary's mother, Gary "always was a mean little boy, forever playing pranks on people and teasing the small animals in the neighborhood. Now he's just a bigger prankster and less easy to control." In view of Gary's history of meanness,

which one of the following courses of action would likely be the *most effective* for the nursing staff to follow initially?

1. Let the patient know the staff has the authority to subdue him if he gets unruly.
2. Keep the patient isolated from the other patients until he is better known by the staff.
3. Provide the patient with a list of rules while emphasizing that he will have to pay for any damages he causes.
4. Observe the patient's behavior on the unit closely to establish a baseline pattern of physical and social functioning.

247. Gary's parents have repeatedly told him that he was a bad, stupid person who would never amount to anything in this world. When Gary confirmed their opinion by dropping out of school and behaving antisocially, which one of the following phenomena is he acting out?

1. Congruency.
2. Double-bind.
3. Consensual validation.
4. Self-fulfilling prophecy.

248. Gary is a short, plump, sloppily dressed young man with a round face, thick glasses, and a stomping walk. He has feelings of inferiority which lead him to pick on others weaker than he. Which one of the following defense mechanisms does his bullying of others exemplify?

1. Fixation.
2. Compensation.
3. Identification.
4. Reaction formation.

249. After Gary has been on the unit for a few days, the nurses notice that he uses his shortness and unattractiveness as an excuse for not attending various unit social functions, such as the weekly dance. Of the following interventions, which one would be *best* for the nursing staff to take *first* to deal with his avoidance of social situations?

1. Tell him he will need a better excuse than his appearance for not participating.
2. Explain to him that everyone's cooperation is necessary to make the program a success.
3. Confront him with the fact that he is using his appearance as an excuse to avoid socializing.
4. Insist that he come up with some alternative ways to spend the time when he should be socializing.

250. Gary often takes pleasure in startling people. His favorite trick

is to loudly expel flatus when in a group and laugh at the discomfort it causes others. The prohibition against passing flatus in public in the American culture is known as a
1. more.
2. norm.
3. taboo.
4. folkway.

251. A staff member said to Gary after one of his more malodorous ejections of flatus, "Do you wonder that people find you repulsive?" Of the following possible effects of the nurse's comment on Gary, the *most likely* one is that it will make him feel
1. defensive and defiant.
2. insulted and indignant.
3. ashamed and remorseful.
4. embarrassed and unhappy.

252. Gary's past history of cruelty and present crass behavior arouse feelings of anxiety and antagonism in both staff and patients. For which one of the following reasons is it *most probable* that this reaction occurs in others?
1. The behavior is beyond comprehension.
2. The behavior is viewed as alien to their value system.
3. The behavior is seen as only too understandable by them.
4. The behavior is easily misinterpreted as to its meaning.

253. The staff member to whom Gary relates best is Mr. Dant, a registered nurse. Even so, Gary sometimes attempts to provoke Mr. Dant by yelling down the hall, "Hey nursie, where's your hat and purse?" In relation to being baited by the patient, which one of the following actions is *best* for the nurse to take?
1. Ignore the patient's kidding to avoid reinforcing it.
2. Smilingly shake the head no at the patient to stop his teasing.
3. Use feminine gestures to indicate acceptance of the patient's ribbing.
4. Challenge the patient to an arm wrestling match to prove the nurse's masculinity.

254. Gary tells the nurse that he likes to call hospitals and make bomb threats. He laughs because, he says, he enjoys watching the patients being evacuated and the police running in and out of the buildings. Of the following replies that the nurse could make, which one would be *least helpful* in encouraging Gary to examine the meaning and effects of such messages?
1. "What does it do for you to tell me that?"
2. "You could be sent to jail for that, you know."

3. "You make bomb threats and everybody hops, is that right?"
4. "You mean to expect me to be shocked by what you are saying?"

255. One evening, Gary takes Mr. Dant aside and whispers, "Don't tell anybody but I'm going to call in a bomb threat to this hospital tonight." Of the following actions the nurse could take, which one would *best* preserve Gary's trust in the nurse and provide the *best* protection for all concerned parties?
1. Warn the patient that his phone privileges will be taken away if he abuses them.
2. Offer to disregard the patient's plan for wrongdoing if he does not go through with it.
3. Say nothing to anyone until the patient has actually completed the call and notify the proper authorities.
4. Explain to the patient that this information will have to be shared immediately with the staff and with his doctor.

256. Each time Gary behaves in a foolhardy or cruel manner, constructive disciplinary action is taken by the staff. At those times, which one of the following ideas is the *most basic* and *most important* for the staff to convey to the patient?
1. He is accepted, although his behavior may not be.
2. No one would bother with him if they did not care about him.
3. If he cannot control his behavior, others will have to control it for him.
4. Everyone must cope with some restriction on his actions.

257. The nursing staff tries hard to provide Gary with corrective emotional experiences that will positively influence his present behavior. Of the following possible interventions, which one would constitute a corrective emotional experience for Gary?
1. The staff gives him gifts to make up for his earlier suffering.
2. The staff treats his misbehavior more objectively than others in his past did.
3. The staff promises him material rewards and extra privileges for good behavior.
4. The staff allows him complete freedom in deciding what available therapies he will utilize.

258. Of the following statements by Gary's mother, which one offers the *best* clue as to why Gary developed into a young adult with impulsive, antisocial tendencies?
1. "He is just like his father, that no-good bum."
2. "His birth entailed a difficult pregnancy for me with a very long labor."
3. "I guess I've just always been a little afraid to say 'no' to him."

    4. "We lived in a poor neighborhood and that's why he turned out so bad."

259. Gary's and the nurse's relationship develops to the point where they are able to delineate and concentrate on a goal for Gary of making friends. To begin the daily conference during which the nurse wishes to assess Gary's progress, which one of the following opening statements by the nurse would be likely to elicit the *least* information from the patient?
    1. "How was your day? Did everything go okay?"
    2. "I noticed you went for a walk by yourself this morning."
    3. "Tell me what you did when people said 'hello' to you today."
    4. "Weren't you going to sit next to someone new at lunch? What happened?"

260. The nurse decides that Gary's problematic behavior stems from feelings of resentment toward his mother. His resentment seems to represent an attempt by Gary to punish his mother for what he perceives as her lack of concern for him. The *best* thing for the nurse to do with this information is to
    1. pass it on to the patient promptly.
    2. assist the patient to gradually discover it for himself.
    3. tell it to the patient's mother so she will better understand him.
    4. record it on the patient's chart so that the psychiatrist can deal with it.

261. Should Gary improve his relationship with his mother and establish his sense of identity as an adult man, which one of the following age-related growth and development tasks would he be expected to master *next*?
    1. A sense of intimacy.
    2. A sense of autonomy.
    3. A sense of integrity.
    4. A sense of productivity.

262. During the latter part of his hospitalization, Gary's progress slows and he seems to be making more enemies than friends. Which one of the following subsequent conjectures of the situation by the nurse is probably *most accurate?*
    1. It is only a temporary setback.
    2. Gary is trying to make the nurse look bad.
    3. Gary has too many shortcomings to overcome.
    4. It means the nurse has been unable to help Gary.

263. Of the following terms, which one *best* describes a patient's sense of self-awareness of his attitudes and defense mechanisms as well as his self-understanding of why he behaves as he does?
    1. Insight.

2. Rapport.
3. Lucidity.
4. Cathexis.

Monica Moore, who is 14 years old, was readmitted to the adolescent unit of the psychiatric hospital. She recently had run away from home for the fifth time that year and was picked up by the police while hitchhiking in a state of drug-induced euphoria on the freeway. She was accompanied to the unit by her juvenile worker.

Items 264 through 279 relate to this situation.

264. "Hi, gang, I'm back," Monica says cheerfully to the unit at large. Which one of the following statements that Monica could make about her readmission would show the *best* prospects for her eventual success in therapy?
1. "I'm here because my parents were bugging me again."
2. "I'm here because my shrink thought it would be best."
3. "I'm here because I made a mess of it on the outside."
4. "I'm here because I missed all the fun we had together."

265. Monica is termed a manipulator by the staff because, in the past, she played one staff member against another for favors and made them angry with each other. Labeling a patient usually functions to
1. stop one from expecting too much of the person.
2. keep one from seeing the person as she really is.
3. prevent one from being made a fool of by the person.
4. help one decide early on how to act toward the person.

266. Monica is assigned to the care of an overweight nurse on the evening shift. The nurse recalls that, after finding Monica in bed with a young male patient during her last admission, she became the butt of some of Monica's jokes. Which one of the following courses of action would be *best* for the nurse to take concerning such previous negative experiences with a patient?
1. Forget them as quickly as possible.
2. Accept them as unpleasant but past experiences.
3. Excuse them as part of the patient's poor upbringing.
4. Remember them as significant examples of the patient's present capacity for mischief.

267. The nurse initiates a conversation with Monica. Monica tries to put the nurse at ease, graciously telling her to sit down and inquiring what she could do for her. Monica leads the discussion and informs the nurse how much time she can spend with

her. Which one of the following phenomena is illustrated by this interaction?
1. Denial.
2. Incongruency.
3. Role reversal.
4. Self-fulfilling prophecy.

268. The nurse recognizes that she is having difficulty maintaining control in her relationship with Monica. Which one of the following actions would be *best* for the nurse to take in relation to being outmaneuvered by this patient?
1. Try to handle the situation alone.
2. Request to be assigned to a different patient.
3. Seek help from the supervisor with the relationship.
4. Discuss feelings of frustration with the patient.

269. In the course of their conversation, Monica tells the nurse bitterly, "My parents are mean. They don't care about me at all." Which one of the following responses by the nurse would be the *least* therapeutic?
1. "You feel your parents don't care about you."
2. "What would be a sign to you that your parents cared?"
3. "I am sure your parents have your best interests at heart."
4. "Tell me more about your parents being mean and not caring."

270. Monica is quick to learn what the problems of other people are and to utilize this knowledge for her own amusement. She makes a target of a 15-year-old withdrawn girl and has the other patients tease and play tricks on her. Of the following people, who would probably have the *most* influence in getting Monica to change her behavior?
1. Her physician.
2. Her peer group.
3. Her juvenile worker.
4. Her religious counselor.

271. Which one of the following interventions would be *best* for the nursing staff to make when Monica uses others for her amusement?
1. Transfer the withdrawn patient to another unit until Monica leaves.
2. Reprimand Monica and confine her to her room until her behavior improves.
3. Transfer Monica to another unit and explain to her why it was necessary to do so.
4. Confront Monica with her behavior and let her know what is expected of her and the consequences of misbehaving.

272. Which one of the following statements that could be made by a

staff member would be *best* in explaining to Monica why she must abide by hospital regulations?

1. "If you do not follow the rules, your privileges will be taken away."
2. "It is not always easy, but the rules must be followed so everyone will get a fair shake."
3. "You are not the only person around; the rest of us have rights too, that must be respected."
4. "You may break the rules as you want, but don't expect any sympathy from us if you get caught."

273. It did not bother Monica that her trick-playing, teasing, and running away from home may have caused suffering to others. This lack of remorse is due to a defect in the functioning of the

1. id.
2. ego.
3. superego.
4. nervous system.

274. Which one of the following traits would Monica also be *most likely* to display?

1. Poor judgment.
2. Faulty memory.
3. Low intelligence.
4. Disordered thinking.

275. Which one of the following qualities would be *especially important* for the nursing staff to show when taking disciplinary measures with a patient such as Monica?

1. Strictness.
2. Acceptance.
3. Consistency.
4. Permissiveness.

276. At the weekly dance, Monica flirts with a staff member and while dancing, rubs up against him suggestively. Which one of the following responses by the staff member would be the *most appropriate?*

1. "You shouldn't do that. People are watching us."
2. "Let me show you how to do this new dance. It's a lot of fun."
3. "You look thirsty. I'll go get us some punch from the dining room."
4. "It makes me feel very uncomfortable when you do that. Please stop."

277. In the situation described in item 276, it would be *most important* that the nurse try to avoid making Monica feel

1. unhappy.
2. rejected.

3. punished.

4. unfeminine.

278. The structured program of the unit helps Monica modify her behavior in a positive direction although she still occasionally reverts to her old habits. For example, Monica explains that she did not sign out when she left the unit for a walk because the sign-out sheet was full. Also, she says, the other patients knew where she was going and could have told the staff. Which one of the following defenses is Monica using?

1. Isolation.

2. Confabulation.

3. Rationalization.

4. Intellectualization.

279. One month after her admission, Monica is to be discharged home. As the nurse walks with her to the door, Monica says in an offhand manner, "I'll probably be back." Which one of the following actions would be *best* for the nurse to take in relation to this situation?

1. Ask what she meant by the remark.

2. Agree with her assessment of the situation.

3. Ignore the comment as a play for attention.

4. Consult the physician concerning readmission for more therapy.

Ms. Alice Choates, who is 22 years old, was brought by her parents' limousine from the cold-water flat where she had been living with several other drug addicts to the emergency room of a psychiatric hospital. The admitting diagnosis was depression and drug toxicity. However, it was known that Ms. Choate is a heroin addict.

Items 280 through 297 are related to this situation.

280. The purposeful provision of a relatively nonspecific and vague admitting diagnosis for a patient with known drug addiction *most likely* represents a misguided and generally unnecessary effort on the part of the physician to

1. test the observation skills of the nurses.

2. ensure payment by the patient's insurance company.

3. safeguard the patient's reputation in the community.

4. give himself additional time to evaluate the patient's condition.

281. Earlier on the day of her admission, Ms. Choate gave herself her usual dose of heroin. However, it came from a purer-than-usual supply of heroin, sending her into a light coma. Her

respirations were shallow and her blood pressure was low. A narcotic antagonist, naloxone (Narcon), is administered to the patient. When compared with the narcotic antagonists, N-allynormorphine (Nalline) and levallorphan (Lorfan), the duration of action of naloxone is

1. much shorter.
2. about the same length.
3. about twice as long.
4. about five times as long.

282. For which one of the following conditions should the patient who has received naloxone be carefully and continuously observed?

1. Cerebral edema.
2. Kidney failure.
3. Seizure activity.
4. Recurrence of coma.

283. Which one of the following "street" techniques tried by Ms. Choate's friends to combat her heroin overdose was *least likely* to have worsened or complicated her physical condition?

1. Giving milk intravenously.
2. Infusing salt intravenously.
3. Injecting an amphetamine intramuscularly.
4. Administering mouth-to-mouth resuscitation.

284. In the past, Ms. Choate occasionally used cocaine. For which one of the following telltale signs should the nurse look to help detect whether the patient had recently abused this drug?

1. Red, excoriated nostrils.
2. Clear, constricted pupils.
3. White patchy areas on the tongue.
4. Lumpy abscesses in intramuscular areas.

285. Ms. Choate is transferred to the chemical dependency unit when her condition becomes stable. Twelve hours later, she develops signs of heroin withdrawal. Of the following signs/symptoms of opiate withdrawal, which ones occur *late*, rather than early, in the course of withdrawal?

1. Vomiting and diarrhea.
2. Yawning and diaphoresis.
3. Lacrimation and rhinorrhea.
4. Restlessness and nervousness.

286. Ms. Choate has numerous complaints of discomfort while abstaining from heroin. Which one of the following nursing orders that appear on the patient's care plan would be the *least* advisable and effective?

1. Be sympathetic but firm with her complaints.
2. Promise to reevaluate her withdrawal plan to ease her discomfort.
3. Prepare her in advance for the minor discomforts that might occur.
4. Inform her of alternative methods, such as warm baths, for dealing with aches and pains.

287. Mr. Choate is 5 months pregnant. Starting about 48 hours after birth, an infant born to a mother dependent on heroin would be *most likely* to show *all* of the following symptoms *except*
1. hypertonicity.
2. urinary retention.
3. hyperbilirubinemia.
4. respiratory distress.

288. Ms. Choate's mother, a fashionably dressed woman, complains to the nurse, "Can you imagine, *my* daughter, so educated and well brought up, getting pregnant by one of those revolting, illiterate nobodies she was living with? I'll never live it down." Which one of the following possible replies by the nurse would be *best?*
1. "It must be very difficult for you to accept."
2. "I guess everyone has to have a share of problems."
3. "Is this the first time something like this has happened with your daughter?"
4. "I wonder if perhaps you aren't more concerned with yourself than with your daughter."

289. Although Ms. Choate feels she was forced into the hospital, she nevertheless reluctantly says she will give the unit program a try. Which one of the following explanations provides the *most likely* reason for her seeming willingness to change?
1. She is bending to staff pressure to alter her ways.
2. She is at a crisis point in her life and, thus, is more receptive to new ideas.
3. She has reached a stage in her pregnancy when her maternal instincts have taken over.
4. She has had the time and opportunity to examine her former life style and has logically made the decision to reject it.

290. Ms. Choate's physician orders a methadone substitution program for the patient. Which one of the following agencies regulates and restricts the use of methadone in detoxification programs?
1. The Food and Drug Administration.
2. The Commission on Marijuana and Drug Abuse.
3. The Department of Health, Education and Welfare.

4. The National Conference for Methadone Treatment.

291. If Ms. Choate becomes intoxicated from a dose of methadone, which one of the following nursing actions is indicated?
1. Withhold her next dose of methadone.
2. Search her belongings for hidden drugs.
3. Stay with her when she is up and about.
4. Keep her actively involved in a fast-paced sport.

292. Which one of the following characteristics of methadone offers the *most* potential for its abuse?
1. It blunts the craving for heroin.
2. It prevents the suffering of withdrawal symptoms.
3. It blocks the pleasurable effects of heroin.
4. It is equally effective at a low dose or a high dose.

293. In order to comply with official guidelines for a methadone maintenance program, which one of the following policies is *most often* specified as necessary?
1. Clients should not be identified by name.
2. Clients should not take methadone off the premises when they receive it.
3. Regular blood test checks should be made on the clients.
4. Social and rehabilitation services are to be made available to the clients.

294. In relation to Ms. Choate's drug habit, the *primary* reason she will need to learn new living and social skills from the health team members is that she formerly lived in a world dominated by
1. false sensory data.
2. fear of the authorities.
3. minimal contact with others.
4. preoccupation with obtaining and taking drugs.

295. Ms. Choate says she will ask for help from Synanon if nothing else works for her. Which one of the following concepts will the newly arrived addict at Synanon *most likely* encounter?
1. A member is expected to make a lifelong home with the Synanon community.
2. A member cannot leave the Synanon community for at least 3 months after entering it.
3. The narcotic addict will learn containment of his emotions in informal group sessions.
4. The narcotic addict can eventually be cured of his addiction with the help of the Synanon members.

296. Ms. Choate's eventual success or progress when out of the hospital can probably *best* be measured by the
1. kinds of friends she makes.

2. number of drug-free days she has.

3. way she gets along with her parents.

4. degree of responsibility her job entails.

297. Which one of the following physical disorders is the heroin addict *least* prone to develop?

1. Hepatitis.

2. Pneumonia.

3. Tuberculosis.

4. Cholelithiasis.

Ms. Lola Albert, a 36-year-old mother of two children, was brought by ambulance to the emergency room of the hospital after taking an overdose of barbiturates. A male friend arrived a short time later carrying some of her personal belongings. Items 298 through 317 relate to this situation.

298. Ms. Albert went into a state of shock at home and is in a semicoma on admission. Should death occur shortly, to which one of the following causes would it *most likely* be due?

1. Kidney failure.

2. Internal hemorrhage.

3. Cardiac standstill.

4. Respiratory depression.

299. Ms. Albert's acquaintance says she has been taking about eight "reds" (800 mg. of secobarbital [Seconal]) daily besides drinking more alcohol than she usually does. Of the following terms, which one *best* describes the interaction of barbiturates and alcohol?

1. Additive.

2. Suppressive.

3. Potentiating.

4. Antagonistic.

300. After about 20 minutes, Ms. Albert's friend asks anxiously, "Do you think she will live?" Which one of the following replies would be *best*?

1. "We can only wait and see."

2. "You had better ask the doctor about that."

3. "If she doesn't, it will be her own fault."

4. "Her condition is serious. You are worried, aren't you?"

301. The nurse talks further with Ms. Albert's friend and tries to determine the nature of their relationship. Which one of the following motivations provides the *best* justification for the nurse's inquiries?

1. To satisfy the nurse's curiosity about the patient's life style.

2. To ascertain the friend's capabilities as a source of support for the patient.

3. To establish how much financial responsibility the friend will assume for the patient.

4. To determine whether the friend can be trusted with confidential information about the patient.

302. Prior to her hospitalization, Ms. Albert needed increasingly larger doses of barbiturates to achieve the same euphoric effect she initially realized from their use. This decreased response to a drug is known as

1. tolerance.
2. addiction.
3. dependence.
4. habituation.

303. By which one of the following symptoms could Ms. Albert probably have been identified as a chronic user of barbiturates in the days before her hospitalization?

1. Her drooling, fainting, and illusions.
2. Her diaphoresis, twitching, and sneezing.
3. Her suspiciousness, tachycardia, and edema.
4. Her sluggishness, ataxia, and irritability.

304. After gastric lavage, Ms. Albert's vital signs stabilize and she later awakens in a confused state. Which one the following measures would be *least desirable* for the nurses to take while Ms. Albert is recovering from the overdose of sedatives?

1. Maintain seizure precautions with the patient.
2. Close the windows in the vicinity of the patient.
3. Use short, complete sentences when speaking to the patient.
4. Obtain a prn order for a medication for anxiety and agitation.

305. Following a dose-response test, Ms. Albert receives pentobarbital sodium (Nembutal) at a nonintoxicating maintenance level for 2 days, and at decreasing doses thereafter. This regimen is prescribed for the patient *primarily* to help prevent the possibly fatal occurrence of

1. psychosis.
2. convulsions.
3. hypotension.
4. hypothermia.

306. By how many mg. is the maintenance dose of the barbiturate pentobarbital sodium usually reduced daily?

1. 50 mg.
2. 100 mg.
3. 150 mg.
4. 200 mg.

307. Which one of the following phrases *best* describes the duration of activity of pentobarbital sodium in the body?
    1. Long-acting.
    2. Short-acting.
    3. Intermediate-acting.
    4. Of indeterminate duration.

308. When Ms. Albert becomes more alert and responsive, she says to her physician, "It was an accident. I must have forgotten how many sleeping pills I had already taken and just downed a few more." Accidental overdose is a common occurrence even with those who do not abuse the drugs and can *best* be prevented by
    1. jotting down an "X" and the time for every capsule taken.
    2. keeping the capsules in a place inconvenient to the bedside.
    3. using packaged unit-dose capsules rather than a container jar.
    4. turning on a light by which to read the medication label each time before a capsule is taken.

309. Laboratory data and further discussions of Ms. Albert with her psychiatrist reveal that she is also taking the amphetamine phenmetrazine hydrochloride (Preludin) as an "upper" daily. Ms. Albert can be expected to show *all* of the following symptoms during amphetamine withdrawal *except*
    1. hunger.
    2. fatigue.
    3. depression.
    4. lacrimation.

310. Which one of the following disadvantages associated with a continuous high intake of amphetamines poses the *greatest* danger for the drug abuser?
    1. The person may become psychologically dependent on the drug.
    2. The person may become paranoid and violent from taking the drug.
    3. The person may become depressed and suicidal between doses of the drug.
    4. The person may develop an infection from self-administration of the drug.

311. For which one of the following conditions is the use of amphetamines legally and medically approved?
    1. Fatigue.
    2. Narcolepsy.
    3. Depression.
    4. Long-term weight reduction.

312. In view of Ms. Albert's chemical dependencies, toward which

one of the following ends in particular should her nursing care
be directed during her first few days on the mental health unit?
1. Toward increasing her level of physical activity.
2. Toward renewing her optimism and faith in herself.
3. Toward correcting her fluid and electrolyte imbalance.
4. Toward getting her legal entanglements, if any, straightened
   out.

313. Which one of the following items of information will Ms. Albert's
     physician probably be *most concerned* with obtaining during
     the initial interview sessions with the patient?
     1. The effects of her drug dependency on her children.
     2. The positive and negative ways she views her drug depen-
        dency.
     3. The personal and social drives that led to her drug depen-
        dency.
     4. The length of time she thinks she will need to recover from her
        drug dependency.

314. In the opinion of one staff member, Ms. Albert is rich, pampered,
     and spoiled. When trying to influence that staff member to
     perceive the patient in a more positive light, which one of the
     following statements that the nurse could make would be
     best?
     1. "It sounds to me as though you're a bit jealous of her."
     2. "She is a very likeable person once you get to know her."
     3. "If you knew all the trouble she's had, you'd be less quick to
        judge."
     4. "I find her to be a frightened and lonely woman beneath that
        indulged exterior."

315. At which time of the day during the drug withdrawal period can
     the nurse anticipate that Ms. Albert will probably become the
     most demanding and have the most complaints?
     1. At night when she cannot sleep.
     2. In the evening when she is bored.
     3. After lunch when her visitors arrive.
     4. In the morning when she wakes up trembling.

316. The staff notices that Ms. Albert spends most of her time with the
     young adult patients, most of whom have also misused drugs.
     This group of patients is a dominant force on the unit, keeping
     the nondrug users entertained with stories of their "highs."
     In which one of the following ways is this problem *best* dealt
     with by the staff?
     1. By providing additional recreation for the patients.
     2. By breaking up drug-oriented discussions whenever possible.
     3. By speaking with the patients individually about their
        behavior.

4. By bringing up for discussion staff observations of the patients' drug-oriented conversations at the weekly patient group meetings.

317. Of the following factors, which one has probably contributed *most* to the widespread abuse of drugs in the American culture today?
1. The lax moral standards of the present generation.
2. The negligible legal penalties imposed for illicit drug possession.
3. The abundant, inexpensive, and readily available supply of drugs on the market.
4. The socially acceptable, routine use of drugs for the relief of minor ailments.

Ms. George, Ms. Salter, and Mr. Victor are nurse counselors at a crisis shelter. The length of their experience in crisis counseling ranges from 3 weeks to 2 years. Several patients arrived at the shelter one evening simultaneously.
Items 318 through 339 relate to this situation.

318. For the inexperienced members of the crisis team, *all* of the following job requirements are immediately essential for effective nursing practice *except*
1. formal classes in crisis theory and intervention.
2. close supervision by a qualified member of the team.
3. a complete orientation to the shelter policies and procedures.
4. an interest in working with disturbed individuals on a short-term basis.

319. Ms. George brings Cari, an anxious-looking, pretty blonde teenager, to an interviewing room. The girl, sobbingly, relates that she thinks she is pregnant but does not know what to do. Which one of the following possible interventions would be the *most appropriate* at this point?
1. Ask the patient what she wishes to do next.
2. Give the patient some ideas about what to do next.
3. Summarize what the patient was heard to say and ask her to confirm or correct the nurse's perceptions.
4. Question the patient in more detail about her feelings and about what her parents' reactions are likely to be.

320. Cari says she and her boy friend have engaged in "mostly heavy petting and necking." For which one of the following reasons is the nurse *least likely* to ask the girl to define what she means by "heavy petting and necking" and "mostly?"
1. To try to gain a shared meaning for vague words.

2. To determine the extent of the couple's sexual activities.
3. To establish a relationship based on mutual understandings.
4. To pinpoint discrepancies or contradictions in the patient's story.

321. Tests for pregnancy indicate that Cari is not pregnant. The *most likely* reason for the patient's temporary menstrual cessation is
1. inflammation of the endometrium.
2. anxiety related to personal concerns.
3. diminishing levels of estrogen in the blood.
4. minor damage to the fallopian tubes during strenuous physical activity.

322. Ms. George teaches Cari about sexual intercourse, contraceptives, and the like. For which one of the following behaviors will the nurse *most probably* be indirectly responsible for increasing in Cari?
1. Her promiscuity.
2. Her antagonism toward men.
3. Her rejection of the female role.
4. Her preparedness for sexual encounters.

323. Cari states that although she is grateful for the information she has received from Ms. George, she does not believe she needs it. "No more fooling around for me!" she states. Which one of the following replies by the somewhat skeptical nurse would be *best?*
1. "The last person who said that ended up having a baby."
2. "Just in case, why don't you try the pills for a while."
3. "It's up to you, but if you should change your mind, come back and we'll try to help you."
4. "Aren't you being a little bit overconfident about it, as attractive as you must be to the fellows?"

324. The state law, as well as the crisis shelter where Ms. George is employed, follows a current trend in relation to releasing information when the patient is a minor. If Cari's parents ask that the content of the nurse-patient interviews be revealed to them, it would be best for the nurse to be guided by knowledge that the information
1. may be obtained by the parents only through a court order.
2. is confidential and should be released only with the patient's consent.
3. must be given to the parents of the underage patient upon the parents' request.
4. is available to the parents with the signed approval of the director of the crisis shelter.

325. Mr. Victor talks to two 11-year-old boys on the telephone who

think a friend of theirs sniffs. They say his breath sometimes smells like glue and he acts "drunk." They ask if glue-sniffing could do him any harm. When formulating a reply, the nurse should be guided by knowledge that the body organs *most often* damaged by inhalants are the

1. lungs and the liver.
2. heart and the aorta.
3. pancreas and the spleen.
4. gallbladder and the stomach.

326. Mr. Victor urges the boys to seek help for their friend and warns them that delayed treatment could result in the boy's death. A person who inhales noxious substances is *most likely* to die from

1. anemia.
2. fat embolus.
3. malnutrition.
4. brain lesions.

327. Ms. Salter is caring for a 19-year-old patient who was accompanied to the crisis shelter by two female friends. His name is Fred and he is frightened and hallucinating. The nurse learns that he "dropped acid" about 3 hours ago. The psychedelic substance Fred took was lysergic acid diethylamide (LSD). Which of the following names are also used for psychedelics or hallucinogens?

1. Skag, junk, H.
2. Rainbows, downs, M.
3. Bennies, speed, APC.
4. Cactus, psilocybin, DMT.

328. Which one of the following statements about the usual effects of LSD is *incorrect?*

1. It increases one's creativity.
2. It makes time seem to pass more slowly.
3. It causes sounds to be portrayed in color.
4. It gives rise to vivid visual hallucinations.

329. Fred is having an adverse reaction to LSD known as a "bad trip" and he shows extreme anxiety and loss of touch with reality. His *greatest* need at this time will *most likely* be for

1. physical contact with others.
2. privacy and isolation from others.
3. involvement in a physical activity.
4. reassurance and a soothing atmosphere.

330. To help Fred reestablish his self-control and orientation, which one of the following comments would be *most useful* for the nurse to make to him?

1. "You have no need to be concerned; you are going to be all right."
2. "You have taken a drug you should not have and it is making you sick."
3. "You are coming down from an acid trip and will soon be past the main drug reaction."
4. "You have a temporary psychosis from ingesting a psychedelic; let's watch some television while we wait for it to pass."

331. The use of tranquilizing drugs, such as chlorpromazine hydrochloride (Thorazine), to shorten the hallucinogenic drug reaction should be *avoided* because
1. the hallucinations might stem from an entirely different source than the psychedelic drug.
2. the major tranquilizers can cause a re-uptake of the hallucinogen in the brain.
3. flashbacks increase in severity when mediating drugs are used to treat the initial reaction.
4. other incompatible drugs might have been combined with the hallucinogen that, together with the tranquilizer, might be fatal.

332. If Fred continues to use hallucinogens, such as LSD, on a long-term basis, which one of the following events would be very likely to happen?
1. He might die from an overdose.
2. He might develop pericarditis.
3. He might become physically addicted.
4. He might have children with birth defects.

333. Sheila, a rather heavy, long-haired, buxom girl of 17 has come to the crisis shelter. She shares a coke with Mr. Victor during his break and asks him, seemingly casually, "How would you feel if your girlfriend had been raped?" Mr. Victor suspects the question was a personal one not rhetorical. Which one of the following replies that the nurse could make would be *best?*
1. "Before I answer, tell me what's really on your mind, okay?"
2. "I have not thought about it. How would you expect me to feel?"
3. "Probably I'd be upset and angry. Do you have a special reason for asking?"
4. "It wouldn't bother me too much. But don't you think there is too much violence these days?"

334. Sheila has been ambivalent about telling anyone of a recent sexual assault on her. Which one of the following beliefs about the rape experience is probably the *most widely* held in

this society and no doubt has contributed to the patient's reluctance to speak about being raped?

1. The woman is somehow to blame for the rape.
2. The woman is probably out to "get" the man involved.
3. The woman must show physical injury to prove her innocence.
4. The woman gets more enjoyment than pain from the experience.

335. Mr. Victor tells Sheila that even if she was protected against pregnancy by a contraceptive and has no intention of taking any legal action against her assailant, she should still be checked by a physician. This postrape physical examination is indicated for the early detection of

1. venereal disease.
2. neurotic reaction.
3. periurethral tears.
4. menstrual difficulties.

336. Since the rape, Sheila has constantly sought out brightly lit places and the company of friendly people. In addition, she plans to move to another part of the city. At which one of these unconscious goals are her maneuvers *most* probably aimed?

1. Self-defense.
2. Self-assertion.
3. Self-deception.
4. Self-gratification.

337. In which one of the following instances can the nurse anticipate that Sheila will have future adjustment problems and a need for additional counseling in relation to being sexually assaulted?

1. When she becomes upset when talking about the rape to anyone.
2. When she seeks support from formerly ignored relatives and friends.
3. When her parents show shame and suspicion over her part in the rape.
4. When her life becomes focused on helping other rape victims like herself.

338. When a rape victim arrives at an emergency room for treatment, which one of the following activities should the nursing staff be *especially* sure to carry out for its own and the client's legal protection?

1. Keep prying, insensitive personnel away from the victim.
2. Record the victim's account of the assault in her own words.
3. Arrange for the victim to be escorted home by a trustworthy party.

4. Hand-carry any evidence from the victim's person to the pathology laboratory.
339. Which one of the following actions should a nurse involved in a rape prevention program encourage both women and children to take on their own behalf?
1. Strive to physically incapacitate the attacker.
2. Plead with the attacker to be let go unharmed.
3. Try to avoid areas where potential assailants may be lurking.
4. Threaten the assailant by saying that he will go to jail for his crime.

A friend accompanied Mr. Peter Willard to the substance abuse unit of the hospital where he is to be admitted for detoxication from alcohol.
Items 340 through 359 relate to this situation.

340. Mr. Willard consumed about 6 ounces of alcohol just before coming to the hospital. Of the following methods, which one would be *best* for the nursing staff to use in promoting the rate of alcohol destruction in the patient's body?
1. Walk him around the unit following a cold shower.
2. Have him breathe pure oxygen through a face mask.
3. Give him copious amounts of black coffee to drink.
4. Provide him with a restful room so that he can sleep off the effects of alcohol.
341. Hospital policy requires that the patient's belongings be searched for contraband on admission. In view of Mr. Willard's drinking problem, which one of the following possessions of his is *most likely* to be confiscated by the nursing staff?
1. Hair oil.
2. Shaving cream.
3. Electric razor.
4. Antiseptic mouthwash.
342. When obtaining a nursing history, the nurse questions Mr. Willard regarding the amount of alcohol he consumed daily. The nurse can expect that Mr. Willard will probably answer the question by
1. exaggerating the amount.
2. being untruthful about the amount.
3. underestimating the amount.
4. expressing uncertainty about the amount.
343. Of the following basic needs of Mr. Willard, which two will probably require the *most* attention from the nursing staff during the early detoxication period?

1. Rest and nutrition.
2. Comfort and hygiene.
3. Safety and security.
4. Aeration and elimination.

344. The nurse who could probably relate *most effectively* with an alcoholic patient like Mr. Willard is one who has an attitude of
1. hearty optimism.
2. strict morality.
3. tolerant acceptance.
4. sympathetic indulgence.

345. The nurse learns that Mr. Willard was once arrested for driving while intoxicated. Most laws in this country state that a person is considered to be legally intoxicated when his blood alcohol level is above
1. 0.05 percent.
2. 0.15 percent.
3. 0.25 percent.
4. 0.40 percent.

346. Which one of the following medications, administered intramuscularly, would the physician *most likely* prescribe for Mr. Willard to provide sedation and to ease some of the anxiety and discomfort of the alcohol withdrawal process?
1. Paraldehyde (Paral).
2. Chlordiazepoxide (Librium).
3. Phenobarbital sodium (Luminal).
4. Diphenylhydantoin sodium (Dilantin).

347. Mr. Willard could not remember the events of the past weekend although he had receipts in his pockets from several shops where he made purchases on Saturday. This problem is illustrative of a condition known as
1. a blackout.
2. a hangover.
3. a dry drunk syndrome.
4. an alcoholic hallucinosis.

348. After a day of abstinence, Mr. Willard has coarse tremors of the hands which make it hard for him to feed himself. He asks the nurse how long it will be before his "shakes" go away. On which one of the following facts should the nurse base her reply?
1. The tremors can only be relieved by a further intake of alcohol.
2. The tremors usually are relieved after 2 days of abstinence from alcohol.
3. The tremors are a permanent condition due to irreversible central nervous system damage.

4. The tremors may persist for several days or even longer after alcohol intake has stopped.

349. Mr. Willard starts to crave a drink while withdrawing from alcohol. Which one of the following controls constitutes the *best* way to prevent the patient from obtaining alcoholic beverages at this time?
1. A locked door policy.
2. A routine search of visitors.
3. One-to-one supervision by the staff.
4. Support from other alcoholic patients.

350. Mr. Willard ashamedly told the nurse that he had hit his wife during a recent argument and asked the nurse if she thought his wife would ever forgive him. Which one of the following replies by the nurse would be *best* to make?
1. "Do you think she will?"
2. "I wouldn't, if I were she."
3. "Perhaps you could call her up and find out."
4. "It would depend on how much she really cares for you."

351. Mr. Willard's wife agrees to meet with her husband's therapist but says she has "about had it with his foolishness and bad temper." Which one of the following organizations would probably be the *most helpful* to her in obtaining additional assistance and support in coping with her alcoholic spouse?
1. Al-Anon.
2. Alateen.
3. The Salvation Army.
4. Alcoholics Anonymous.

352. After his physical condition stabilizes, Mr. Willard begins to attend daily group therapy sessions. Which one of the following descriptions *best* fits the group's members, who are "typical" victims of alcoholism?
1. They are members of evangelistic-type religions.
2. They are individuals from a low socioeconomic class.
3. They are persons with male or mannish characteristics.
4. They are individuals representative of the general adult population.

353. The members of Mr. Willard's group try to give each other feedback on their behavior. Of the following statements, which one is illustrative of *constructive* feedback?
1. "I think you are a real con artist."
2. "You are dominating the conversation."
3. "You interrupted John twice in four minutes."
4. "You don't give anyone a chance to finish talking."

354. Toward which one of the following ends should an inpatient

alcoholism program be geared to *best* assist a chemically dependent individual toward a state of health?
1. Changing the family interaction and communication patterns.
2. Determining the underlying intrapsychic problem of the person.
3. Rebuilding the person's life around satisfying substitutes for alcohol.
4. Withdrawing the person from alcohol to a plateau of physiological stability.

355. Mr. Willard was started on a regimen of disulfiram (Antabuse). A valuable asset of disulfiram therapy is that it
1. reminds the problem drinker of his misbehavior.
2. helps curb the impulsiveness of the problem drinker.
3. improves the capacity of the alcoholic for logical drinking.
4. creates a nerve block so the effects of the alcohol are not felt.

356. If Mr. Willard were to drink alcohol while receiving disulfiram, the nurse might expect him to show *all* of the following symptoms *except*
1. flushing.
2. palpitations.
3. muscular flaccidity.
4. nausea and vomiting.

357. A daily lecture series on alcoholism is conducted by the therapists on the substance abuse unit. When considering the following symptoms of alcoholism, it should be explained by the therapists that later, during the more chronic stage of the disease, the patient will *most likely* experience.
1. increased alcohol tolerance.
2. feelings of grandiosity and increasing combativeness.
3. the desire to switch to a different form of alcoholic beverage.
4. vague feelings of apprehension and doom.

358. Which one of the following instructions should be given to members of Mr. Willard's family who are concerned about helping him to maintain his sobriety after his release from the hospital?
1. "Warn others not to serve him drinks."
2. "Refrain from bringing up his past mistakes."
3. "Destroy his liquor supply before he comes home."
4. "Use whatever means you have to make him get needed help."

359. Prior to Mr. Willard's being discharged, which one of the following remarks that he might make would show the *most* realistic assessment of his situation in relation to avoiding future drinking problems?

1. "I promise I will never get drunk again."
2. "I am going to try hard to stay away from that first drink."
3. "I will just have one or two drinks at the most, now and then."
4. "I can whip this drinking business if my wife keeps off my back."

Ms. Gena Baxter, a 44-year-old housewife, entered the hospital for treatment of cirrhosis of the liver. She was accompanied by her husband.
Items 360 through 380 relate to this situation.

360. The nursing assistant who admitted Ms. Baxter comments to the nurse, "Cirrhosis, huh? She must be a lush." The practice of automatically attributing an overindulgence in alcohol to people with cirrhosis is an example of
1. an ideology.
2. a stereotype.
3. a mental set.
4. a halo effect.

361. By which one of the following methods can nurses *best* avoid developing premature, biased views of patients?
1. By reading about the person's illness.
2. By personally getting to know what the person is really like.
3. By asking others for their opinions of the person.
4. By acquainting oneself with others of the person's kind.

362. The physician noted on the medical record that Ms. Baxter has a 7-year history of drinking a 6-pack of beer and some wine every day. In which one of the following ways did the cirrhosis *most likely* result from the consumption of alcohol?
1. Directly from the poisonous effects of alcohol on liver cells.
2. Directly from the dilating effects of alcohol on the arteries and veins in the portal circulation.
3. Indirectly from deficiencies in nutrients and vitamin intake over a long period of time.
4. Indirectly from the buildup of glycogen in the liver from excess carbohydrate ingestion.

363. The unit secretary reads the physician's notes about Ms. Baxter's drinking habits and exclaims, "I have a friend who drinks more than that! Would he be considered an alcoholic?" Which one of the following possible replies by the nurse shows the *best* understanding of alcoholism as a social disease?
1. "Not if he drinks with others and not alone."
2. "Not if he sticks to beer and avoids the hard liquor."
3. "Not if he drinks only in the evening or on weekends."

4. "Not if he is able to get along well at work and at home."

364. Most of the information concerning Ms. Baxter has come from her husband who says his wife sees no connection between her liver disorder and her intake of alcohol. He reports that she felt she drank very little and that her family was making something out of nothing. Which one of the following defense mechanisms was she utilizing?
   1. Denial.
   2. Displacement.
   3. Rationalization.
   4. Reaction formation.

365. To which one of the following conditions might attempts by health team members to force Ms. Baxter to face up to the fact that she is an alcoholic and to break down her defenses *most likely* lead?
   1. Insight and rehabilitation.
   2. Hallucinations and psychosis.
   3. Restlessness and hyperactivity.
   4. Disorganization and depression.

366. Medications for Ms. Baxter include niacin (nicotinic acid). Of the following effects, which one is *least likely* to occur after the administration of large doses of niacin?
   1. Pruritis.
   2. Glossitis.
   3. A sensation of body warmth.
   4. Flushing of the face and neck.

367. Cyproheptadine hydrochloride (Periactin) is often ordered for those addicted to alcohol to combat the side effects of niacin. For which of the following properties in particular is the cyproheptadine hydrochloride useful?
   1. Its anticonvulsant and antiemetic properties.
   2. Its antipruritic and antihistaminic properties.
   3. Its antidepressant and antispasmodic properties.
   4. Its antibacterial and antihemorrhagic properties.

368. Besides her cirrhosis, Ms. Baxter suffers from numbness, itching and pain in her extremities and is prone to footdrop. This disorder of the nervous system is termed
   1. neuralgia.
   2. neurasthenia.
   3. Bell's palsy.
   4. peripheral neuritis.

369. When a patient has neurological damage, such as Ms. Baxter has, a precautionary nursing measure that would be indicated would be to give special attention to

1. cleansing the patient's skin.
2. massaging the patient's feet.
3. turning the patient from side to side.
4. applying heat to the patient's lower legs.

370. During Ms. Baxter's hospitalization, a noncaffeinated beverage is substituted for her usual morning coffee. This measure is taken because
1. patients transfer their oral dependency needs symbolically to coffee.
2. patients tend to abuse coffee in the same way that they once turned to alcohol.
3. regular coffee aggravates tremors and interferes with the sleep of the patient.
4. regular coffee has a diuretic effect that interferes with the hydration of the patient.

371. Ms. Baxter receives the appropriate medical and nursing treatment for her liver disorder and neurological ailments and her condition improves slightly. However, after 5 days in the hospital, she begins to thrash about in bed, hitting the sheets and yelling, "Go away, bugs, go away!" Several times she was overheard asking, "What? What did you say?"—when alone in her room. Which one of the following nursing notes *best* sums up Ms. Baxter's behavior?
1. Restless and disoriented; hallucinating.
2. Agitated; having auditory and visual hallucinations.
3. Fidgety; out of contact with reality; overheard talking to herself in her room.
4. Seeing "bugs" in her bedclothes and slapping at them; responding to unseen voices with "What?"

372. While Ms. Baxter has delirium tremens (d.t.'s), which of these measures should be included in her nursing care?
1. Stay with her and keep the room well lit.
2. Restrain her and keep the room dark and well-ventilated.
3. Touch her before saying anything to her and telling her where she is.
4. Tell her she is having nightmares and that she will be better soon.

373. The unit coordinator conducts a class on alcoholism to prepare for the time when Ms. Baxter returns to optimal physical functioning. The nursing assistant asks the coordinator which area of the brain causes people to lose their inhibitions and become euphoric. The area of the brain responsible for that function is the
1. cerebellum.
2. hypothalamus.

3. cerebral cortex.

4. medulla oblongata.

374. The *chief* purpose in promoting the idea that alcoholism is a disease is to influence others to
1. treat the alcoholic rather than to jail him.
2. acknowledge the physiological factors involved in alcoholism.
3. support research on the constitutional and biochemical causes of alcoholism.
4. appreciate the humanness and sensitivity of the alcoholic and to judge him less harshly.

375. Which one of the following statements *best* explains why Ms. Baxter's husband might have difficulty adjusting to his wife's projected future sobriety?
1. Her drinking focuses family attention away from his inadequacies.
2. He is a selfish person and would unconsciously resent her success.
3. Her drinking meets his needs for dominance as well as for the victim role.
4. She is less demanding of his time and attention when inebriated than when sober.

376. From which one of the following disorders is the alcoholic or his partner suffering when he derives unconscious satisfaction, or relief of guilt, from the misery and distress imposed by alcoholism?
1. Sadism.
2. Hedonism.
3. Masochism.
4. Autoerotism.

377. After spending time conversing with his wife, Mr. Baxter tells the nurse that he also drinks heavily in the evenings and would like to stop. The nurse suggests that he attend Alcoholics Anonymous (AA), but he said, "I went to one men's meeting and all they did was swear and brag about how drunk they got." Of the following responses, which one would be *best* for the nurse to make?
1. "Not all people are suited to that kind of therapy. Perhaps you are one of them."
2. "If you really wanted to help yourself, you would go whether you liked it or not."
3. "That's too bad. I can see how you might have been turned off by the experience."
4. "A different group might be more to your liking. You owe it to yourself to give it another try."

378. Mr. Baxter is unsure what requirements he must meet to be a

member of Alcoholics Anonymous. To become a member of the organization the alcoholic *first* must

1. resolve to abstain from alcohol and help others to do so.
2. admit he is powerless over alcohol and that he needs help.
3. analyze the wrongs he has done while drinking and try to make amends for them.
4. turn his life over to the care of a greater power and seek through meditation to improve contact with that power.

379. Even after Ms. Baxter overcomes her toxic state and regains her physical strength, she refuses to consider meeting with a therapist from the substance abuse unit, saying angrily, "You have a lot of nerve suggesting that I drink too much!" In relation to untreated alcoholism, which one of the following conditions *best* describes the type of mental disturbance the person who chronically abuses alcohol is *most likely* to develop in the future?

1. Alcoholic stupor.
2. Organic brain disorder.
3. Pathologic intoxication.
4. Alcoholic hallucinosis.

380. On discharge, Ms. Baxter is to be followed by a nurse from the public health department. What knowledge is *most essential* for the community health nurse to have in order to work effectively with alcoholic patients and their families?

1. A clear picture of ethnic patterns and a solid grasp of dietetic principles.
2. A thorough knowledge of relationship therapy and psychotherapeutic techniques.
3. A familiarity with a broad spectrum of local health and social service agencies.
4. An understanding of principles of addiction and of the effects various drugs have on the body.

Ms. Mary Silver, a 72-year-old widow, was brought by ambulance to the psychiatric hospital from a nursing home where she had been a patient for 3 months. Transfer data indicate that she had become increasingly confused and disoriented, and a "management problem." The tentative diagnosis for Ms. Silver is chronic organic brain syndrome.
Items 381 through 402 relate to this situation.

381. In which one of the following ways should the hospital admission routine be modified for an older, confused person like Ms. Silver?

1. The patient should be left alone to promote recovery of her faculties and composure.
2. The patient should be medicated to ensure her calm cooperation during the admission procedure.
3. The patient should be allowed extra, sufficient time, in which to gain an understanding of what is happening to her.
4. The patient should be given a detailed, complete tour of the unit to acquaint her with the furniture placement in the various rooms.

382. Chronic organic brain syndrome differs from acute organic brain syndrome in that chronic organic brain syndrome is a
1. painful condition.
2. permanent condition.
3. reversible condition.
4. potentially fatal condition.

383. Of the following phrases, which one *best* describes the typical onset of a chronic organic brain disorder?
1. Abrupt, with no forewarning.
2. Rapid, with many precursory signs.
3. Slow, with obvious symptomatology.
4. Gradual, with lucid intervals interspersed throughout.

384. Ms. Silver is to undergo a series of diagnostic tests to determine whether or not her organic brain disorder is treatable. Treatable forms of dementia (those with symptoms that can be arrested or reversed) include *all* of the following disorders *except* those caused by
1. cerebral abscess.
2. multiple sclerosis.
3. electrolyte imbalance.
4. syphilitic meningitis.

385. An electroencephalogram (EEG) is ordered for Ms. Silver. Which one of the following statements concerning the procedure is *accurate?*
1. It is a somewhat painful but short procedure.
2. It does not involve the use of electrical shock.
3. It tests the patient's intelligence but not her sanity.
4. It enables the examiner to know what the patient is thinking.

386. Which one of the following beverages should the nurse make sure is omitted from Ms. Silver's diet at the meal prior to the patient's electroencephalogram?
1. Milk.
2. Coffee.
3. Lemonade.
4. Orange juice.

387. On the night before her electroencephalogram, which one of the following preparations will *most probably* be required for Ms. Silver?
   1. Washing her hair.
   2. Taking a laxative.
   3. Going to bed early.
   4. Providing a sample of her handwriting.
388. After the diagnostic tests on Ms. Silver are completed, her organic condition is found to be due to cerebral arteriosclerosis. Since no known cure exists for this disorder, which one of the following attitudes should the nursing staff try to influence the patient (and each other) to adopt?
   1. A hopeful attitude.
   2. A resigned attitude.
   3. A concerned attitude.
   4. A nonchalant attitude.
389. Which one of the following factors has the *most* bearing on the present severity of Ms. Silver's mental symptoms?
   1. Her age and socioeconomic level.
   2. The specific areas of her brain that are damaged.
   3. Her psychological response to the organic changes.
   4. The amount of her brain damage inflicted by the causative illness.
390. In addition to disturbances in her mental awareness and in her orientation to reality, Ms. Silver is also likely to show loss of ability in her
   1. hearing, vocalizing, and seeing.
   2. endurance, strength, and mobility.
   3. learning, creativity, and judgment.
   4. balance, flexibility, and coordination.
391. Of the following comments the nurse could make, which one would provide the *best* reality orientation for Ms. Silver when the patient first awakens in the morning?
   1. "Do you remember who I am, Ms. Silver, or what day it is today?"
   2. "Hello, Ms. Silver, did you sleep well? Which dress would you like to wear today, the yellow or the green one?"
   3. "Here I am again, Ms. Silver, your favorite nurse. Today is Tuesday so there will be pancakes for breakfast this morning."
   4. "Good morning, Ms. Silver. This is your second day in the Jonestown Hospital and I am your nurse for today. My name is Ms. Daly."
392. Because of Ms. Silver's age and organic impairment, which one of the following items should *most certainly* be included in

the plan of care for her?

1. Have two people accompany her when she is up and about.
2. Make sure objects she may trip over are removed from her path.
3. Check her mouth to make certain she has swallowed her medications.
4. Put her favorite belongings in a safe place so she will not lose them.

393. Ms. Silver is placed on a low cholesterol diet. Which one of the following principles should the nursing team *especially* adhere to in adapting the diet order for this elderly patient's needs?
   1. The patient's religious affiliation should be considered when making dietary changes.
   2. The patient's cultural background should be explored before deciding on food substitutes.
   3. The patient should not have to buy expensive ingredients or products to meet the dietary demands.
   4. The patient should not be expected to alter her lifelong eating habits to satisfy the requirements of the diet.

394. Ms. Silver roams about the hospital unit at night, disturbing the sleep of other patients. When asked why she walks about, she complains of being lost and unable to sleep. A large sign is posted on the door of her room to help her locate it. Which one of the following programs would be *best* for dealing with the patient's insomnia?
   1. A daily afternoon nap to prevent overtiredness at night.
   2. A brisk nightly massage so her muscles will not be tense.
   3. Enough active exercise daily so she will be comfortably tired at night.
   4. A cup of hot tea with lemon before bed to promote a feeling of well-being.

395. Phenothiazines rather than barbiturates are commonly used to treat insomnia or agitation for a patient with organic brain syndrome *primarily* because barbiturates tend to cause
   1. habituation and addiction.
   2. chronic poisoning and renal damage.
   3. respiratory and cardiac depression.
   4. delirium and paradoxical excitement.

396. Ms. Silver's daughter says that her mother wore the same dirty, worn-out undergarments for weeks at home. Of the following techniques, which one would be best for the nursing staff to follow with Ms. Silver while she is hospitalized to prevent further regression in her personal hygiene habits?

1. Accept her need to go without bathing if she so desires.
2. Make her assume responsibility for her own physical care.
3. Encourage her to do as much self-care as she is capable of doing.
4. Do most of her physical care while letting her think she did it herself.

397. Projects and activities for Ms. Silver, selected by the nurses from those available on the unit, should be *especially* directed toward giving the patient a chance to
1. succeed at a task.
2. compete with others.
3. socialize with others.
4. concentrate on a task.

398. Because of Ms. Silver's age and organicity, which one of the following practices in relation to activities of daily living should the nurses *avoid* for Ms. Silver?
1. Making demands on her abilities.
2. Monitoring her food intake and output.
3. Arousing strong positive feelings in her.
4. Changing her physical surroundings periodically.

399. A 35-year-old nurse on the unit often avoided Ms. Silver's company, preferring to associate with patients of her own age group or younger. Which one of the following factors is *most likely* responsible for the nurse's extreme discomfort with older patients and her unconscious avoidance of them?
1. Her own fears and conflicts about aging.
2. Her dislike of physical contact with others.
3. Her desire to be surrounded by beauty and perfection.
4. Her recent experiences with her mother's elderly friends.

400. To deal with a nurse's avoidance and discomfort with the aged patient, which one of the following actions that the nursing supervisor could take would be *most helpful?*
1. Transfer the nurse to a young adult unit.
2. Provide inservice classes for the nurse on the rewards of caring for the elderly.
3. Continue to assign the nurse to older patients until she has overcome her dislike for them.
4. Give the nurse an opportunity in staff and individual conferences to voice her feelings about the aged.

401. One day, when she is more alert than usual, Ms. Silver asks the nurse to help her make out her will. Which one of the following possible responses by the nurse would be *best?*
1. "I am not a lawyer but I will do what I can for you."
2. "You have a long way to go before you will need to do that.

Let's wait on it a while, shall we?"
3. "I don't believe in getting involved in legal matters but maybe I can find another nurse who will help you."
4. "You need to consult an attorney since I am not trained in such matters. Is there a family lawyer I could call for you?"

402. Ms. Silver is allowed to reminisce about her past life. Which one of the following effects can the nurses *most likely* expect reminiscing to have on the patient's functioning in the hospital?
1. It will decrease her isolation and loneliness.
2. It will increase her confusion and disorientation.
3. It will subject her to the impatient responses of others.
4. It will keep her from participating in more therapeutic activities.

A community health nurse has visited the Steven's home regularly to help with the personal care of their severely retarded daughter, Patty, who is 10 years old. Patty's mother has a back ailment of recent origin that has prevented her from assuming responsibilities for Patty's care.
Items 403 through 418 relate to this situation.

403. Patty has mongolism, or Down's syndrome. The majority of cases of mental retardation result from
1. hydrocephalus.
2. unknown causes.
3. phenylketonuria.
4. muscular dystrophy.

404. Patty's disability was apparent at birth and she was slow to develop as an infant. *All* of the following behaviors describe delays in the early development common to mentally deficient children *except*
1. not using expressive language.
2. not responding to verbal commands.
3. starting to walk at 20 months of age.
4. being able to sit up at 6 months of age.

405. Patty has had extensive testing. Which one of the following pieces of information can psychological tests realistically provide about a patient?
1. The patient's response to drug and other therapies.
2. The exact location of the patient's organic lesions.
3. The intelligence and vocational aptitude of the patient.
4. A differential diagnosis from other forms of psychopathology.

406. Patty has an intelligence quotient (I.Q.) of approximately 35.

The kind of environment and interdisciplinary program from which Patty is likely to profit *most* would *best* be described as

1. custodial.
2. educational.
3. habit training.
4. sheltered workshop.

407. By which one of the following means can the intelligence quotient of a mentally subnormal child like Patty *most likely* be raised?

1. By serving her hearty, nutritious meals.
2. By giving her vasodilating medications as prescribed.
3. By letting her play with children more able than herself.
4. By providing her with interesting, nonthreatening life experiences.

408. Patty has no major physical defects. When instructing her parents about physical problems associated with mongolism, to which one of Patty's vital signs should the nurse *most likely* teach the family to pay *special* attention?

1. To her pulse rate.
2. To her temperature.
3. To her respirations.
4. To her blood pressure.

409. The *basic* aim of the nurse working with the parents of a mentally retarded child is to increase their sense of

1. liking for their child.
2. responsibility for their child's welfare.
3. understanding of their child's disabilities.
4. confidence in their abilities to care for their child.

410. Ms. Steven's childbearing days are over, but she inquires about genetic counseling for her younger sister. The *primary* role of the genetic team working with a family is to

1. provide the parents with the facts about their birth defect risks.
2. report to the family on chromosome analysis of the amniotic cells.
3. prepare the parents psychologically for the birth of a defective child.
4. prescribe birth control or abortion measures for parents to take as needed.

411. The nurse mentions to Ms. Steven that a group meeting for the mothers of retarded children is to be held soon. "Not retarded!" blazes Ms. Steven, "exceptional!" In response to this outburst by the mother, which one of the following possible replies by the nurse would be *best*?

1. "What do you not like about the word 'retarded'?"

2. "I'm sorry if I offended you by my thoughtless remark."
3. "No matter what it's called, the condition is still the same, isn't it?"
4. "I'd like to hear more of your thoughts and feelings on that, if I may."

412. Ms. Steven is aware that her child needs play activities. Which one of the following age levels should the toys selected for Patty ultimately reflect?
1. Her language level of 3 years.
2. Her development level of 4 years.
3. Her chronological age of 10 years.

413. In relation to teaching goals, Ms. Steven's desire for Patty to be able to dress herself would *best* be written in a nursing care plan as
1. a single attainable goal.
2. a goal that may be postponed.
3. a series of small short-term goals.
4. a part of the overall larger goal of optimal functioning.

414. Sometimes Patty seems to deliberately do things that cause her mother to become displeased and upset, such as taking off her clothes. Which one of the following reasons probably *best* explains why Patty tends to act this way?
1. To annoy her mother.
2. To get attention from her mother.
3. To express anger with her mother.
4. To relieve her boredom with herself.

415. The community health nurse has occasion to observe the Steven family at mealtime. She notes that Patty is messy and eats noisily. Which one of the following approaches that the nurse could recommend to decrease the undesirable eating habits would provide the *most positive* reinforcement for Patty's desirable table manners?
1. Praising her when she chews quietly.
2. Scolding her when she smacks her lips.
3. Ignoring her when she plays with her food.
4. Making her leave the table when she spills her milk.

416. It is possible that a decision might be made to institutionalize Patty. An *undesirable* element that sometimes appears in a program for mentally deficient persons living in an institutional setting is the element of
1. stimulating interest.
2. competing successfully.
3. providing homelike surroundings.
4. developing individual responsibilities.

417. In the past, the trend of putting mentally retarded persons in institutions was based on *all* of the following beliefs about the mentally retarded *except* that they
1. could learn new behaviors and skills.
2. were prone to be violent and emotionally unstable.
3. had hopeless and burdensome outcomes of impairment.
4. had a high rate of fertility and inherited disorders.

418. Which one of the following percentages *best* approximates that part of the population in the United States that is mentally retarded?
1. 1 percent.
2. 3 percent.
3. 5 percent.
4. 7 percent.

Thirteen-year-old Greg Shaw was admitted to the hospital for the third time. His diagnosis is acute lymphatic leukemia. The liaison psychiatric nurse was asked by the team leader to help the nursing staff work more effectively with this terminally ill child and his family.
Items 419 through 439 relate to this situation.

419. At a nursing care conference, one of the nurses says to the liaison nurse, "Whenever I go to Greg's room, I feel like I have to smile and act happy even though I want to cry when I see him." Which one of the following responses that the liaison nurse could make would be *best?*
1. "Keep smiling; you will only upset him if you cry."
2. "Try not to show emotion; pinch yourself, if necessary."
3. "Tell him that you feel bad when he is ill; it offers you time to regain your composure."
4. "Go ahead and cry; tears are nothing to be ashamed of when you are sharing an experience with the patient."

420. Greg suspects that he will not live. However, others talk about only pleasant matters with him and have a persistently cheerful manner around him in the face of his suspicions. Which one of the following feelings is Greg *most likely* to develop as a result of such behavior?
1. Feelings of relief.
2. Feelings of isolation.
3. Feelings of hopefulness.
4. Feelings of independence.

421. Most authorities would agree that Greg's parents should be told as much about Greg's disease and its prognosis as

1. they insist on knowing.
2. they are able to understand.
3. the physician can tell them.
4. their clergyman thinks it is advisable for them to know.

422. Greg is told that he was not responding well to treatment and that everything possible has been tried. Greg then tells his parents that he wants all of his friends to come to his funeral. At approximately what age are children (especially terminally ill children) first thought to become concerned with the idea of death?
1. Between 4 and 6 years of age.
2. Between 6 and 8 years of age.
3. Between 8 and 10 years of age.
4. Between 10 and 12 years of age.

423. Greg starts refusing to take his medications, saying belligerently, "You can't make me take them. They are not doing me a bit of good. Being in the hospital isn't helping me either. It's a stupid place to come for help." Which one of the following stages of adaptation to dying is Greg *most likely* experiencing at this time?
1. Anger.
2. Denial.
3. Bargaining.
4. Depression.

424. Since Greg is increasingly prone to outbursts concerning his treatments, which one of the following approaches by the nurses when treatments are to be done would likely be *most helpful* in gaining his cooperation?
1. Tell him how the treatment can be expected to help him each time.
2. Describe the probable effect on his body that missing each treatment would have.
3. Ask him to be a good boy and not make the treatment any harder for himself or the staff.
4. Promise to give him a backrub every 2 hours if he does not make a fuss about the treatment.

425. Which one of the following behaviors if displayed by Greg would indicate *most clearly* his need for emotional support?
1. He teases his sister about her new boyfriend.
2. He wants to have someone with him at all times.
3. He has the nurse wait with his bath while he makes a phone call.
4. He complains about the limited number of choices on the dietary list.

426. Projective techniques are sometimes used by health professionals to assist in exploring the thoughts of dying children. When
asked to make up stories related to pictures he is shown or
asked to draw, the dying child most often describes central
characters in a picture as being
1. monsters.
2. a favorite nurse.
3. a dying child like himself.
4. healthy friends and relatives.

427. The liaison nurse suggests that some recreational diversion be
planned for Greg. Which one of the following guidelines *in
particular* should the recreational activities selected for Greg
reflect?
1. They should be of a nonviolent nature.
2. They should require some physical effort.
3. They should stimulate the imagination.
4. They should be geared to early adolescent interests.

428. An environment on the nursing unit from which Greg would be
least likely to benefit would be one in which
1. limits are set on Greg's activities.
2. hospital rules are firmly enforced.
3. Greg knows his wishes will be gratified.
4. behavioral expectations are clearly defined.

429. During a nursing report, the team leader makes no comments
about Greg, other than to list tasks and routines completed for
him. Which one of the following kinds of behavior is a nurse
most likely demonstrating when she emphasizes the scientific
aspects of caring for a dying patient?
1. Tactful behavior.
2. Defensive behavior.
3. Efficient behavior.
4. Objective behavior.

430. The nurse who usually is *most effective* when helping patients
and their families cope with death is one who demonstrates
that she
1. has contemplated her own death and mortality.
2. has a strong attachment to her pets and material possessions.
3. dislikes reminders of the passage of time, such as birthdays.
4. views dying persons as a separate, distinct clinical population
in need of comfort.

431. The liaison nurse explains to the staff that because Greg's
mother's best friend recently died after a brief illness, Ms.
Shaw can be expected to react to the impending loss of her son
even more intensely than is usually expected. Which one of

the following concepts *best* explains this expected grief experience?
1. Losses are cumulative in effect.
2. Losses take time to become resolved.
3. Losses affect one's emotional reserves.
4. Losses involve objects or people that are significant to oneself.

432. After a period of depression and preoccupation with his son's death, Mr. Shaw has started to adjust to the idea of life without Greg. This phenomenon of emotionally reacting to a person's death before it actually occurs is known as
1. neurotic depression.
2. acute grief reaction.
3. anticipatory mourning.
4. pathological mourning.

433. If Greg were not terminally ill, with which one of the following psychosocial issues would he be expected to be resolving, according to Erik Erikson's theory?
1. A social conscience.
2. A lifetime vocation.
3. A personal and sexual identity.
4. A sense of initiative and industry.

434. Of the following attitudes that Greg could display toward himself, which one indicates that he has come to healthy terms with his death and dying?
1. He is bitter.
2. He is resigned.
3. He is accepting.
4. He is optimistic.

435. Which one of the following philosophies that could be adopted by Greg and his family would most likely help them cope *best* during the final stages of Greg's illness?
1. To relive the pleasant memories of days gone by.
2. To live each day as it comes as fully as possible.
3. To expect the worst and be grateful when it does not happen.
4. To plan ahead for the remaining good times that will be spent together.

436. Greg's physician and parents contemplate discontinuing chemotherapy and blood transfusions that are keeping Greg alive and in a state of suffering. They are contemplating the act of
1. homicide.
2. euthanasia.
3. pedophilia.
4. decerebration.

437. Greg dies quietly one morning. Nursing intervention to assist the family at this time should include *all* of the following measures *except*
1. providing an unobtrusive place for the family to gather.
2. encouraging the family members to express their feelings.
3. supporting the defense mechanisms in use by the family members.
4. staying with the family while they make the funeral arrangements.

438. The time of death for Greg was recorded as 5:48 A.M. While there is no universally accepted definition of death, the current trend in the United States is to define death as occurring at the time when there is cessation of the person's
1. lung function.
2. brain function.
3. heart function.
4. kidney function.

439. Which one of the following behaviors that Greg's parents might show after his death would be considered a part of the *normal* sequence of grief and mourning, as opposed to being a sign of pathological mourning?
1. Mourning for him for as long as 1 year.
2. Refusing to acknowledge any negative memories of him.
3. Becoming upset as the anniversary of his death approaches.
4. Developing his symptoms in chronic identification with him.

answer sheet for psychiatric nursing

Read each question in the examination carefully and select which one of the options is the *best* or *correct* answer. If the answer you would prefer is not given, select the one which seems *most appropriate*.

Locate on the answer sheet the number of the item you are answering. With a pencil, blacken the circle corresponding to the answer you have selected. Be sure you are recording your answer in the proper space.

	1 2 3 4		1 2 3 4		1 2 3 4		1 2 3 4
1	○○○○	18	○○○○	35	○○○○	52	○○○○
2	○○○○	19	○○○○	36	○○○○	53	○○○○
3	○○○○	20	○○○○	37	○○○○	54	○○○○
4	○○○○	21	○○○○	38	○○○○	55	○○○○
5	○○○○	22	○○○○	39	○○○○	56	○○○○
6	○○○○	23	○○○○	40	○○○○	57	○○○○
7	○○○○	24	○○○○	41	○○○○	58	○○○○
8	○○○○	25	○○○○	42	○○○○	59	○○○○
9	○○○○	26	○○○○	43	○○○○	60	○○○○
10	○○○○	27	○○○○	44	○○○○	61	○○○○
11	○○○○	28	○○○○	45	○○○○	62	○○○○
12	○○○○	29	○○○○	46	○○○○	63	○○○○
13	○○○○	30	○○○○	47	○○○○	64	○○○○
14	○○○○	31	○○○○	48	○○○○	65	○○○○
15	○○○○	32	○○○○	49	○○○○	66	○○○○
16	○○○○	33	○○○○	50	○○○○	67	○○○○
17	○○○○	34	○○○○	51	○○○○	68	○○○○

	1 2 3 4		1 2 3 4		1 2 3 4		1 2 3 4
69	○○○○	91	○○○○	113	○○○○	135	○○○○
70	○○○○	92	○○○○	114	○○○○	136	○○○○
71	○○○○	93	○○○○	115	○○○○	137	○○○○
72	○○○○	94	○○○○	116	○○○○	138	○○○○
73	○○○○	95	○○○○	117	○○○○	139	○○○○
74	○○○○	96	○○○○	118	○○○○	140	○○○○
75	○○○○	97	○○○○	119	○○○○	141	○○○○
76	○○○○	98	○○○○	120	○○○○	142	○○○○
77	○○○○	99	○○○○	121	○○○○	143	○○○○
78	○○○○	100	○○○○	122	○○○○	144	○○○○
79	○○○○	101	○○○○	123	○○○○	145	○○○○
80	○○○○	102	○○○○	124	○○○○	146	○○○○
81	○○○○	103	○○○○	125	○○○○	147	○○○○
82	○○○○	104	○○○○	126	○○○○	148	○○○○
83	○○○○	105	○○○○	127	○○○○	149	○○○○
84	○○○○	106	○○○○	128	○○○○	150	○○○○
85	○○○○	107	○○○○	129	○○○○	151	○○○○
86	○○○○	108	○○○○	130	○○○○	152	○○○○
87	○○○○	109	○○○○	131	○○○○	153	○○○○
88	○○○○	110	○○○○	132	○○○○	154	○○○○
89	○○○○	111	○○○○	133	○○○○	155	○○○○
90	○○○○	112	○○○○	134	○○○○	156	○○○○

	1 2 3 4		1 2 3 4		1 2 3 4		1 2 3 4
157	○○○○	179	○○○○	201	○○○○	223	○○○○
158	○○○○	180	○○○○	202	○○○○	224	○○○○
159	○○○○	181	○○○○	203	○○○○	225	○○○○
160	○○○○	182	○○○○	204	○○○○	226	○○○○
161	○○○○	183	○○○○	205	○○○○	227	○○○○
162	○○○○	184	○○○○	206	○○○○	228	○○○○
163	○○○○	185	○○○○	207	○○○○	229	○○○○
164	○○○○	186	○○○○	208	○○○○	230	○○○○
165	○○○○	187	○○○○	209	○○○○	231	○○○○
166	○○○○	188	○○○○	210	○○○○	232	○○○○
167	○○○○	189	○○○○	211	○○○○	233	○○○○
168	○○○○	190	○○○○	212	○○○○	234	○○○○
169	○○○○	191	○○○○	213	○○○○	235	○○○○
170	○○○○	192	○○○○	214	○○○○	236	○○○○
171	○○○○	193	○○○○	215	○○○○	237	○○○○
172	○○○○	194	○○○○	216	○○○○	238	○○○○
173	○○○○	195	○○○○	217	○○○○	239	○○○○
174	○○○○	196	○○○○	218	○○○○	240	○○○○
175	○○○○	197	○○○○	219	○○○○	241	○○○○
176	○○○○	198	○○○○	220	○○○○	242	○○○○
177	○○○○	199	○○○○	221	○○○○	243	○○○○
178	○○○○	200	○○○○	222	○○○○	244	○○○○

psychiatric nursing answer sheet   3

	1 2 3 4		1 2 3 4		1 2 3 4		1 2 3 4
245	○○○○	267	○○○○	289	○○○○	311	○○○○
246	○○○○	268	○○○○	290	○○○○	312	○○○○
247	○○○○	269	○○○○	291	○○○○	313	○○○○
248	○○○○	270	○○○○	292	○○○○	314	○○○○
249	○○○○	271	○○○○	293	○○○○	315	○○○○
250	○○○○	272	○○○○	294	○○○○	316	○○○○
251	○○○○	273	○○○○	295	○○○○	317	○○○○
252	○○○○	274	○○○○	296	○○○○	318	○○○○
253	○○○○	275	○○○○	297	○○○○	319	○○○○
254	○○○○	276	○○○○	298	○○○○	320	○○○○
255	○○○○	277	○○○○	299	○○○○	321	○○○○
256	○○○○	278	○○○○	300	○○○○	322	○○○○
257	○○○○	279	○○○○	301	○○○○	323	○○○○
258	○○○○	280	○○○○	302	○○○○	324	○○○○
259	○○○○	281	○○○○	303	○○○○	325	○○○○
260	○○○○	282	○○○○	304	○○○○	326	○○○○
261	○○○○	283	○○○○	305	○○○○	327	○○○○
262	○○○○	284	○○○○	306	○○○○	328	○○○○
263	○○○○	285	○○○○	307	○○○○	329	○○○○
264	○○○○	286	○○○○	308	○○○○	330	○○○○
265	○○○○	287	○○○○	309	○○○○	331	○○○○
266	○○○○	288	○○○○	310	○○○○	332	○○○○

4   psychiatric nursing answer sheet

	1 2 3 4		1 2 3 4		1 2 3 4		1 2 3 4
333	◯◯◯◯	355	◯◯◯◯	377	◯◯◯◯	399	◯◯◯◯
334	◯◯◯◯	356	◯◯◯◯	378	◯◯◯◯	400	◯◯◯◯
335	◯◯◯◯	357	◯◯◯◯	379	◯◯◯◯	401	◯◯◯◯
336	◯◯◯◯	358	◯◯◯◯	480	◯◯◯◯	402	◯◯◯◯
337	◯◯◯◯	359	◯◯◯◯	381	◯◯◯◯	403	◯◯◯◯
338	◯◯◯◯	360	◯◯◯◯	382	◯◯◯◯	404	◯◯◯◯
339	◯◯◯◯	361	◯◯◯◯	383	◯◯◯◯	405	◯◯◯◯
340	◯◯◯◯	362	◯◯◯◯	384	◯◯◯◯	406	◯◯◯◯
341	◯◯◯◯	363	◯◯◯◯	385	◯◯◯◯	407	◯◯◯◯
342	◯◯◯◯	364	◯◯◯◯	386	◯◯◯◯	408	◯◯◯◯
343	◯◯◯◯	365	◯◯◯◯	387	◯◯◯◯	409	◯◯◯◯
344	◯◯◯◯	366	◯◯◯◯	388	◯◯◯◯	410	◯◯◯◯
345	◯◯◯◯	367	◯◯◯◯	389	◯◯◯◯	411	◯◯◯◯
346	◯◯◯◯	368	◯◯◯◯	390	◯◯◯◯	412	◯◯◯◯
347	◯◯◯◯	369	◯◯◯◯	391	◯◯◯◯	413	◯◯◯◯
348	◯◯◯◯	370	◯◯◯◯	392	◯◯◯◯	414	◯◯◯◯
349	◯◯◯◯	371	◯◯◯◯	393	◯◯◯◯	415	◯◯◯◯
350	◯◯◯◯	372	◯◯◯◯	394	◯◯◯◯	416	◯◯◯◯
351	◯◯◯◯	373	◯◯◯◯	395	◯◯◯◯	417	◯◯◯◯
352	◯◯◯◯	374	◯◯◯◯	396	◯◯◯◯	418	◯◯◯◯
353	◯◯◯◯	375	◯◯◯◯	397	◯◯◯◯	419	◯◯◯◯
354	◯◯◯◯	376	◯◯◯◯	398	◯◯◯◯	420	◯◯◯◯

	1	2	3	4		1	2	3	4		1	2	3	4		1	2	3	4
421	○	○	○	○	426	○	○	○	○	431	○	○	○	○	436	○	○	○	○
422	○	○	○	○	427	○	○	○	○	432	○	○	○	○	437	○	○	○	○
423	○	○	○	○	428	○	○	○	○	433	○	○	○	○	438	○	○	○	○
424	○	○	○	○	429	○	○	○	○	434	○	○	○	○	439	○	○	○	○
425	○	○	○	○	430	○	○	○	○	435	○	○	○	○					

answer sheet for psychiatric nursing

Read each question in the examination carefully and select which one of the options is the *best* or *correct* answer. If the answer you would prefer is not given, select the one which seems *most appropriate*.

Locate on the answer sheet the number of the item you are answering. With a pencil, blacken the circle corresponding to the answer you have selected. Be sure you are recording your answer in the proper space.

	1 2 3 4		1 2 3 4		1 2 3 4		1 2 3 4
1	○○○○	18	○○○○	35	○○○○	52	○○○○
2	○○○○	19	○○○○	36	○○○○	53	○○○○
3	○○○○	20	○○○○	37	○○○○	54	○○○○
4	○○○○	21	○○○○	38	○○○○	55	○○○○
5	○○○○	22	○○○○	39	○○○○	56	○○○○
6	○○○○	23	○○○○	40	○○○○	57	○○○○
7	○○○○	24	○○○○	41	○○○○	58	○○○○
8	○○○○	25	○○○○	42	○○○○	59	○○○○
9	○○○○	26	○○○○	43	○○○○	60	○○○○
10	○○○○	27	○○○○	44	○○○○	61	○○○○
11	○○○○	28	○○○○	45	○○○○	62	○○○○
12	○○○○	29	○○○○	46	○○○○	63	○○○○
13	○○○○	30	○○○○	47	○○○○	64	○○○○
14	○○○○	31	○○○○	48	○○○○	65	○○○○
15	○○○○	32	○○○○	49	○○○○	66	○○○○
16	○○○○	33	○○○○	50	○○○○	67	○○○○
17	○○○○	34	○○○○	51	○○○○	68	○○○○

	1 2 3 4		1 2 3 4		1 2 3 4		1 2 3 4
69	○○○○	91	○○○○	113	○○○○	135	○○○○
70	○○○○	92	○○○○	114	○○○○	136	○○○○
71	○○○○	93	○○○○	115	○○○○	137	○○○○
72	○○○○	94	○○○○	116	○○○○	138	○○○○
73	○○○○	95	○○○○	117	○○○○	139	○○○○
74	○○○○	96	○○○○	118	○○○○	140	○○○○
75	○○○○	97	○○○○	119	○○○○	141	○○○○
76	○○○○	98	○○○○	120	○○○○	142	○○○○
77	○○○○	99	○○○○	121	○○○○	143	○○○○
78	○○○○	100	○○○○	122	○○○○	144	○○○○
79	○○○○	101	○○○○	123	○○○○	145	○○○○
80	○○○○	102	○○○○	124	○○○○	146	○○○○
81	○○○○	103	○○○○	125	○○○○	147	○○○○
82	○○○○	104	○○○○	126	○○○○	148	○○○○
83	○○○○	105	○○○○	127	○○○○	149	○○○○
84	○○○○	106	○○○○	128	○○○○	150	○○○○
85	○○○○	107	○○○○	129	○○○○	151	○○○○
86	○○○○	108	○○○○	130	○○○○	152	○○○○
87	○○○○	109	○○○○	131	○○○○	153	○○○○
88	○○○○	110	○○○○	132	○○○○	154	○○○○
89	○○○○	111	○○○○	133	○○○○	155	○○○○
90	○○○○	112	○○○○	134	○○○○	156	○○○○

2   psychiatric nursing answer sheet

	1 2 3 4		1 2 3 4		1 2 3 4		1 2 3 4
157	○○○○	179	○○○○	201	○○○○	223	○○○○
158	○○○○	180	○○○○	202	○○○○	224	○○○○
159	○○○○	181	○○○○	203	○○○○	225	○○○○
160	○○○○	182	○○○○	204	○○○○	226	○○○○
161	○○○○	183	○○○○	205	○○○○	227	○○○○
162	○○○○	184	○○○○	206	○○○○	228	○○○○
163	○○○○	185	○○○○	207	○○○○	229	○○○○
164	○○○○	186	○○○○	208	○○○○	230	○○○○
165	○○○○	187	○○○○	209	○○○○	231	○○○○
166	○○○○	188	○○○○	210	○○○○	232	○○○○
167	○○○○	189	○○○○	211	○○○○	233	○○○○
168	○○○○	190	○○○○	212	○○○○	234	○○○○
169	○○○○	191	○○○○	213	○○○○	235	○○○○
170	○○○○	192	○○○○	214	○○○○	236	○○○○
171	○○○○	193	○○○○	215	○○○○	237	○○○○
172	○○○○	194	○○○○	216	○○○○	238	○○○○
173	○○○○	195	○○○○	217	○○○○	239	○○○○
174	○○○○	196	○○○○	218	○○○○	240	○○○○
175	○○○○	197	○○○○	219	○○○○	241	○○○○
176	○○○○	198	○○○○	220	○○○○	242	○○○○
177	○○○○	199	○○○○	221	○○○○	243	○○○○
178	○○○○	200	○○○○	222	○○○○	244	○○○○

	1 2 3 4		1 2 3 4		1 2 3 4		1 2 3 4
245	○○○○	267	○○○○	289	○○○○	311	○○○○
246	○○○○	268	○○○○	290	○○○○	312	○○○○
247	○○○○	269	○○○○	291	○○○○	313	○○○○
248	○○○○	270	○○○○	292	○○○○	314	○○○○
249	○○○○	271	○○○○	293	○○○○	315	○○○○
250	○○○○	272	○○○○	294	○○○○	316	○○○○
251	○○○○	273	○○○○	295	○○○○	317	○○○○
252	○○○○	274	○○○○	296	○○○○	318	○○○○
253	○○○○	275	○○○○	297	○○○○	319	○○○○
254	○○○○	276	○○○○	298	○○○○	320	○○○○
255	○○○○	277	○○○○	299	○○○○	321	○○○○
256	○○○○	278	○○○○	300	○○○○	322	○○○○
257	○○○○	279	○○○○	301	○○○○	323	○○○○
258	○○○○	280	○○○○	302	○○○○	324	○○○○
259	○○○○	281	○○○○	303	○○○○	325	○○○○
260	○○○○	282	○○○○	304	○○○○	326	○○○○
261	○○○○	283	○○○○	305	○○○○	327	○○○○
262	○○○○	284	○○○○	306	○○○○	328	○○○○
263	○○○○	285	○○○○	307	○○○○	329	○○○○
264	○○○○	286	○○○○	308	○○○○	330	○○○○
265	○○○○	287	○○○○	309	○○○○	331	○○○○
266	○○○○	288	○○○○	310	○○○○	332	○○○○

	1 2 3 4		1 2 3 4		1 2 3 4		1 2 3 4
333	○○○○	355	○○○○	377	○○○○	399	○○○○
334	○○○○	356	○○○○	378	○○○○	400	○○○○
335	○○○○	357	○○○○	379	○○○○	401	○○○○
336	○○○○	358	○○○○	480	○○○○	402	○○○○
337	○○○○	359	○○○○	381	○○○○	403	○○○○
338	○○○○	360	○○○○	382	○○○○	404	○○○○
339	○○○○	361	○○○○	383	○○○○	405	○○○○
340	○○○○	362	○○○○	384	○○○○	406	○○○○
341	○○○○	363	○○○○	385	○○○○	407	○○○○
342	○○○○	364	○○○○	386	○○○○	408	○○○○
343	○○○○	365	○○○○	387	○○○○	409	○○○○
344	○○○○	366	○○○○	388	○○○○	410	○○○○
345	○○○○	367	○○○○	389	○○○○	411	○○○○
346	○○○○	368	○○○○	390	○○○○	412	○○○○
347	○○○○	369	○○○○	391	○○○○	413	○○○○
348	○○○○	370	○○○○	392	○○○○	414	○○○○
349	○○○○	371	○○○○	393	○○○○	415	○○○○
350	○○○○	372	○○○○	394	○○○○	416	○○○○
351	○○○○	373	○○○○	395	○○○○	417	○○○○
352	○○○○	374	○○○○	396	○○○○	418	○○○○
353	○○○○	375	○○○○	397	○○○○	419	○○○○
354	○○○○	376	○○○○	398	○○○○	420	○○○○

```
     1 2 3 4           1 2 3 4           1 2 3 4             1 2 3 4
421 ○ ○ ○ ○      426 ○ ○ ○ ○      431 ○ ○ ○ ○      436 ○ ○ ○ ○
     1 2 3 4           1 2 3 4           1 2 3 4             1 2 3 4
422 ○ ○ ○ ○      427 ○ ○ ○ ○      432 ○ ○ ○ ○      437 ○ ○ ○ ○
     1 2 3 4           1 2 3 4           1 2 3 4             1 2 3 4
423 ○ ○ ○ ○      428 ○ ○ ○ ○      433 ○ ○ ○ ○      438 ○ ○ ○ ○
     1 2 3 4           1 2 3 4           1 2 3 4             1 2 3 4
424 ○ ○ ○ ○      429 ○ ○ ○ ○      434 ○ ○ ○ ○      439 ○ ○ ○ ○
     1 2 3 4           1 2 3 4           1 2 3 4             1 2 3 4
425 ○ ○ ○ ○      430 ○ ○ ○ ○      435 ○ ○ ○ ○
```

psychiatric nursing examination

correct answers and rationales

JOHN SOUTH

1. 3. Option 3 shares the nurse's observation and focuses on the patient. Questions using the word why tend to intimidate, and questions that can be answered with a "yes" or a "no" tend to elicit little information. Option 4 has a note of sarcasm about it.

2. 4. In order to gain the patient's attention, option 4 offers the best choice. Interrupting the patient may antagonize or startle him.

3. 4. For this patient, it is especially desirable that his environment be as free from anxiety-producing situations as possible. A hygienic environment is indicated but is not of the same priority as a nonstressful environment.

4. 3. Rewards and reprimands are not as effective as helping the patient to help himself. Option 1 should be used only if option 3 fails.

5. 4. The term narcissm is best defined by this stem. The term cathexis refers to the investment of emotions and significance in an idea or object but most commonly another person. Blocking refers to difficulty in recalling a train of thought or speech due to emotional factors. Imprinting refers to the process of rapid learning and behavioral patterning which occurs at critical points in very early stages of development in animals and possibly humans.

6. 3. The withdrawal of this patient most accurately reflects a weak or fragmented ego. The ego is concerned with negotiating the realities of the external world whereas the id operates in terms of the pleasure principle and the superego in terms of right and wrong.
7. 2. Déja vu is best described by this stem. This is the experience of feeling that the situation at hand has happened to the person before. With depersonalization, there would be feelings of strangeness or unreality concerning the environment. Hypnagogic imagery refers to the mental images that may occur just before sleep. Autism is thinking unduly directed toward the self to the exclusion of others.
8. 1. Gaining the patient's trust is of most importance during the early stages of a one-to-one relationship. The person must feel safe with the therapist before he will relinquish any of his symptoms or become more self-sufficient.
9. 4. It is best to remove the patient from the lounge where his behavior may offend others. Being critical of the patient is contraindicated. The behavior is best viewed as an outlet for anxiety.
10. 4. Masturbation will not lead to consequences described in options 1 and 2, and authorities do not accept option 3 as accurate. Some lay persons may hold to opinions in these first three options. Option 4 is the best answer, although masturbation is not necessarily contraindicated for married persons or older persons.
11. 4. Although there may be some elements of truth in options 1, 2, and 3, the primary reason for using personnel of the same minority racial group as the patient is best described in option 4.
12. 3. The patient's comment is best described as the tendency to view one's own group members as inferior.
13. 4. Nortriptyline hydrochloride is classified as an antidepressant. It is often used to initiate treatment of patients with moderate to severe depression.
14. 1. Option 1 describes the gravest implications when adverse effects occur. Adverse effects described in options 2, 3, and 4, if they occur, can be more easily handled.
15. 4. Simple, concrete subjects for conversation in remotivational group sessions are best. In general, it would be best to avoid subjects involving love, religion, sex, parental relationships, and the like.
16. 3. Generally, every chronic patient is assumed to have potential for improvement. Negative predictions of outcome, the so-

called hopeless patient, with an implied passivity in treatment are not held as valid. Some improvement is always seen as possible.

17. 1. The purpose of remotivation group therapy is to stimulate interaction centered around reality-oriented topics. This has been found to be occurring when patients increase eye contacts among themselves.

18. 4. There may be some element of truth in options 1 and 2. Anxiety is least likely to increase when remotivational techniques are used effectively. However, the most frequently noted observation is that staff members find their jobs more rewarding as the patients respond to the remotivational therapy. The staff, in turn, becomes more hopeful and satisfied.

19. 3. Behavior described in options 1, 2, and 4 may occur as a result of participating in music and dance therapy. However, the primary benefit of this type of therapy is to allow for open expression of feelings.

20. 4. Option 1 offers little if any help. The nurse is shunning her responsibility when she uses option 2. Option 3 is belittling. Option 4 is a simple statement of fact and reminds the patient of reality, that is, his discharge.

21. 2. This patient can be expected to function as well after discharge as he did before he became ill, that is, he can be expected to return to about the same level of functioning as he had previously.

22. 2. Statistics show that approximately 50 percent of the mental hospital population consists of patients diagnosed as schizophrenic.

JERRY RAND

23. 2. Option 2 offers the least threat to the patient. Options 1, 3, and 4 are less desirable since they involve secrecy, dishonesty, and threat.

24. 1. Option 1 allows the nurse to understand behavior better and is least demanding on the patient. Options 2 and 3 are very unlikely to be accepted by the patient.

25. 3. The patient's behavior is likely to be reinforced when the nurse takes steps to agree with it. Options 1, 2, and 4 are possibilities but not likely and deserve little consideration when deciding whether or not to comply with the patient's requests.

26. 4. The patient's thought process is best defined as a delusion of persecution. A delusion of grandeur involves an exaggerated idea of one's importance or identity. An idea of reference

assumes that the remarks or behavior of others apply to self.

27. 2. Options 1 and 3 are often impractical. Option 4 is unlikely to convince the patient. Option 2 offers the best solution in this situation.

28. 1. The assistant's question places the patient on the defensive. Her question is most unlikely to lead to behavior described in options 2, 3, and 4.

29. 4. The suspicious patient characteristically considers others as part of the conspiracy against him. The behaviors in options 1, 2, and 3 are more easily managed by the nurse and are not central to the core problem of suspicion.

30. 1. It is generally best to try giving the medication in its liquid form if the patient is "fighting" taking the medication. If he refuses to swallow or expectorates the medication, the intramuscular route then should be used but will probably meet with more resistance by the patient.

31. 2. The patient's behavior is best defined as akathisia. Dyskinesia is marked by twitching or involuntary muscular movement. Dystonia is characterized by uncoordinated spasmotic movements, such as torticollis, opisthotonas, or oculogynic crisis.

32. 2. The drug of choice is bentropine mesylate for its anticholinergic properties. Option 1 is a minor tranquilizer or antianxiety agent. Option 2 is an antidepressant. Option 4 is a major tranquilizer or antipsychotic agent.

33. 4. Option 1 illustrates appropriate affect. Option 2 is a positive, direct action toward a bothersome situation. Option 3 needs follow-up with the patient but may be due to any number of unknown reasons. In option 4, the patient may show some aggression against his perceived adversary so that the staff will need to watch him carefully for signs of impending violent action and perhaps protect the other patients from bodily harm by this patient.

34. 2. The patient's behavior is best described as projection. An element of denial exists in projection but it is not the primary or total mechanism. Idealization would prevent the patient from seeing another person's faults. Introjection involves turning feelings and responses inward against the self.

35. 2. Just as patients, health personnel have feelings and rights also. The nurse allows the assistant her rights by making a statement that allows her to be angry without scolding her or dismissing her feelings.

36. 1. The suspicious patient is especially sensitive to authority symbols and figures, and more so when he learns that accord-

ing to policy, he cannot leave without an escort. Regulations described in options 2, 3, and 4 are less likely to arouse his antagonism and status fears.

37. 4. Typically, the suspicious person projects his distrust onto others and tends, in turn, not to see others as trustworthy in business or social interactions.

38. 4. Statistics have shown that signs of a paranoid reaction commonly first appear after the age of about 30.

39. 4. The most likely interpretation that this suspicious person will make is that the nurse's behavior was an aggressive move.

40. 2. Option 2 involves team effort and competition. Solitary, intellectual persuits are considered best and least threatening for the suspicious person.

41. 4. Behaviors described in options 1, 2, and 3 are least likely to arouse feelings of suspicion and conspiracy. Option 4 describes behavior that may arouse paranoid ideation.

DINAH WALLACE

42. 1. Actions described in options 2 and 3 are not likely to be helpful upon admission. Behavior described in option 4 may be desirable but it would be of most importance to help this patient feel safe and accepted.

43. 3. The best charting describes exactly what the patient did and said in a particular situation. Options 1, 2, and 4 do not follow this basic principle of charting.

44. 4. The most outstanding characteristic of this drug is that it can be used effectively while being administered relatively infrequently.

45. 3. Option 1 is indicated because a side effect of fluphenazine decanoate is peripheral edema with weight changes. The patient should be monitored for blood dyscrasias (option 2). Blood pressure may fluctuate while using this agent. Of least importance is to conduct pulmonary function tests.

46. 3. The patient's behavior is best described as waxy flexibility. Echolalia means repeating or parroting the words of another. Neurasthenia refers to feeling weak. Reaction formation is a defense mechanism.

47. 3. Option 3 shares the nurse's observations with the patient and may stimulate the patient to agree, disagree, or clarify thoughts, feelings, and actions for the nurse.

48. 3. Punishment (option 1) or reward (option 4) are likely to be of little value. The patient simply may not eat if option 2 is followed. The best course of action is to lead the patient firmly to the dining room.

49. 1. The type of parenting this patient received was most probably ambiguous. Given chronically conflicting or ambivalent cues, a person becomes confused and/or frustrated and finds it safer to avoid communicating with others. This usually causes withdrawing from reality and communicating mostly nonverbally or symbolically.

50. 2. The patient's behavior is best described as regression. Fixation means not progressing beyond a given level of development. Substitution means replacing unacceptable ideas with more acceptable ones. Symbolization means one idea or object comes to stand for another.

51. 1. It has been shown that nonverbal communications convey feelings more accurately than do spoken words. Words very often are used to cover feelings. Options 2, 3, and 4 are false statements in relation to nonverbal communications.

52. 3. The recommended first course of action is to prevent accidents and injuries when a patient becomes violent. Other courses of action may be followed later once safety is assured.

53. 3. The indiscriminate use of restraints can lead to charges of false imprisonment which is defined as unjustifiable retention without proper consent. Fraud is willful and purposeful misrepresentation that could cause or has caused harm. Assault refers to a threat or an attempt to make bodily contact with another person without consent. Invasion of privacy is a wrong that invades the right of a person to be let alone.

54. 1. Option 1 illustrates the nurse's interest in the husband's feelings and provides opportunity to discuss them. The other three options give the husband no assurance and ignore his feelings by offering answers that are unlikely to be of any help.

55. 2. The nurse needs to know to whom the patient is referring and should elicit from the patient more description about the conclusive statement and situation. Options 1 and 3 are premature although they may be indicated later; however, the danger implied in option 3 is unlikely. Option 4 would not be helpful in gaining an understanding of the situation.

56. 4. Good premorbid social adjustment is a clinical factor on the favorable prognostic side. Options 1, 2, and 3 are clinical factors on the unfavorable prognostic side.

MELISSA CORNING

57. 4. Although the therapist *may* make subjective judgments concerning this patient in relation to factors described in options 1, 2, and 3, the patient's interpersonal difficulties are most open to the therapist's scrutiny during play therapy.

58. 3. Play techniques are used for the reason given in option 3. Options 1 and 2 are inaccurate statements. The first half of option 4 is inaccurate.

59. 3. Both verbal and nonverbal messages should be sent by the nurse during therapy sessions. However, it is essential that they be genuine and congruent.

60. 1. The initial or original contract or schedule set up with a child should be adhered to, to promote trust and in the interests of limit setting.

61. 3. Option 3 suggests and shares an emotional response to the behavior. Questions using the word, why, are likely to place the patient on the defensive. Options 1 and 4 read too much into the placement of the doll and the interpretations implied may be incorrect.

62. 4. It would be best for the therapist to acknowledge the patient's behavior. Interpreting to the patient is inappropriate for the nurse therapist unless such interpreting reflects present behavior, feeling tone, or action to the child. Agreement tends to block further communications.

63. 3. Collaboration is a tool developed in the preadolescent era (9 to 12 years of age). Competition is a tool of the juvenile era (6 to 9 years of age). The self and language are tools of childhood (1½ to 6 years of age).

64. 3. Information described in options 1, 2, and 4 is positive, direct, and supportive. However, when staff members have disagreements and in-fighting, their behavior can be very destructive in terms of the patient's progress, especially if the patient senses the intrastaff conflict.

65. 1. Although a child has other needs, his dependency needs are best met when the nurse acts the mother surrogate role.

66. 1. The patient's behavior needs to be stopped by physical means if necessary. Other actions may be taken but they are less satisfactory when out-of-control behavior, such as flailing arms, has occurred.

67. 2. Option 2 is the least competitive and the most positive and direct response in this situation. It also offers some support for the child. The best procedure is to be calm and unaccusing.

68. 1. Option 1 describes a physical deformity that is unrelated to child abuse, which inflicts mistreatment resulting in physical and mental signs/symptoms.

69. 2. Of prime importance is the right of the child to be treated humanely; other rights are of secondary importance, when compared with the child's rights.

70. 4. Option 4 is likely to result in better rapport with the parents since the focus is on needs of the parents. The nurse overextends herself when using option 3. Option 2 almost invites not calling for help. Option 1 is threatening and, therefore, contraindicated.
71. 2. A characteristic behavior of parents who abuse children is that they are unaware of how their child feels. Factors described in options 1, 3, and 4 are often observed in parents who abuse children.
72. 1. Parents generally learn parenting from their own mothers and fathers. Abuse-prone parents can be expected to have been treated critically and punitively as children.
73. 2. Only option 2 describes a form of prevention. Options 1, 3, and 4 are after-the-fact measures.
74. 2. To best meet the problems in this situation, the parents as well as the children need help. It will be of little value to help either the parents alone or the children alone with therapy.
75. 2. Although information described in options 1, 3, and 4 may be helpful, records of nurse participant observations are most likely to contain information concerning interactional or behavioral problems of the patient which will serve as a basis for future intervention and, hence, will be most useful.
76. 3. While all of the qualities given here are important, the most likely quality lacking in this situation is that of consistency in relating with the patient.
77. 3. Options 1, 2, and 4 describe desirable long-range aims of therapy. Although some routine is desirable, it is of least importance to aim toward helping this patient tolerate strict routines of daily living.
78. 3. When a child starts to care about herself, she will take better care of her personal needs, such as the one described in option 3.

STEPHANIE JAMET

79. 1. The very active patient is usually best placed in a quiet atmosphere in order to decrease stimuli for actions.
80. 3. The best response is expressed in option 3. It focuses on the husband's feelings. Option 2 ignores the husband's feelings. So also does option 2. Option 4 is critical of the patient's behavior and agrees to what might be an inaccurate assessment of the patient's behavior by the husband.
81. 1. Options 2 and 3 are inappropriate; the patient needs some explanation but details are unnecessary. There is no indication for additional help being needed for this patient.

82. 1. Since the patient is very active, it would be best to give her food she can carry with her and eat as she moves about. Option 4 is generally impractical and the patient would most probably be too busy to eat anyway. Options 2 and 3 do not meet the problem of seeing to it that the patient has proper nourishment while being very active.

83. 2. Explanations and illustrations are unlikely to be of value for helping this patient. It is best to assist her into proper attire in a matter-of-fact way.

84. 2. The patient is demonstrating flight of ideas. Concreteness is interpreting another person's words literally. Depersonalization refers to feelings of strangeness concerning the environment or the self. A neologism is a word coined by a patient.

85. 1. The anxiety the patient feels gives rise to the distorted thinking displayed in the speech pattern, as flight of ideas. The other options have little, if any, relation to the thought disorder expressed.

86. 4. In option 4, the nurse takes responsibility for not being able to understand the patient; this is least likely to arouse anxiety in the patient. While helping the patient make adequate connections between events is desirable, the manner in which it is being done, as described in option 2, offers more threat by requiring that the patient analyze thoughts by describing why they occur.

87. 4. Of those given here, ping pong is likely to be best since the patient is very active and would probably not be able to concentrate or sustain interest in the more sedentary activities.

88. 4. The patient during a manic episode is unlikely to evidence feelings of guilt, anger, or distrust. Hostility is a more characteristic feeling.

89. 3. The most attractive compromise is to grant partial fulfillment of this patient's request. Options 1 and 2 are ill-advised and the patient does not need 30 bars of soap.

90. 4. Initial mild forms of the ensuing manic phase are called hypomania. Typically, the person looks and acts cheerful, is restless and overactive, and his speech is overproductive. In other words, the patient appears extroverted.

91. 2. During periods of euphoria and extreme activity, the patient should be observed for physical exhaustion which predisposes to infections.

92. 1. Patients who do not maintain adequate sodium intake may quickly become toxic. Sodium is necessary for the renal excretion of lithium. A low sodium intake results in the retention of lithium and lithium toxicity.

93. 4. Behavior is caused. Options 1, 2, and 3 serve only to ignore the cause. Option 4 is the best way to approach the problem since it recognizes the cause of the behavior.

94. 4. The patient's anger and her manner of expressing it are likely to decrease as the patient improves and gains more control over her behavior. Options 1, 2, and 3 do not offer sound guidelines for nursing intervention. Option 1 is true but is of secondary importance and can be managed on an individual basis. Option 2 is an inaccurate statement. Option 3 focuses on the nurse's needs and does not accept the patient's behavior.

95. 2. Research has shown that this patient's symptoms of her mood disorder are likely to recur periodically.

96. 1. Options 2, 3, and 4 describe desirable ways that family members can help this patient. It is unrealistic and impractical to attempt to eliminate worry and anxiety from the environment.

97. 2. Options 1, 3, and 4 have not been found to be of eiological significance for manic-depressive psychoses; a family history of the illness often is present.

MAY BULLEN

98. 2. Only option 2 describes a situation that makes this patient legally committable.

99. 4. A person who has had to be committed to a mental hospital loses the right to leave the hospital of his own accord. He does not lose the rights described in options 1, 2, and 3.

100. 3. A writ of habeus corpus is defined as an order requiring that a prisoner (in this case, the patient) be brought before a judge or into court to decide whether he is being held lawfully. Its purpose is to obtain liberation of a person being held without just cause.

101. 4. The patient has an inadequate self-concept and develops an unconscious feeling that she is personally inadequate, that is, a failure. The grandiose delusion is an attempt to relieve anxiety and her intolerable sense of personal and social inadequacy.

102. 3. Although some persons are likely to experience factors described in options 1, 2, and 4, the suspicious person characteristically views others as wishing to attack him.

103. 4. Doing something with or to the patient is unlikely to help a restless and incoherent patient. It is best to sit by quietly until the medication takes effect. A warm bath might be used but not a cold shower.

104. 2. The correct option offers help calmly. Option 1 directs atten-

tion to the nurse and not to the patient. Option 3 is very impersonal and offers no help. Option 4 adds to the patient's delusions.

105. 2. Estrogens enhance bone formation and when lacking, osteoporosis may develop. There is no known contraindication for estrogens when emphysema is present. These agents tend to cause increased edema, increased blood calcium levels, and increased growth of tumors.

106. 3. Nausea, weight gain (due to water retention), and breast tenderness (due to continuous breast stimulation) are commonly reported. Hypotension is not associated with estrogen therapy.

107. 2. The negative impact of menopause is most often considered due to the woman's feelings of worthlessness, once childbearing years have passed. These feelings are not believed due to physical reasons (options 1 and 4) nor to financial problems associated with aging.

108. 1. It has been found that in men the involutional period is much less clearly marked than for women but some changes usually do take place, commonly some 10 to 15 years later than in women.

109. 4. The personality of the patient prior to the illness is often stated to be rigid, overconscientious, and emotionally constricted. Life histories reveal that involutional melancholia usually appears in people who have been over meticulous, sensitive, and rigid in their daily habits.

110. 1. The best way to answer the patient and her family is by the comment in option 1. Options 2 and 3 are not entirely accurate; some patients find it unpleasant and do not become accustomed to the sensations they may feel. Option 4 offers little support to the patient and the family.

111. 3. Preparation as described in options 1, 2, and 4 is not indicated before therapy can be administered. It is essential to have a signed consent for the procedure. Chest x-rays and an EKG are indicated also.

112. 2. The best course of action is described in option 2. Option 1 may cause the patient to lose confidence in the treatment. Option 3 is a dishonest way to handle the problem. Option 4 offers little help and is too impersonal; nursing responsibilities are being transferred.

113. 2. The patient's dentures should be removed in order to help prevent injury or damage should the dentures slip out of place during therapy.

114. 2. Thiopental sodium renders the patient unconscious but lacks

good muscle-relaxing qualities. Atropine acts to relax smooth muscles and is often used for its antispasmodic and antisecretory effects.

115. 1. Options 2, 3, and 4 describe undesirable results which can occur when electroconvulsive therapy is used. Residual epilepsy has not been reported.

116. 2. Observations have shown that this patient's recovery is most likely to be gradual. The course of involutional melancholia tends to be prolonged and recovery may take as long as 8 years if untreated.

117. 4. Options 1, 2, and 3 are unlikely to help prevent involutional problems. See item 107 also. Supporting women toward role satisfaction will help to substitute feelings of worthlessness with feelings of self-respect and self-esteem.

ARCHIE ROWLAND

118. 4. Excess elimination of carbon dioxide from the lungs by hyperventilating will cause respiratory alkalosis. Poor elimination of carbon dioxide from the lungs will cause respiratory acidosis. HCO_3 and Base Excess levels help to determine whether nonrespiratory (metabolic) alkalosis or acidosis is present.

119. 1. The best measure is to have the patient rebreathe into a paper bag. He will be inhaling air higher in carbon dioxide and lower in oxygen content than normal air; this is desirable since his body has been eliminating more than normal amounts of carbon dioxide while hyperventilating. Placing the head down will accomplish nothing in relation to the effects of hyperventilating. Options 3 and 4 are likely to aggravate the situation.

120. 2. The patient needs support which option 2 offers him. Options 1 and 3 are likely to aggravate this condition and option 4 offers no support.

121. 3. Option 1 has a combination of mild anxiety symptoms (attention and sensitivity) and severe anxiety symptoms (emotional and stereotyped behaviors). Options 2 depicts a moderate level of anxiety. Option 4 depicts a severe level of anxiety.

122. 1. Neurotic anxiety is out of proportion to its cause. Options 2, 3, and 4 are inaccurate statements in relation to neurotic anxiety but are often noted when normal anxiety is present.

123. 1. Responding for a patient encourages dependence. Options 2, 3, and 4 are constructive and encourage independence.

124. 3. The patient with neurotic anxieties experiences feelings of inadequacy and inferiorities. Distrust, alienation, and

superiority are not associated with neurotic anxiety.

125. 2. The defense mechanism, repression, operates to banish unacceptable ideas from conscious awareness. It occurs automatically and involuntarily. Projection occurs when feelings and wishes from within oneself are attributed to others. Regression denotes a return to more infantile patterns of reacting. Sublimation involves diverting instinctual drives into socially acceptable channels.

126. 4. Using optimistic verbalizations avoids the patient's feelings and, therefore, offers no help. The nurse's presence, respecting how the patient feels, and demonstrating competence are helpful measures.

127. 2. Feelings of anxiety causes the body to secrete epinephrine which is a vasconstrictor. One of the effects of vasoconstriction is a cold, clammy skin. Other effects of epinephrine on the body include a rapid heartbeat, a decrease in salivation, and muscular tenseness.

128. 1. The nurse has the right to her feelings also. The best practice in this situation is for the nurse to leave if her anxiety level is too high for her to function effectively.

129. 2. The neurotic patient tends to be self-centered and needs a range of outside interests to help divert attention from himself.

130. 2. Not making sexual advances for fear of being turned down best illustrates the tendency of the neurotic patient to expect ineffective reactions from others. No physical complaint or ineffective method is depicted in the illustration. The goal (marital sexual relations) would not seem unattainable.

131. 3. Although all of the effects given here may result when antianxiety agents are used, the primary reason for some persons preferring not to use them during psychotherapy is that they tend to reduce motivation for change. Psychotherapy is most effective when the patient's motivation for change is high.

132. 3. Through role-playing, role reversal and doubling techniques, the patient learns to see his behavior in a different light and more objectively. He can then practice responding differently to problematic situations, with group support, input, and feedback. Options 1, 2, and 4 are not major goals of psychodrama and may even be undesirable as aims.

133. 1. The feelings of inadequacy that occur for patients with an anxiety neurosis are usually traceable to the inability to win parental approval during childhood.

134. 3. Even though the patient may be able to carry out behavior described in options 1, 2, and 4, he is still going to experience neurotic symptoms unless he has learned to alter his methods

of behaving in a way that handles his anxiety successfully.

135. 1. The drugs given in options 2, 3, and 4 are generally classified as major tranquilizing (antipsychotic) agents.

136. 2. Minor tranquilizers are prescribed when possible because they are characteristically freer of undesirable side effects.

137. 4. It is generally agreed that some anxiety is necessary to help develop adaptive behavior. Increasing one's alertness to the environment is adaptive behavior. For example, the anxiety associated with taking an examination alerts one to study.

NED PACKARD

138. 4. The nurse most likely refrains from using the patient's first name because it implies an equal status with which she is uncomfortable. Using the patient's first name has no bearing on the nurse's professionalism or the patient's age.

139. 3. The nurse counselor, unless trained in psychoanalytic techniques, deals mostly with the current life experiences of the patient on which she can exert a positive influence in a limited amount of time.

140. 4. Option 4 uses the therapeutic technique of restatement. Option 1 is impersonal and implies the patient is being uncooperative. Option 2 implies that perhaps the other patients do not have potential. Option 3 challenges and requests an explanation.

141. 3. In this situation, the nurse should focus on the simplest type of behavior, that which would require the least effort for the patient. The relationship is still in an early exploratory stage when self-expression and verbalization are the more appropriate goals.

142. 2. In option 2, the patient has gone beyond testing and acquainting himself with a new relationship and is now working on his problems. Option 1 describes an exploratory phase of the relationship. Option 3 illustrates a termination phase of the relationship. Option 4 describes an initial phase in the relationship.

143. 1. The stem best defines the word empathy. Climate refers to environmental conditions characterizing a relationship. Rapport is defined as the harmonious feeling experienced by two people who hold one another in mutual respect. Sympathy implies a warmth or urge to act to alleviate the distress of another.

144. 3. The responsibility for maintaining the relationship rests with the nurse. In option 3, the nurse assumed this responsibility

and the patient is also given a nonthreatening opportunity to respond. Option 2 prematurely interprets the patient and is nontherapeutic. Option 4 does not keep to the limits of the contract and offers little help to the patient.

145. 1. Although the nurse's behavior may help accomplish goals described in all 4 options, the primary reason is that the nurse will not wish to create distrust. Distrust will be most destructive of a therapeutic relationship.

146. 4. The defense mechanism, reaction formation, is described in the stem. Sublimation is directing unacceptable impulses into constructive channels. Suppression is a conscious effort to overcome unacceptable thoughts or desires. Rationalization is utilizing a more acceptable or plausible reason for a behavior than the real one.

147. 1. Comments described in options 2, 3, and 4 are not supportive and options 2 and 3 could add to the patient's negative feelings. Option 1 describes a comment that will help the patient most to explore his feelings further and demonstrates understanding on the part of the other members of the group.

148. 4. Tranylcypromine sulfate is a monamine oxidase inhibitor.

149. 3. When taken with foods or beverages rich in amines or amino acids, a hypertensive crisis may result because amines and amino acids form pressor amines that are inactivated by monamine oxidase. Foods to be avoided include wine, beer, cheese, yogurt, chocolate, sardines, chicken livers, bananas, and avocados.

150. 4. Option 4 offers the best understanding of the patient's needs. There are no indications for extra rest or for unusual activities and the patient has not demonstrated suicidal tendencies.

151. 2. Terminating a relationship is a weaning process. Options 1, 3, and 4 do not provide for this while option 2 does. Future-oriented conversations would focus, for example, on how the patient might apply the skills he learned in the relationship.

152. 3. While keeping verbatim records may help reach the goals described in all of these options, this type of record is generally used for helping the nurse improve her communication skills.

153. 4. Regret is a direct and appropriate response to termination of a positive relationship and indicates acceptance of termination. Anger is healthy when openly expressed but is a less healthy grief reaction than regret. A lack of response may be interpreted as indifference but it represents a profound emotional reaction which the patient is unable to express. Humor may be a defense against feelings of loss.

154. 3. Options 1, 2, and 4 are conclusions or value judgments based on insufficient data. Option 3 acknowledges that the behavior is meaningful but not yet fully understood.

155. 2. The nurse should take the initiative initially in this relationship and, therefore, remaining silent until the patient speaks is least therapeutic. The other options allow for ventilation of anger or other feelings and thoughts of the patient.

156. 3. A good rule-of-thumb is to let the patient bring up his own topics for discussion and to explore given clues more fully, especially if they relate to the patient's feelings about the nurse. Option 4 suggests that the nurse is reading the patient's mind and interpreting behavior without sufficient evidence. Option 2 is impersonal.

157. 1. Studies have shown that bringing up the subject of suicide when there is reason to suspect the patient may be considering it has not harmed anyone and has helped a great many. Option 2 is unwise—the safest procedure is to investigate. Option 3 is premature. Option 4 is premature and too indirect.

158. 2. The patient is expressing a fear of being stigmatized or discredited, should others discover his socially undesirable tendencies.

159. 1. The patient is exhibiting conflict. An impulse is a sudden inclination to take some unpremeditated action. Regression is a return to earlier, more satisfying ways of behaving. An ego break would be manifested as a severe personality disturbance.

160. 3. The patient is utilizing introjection. Conversion occurs when repressed ideas are converted into a variety of somatic symptoms. Restitution is a coping mechanism whereby an individual atones for his unacceptable ideas, feelings, or actions. When substitution is present, an unacceptable or unattainable goal is replaced by one which is more acceptable or attainable.

161. 3. In the depressive syndromes, loss is of most importance. Options 1 and 2 may lead to feelings of loss but option 3 is a broader concept and more universally applicable.

162. 4. Decision-making is difficult for the depressed person because of feelings of ambivalence and thought retardation. Options 1 and 2 are in error because when depression is present, alimentary tract motility is retarded, causing delayed emptying of the stomach, a feeling of fullness, loss of appetite, weight loss, and constipation.

163. 3. Cheerfulness and gaiety have a tendency to make a depressed

person feel more guilty and unworthy. It is helpful to be firm and businesslike or serious with depressed persons and to behave naturally and spontaneously.

164. 3. It ordinarily takes from approximately 1 to 3 weeks before this drug can be expected to have a favorable effect.

165. 4. This patient is not ready for activity described in options 1, 2, and 3, but is ready for observing simple daily routines.

166. 1. Depressed patients are difficult to relate to because of their expressed feelings of hopelessness and general apathy. The concomitant feelings of hopelessness and lack of success experienced by the nurse with these patients may lead the nurse to withdraw or feel angry with the patient. Option 2 may be a factor in this situation but can be more easily and directly managed by the nurse. Depressed persons are typically dependent on others. They are not motivated by laziness and are usually conscientious and dependable.

167. 1. Suicide attempts are more likely to occur soon after the depression lifts and the patient has more energy to act on her thoughts and impulses. The patient does not have the energy to commit suicide during times of greatest depression. The energy level of the patient, rather than her status, is related to the danger involved.

168. 2. The measures described in options 1, 3, and 4 will help relieve mouth dryness. Sucking hard candy will not and it also predisposes to dental caries and feelings of thirst.

169. 3. Depressed patients have sleep disturbances and, hence, the property of sedation is a valuable one. Very often, a patient is treated with antipsychotic, antidepressant, and antiparkinson agents simultaneously. An additive effect very often leads to urinary retention and paralytic ileus, either of which can lead to death.

170. 1. When the nurse accepts the patient's gift, she renders herself powerless in the relationship with the patient. Patients do expect some reciprocation from the nurse who accepts their gifts.

171. 4. The option 4 comment points out specific progress that has been made. The other three options may prove more frustrating than helpful for the patient who is already finding fault with herself. Option 3 changes the subject.

JAY BONNER

172. 2. The necessary factual data must be collected before the problem-solving process inherent in crisis intervention can be implemented. The patient may have some ideas concerning

what would help him but intervention described in option 1 would come at a later point in the problem-solving process. Option 3 is an overoptimistic statement since possibly, the patient may not be in the "right place." Option 4 is incorrect since the focus should be on the patient's thoughts and feelings. Patients such as the one described here are generally aware of their symptoms.

173. 4. The comment in option 4 responds to the feelings of the patient and also gives proper reassurance. Option 1 is belittling. In option 2, the nurse is trying to make a judgment which is contraindicated. Option 3 does not get at the patient's feelings or the problem involved; sane is a legal term and not used in psychiatric practice.

174. 1. When obsessive-compulsive reactions are present, the patient is attempting to control his anxiety. The compulsive part of the behavior is an act that is performed by the individual to avoid anxiety.

175. 2. A patient who is able to take care of his basic nutritional and hygiene needs is probably not severely incapacitated by his illness to the point of requiring hospitalization. The ability to behave normally is of lesser importance in this decision, depending on the tolerance of the patient's family or significant others for the behavior. Options 1 and 4 may be considered in making the decision but are not valid criteria for hospitalization.

176. 4. The dynamics of compulsive activity involve a defense against anxiety by persistently doing something else, that is a substitutive activity, each time threatening thoughts or impulses make their appearance. Option 1 is a healthy defense mechanism (sublimation). Option 2 and 3 are based on insufficient data and oversimplify the problem.

177. 4. Displacement is the mechanism employed here. Fixation is the arrest of psychosocial maturation. Projection occurs when emotionally unacceptable self-traits are unconsciously rejected and attributed to others. Conversion occurs when repressed ideas or impulses are converted into a variety of somatic symptoms.

178. 2. The disturbance described is an obsession or unwanted idea or thought. A phobia is a persistent, unrealistic fear of an external object or situation through the mechanism of displacement. A compulsion is an unwanted urge to perform an act. Dissociation is an unconscious process of separating and detaching emotional significance and affect from an idea, situation, or effect.

179. 2. Option 2 is realistic and truthful. While option 1 may be true, it is a negative approach and will likely be discouraging to the mother. Option 3 is not necessarily true. Option 4 is discouraging and not necessarily true.

180. 4. It is best to accept compulsive behavior in a comparatively permissive manner. The patient may become restless or anxious if the ritualistic activity is denied him. Option 2 is an incorrect statement. Option 2 is unwarranted. Isolation (option 1) will make the patient feel more alone and unworthy.

181. 1. While all qualities given here may have some degree of desirability, it is considered to be most important that the nurse demonstrate patience. It takes these patients a long time to complete necessary tasks. Unless the nurse is patient, she can easily become frustrated, upset, or even angry. The obsessive-compulsive patient cannot be hurried.

182. 4. The patient derives the most benefit from keeping in contact with his family and social group while receiving therapeutic help. This plan decreases social isolation, rejection, and dependency.

183. 1. The group has used the staff as role models. Other patients are likely to devalue him as he devalues himself when he uses self-effacing mannerisms. Also, they are likely to resent an expensive wardrobe. Telling stories is unlikely to be sustained as a basis for acceptance and may irritate depressed patients.

184. 4. Option 1 and 3 are likely to increase the patient's dependency and option 2 belittles the patient. Option 4 promotes independence.

185. 2. Letting the patient eat earlier meets both his needs for more time and the group's need for prompt departure. It also protects the patient from being resented by others and lets him be included in group activity. Option 1 is undesirable and may be impractical as well.

186. 2. Drama clubs are good for their social and self-expressive qualities. These patients need outlets that are creative and other-oriented.

ROGER CRANST

187. 3. In order to help the patient, the nurse should first plan to get the facts before she plans, implements, or evaluates. This can best be accomplished by actions described in option 3.

188. 1. School-refusal or phobia is associated with intense anxiety, usually over separation from the mother. It is related to the

parents' inability to allow the child to be separated or independent.

189. 3. Option 3 helps the patient look at and think for himself. Option 1 makes the nurse seem uncertain and could lead the patient to deny seductiveness. Option 2 serves as a type of hedge and does not face the problem. Option 4 puts the patient down.

190. 3. The defense mechanism described is reaction formation. Sublimation diverts instinctual drives into socially acceptable channels. Introjection takes loved or hated external objects within oneself symbolically. Insulation is reducing ego involvement and withdrawing into passivity to protect the self from hurt.

191. 2. In order to change behavior, the patient must be motivated to do so. Factors described in options 1, 3, and 4 are of less significance.

192. 2. Taking sides limits the nurse's effectiveness and does not help either party. It is more destructive than the other options and also less easily recognized because the nurse's personal values are involved. This makes the counseling situation harder to manage.

193. 2. The counselor must be responsive to the needs of the couple and be especially flexible. The personality of the family therapist is an important consideration. Attempts to imitate another therapist or to adhere rigidly to a particular professional stereotype will result in a loss of spontaneity and effectiveness as a family therapist. There are many unpredictables in family therapy. The counselor may need to be a parent figure, an advocate, and interpreter, an innovator, and the like.

194. 2. Authorities do not hold the opinion that a counselor for married couples should be married, male, or female in order to function effectively. Options 1, 3, and 4 do not express authoritative opinion.

195. 4. For present family relationships to be overt and productive, it is helpful for the couple to explore the relationship between present patterns of interacting and the previous functioning of parental models. Unperceived parental behavioral patterns are continued in present relationships unless uncovered in therapy. Thus, data collecting is important.

196. 4. Verbalizing expectations minimizes the possibility that unrealistic images will be projected on a marital partner. In order for acceptance to occur, expectations must first be made known through verbalization.

197. 3. Unmet expectations create anxiety and frustration in the individual and can lead to withdrawal or other negative behaviors. Compromise and cooperation are more likely to result from shared expectations.

198. 3. The use of power in transacting family life is a coercive mode and can lead to conflict and crisis. The other modes are more likely to resolve conflicts within the family.

199. 2. The patient is speaking negatively by saying what he does not want. Appropriate intervention is to help him to say what he does want, and to his wife directly.

200. 4. The focus in family/couple therapy is on understanding and responding to each others' messages. Personal needs and lacks are not treated as individual problems but as issues affecting the relationship. The past is taken up primarily in terms of clarifying how it distorts the ability to hear each other now. There is less need in couple therapy than in individual therapy to promote and use transference to the therapist in order to re-experience the conflict in therapy and make it amenable to resolution.

201. 3. Hard-of-hearing persons report feelings described in options 1, 2, and 4. It is the rare hard-of-hearing person who has experiences as described in option 3.

202. 4. Good eye contact is important in talking with the deaf. It is annoying to shout and most uncomfortable for the hard-of-hearing person wearing a hearing aid. It is better to slow the rate of talking than using exaggerated lip movements. The glare behind the speaker strains the eyes and casts a shadow over the face of the speaker (option 4).

203. 4. Coalition refers to the pathological ways family members align themselves within the family system when subgroups are more intense than those of the whole family. Myths are passed on by each generation without reason or explanation and without tolerance of deviation. When a rule is used, members behave in an organized, repetitive manner.

204. 1. Adult to adult transactions are most likely to solve problems. Communications break down when a transaction is crossed, that is, when a stimulus evokes a response from an ego state other than the one addressed.

205. 4. When a couple has solved urgent problems and learned ways of coping without conflict, termination is to be considered. Not all problems need to be solved nor is counseling able to guarantee happiness. It is rare to encounter profound dependency on the therapist and termination is often instigated by the couple.

206. 3. Option 3 acknowledges an accurate situation and gives the patient an opportunity to express his feelings. Option 1 serves little purpose except as a social comment. Option 2 could be interpreted as rude and challenging. Option 4 expresses an unwarranted assumption.

207. 1. The defense mechanism being utilized is fantasy. Repression is preventing painful thoughts from entering consciousness. Projection is attributing one's own unacceptable traits to others. Compensation covers up a weakness by emphasizing a desirable trait.

208. 3. Nonverbal behavior is most likely to express a person's true feelings. The other options which describe verbal communications are likely to be less accurate expressions of the nurse's feelings.

209. 4. The nurse who pities a patient tends to dehumanize him and to see him as if he were an object or inferior being. It involves an act of condescension.

210. 4. Using people as therapy (option 4) rather than manipulating the environment, as described in options 1, 2, and 3, is usually more helpful in situations such as this. Tension is less likely to build when the patient is interpersonally involved than when the time element in relation to eating has been altered.

211. 1. Activity within physical limits is desirable but the emphasis of treatment lies in providing rest and freedom from emotional stress to the extent possible. These goals are best met by option 1 and less well met by activities described in the other three options.

212. 2. The most frequently observed personality characteristics noted in patients with ulcerative colitis are those described in option 2.

213. 1. Patients with ulcerative colitis need strong emotional support. It is generally recommended that no attempts at interpretive or deep psychotherapy be used. These patients do not usually have sufficient flexibility to change without further disruption of the personality and may become suicidal or psychotic if their defenses are broken down or exposed.

214. 3. Options 1, 2, and 4 are true statements but option 3 is an inaccurate statement in relation to the gastrointestinal tract.

215. 2. The body systems and organs affected by psychophysiological disorders are usually innervated by the autonomic nervous system. In reaction to stress, the autonomic nervous system prepares the gastrointestinal tract for the body's reaction with hyperemia, hypermotility, and hypersecretion. Lesions in

the form of ulcers may result in the lining of the intestine from chronic irritation.

216. 1. Options 2, 3, and 4 are inaccurate in relation to psychophysiological disorders. Option 1 may well occur. For example, if a patient is untreated for ulcerative colitis, the intestine may perforate. Perforation is the most frequent cause of death when ulcerative colitis is present.

217. 1. Of the illnesses given here, only asthma is considered to be at least partly due to psychobiological factors. One's way of life may contribute to, but not cause, epilepsy.

218. 1. Option 1 gives the patient an opportunity to express his feelings. Option 2 ignores the patient's comment. Option 3 suggests criticism of the patient for his feelings and is defensive of the physician. Option 4 tends to make an unwarranted assumption; one should let the patient explore his feelings in his own way.

219. 3. Option 3 gives the patient an opportunity to express his feelings in an emotionally charged situation. It serves as a release valve. Option 1 is contraindicated; it will tend to aggravate the patient's anger and he is entitled to his feelings. Scolding will not help (option 2) nor will ignoring the situation assist the patient (option 4).

220. 4. The patient's behavior is typical of emotional lability which is a readily changeable or unstable emotional affect. Punning is using a word when it can have two or more meanings; a play on words. Confabulation is replacing memory loss by fantasy to hide confusion; it is unconscious behavior. Flight of ideas refers to a rapid succession of verbal expressions that jump from one topic to another and are only superficially related.

221. 1. From information given about this patient, it is most likely that he has not accepted the idea of having surgery. Hence, he is not in a state of readiness for learning. The factors given in options 2, 3, and 4 influence learning but are unlikely to be the basic reasons for this patient's failure to grasp what the nurses were teaching.

222. 3. Preoperative visits and talks with patients who have made successful adjustments to ileostomies are helpful and tend to make the patient less fearful of the operation and its consequences.

223. 1. Feelings of guilt and domination would tend to cause the most amount of intrapsychic conflict. Also they involve feelings that are least easy to express and communicate openly. Hence, feelings of guilt and domination would tend to have the most negative and destructive effect on interrelationships

in terms of behavioral symptomatology.

224. 4. Surgical intervention for this patient only helps to solve a physical problem. In order to stay healthy, the patient will need to find emotionally satisfying substitutes for his physical symptoms. Strict dietary therapy is no longer treatment of choice for patients with ulcerative colitis.

GROUP THERAPY IN PROBLEMS OF OVERWEIGHT

225. 3. Although there may be benefits described in all of the options when a co-leadership approach in a group is used, the most immediate benefit is that it allows the leaders to demonstrate model patterns of relating to each other and to the clients. Options 1, 2, and 4 benefit the therapists most while option 3 most directly benefits the clients.

226. 1. Before seeking psychiatric help, it would be best for the nurse to talk out her feelings in a staff meeting. Using actions described in option 3 may prove to be detrimental to the members. Option 4 may be satisfactory but is not indicated until her perspective has altered.

227. 1. Sustained weight loss occurs when the individual has the will and determination to reduce. Other motivations, expressed in options 2, 3, and 4, usually are not of significant value or effectiveness in a weight reduction program. The person must be self-motivated.

228. 3. Of the conditions given, hypervitaminosis and hypotension are least likely to be related to obesity. Hypertension is more likely. The obese person ordinarily does not eat a balanced diet and, hence, hypervitaminosis is unlikely. One can be obese and malnourished.

229. 2. According to one study, statistics have shown that extreme overweight was seven times more frequent among women of the lower socioeconomic class than those of a higher class. The same finding was noted among men but to a lesser degree.

230. 2. Studies have shown that authoritarianism tends to produce group behavior that is apathetic and that uses others as scapegoats. These behaviors are demanding of attention from the leaders and are disruptive and nonproductive, especially when the leaders are absent.

231. 1. Asking for the opinion of others involves the members in a nonthreatening, noncoercive way. It does not reprimand the asker. Options 2, 3, and 4 might lead to group problem solving but they are not supportive of the members and might

more readily lead to resentment and dissatisfaction among the group members.

232. 1. Option 1 encourages self-evaluation. Option 2 challenges the client and is not supportive. Option 3 reinforces the client's hopelessness. Option 4 makes a judgment about the client that might cause resentment.

233. 4. The quality described is known as group cohesiveness. Mutuality is having the same or reciprocal feelings for the other person. Dependency is relying on another for emotional or physical support. Genuineness is being true to one's character and expressing oneself sincerely and honestly.

234. 4. The member described in option 4 is utilizing the role of a contributor and a group maintenance provider. Individual roles, irrelevant to the group task or solving individual needs, are being utilized in the other options. Option 1 describes a "blocker" for progress. Option 2 describes a special interest pleader. Option 3 describes a withdrawer.

235. 4. The group members were using identification with the successful dieter. Imitation is consciously assuming or copying the modes of behavior observed in others. Sublimation is diverting instinctual drives into socially acceptable channels. Incorporation is figuratively ingesting (taking on) the psychic representation of a person.

236. 2. Plateaus in dieting and weight loss programs are related to the accumulation of water as fat is lost.

237. 2. Option 2 gives the members the truth in relation to fad diets in a noncondemning way. The other three options are true but are stated judgmentally and would arouse defensiveness in the dieters.

238. 2. Option 2 describes the most frequently recommended method. Options 1, 3, and 4 describe practices that are often impractical or are likely to be discouraging to the person on a diet.

239. 2. Option 2 is least rejecting and punitive. It demonstrates that the speaker is taking the burden and responsibility for her own feelings. Option 1, 3, and 4 are almost rude statements that may add to interpersonal problems between these two people.

240. 1. Obesity most often is the result of taking in more calories than the body uses. The excess intake is stored in the body as fat.

241. 2. There may be some persons who feel a sense of invulnerability because of their size. However, the most frequently reported feeling is that of isolation. Most often, society tends to stigmatize people with any characteristic it considers undesirable.

242. 2. Through the ages, we have communicated with food: honor is extended through food; punishment is given by withholding food; and the like. Food is recognized as giving comfort, since food often serves this purpose during childhood. Hence, food is very often equated with love and affection in this culture.

243. 4. Bariatrics deals with obesity. Podiatry is related to the care of the feet. Cryogenics refers to the freezing of dead bodies. Lithology is the scientific study of calculi.

244. 2. Adverse side effects when using amphetamines include those described in options 1, 3, and 4. Gastritis is not associated with the use of amphetamines.

245. 2. Habits are ingrained and obesity is rampant in the general population. It would be best to teach prospective and new mothers to avoid overweight in their children, by teaching proper nutrition, and the like. Obesity would then be controlled in that generation with sound habits of eating.

GARY ORD

246. 4. The best first course of action is to observe a patient in order to learn to know him and establish baseline information. It is not recommended that patients be isolated unless there is very good reason for it. An example would be the very active, combative patient who becomes a danger to himself and others. Options 1 and 3 threaten the patient and are more likely to promote trouble.

247. 4. The self-fulfilling prophecy is described here, which is a tendency to behave according to the views and expectations that significant others have of the individual. Congruency refers to consistence in thinking, feeling, and acting. Double-bind is a type of interaction demanding a response to a message that has contradictory signals. Consensual validation is the process of checking out words and events to ensure a shared meaning.

248. 2. The defense mechanism given here is (over) compensation. Fixation refers to remaining (fixing) at a comfortable level of emotional development. Reaction formation is preventing dangerous desires from being expressed by exaggerating opposed attitudes and behavior.

249. 3. The antisocial person needs to be confronted by his behavior, to learn what is expected of him, and how to achieve what is expected. Option 1 encourages the use of excuses and belittles the patient. Option 2 is unlikely to elicit participation.

Option 4 avoids dealing with the problem and would not be a "first choice."

250. 3. A taboo is a cultural prohibition banning behavior on the basis of morality or taste. There is a taboo against passing flatus in public in this culture. A more is a norm that specifies behavior of vital importance to the society and embodies basic moral values. A norm is a rule of behavior for a group and specifies rewards for adherence; norms include folkways and mores. A folkway is a cultural norm that specifies behavior regarded by society as of relatively minor importance.

251. 1. The comment is likely to make the patient feel defensive and defiant. It is belittling and a natural tendency is to counterattack the threat to the self-image. Since the person with an antisocial personality is egocentric and unconcerned about his effect on others, he is unlikely to feel shame, remorse, or embarrassment.

252. 2. Just as was true in the case of obesity (item 241), society tends to stigmatize those who vary from its value system. Therefore, this patient's behavior was a source of anxiety because it was alien to the staff's and patients' value systems.

253. 1. The patient wants a reaction from the nurse and if he receives it, the behavior is reinforced. Reward is the best reinforcement for behavior and the patient would be rewarded if he receives a reaction from the nurse. Hence, option 1 describes the best course of action. The other options describe responses to the patient's behavior, any one of which would tend to reinforce it.

254. 2. Option 2 moralizes and is very unlikely to help the patient. Options 1, 3, and 4 attempt to validate and clarify the meaning of the message. They give feedback to the patient and promote self-evaluative responses.

255. 4. In a situation such as this, the results can be too serious to risk bargaining with the patient. The best course of action and the one that is likely to promote trust, is to tell the patient honestly what must be done about the bomb threat. It is possible that the patient is also asking to be stopped and that he is probably crying for help.

256. 1. The most basic and important idea to convey to this patient is that as a person, he is accepted although his behavior may not be. None of the other options convey acceptance of the patient as a person.

257. 2. Only option 2 constitutes a corrective emotional experience. There is a planned regulation of staff responses to the patient's behavior in such a way as to counteract the harmful effects of

the parental attitudes, in this case, the mother's lack of limit setting and overindulgence. Giving the patient gifts, privileges, or freedom would not help provide the corrective, structured, disciplined environment this patient needs.

258. 3. The developing child needs limits set on his antisocial or destructive tendencies in order to learn right from wrong. Being afraid to say "no" provides no limits. Heredity, birth trauma, and poverty are not significant factors in the development of an antisocial personality.

259. 1. Option 2, 3, and 4 offer the patient an opportunity to discuss his feelings. Option 1 is a stereotype question that almost begs for no response. Questions that can be answered with "yes" or "no" are poor for helping the patient express himself.

260. 2. Therapy is usually most effective when the patient is helped to understand why he behaves as he does. The therapist's insight is not likely to be accepted by the patient until he understands himself (option 1). Option 3 focuses on someone other than the patient. Option 4 delegates a nursing responsibility to the physician.

261. 1. Intimacy is a growth and development task of adulthood (18 to 45 years of age). It is mastered after a sense of identity is established, usually in adolescence. A sense of autonomy is usually developed in early childhood (1 to 4 years of age), a sense of integrity in later life (over 65 years of age), and a sense of productivity in the middle years (45 to 65 years of age).

262. 1. Regression happens even in the best of relationships since the process of behavior change is not without its plateaus and spurts.

263. 1. The term insight best describes the patient's self-awareness and self-understanding. Rapport is the manner in which the patient and nurse perceive each other and relate to each other; it is a positive feeling. Lucidity is the state of being intelligible or clear to the understanding of others. Cathexis refers to an emotional investment in a person, object, or idea.

MONICA MOORE

264. 3. Option 3 indicates that the patient has insight into her behavior. Options 1 and 2 seek to blame others instead of looking at oneself. Option 4 suggests that the patient is dependent on the hospital environment and still unable to understand her own behavior.

265. 2. Labeling a patient keeps one from seeing a person objectively; labels devalue people and may be highly detrimental in their effects. For example, it could keep one from forming a posi-

tive relationship with the patient.

266. 2. Previous negative experiences with a patient should not be suppressed, as in option 1, be excused on the basis of the patient's past (option 3); nor should they constitute a basis for present intervention with the patient, as in option 4. They should be reviewed and accepted as unpleasant but past realities. A new relationship should be initiated with the patient based on present behavior and concerns.

267. 3. Role reversal is illustrated in the interaction. Incongruency is inconsistency in thinking, feeling, and acting. Denial is a mechanism by which the mind refuses to acknowledge a reality factor. Self-fulfilling prophecy is the tendency to behave according to the views and expectations significant others have of one and according to one's own views of the self.

268. 3. The best course of action is to seek suitable help. There would seem to be little point in continuing, as suggested in option 1, and option 2 avoids the problem. The patient is unlikely to be able to help and the course of action described in option 4 is likely to increase the problem. It is usually best policy to admit that one does not know and then seek proper help or information.

269. 3. It would be least therapeutic to try to tell the patient that she is wrong and her feelings are unjustified. Options 1, 2, and 4 give the patient openings to discuss her feelings further and to be most specific about her sweeping conclusion.

270. 2. Most teenagers respond best to their peers and less well to persons such as those described in options 1, 3, and 4.

271. 4. Confronting the patient with her behavior gives her direct feedback and helps her learn what is expected of her. Scolding and confining the patient provides no learning for her and also promotes anger. The problem is not solved or directly attacked by transferring either the patient or her victim.

272. 2. Option 2 acknowledges efforts and it is not a punitive nor threatening statement, as those described in options 1, 3, and 4.

273. 3. A lack of remorse is due to a defect in the functioning of the superego, the conscience of the person. No organic defect is involved. The id strives to satisfy basic instinctual drives; the ego mediates in a reasonable way between the other components of the personality and the realities of the external world.

274. 1. The person with antisocial attitudes frequently uses extremely poor judgment. The person is often above average in intelligence, has an intact memory and intelligence, and is usually a clever rather than disordered thinker.

275. 3. Consistency by the staff in enforcing limits with a person with antisocial attitudes is an especially important policy to observe. Options 1, 2, and 4 are undesirable qualities in the staff: acceptance and permissiveness would reinforce the patient's problem which is related to her self-control; and strictness is likely to provoke anger and acting out, although firmness is indicated in enforcing rules and standards.

276. 4. It is most appropriate for the nurse to state his own feelings and reactions to the patient's behavior and bear the responsibility for them. Option 1 indicates falsely that the behavior would be satisfactory under other circumstances; and options 2 and 3 avoid the issue.

277. 2. The patient should not be made to feel rejected. The basis of all helping relationships is acceptance of the patient as an important person. In addition, this patient's problems may stem from parental rejection and criticism. Options 1, 3, and 4 are undesirable effects also, but they would be likely to result in behaviors by the patient that are more overt and, therefore, more easily managed by the nurse.

278. 3. The patient was using rationalization, that is, substituting one reason for behavior for the real one. Isolation is separating thought and effect with only the former in consciousness. Confabulation is filling in memory gaps with made-up stories believed to be true. Intellectualization is employing reasoning and logic to defend against uncomfortable feelings.

279. 1. Before making a judgment (options 2 and 3), it would be best to learn more about what the patient meant by her remark. Option 4 may or may not be necessary, depending on the patient's comment.

ALICE CHOATES

280. 3. The most frequent reason for using a vague admitting diagnosis in the case of the heroin addict is to help safeguard the patient's reputation. Society stigmatizes the heroin addict but is more accepting of a person with a diagnosis of depression and drug toxicity.

281. 1. The action of naloxone is much shorter than the action of other drugs named. This characteristic of naloxone is important since the patient may relapse into respiratory depression, once the effects of the drug have ended.

282. 4. See item 281.

283. 4. The patient would have been least likely to have serious effects if her friends used mouth-to-mouth resuscitation. Option 1 can lead to lipoid pneumonia. Option 2 can cause

serious electrolyte imbalances. Option 3 could lead to convulsions.

284. 1. Cocaine is usually sniffed by inhaling the drug through the nostrils. This procedure is likely to cause red, excoriated nostrils due to local irritation.

285. 1. Vomiting and diarrhea are usually late, rather than early, signs of heroin withdrawal.

286. 2. Option 2 describes a course of action that "waffles" on the plan of therapy. It may only serve to aggravate the situation. Options 1, 3, and 4 are indicated during a withdrawal program.

287. 2. Of the symptoms given, only urinary retention is not associated with heroin withdrawal in the newborn infant.

288. 1. Option 1 describes the best response. Option 2 is impersonal and does not offer help to the mother. Option 3 does not focus on the mother's concern. Option 4 is judgmental and has a hostile tone.

289. 2. It has been observed that it is during a crisis situation when a person is most susceptible to change, and compassionate help can provide the opportunity to change. Options 1, 3, and 4 play little effective part in behavior modification.

290. 2. The Commission on Marijuana and Drug Abuse regulates methadone detoxification programs.

291. 3. The intoxicated patient should be accompanied by a staff member when moving about to protect her from injuring herself. Option 4 is contraindicated for the aforementioned reason. Searching her belongings is not necessarily indicated. The next dose of methadone would probably be reduced rather than withheld.

292. 4. Methadone is equally effective for the patient at a low dose or a high dose. The danger is that the patient may take small doses and sell the excess to drug abusers.

293. 4. Guidelines indicate that the patient should have social and rehabilitation services available. Guidelines require complete records, including the client's name, and allow methadone to be taken at home. Regular urine testing is part of the program; narcotics are excreted through the urine and testing will quickly reveal whether the patient is taking drugs.

294. 4. Obtaining and taking drugs is a full-time job for the drug addict and, hence, the person needs help with learning new skills and interests. Options 1, 2, and 3 are true but are not the main reason the patient needs to learn a new life style.

295. 1. In line with the belief that an addict is never cured, a member is expected to stay permanently affiliated with the Synanon organization. An open-door policy exists at Synanon. A

member is free to leave at any time. The addict has difficulty expressing his emotions and is forced to expose his feelings and defenses in the group sessions.

296. 2. Although factors described in options 1, 3, and 4 could possibly influence the patient's success, the best judgment rests with the number of days the patient remains free of drugs.

297. 4. The heroin addict is least likely to develop cholelithiasis. Drug addicts are prone to develop illnesses described in options 1, 2, and 3.

LOLA ALBERT

298. 4. Of the causes given, the patient is most likely to succumb because of respiratory failure. Cardiac arrest is not common but circulatory depression also may occur.

299. 1. It is the combination of barbiturates and alcohol that becomes dangerous because the two act as depressants. An additive effect results. The agents do not enhance the effects of each other (option 3), nor do they suppress or act as antagonists.

300. 4. Option 4 acknowledges the seriousness of the situation and will not arouse false hopes. Option 1 is a stereotype remark and offers no help. Option 2 transfers responsibility and does not deal with the issue. Option 3 is punitive.

301. 2. The purpose of the conversation should focus on the patient and her needs; this is best expressed in option 2. Option 1 is indefensible behavior. Option 3 and 4 are irrelevant at this time.

302. 1. The patient's behavior describes tolerance to a drug. Addiction is the highest degree of physical and psychological dependence, and withdrawal is accompanied with severe physical symptoms. The drug dependent person cannot keep drug intake under control and finds it hard to function without its effects. Habituation is defined as a mild degree of dependence.

303. 4. Typical signs/symptoms of barbiturate abuse include sluggishness, difficulty in walking, and irritability. Judgment and understanding are impaired and speech is slurred and confused. The patient acts drunk as from alcohol but will not have the odor of alcohol on his breath. Symptoms described in option 2 are typical of heroin withdrawal.

304. 4. Options 1, 2, and 3 are indicated. Using a medication for reducing anxiety and agitation may add to the depressant effects of the barbiturates which the patient took.

305. 2. Generalized convulsions may appear on the second or third

day of withdrawal. Without treatment of the described nature, the convulsions may be fatal. Postural hypotension and psychoses are possibilities but unlikely to be fatal; they are unrelated to the Nembutal regimen. Hyperthermia rather than hypothermia occurs during withdrawal.

306. 2. It is recommended that maintenance doses of pentobarbital be reduced by about 100 mg. daily. This may need to be modified if the patient develops signs of intoxification or withdrawal.

307. 2. Pentobarbital is classified as a short-acting barbiturate.

308. 2. Although options 1, 3, and 4 may help to a certain extent to prevent an accident of the nature this patient described, the safest procedure would be to keep medications away from the bedside. This practice would make it more difficult to obtain additional medication when the person is drowsy and unaware of what she might be doing.

309. 4. The only symptom given here that is not ordinarily associated with amphetamine withdrawal is lacrimation. Dryness of the mouth is more likely to occur.

310. 2. The greatest danger to self and others is believed to be posed by the patient's tendencies to act out violently and aggressively. It is recommended that this type of drug abuser be treated on an inpatient unit where appropriate sedation and restraint can be provided.

311. 2. Narcolepsy is a neurological disorder in which the patient is frequently overcome by uncontrollable drowsiness. The desire for sleep becomes overwhelming. Amphetamines are frequently prescribed for patients with narcolepsy. The FDA has not approved the use of amphetamines for the disorders given in options 1, 3, and 4 although there is approval for early and limited treatment of obesity with this drug.

312. 3. During the first few days, of most concern are the patient's associated medical problems, commonly sequels of poor nutrition and the self-administration of drugs. The patient should be allowed to sleep if desired. When the toxic syndrome subsides, the other options assume more importance in the nursing care of the patient.

313. 3. Before beginning therapy, the physician will wish to obtain baseline information which will include learning what brought the patient to a stage of drug dependency. Options 1, 2, and 4 describe areas of concern which may become important as therapy proceeds.

314. 4. Option 4 offers the staff member a new viewpoint to consider. Option 1 verges on the point of attacking the staff member.

Options 2 and 3 defend the patient and will offer the staff member little if any insight.

315. 1. It has been observed that the majority of patients tend to complain most at night.

316. 4. Option 4 offers the best method of dealing with the problem because the problem involves all of the patients and they should have a chance to express their opinions concerning what should be done. Option 2 is likely to be futile. Additional recreation does not directly attack the problem.

317. 4. There may be some elements of truth in factors described in options 1, 2, and 3 although option 3 is possibly least accurate since illicit drugs are generally very expensive. However, experts hold the opinion that the socially acceptable use of drugs for minor ailments contributes most to drug abuse in the American culture.

CRISIS SHELTER COUNSELING

318. 1. For immediate effective nursing practice in this crisis center, it is vital that the nurse is interested, oriented to her work, and properly supervised. Certainly classes in crisis theory and intervention are important but they can safely be undertaken later provided the other factors are present.

319. 3. Option 3 describes what the nurse should do in order to obtain accurate information concerning this patient. Option 1 ignores the patient's request for help. Option 2 gives advice but no help. Option 4 asks the patient to mind-read her parent's reactions and focuses on them rather than on the patient.

320. 4. Option 4 implies that the nurse may think the patient is dishonest. The other options describe action that aims to clarify and help improve communications.

321. 2. It has been observed that anxiety can influence the normal menstrual cycle. This patient has reported concern and appeared anxious and there is no indication that she may have a physical illness which may be interfering with menstruation.

322. 4. Sex education has the goal of increasing one's knowledge about sex and this ordinarily leads to the person's taking more responsibility for his/her sexual behavior.

323. 3. Option 3 leaves the door open for the patient to return and leaves the decision-making up to her. The response does not threaten, as does option 1, or push the nurse's point of view onto the patient.

324. 2. This item deals with the rights of minors to confidential health care, rights increasingly being sanctioned by state legislatures. Options 1, 3, and 4 are not necessarily true. The nurse

should familiarize herself with local laws and customs before releasing the information to the parents.

325. 1. Inhalants most often damage lung tissue by their local effects, and liver tissue which results in impaired liver functioning.

326. 1. Of the causes of death that are given, anemia is most often the culprit. Blood dyscrasias occur frequently when inhalants are used extensively. Deaths have also been observed to occur from respiratory or cardiac failure.

327. 4. The names in option 1 refer to heroin. Downs and rainbows are barbiturates and M is the narcotic, morphine. Bennies and speed refer to amphetamines and APCs, to aspirin.

328. 1. Options 2, 3, and 4 describe common effects of LSD. LSD has not been proven to increase one's creativity although some persons have believed it would.

329. 4. Most bad trips respond to supportive management in a friendly, protective environment. Isolation aggravates the panic, as do physical contact and activity.

330. 3. Option 3 is a truthful statement and prepares the patient for what to expect. Option 1 offers false reassurance. Option 2 moralizes and offers no help. The terminology is too technical for a lay person in option 4 and watching television is generally contraindicated.

331. 4. Major tranquilizers should not be given to shorten the LSD reaction because of the danger, possibly fatal, of drug incompatability. Hallucinogens are often combined with other substances, atropine being present in a few cases when death has occurred.

332. 4. There is evidence to indicate that the children of people who use LSD are predisposed to birth defects. LSD is not addictive and if death occurs, it occurs from reasons other than an overdose of LSD.

333. 3. Option 3 is straightforward and focuses on the client. Option 1 probes and the patient is not likely to answer correctly. Option 2 asks the patient to analyze the nurse's feelings, rather than her own. Option 4 changes the subject and, hence, ignores the patient's problem.

334. 1. Many people believe that the woman is most often responsible for the rape. Beliefs described in options 2 and 4 are not widely held and option 3 is untrue.

335. 1. Venereal diseases can be spread through the act of rape. Other conditions given here may be associated with rape in some instances but are not the main reason for the examination.

336. 1. The patient's unconscious goal is most likely to be that of

self-defense. After a rape, the reorganization process calls into play self-protective, or self-preservation, instincts and behavior; hence, the maneuvers described are most likely self-defensive in nature.

337. 3. When those around the victim treat her as though she is to blame for the rape and she already has some guilt and shame about it, the potential for problems and difficulty in adjusting after the rape will be increased. Options 1, 2, and 4 describe adjustive behaviors.

338. 2. It is most important to have an account of the person's description of the assault. Option 4 may be desirable but it is not vital. Option 1 is also desirable but not a legal necessity. Option 3 may be desirable but not necessary legally for the client or nursing staff.

339. 3. Option 3 gives the best protection. Options 1, 2, and 4 are contraindicated and may even excite some attackers.

PETER WILLARD

340. 4. Alcohol is destroyed/oxidized in the body at a low, steady rate. Thus, the rate of destruction would not be influenced by the measures described in options 1, 2, and 3.

341. 4. Antiseptic mouthwash may contain drinkable alcohol and, therefore, may have to be confiscated.

342. 3. It is likely that he will underestimate the amount, since he may possibly be unaware of how much he really drinks or he fails to admit, even to himself, how much he really drinks.

343. 1. Although all factors named are important, most alcoholics are undernourished and need extra nourishment and rest. Alcoholism disrupts both eating and sleeping habits.

344. 3. It has been found that the best way to deal with an alcoholic is to be tolerant and understanding of him. The other approaches mentioned have been shown to be ineffective.

345. 2. Most states use the percentage of 0.15 to describe intoxication.

346. 2. Tranquilizers, particularly chlordiazepoxide, are currently the drugs of first choice. The intramuscular route for paraldehyde should be avoided to prevent sterile abscesses and damage to nerves. Option 4, an anticonvulsant, does not relieve anxiety. Barbiturates are contraindicated; see item 299.

347. 1. The condition described is a blackout. A hangover is manifested by headaches, gastrointestinal distress, and the like, following heavy consumption of alcohol. Dry drunk syndrome means the patient has not been drinking but acts grandiose, impatient, and uses many defense mechanisms.

348. 4. Tremors may continue for several days or even longer after

alcohol intake has stopped. Options 1, 2, and 3 are inaccurate statements.

349. 4. Group support has proven to be more successful than individual attention from the staff in influencing positive behavior in alcoholics. Locked doors do not help patients to change or develop their own controls. Searching visitors is also impractical and externally oriented.

350. 1. The therapeutic technique used in option 1 is reflective and acknowledges the patient's right to think for himself. Option 2 focuses on the nurse's point of view, rather than the patient's. Option 3 gives advice prematurely. Option 4 hedges and gives no help.

351. 1. Al-Anon is for the mates of alcoholics. Alateen is for the children of alcoholics. The Salvation Army does not have a program for alcoholics. Alcoholics Anonymous is for the alcoholic.

352. 4. Alcoholics are representative of the general public. No one group, such as those described in options 1, 2, and 3, is likely to have a more than average number of alcoholics.

353. 3. Option 3 states specifically what was seen and heard and is descriptive rather than judgmental.

354. 3. Although other methods have been tried, it has been found that the best and most practical way to help the alcoholic is by assisting him to rebuild his life around substitutes for alcohol.

355. 2. Disulfiram helps curb the impulsiveness of the problem drinker. As long as there is any of the drug in the body, it reacts with the alcohol to produce marked discomfort. Typical symptoms include headaches, nausea and vomiting, breathing difficulties, and skin irritation.

356. 3. See item 355. Muscular flaccidity is not associated with the use of disulfiram.

357. 4. Vague feelings of apprehension and doom appear during the chronic phase of alcohol addiction. The other symptoms appear at an earlier stage of the disease.

358. 2. Option 2 offers the best course of action. The alcoholic learns to refuse drinks and is not bothered by the presence of alcohol after successful therapy. Option 4 is impractical; the alcoholic must want to receive therapy before it will be successful.

359. 2. The most realistic assessment is described in option 2. The alcoholic is taught that he cannot take even one drink without returning to his old habits of drinking. Option 4 suggests that the patient did not see the problem as his but blames his wife; continued abstinence would be doubtful. Option 1 does not

describe the philosophy of taking one day at a time and it is unrealistic to make such a promise.

GENA BAXTER

360. 2. A stereotype is the concept described. Ideology is a manner of thinking that is characteristic of an individual. A mental set is a readiness to organize an individual's perceptions in a particular way. The halo effect is a tendency to be influenced by one's general impression of a person (favorable or unfavorable) when rating one of his specific traits.

361. 2. The best way to learn to know a person is to get to know the individual personally. Depending on others or books is a poor substitute.

362. 3. The pathology of cirrhosis of the liver due to alcohol are the result of deficiencies in nutrients and vitamin intake. Alcohol is used in place of food and liver tissues become damaged.

363. 4. The alcoholic is usually differentiated from the person who consumes more-than-average quantities of alcohol by his inability to get along in his social relationships at work and at home. Comments described in options 1, 2, and 3 do not differentiate alcoholics from nonalcoholics.

364. 1. The patient is utilizing denial. Displacement is the transfer of a feeling to a more acceptable substitute object. Rationalization is substituting one reason for a behavior for the real one motivating the behavior. Reaction formation refers to an opposite attitude taking the place of the real attitudes or impulses the individual harbors.

365. 4. Breaking down the patient's defenses, or her use of denial, will most likely lead to disorganization and depression. Authorities agree that the defense should not be attacked directly; it may prevent complete disorganization in the face of a crisis or there may be a resultant depression if broken.

366. 2. Glossitis is not a side effect of niacin. Pruritis, a burning sensation or a feeling of body warmth, and flushing of the face and neck may occur when the patient receives large doses of niacin.

367. 2. Cyproheptadine hydrochloride is used primarily for properties described in option 2. It does not have properties as described in the other options.

368. 4. Peripheral neuritis is the nervous disorder described. Neurasthenia is neurotic behavior in which the main pattern is motor and mental fatigue. Neuralgia is severe pain along the course of a nerve. Bell's palsy is a type of facial paralysis involving the seventh cranial nerve.

369. 4. A patient with neurological disorders is likely to have sensory changes. Therefore, it is particularly important to guard against burns since the patient may be unaware of the amount of heat present.

370. 3. Coffee contains caffeine which acts as a psychomotor stimulant. Hence, serving this patient coffee may add to her tremors and wakefulness.

371. 4. The nursing notes that offer most help to others are those which describe exactly what the patient did. Medical terms used to describe behavior may be misinterpreted by others.

372. 1. The patient with delirium tremens should not be left unattended; unintentional suicide is a possibility in the attempt to get away from the hallucinations. Shadows created by dim lights are likely to cause illusions. Options 2 and 3 are likely to add to the patient's agitation. Option 4 is untruthful and false reassurance.

373. 3. Research has indicated that the part of the brain involved with persons who are uninhibited and euphoric is the cerebral cortex.

374. 1. For many years, alcoholics were treated as criminals and were jailed. Knowing that alcoholism is a disease has helped to halt this treatment of the alcoholic. Factors described in options 2, 3, and 4 may be influenced by this knowledge but the primary purpose for promoting the idea is to help the patient recover rather than jail him.

375. 3. Emotional needs have top priority in the unconscious motivational realm and, hence, the husband is most likely to use his wife's drinking to meet his needs. Option 1 may be true but is unlikely to be the primary reason for his difficulty. Option 2 is unwarranted. Option 4 is a rather superficial reason.

376. 3. Masochism is the disorder described. Sadism is a form of perversion in which erotic pleasure is experienced in inflicting pain on another person. Hedonism is defined as the constant seeking of pleasure and avoidance of pain. Autoerotism refers to sensual self-gratification by and from one's self.

377. 4. Option 4 promotes the concept of therapy in a nonthreatening way, is supportive of self-help efforts, and does not attack the person. Option 1 is premature and nonhelpful. Option 2 implies the person is at fault and does not take his feelings into account. Option 3 offers sympathy but little help for the person.

378. 2. AA requires that the alcoholic admit to being powerless over alcohol and that he needs help. Options 1, 3, and 4 are true of

AA but not a requisite for initial membership in the organization.

379. 2. The person who abuses alcohol chronically is most likely to develop an organic brain disorder. Pathological intoxication and alcohol stupor are the result of alcohol intoxication. Alcoholic hallucinosis is classified as an abstinence or withdrawal syndrome.

380. 3. While it is important that the nurse have knowledge as described in all options, it is most essential that she be familiar with the many local health and social service agencies that help the alcoholic and his family. This is an illustration of the nurse's role as the coordinator of services available for her patients. She may also serve as an advocate as she obtains other agencies' services for her patient.

MARY SILVER

381. 3. A "don't hurry—take your time" approach is of most importance for the elderly patient. Options 1 and 2 are contraindicated since they do not meet the patient's needs. Option 4 describes orientation that may provoke more confusion rather than less although the patient should be oriented to his surroundings regardless of age.

382. 2. Chronic organic brain syndrome is considered to be a permanent and irreversible condition, whereas acute organic brain syndrome is usually a temporary and reversible condition and is not a painful or fatal condition.

383. 4. Observations have demonstrated that chronic organic brain disorder characteristically produces symptoms gradually and that lucid intervals may be interspersed throughout.

384. 2. Multiple sclerosis is a progressive chronic disease; its course cannot be reversed although patients may experience periods when progression slows or halts temporarily. The disorders given in the other three options are treatable and cure is possible.

385. 2. Electroencephalography records the electrical activity in the brain. It does not involve the use of electrical shock, is not painful, does not test the patient's intelligence, and does not enable others to know what the patient is thinking.

386. 2. Beverages containing caffeine, such as coffee, should be omitted prior to EEG because of the stimulating effects of caffeine which may influence EEG findings.

387. 1. The patient's hair should be free of oils, sprays, and lotion prior to EEG and hence, preparation of the patient includes a shampoo.

388. 1. Humans of all ages need to sense a future for well-being. They must have hope of things to come and believe in growth and change in order to live life to its fullest. Health personnel need to foster this belief and subscribe to it if they wish to be seen as helping people.

389. 3. Symptoms vary widely among patients but it has been demonstrated that factors described in options 1, 2, and 4 are not necessarily related to the severity of symptoms. It is the manner in which the patient responds psychologically that will have the most bearing on symptoms.

390. 3. Basic symptomatology demonstrates that patients with chronic organic brain disorders experience defects in memory, orientation, and intellectual functions, such as judgment and discrimination. Loss of ability in areas described in the other options are not typical.

391. 4. Option 4 is specific and cites time, place, and person to the patient who is likely to be confused or disoriented. Option 1 is a challenging statement and may decrease the patient's self-esteem. Option 2 is a stereotype in nature and gives the patient no basic information. Option 3 gives mostly irrelevant information.

392. 2. It may be necessary to include all items given in these options, but in order to prevent falls, it is most essential to remove objects which are in her path of ambulation.

393. 4. While all the factors discussed here are important to take into consideration, of most importance is that the patient should not have to change long-established eating habits since they have met many of her needs. To make changes may well result in the patient's refusing to make adjustments to a new dietary regimen.

394. 3. The patient is more likely to sleep well if she feels tired at bedtime. Options 1 and 2 are likely to add to her wakefulness. Option 4 may be satisfactory but will not promote sleep if the patient is simply not tired.

395. 4. Delirium, confusion, and excitement are observed signs of barbiturate toxicity. Symptoms described in the other options are not typical.

396. 3. The best procedure for helping the patient remain independent and for helping her observe good habits of hygiene is to encourage her to do as much self-care as she is capable of doing. Option 1 is unacceptable. Option 2 is impractical and unrealistic. Option 4 increases the patient's dependence and is dishonest.

397. 1. If the patient can succeed at a task, her self-esteem and motiva-

tion tend to be increased. Competing with others may have the opposite effect. Concentrating on a task may be beyond her ability and thus become a frustrating experience. Socializing with others is not contraindicated but is unlikely to promote motivation and self-esteem.

398. 4. Activities described in options 1, 2, and 3 are not contraindicated. Elderly patients feel more comfortable and safer when they live in an environment with which they are familiar and can get confused in a strange setting.

399. 1. The most likely reason for this nurse's discomfort is that she has not examined her own fears and conflicts about aging. Until she does, it is unlikely that she will feel comfortable with elderly patients.

400. 4. The nurse should be given an opportunity to explore her feelings. Options 1, 2, and 3 avoid the problem and will not help to solve it.

401. 4. A will is an important legal document and it is best prepared with the help of an attorney. Option 1 describes an unsafe procedure in view of the legal implications. Option 2 avoids the issue. Option 3 is no better than option 1.

402. 1. Reminiscing can help reduce depression in an elderly person and lessens feelings of isolation and loneliness. It gives the person permission to be old.

PATTY STEVEN

403. 2. The cause of Down's syndrome is unknown.

404. 4. Options 1, 2, and 3 are delays in development commonly displayed by a child with retardation. Being able to sit up at 6 months of age is a typical growth and development skill of a normal child.

405. 3. It is unrealistic to expect that psychological testing will provide information in relation to options 1, 2, and 4, but realistic to expect the items of information given in option 3.

406. 3. With recent advances in the care of the mentally retarded, it has been found that persons with an I. Q. of between about 30 and 50 are trainable and can learn to manage their personal hygiene needs. Patients with I. Q.'s of 50 to 70 are considered educable. Custodial care is required for those with I. Q's below 30.

407. 4. Practices described in options 1, 2, and 3 have not been demonstrated to raise I. Q's. However, nonthreatening experiences that are stimulating and interesting to the person have been observed to do so.

408. 3. Since children with Down's syndrome are prone to develop respiratory infections, it is especially important to observe respirations. Observations described in options 1 and 4 are especially important for the child with cardiac defects.

409. 4. The parents must continue to work daily with their retarded child when the nurse is not there. Instructions and counseling are directed toward increasing their ability to confidently handle the child. A sense of liking for, responsibility for, and understanding of the child tends to grow as the former goal is accomplished.

410. 1. The primary aim of genetic counseling is to inform the parents about their birth defect risks. Objectives described in the other options are secondary and vary with the facility. Option 4 involves a decision which is up to the parents to make.

411. 4. Option 4 is exploratory and encourages verbalization of the mother's feeling. Trying to use logic or using apology cannot be expected to be effective for handling this situation.

412. 2. The best guide in this instance is the child's developmental age. The child does not have the necessary motor or intellectual skills for the toys of a 10 year old. He has more physical abilities than are required to satisfactorily utilize toys appropriate for a 3 year old.

413. 3. Goals should be simple because they should be reachable. It is best practice to break skills, such as dressing oneself, into many small parts and have the child repeat each part with slowly advancing variations. Hence, a series of small short-term goals would be the most applicable.

414. 2. The most likely explanation for the child's behavior is that she simply seeks attention from her mother. Often the need to get attention is greater than the fear of being punished and worth the mother's displeasure to the child.

415. 1. It has been found that the best reinforcement for desired behavior is reward, in this case, praise. Other techniques, as described in options 2, 3, and 4, do not serve the purpose of reinforcing desired behavior.

416. 2. Success is desirable for the mentally deficient person but the element of success through competition is not. The progress of the individual can be impeded when comparisons are made with others and can raise anxiety levels. All the other options cite desirable elements of institutional programs.

417. 1. Beliefs described in options 2, 3, and 4 were commonly held and increased the number of institutionalizations. The mentally retarded were previously institutionalized because it was believed they could not learn new behaviors and skills.

418. 2. Statistics indicate that approximately 3 percent of the population in the United States is mentally retarded.

GREG SHAW

419. 3. It would be best for the nurse to verbalize her feelings rather than act them out. It would be dishonest and inappropriate to smile or act indifferently toward the patient. Crying may upset the patient who may then wish to care for the nurse.

420. 2. Studies have shown that children are aware of and show anxieties about death at an earlier age than was once thought and they recognize false cheerfulness. They tend to experience isolation and loneliness when those around them are trying to hide or mask the truth. They are then left to face the realities of death alone.

421. 2. Most authorities now recommend that the parents in this case should be told as much as they can understand and wish to know. The other options do not offer good guidelines.

422. 3. Experience has shown that children tend to become concerned about death when they are approximately 8 to 10 years old.

423. 1. This patient's behavior is typical of the stage of anger; he is hostile and fighting what he knows to be true. The stage of denial is characterized by statements that suggest the patient thinks it cannot be happening to him. Bargaining involves accepting that death is pending but there is still time to exchange death for something else, as a promise to live a better life. Depression is a late stage and is characterized by acknowledgment and general sadness.

424. 1. The best course of action is described in option 1. Option 2 is a negative approach and is threatening. Option 3 is likely to arouse guilt feelings in the patient. Option 4 does not give the patient the necessary information.

425. 2. Wanting to have someone with him at all times is dependent and regressive behavior. Behavior described in options 1, 3, and 4 are normal behavior for a child of this age.

426. 3. Studies have shown that the dying child projects his concerns in that he tends to depict as central characters in his stories a dying child similar to himself.

427. 4. The recreation selected should be interesting and geared to adolescent tastes. Option 2 may be contraindicated. Options 1 and 3 are desirable but it is more important that they be suitable to his age level.

428. 3. A supportive environment for this dying child will be secure and firm while still being nonisolated and warm. To set no

limits by gratifying every wish, as implied in option 3, is likely to result in the child's feeling insecure and with a sense of not knowing what is expected of him.

429. 2. The behavior this nurse is demonstrating may have elements of tactfulness, efficiency, and objectivity but most of all, it would appear that the nurse's behavior is defensive because possibly she has not come to grips with death and dying. See item 430.

430. 1. The nurse who has contemplated her own death and mortality is usually best able to meet the needs of the dying patient. See also item 399 for discussion of a similar nature.

431. 1. Losses tend to be cumulative. Old losses are relived or re-experienced with each new loss and add to the intensity of the present grief experience.

432. 3. The phenomenon described in the stem is called anticipatory grieving or mourning. It is an early "giving up" of the loved one to death.

433. 3. According to Erik Erikson, a child of this age (13) seeks to meet his needs for a personal and sexual identity. Option 1 and 4 occur before adolescence while option 2 ordinarily occurs later.

434. 3. The person's acceptance of death indicates that he has come to terms with his dying and death. It is ordinarily accompanied by signs of being at peace with the circumstances.

435. 2. It is best when supporting the family to focus on the present, the "here and now." This can be accomplished by living each day at a time to its fullest. Families also want to know what to expect and want someone to listen to them as they experience grief with death.

436. 2. The parents are contemplating the act of euthanasia. Pedophilia is defined as a fondness for children and may be used to describe a sexual deviation. Decerebration is a term used in animal experimentation and means brain removal. Homicide means killing another person.

437. 4. The least important role for the nurse is to be present when funeral arrangements are made. Nursing interventions described in options 1, 2, and 3 are indicated.

438. 2. When brain function ceases, it is generally agreed that death has occurred.

439. 1. It is normal to observe that the process of resolution of loss by death can take up to one year. Mourning as described in options 2, 3, and 4 is not ordinarily considered normal.

references

The following references were used most frequently for verifying correct answers.

Aguilera, Donna Conant, *Review of Psychiatric Nursing.* St. Louis, The C. V. Mosby Company, 1977.

Aguilera, Donna C. and Messick, Janice M., *Crisis Intervention: Theory and Methodology.* Edition 2. St. Louis, The C. V. Mosby Company, 1974.

"Anxiety: Recognition and Intervention." Programmed Instruction. *American Journal of Nursing,* 65:129-152, September 1965.

Babcock, Dorothy E., "Transactional Analysis." *American Journal of Nursing,* 76:1152-1155, July 1976.

Barber, Janet Miller, et al, *Adult and Child Care—A Client Approach to Nursing.* Edition 2. St. Louis, The C. V. Mosby Company, 1977.

Barnard, Kathryn E. and Powell, Marcene L., *Teaching the Mentally Retarded Child: A Family Care Approach* St. Louis, The C. V. Mosby Company, 1972.

Bassett, Louise B., "How to Help Abused Children—And Their Parents." *RN,* 37:44, 45, 46, 48, 50, 52, 54, 57, 58, and 60, October 1974.

Beck, Aaron T., *Diagnosis and Management of Depression.* Philadelphia, University of Pennsylvania Press, 1973.

Bellack, Janis Peacock, "Helping a Child Cope with the Stress of Injury." *American Journal of Nursing,* 74:1491-1494, August 1974.

Bergersen, Betty S., *Pharmacology in Nursing.* Edition 13. St. Louis, The C. V. Mosby Company, 1976.

Bradbury, Wilbur, *The Adult Years.* New York, Time-Life Books, 1975.

Brandt, Patricia A., et al, "IM Injections in Children." *American Journal of Nursing,* 72:1402-1406, August 1972.

Breeden, Sue A. and Kondo, Charles, "Using Biofeedback to Reduce Tension." *American Journal of Nursing,* 75:2010-2012, November 1975.

Brunner, Lillian Sholtis and Suddarth, Doris Smith, *Textbook of Medical-Surgical Nursing.* Edition 3. Philadelphia, J. B. Lippincott Company, 1975.

Brunner, Lillian Sholtis, et al, *The Lippincott Manual of Nursing Practice.* Philadelphia, J. B. Lippincott Company, 1974.

Bullough, Bonnie, *The Law and the Expanding Nursing Role.* New York, Appleton-Century-Crofts, 1975.

Burgess, Ann Wolbert and Lazare, Aaron, *Psychiatric Nursing in the Hospital and the Community.* Edition 2. Englewood Cliffs, New Jersey, Prentice-Hall, Inc., 1976.

Burnette, Betty Anne, "Family Adjustment to Cystic Fibrosis." *American Journal of Nursing,* 75:1986-1989, November 1975.

Butler, Robert N. and Lewis, Myrna I., *Aging and Mental Health: Positive Psychosocial Approaches.* Edition 2. St. Louis, The C. V. Mosby Company, 1977.

Carini, Esta and Owens, Guy, *Neurological and Neurosurgical Nursing.* Edition 6. St. Louis, The C. V. Mosby Company, 1974.

Carlson, Carolyn E., coordinator, *Behavioral Concepts and Nursing Intervention.* Philadelphia, J. B. Lippincott Company, 1970.

Chafee, Ellen E. and Greisheimer, Esther M., *Basic Physiology and Anatomy.* Edition 3. Philadelphia, J. B. Lippincott Company, 1974.

Chapman, A. H. and Almeida, Elza M., *The Interpersonal Basis of Psychiatric Nursing.* New York, G. P. Putnam's Sons, 1972.

Chappelle, Mary Lou, "The Language of Food." *American Journal of Nursing,* 72:1294-1295, July 1972.

Chinn, Peggy L. and Leitch, Cynthia Jo, *Child Health Maintenance: A Guide to Clinical Assessment.* St. Louis, The C. V. Mosby Company, 1974.

Clark, Ann L. and Affonso, Dyanne D., *Childbearing: A Nursing Perspective.* Philadelphia, F. A. Davis Company, 1976.

Clausen, Joy Princeton, et al, editors, *Maternity Nursing Today.* New York, McGraw-Hill Book Company, 1973.

Crawford, Annie Laurie and Buchanan, Barbara Boring, *Psychiatric Nursing: A Basic Manual.* Edition 4. Philadelphia, F. A. Davis Company, 1974.

Creighton, Helen, *Law Every Nurse Should Know.* Edition 3. Philadelphia, W. B. Saunders Company, 1975.

Croft, Harriet and Frenkel, Sallie, "Children and Lead Poisoning." *American Journal of Nursing,* 75:102-104, January 1975.

Cullen, Phyllis Palka, "Patients With Colorectal Cancer: How to Assess and Meet Their Needs." *Nursing 76,* 6:42-47, September 1976.

Dickens, Margaret, *Fluid and Electrolyte Balance: A Programmed Text.* Edition 3. Philadelphia, F. A. Davis Company, 1974.

Eppink, Henrietta, "Catheterizing the Maternity Patient." *American Journal of Nursing,* 75:829, May 1975.

Ewy, Donna and Ewy, Rodger, *Lamaze Childbirth.* Boulder, Colorado, Pruett Publishing Company, 1976.

Fagin, Claire M., editor, *Readings in Child and Adolescent Psychiatric Nursing*. St. Louis, The C. V. Mosby Company, 1974.

Falconer, Mary W., et al, *The Drug, The Nurse, The Patient*. Edition 5. Philadelphia, W. B. Saunders Company, 1974.

Fass, Grace, "Sleep, Drugs, and Dreams." *American Journal of Nursing*, 71:2316-2320, December 1971.

Finnegan, Loretta P. and Macnew, Bonnie A., "Care of the Addicted Infant." *American Journal of Nursing*, 74:685-693, April 1974.

Foreman, Nancy Jo and Zerwekh, Joyce V., "Drug Crisis Intervention." *American Journal of Nursing*, 71:1736-1741, September 1971.

Fowler, Roy S., Jr. and Fordyce, Wilbert, "Adapting Care for the Brain-Damaged Patient." *American Journal of Nursing*, 72:2056-2059, November 1972.

French, Ruth M., *Guide to Diagnostic Procedures*. Edition 4. New York, McGraw-Hill Book Company, 1975.

Frobisher, Martin and Fuerst, Robert, *Microbiology in Health and Disease*. Edition 13. Philadelphia, W. B. Saunders Company, 1973.

Fuerst, Elinor V., et al, *Fundamentals of Nursing: The Humanities and the Sciences in Nursing*. Edition 5. Philadelphia, J. B. Lippincott Company, 1974.

Fuhs, Margaret F. and Stein, Alice M., "Better Ways to Cope with C.O.P.D." *Nursing 76*, 6:28-38, February 1976.

Geach, Barbara, "Gifts and Their Significance." *American Journal of Nursing*, 71:266-270, February 1971.

Getty, Cathleen and Shannon, Anna M., "Co-Therapy as an Egalitarian Relationship." *American Journal of Nursing*, 69:767-771, April 1969.

Gilbert, Sarita, "Artificial Insemination." *American Journal of Nursing*, 76:259-260, February 1976.

Greene, Patricia, "Acute Leukemia in Children." *American Journal of Nursing*, 75:1709-1714, October 1975.

Hall, Joanne E. and Weaver, Barbara R., editors, *Nursing of Families in Crisis*. Philadelphia, J. B. Lippincott Company, 1974.

Hardgrove, Carol and Warrick, Louise H., " "How Shall We Tell the Children?" " *American Journal of Nursing*, 74:448-450, March 1974.

Heydman, Abby Hitchcock, "Intestinal Bypass for Obesity." *American Journal of Nursing*, 74:1102-1104, June 1974.

Hudak, Carolyn M., et al, *Critical Care Nursing*. Edition 2. Philadelphia, J. B. Lippincott Company, 1978.

Hyde, Naida D., "Play Therapy: The Troubled Child's Self-Encounter." *American Journal of Nursing*, 71:1366-1370, July 1971.

Irving, Susan, *Basic Psychiatric Nursing*. Philadelphia, W. B. Saunders Company, 1973.

Isolation Techniques for Use in Hospitals. U. S. Department of Health,

Education, and Welfare, Public Health Service, Center for Disease Control, Atlanta, Georgia. Washington, D.C., U. S. Government Printing Office, 1970.

Jensen, J. Trygve, *Physics for the Health Professions.* Edition 2. Philadelphia, J. B. Lippincott Company, 1976.

Justice, Parvin and Smith, George F., "PKU: Phenylketonuria." *American Journal of Nursing,* 75:1303-1305, August 1975.

Kalisch, Beatrice J., "The Stigma of Obesity." *American Journal of Nursing,* 72:1124-1127, June 1972.

Kalkman, Marion E. and Davis, Anne J., *New Dimensions in Mental Health—Psychiatric Nursing.* Edition 4. New York, McGraw-Hill Book Company, 1974.

Karlins, Marvin and Andrews, Lewis M., *Biofeedback: Turning on the Power of Your Mind.* New York, Warner Paperback Library, 1972.

Kelly, Lucie Young, *Dimensions of Professional Nursing.* Edition 3. New York, Macmillan Publishing Company, Inc., 1975.

Kempe, C. Henry and Helfer, Ray E., editors, *Helping the Battered Child and His Family.* Philadelphia, J. B. Lippincott Company, 1972.

King, Joan M., "Denial." *American Journal of Nursing,* 66:1010-1013, May 1966.

Kitzman, Harriet, "The Nature of Well Child Care." *American Journal of Nursing,* 75:1705-1708, October 1975.

Kneisl, Carol Ren and Wilson, Holly Skodol, *Current Perspectives in Psychiatric Nursing: Issues and Trends.* Volume I. St. Louis, The C. V. Mosby Company, 1976.

Kübler-Ross, Elisabeth, *On Death and Dying.* New York, Macmillan Publishing Company, Inc., 1969.

Kukuk, Helen M., "Safety Precautions: Protecting Your Patients & Yourself: Part Three." *Nursing 76,* 6:45-49, July 1976.

Kyes, Joan J. and Hofling, Charles K., *Basic Psychiatric Concepts in Nursing.* Edition 3. Philadelphia, J. B. Lippincott Company, 1974.

Laros, Russell K., et al, "Prostaglandins." *American Journal of Nursing,* 73:1001-1003, June 1973.

LeBow, Michael D., *Behavior Modification: A Significant Method in Nursing Practice.* Englewood Cliffs, New Jersey, Prentice-Hall, Inc., 1973.

Leboyer, Frederick, *Birth Without Violence.* New York, Alfred A. Knopf, 1975.

Lewis, LuVerne Wolff, *Fundamental Skills in Patient Care.* Philadelphia, J. B. Lippincott Company, 1976.

Lindner, Daisy, "The Nurse's Role in a Bariatric Clinic." *RN,* 37:28-33, February 1974.

Lipkin, Gladys B., *Psychosocial Aspects of Maternal-Child Nursing.* St. Louis, The. C. V. Mosby Company, 1974.

Luckmann, Joan and Sorensen, Karen Creason, *Medical-Surgical Nurs-*

ing: A Psychophysiologic Approach. Philadelphia, W. B. Saunders Company, 1974.

Manfreda, Marguerite Lucy, *Psychiatric Nursing.* Edition 9. Philadelphia, F. A. Davis Company, 1973.

Marlow, Dorothy R., *Textbook of Pediatric Nursing.* Edition 4. Philadelphia, W. B. Saunders Company, 1973.

Marram, Gwen D., *The Group Approach in Nursing Practice.* St. Louis, The C. V. Mosby Company, 1973.

Matheney, Ruth V. and Topalis, Mary, *Psychiatric Nursing.* Edition 6. St. Louis, The C. V. Mosby Company, 1974.

Maxwell, Jane E., "Home Care for the Retarded Child." *Nursing Outlook,* 19:112-114, February 1971.

McCaffery, Margo, *Nursing Management of the Patient with Pain.* Philadelphia, J. B. Lippincott Company, 1972.

Mereness, Dorothy A. and Taylor, Cecelia Monat, *Essentials of Psychiatric Nursing.* Edition 9. St. Louis, The C. V. Mosby Company, 1974.

Mezzanotte, E. Jane, "Getting It Together for End-of-Shift Reports." *Nursing 76,* 6:21-22, April 1976.

Mitchell, Helen S., et al, *Nutrition in Health and Disease.* Edition 16. Philadelphia, J. B. Lippincott Company, 1976.

Moidel, Harriet Coston, et al, editors, *Nursing Care of the Patient with Medical-Surgical Disorders.* Edition 2. New York, McGraw-Hill Book Company, 1976.

Morgan, Arthur James and Moreno, Judith Wilson, *The Practice of Mental Health Nursing: A Community Approach.* Philadelphia, J. B. Lippincott Company, 1973.

Morris, Magdalena and Rhodes, Martha, "Guidelines for the Care of Confused Patients." *American Journal of Nursing,* 72:1630-1633, September 1972.

Nalepka, Claire D., "The Oxygen Hood for Newborns in Respiratory Distress." *American Journal of Nursing,* 75:2185-2187, December 1975.

Nordmark, Madelyn T. and Rohweder, Anne W., *Scientific Foundations of Nursing.* Edition 3. Philadelphia, J. B. Lippincott Company, 1975.

Olson, Robert J., "Index of Suspicion: Screening for Child Abusers." *American Journal of Nursing,* 76:108-110, January 1976.

Otte, Mary Jane, "Correcting Inverted Nipples—An Aid to Breast Feeding." *American Journal of Nursing,* 75:454-456, March 1975.

"Pain: Part 1. Basic Concepts and Assessment." Programmed Instruction. *American Journal of Nursing.* 66:1085-1108, May 1966.

"Pain: Part 2. Rationale for Intervention." Programmed Instruction. *American Journal of Nursing.* 66:1345-1368, June 1966.

Peery, Thomas Marin and Miller, Frank Nelson, *Pathology: A Dynamic Introduction to Medicine and Surgery.* Edition 2. Boston, Little, Brown and Company, 1971.

Peplau, Hildegarde E., *Interpersonal Relations in Nursing*. New York, G. P. Putnam's Sons, 1952.

Petrillo, Madeline and Sanger, Sirgay, *Emotional Care of Hospitalized Children: An Environmental Approach*. Philadelphia, J. B. Lippincott Company, 1972.

Plumer, Ada Lawrence, *Principles and Practice of Intravenous Therapy*. Edition 2. Boston, Little, Brown and Company, 1975.

Plummer, Elizabeth M., "The MS Patient." *American Journal of Nursing*. 68:2161-2167, October 1968.

Pritchard, Jack A. and MacDonald, Paul C., *Williams Obstetrics*. Edition 15. New York, Appleton-Century-Crofts, 1976.

Quinn, Joan L., "Triage: Coordinated Home Care for the Elderly." *Nursing Outlook*, 23:570-573, September 1975.

Ray, Oakley S., *Drugs, Society, and Human Behavior*. St. Louis, The C. V. Mosby Company, 1972.

Reeder, Sharon R., et al, *Maternity Nursing*. Edition 13. Philadelphia, J. B. Lippincott Company, 1976.

Roberts, Joyce E., "Suctioning the Newborn." *American Journal of Nursing*, 73:63-65, January 1973.

Robinson, Lisa, *Psychiatric Nursing as a Human Experience*. Philadelphia, W. B. Saunders Company, 1972.

Rodman, Morton J. and Smith, Dorothy W., *Clinical Pharmacology in Nursing*. Philadelphia, J. B. Lippincott Company, 1974.

Rogenes, Paula R. and Moylan, Joseph A., "Restoring Fluid Balance in the Patient with Severe Burns." *American Journal of Nursing*, 76:1952-1957, December 1976.

Rosenbaum, C. Peter and Beebe, John E. III, editors, *Psychiatric Treatment: Crisis, Clinic, and Consultation*. New York, McGraw-Hill Book Company, 1975.

Russin, Ann Woolbert, et al, "Electronic Monitoring of the Fetus." *American Journal of Nursing*, 74:1294-1299, July 1974.

Sana, Josephine M. and Judge, Richard D., editors, *Physical Appraisal Methods in Nursing Practice*. Boston, Little, Brown and Company, 1975.

Scipien, Gladys M., et al, *Comprehensive Pediatric Nursing*. New York, McGraw-Hill Book Company, 1975.

Seitz, Pauline M. and Warrick, Louise H., "Perinatal Death: The Grieving Mother." *American Journal of Nursing*, 74:2028-2033, November 1974.

Shader, Richard I., editor, *Manual of Psychiatric Therapeutics*. Boston, Little, Brown and Company, 1975.

Shafer, Kathleen Newton, et al, *Medical-Surgical Nursing*. Edition 6. St. Louis, The C. V. Mosby Company, 1975.

Shaw, Bernice L., "When the Problem is Rape." *RN*, 35:27, 28, 29, 74, and 76, April 1972.

Shearer, Donald, et al, "Preparing a Patient for EEG." *American Journal of Nursing*, 75:63-64, January 1975.

Shepard, Katherine F. and Barsotti, Louise M., "Family Focus—

Transitional Health Care." *Nursing Outlook,* 23:574-577, September 1975.

Slaby, Andrew E., et al, *Handbook of Psychiatric Emergencies.* Flushing, New York, Medical Examination Publishing Company, Inc., 1975.

Smith, Dorothy W. and Germain, Carol P. Hanley, *Care of the Adult Patient: Medical-Surgical Nursing.* Edition 4. Philadelphia, J. B. Lippincott Company, 1975.

Solomon, Philip and Patch, Vernon D., editors, *Handbook of Psychiatry.* Edition 3. Los Altos, California, Lange Medical Publications, 1974.

"Standards for Cardiopulmonary Resuscitation (CPR) and Emergency Cardiac Care (ECC)." (Supplement) *The Journal of the American Medical Association,* 227:833-868, February 18, 1974.

Staudt, Annamay Ricco, "Femur Replacement." *American Journal of Nursing,* 75:1346-1348, August 1975.

Sterman, Lorraine Taylor, "Clinical Biofeedback." *American Journal of Nursing,* 75:2006-2009, November 1975.

Sundeen, Sandra J., et al, *Nurse-Client Interaction: Implementing the Nursing Process.* St. Louis, The C. V. Mosby Company, 1976.

Sutterley, Doris Cook and Donnelly, Gloria Ferraro, *Perspectives in Human Development: Nursing Throughout the Life Cycle.* Philadelphia, J. B. Lippincott Company, 1973.

Taylor, E. Stewart, *Obstetrics.* (Condensed from *Beck's Obstetrical Practice.* Edition 9.) Baltimore, The Williams & Wilkins Company, 1972.

Townley, Charles and Hill, Leslie, "Total Knee Replacement." *American Journal of Nursing.* 74:1612-1617, September 1974.

Travelbee, Joyce, *Interpersonal Aspects of Nursing.* Edition 2. Philadelphia, F. A. Davis Company, 1974.

"Understanding Hostility." Programmed Instruction. *American Journal of Nursing,* 67:2131-2150, October 1967.

Ungvarski, Peter J., et al, "CPR: Current Practice Revised." *American Journal of Nursing,* 75:236-247, February 1975.

Volk, Wesley A. and Wheeler, Margaret F., *Basic Microbiology.* Edition 3. Philadelphia, J. B. Lippincott Company, 1973.

Waechter, Eugenia H. and Blake, Florence G., *Nursing Care of Children.* Edition 9. Philadelphia, J. B. Lippincott Company, 1976.

Wallach, Jacques, *Interpretation of Diagnostic Tests: A Handbook Synopsis of Laboratory Medicine.* Edition 2. Boston, Little, Brown and Company, 1974.

Wasserman, Edward and Slobody, Lawrence B., *Survey of Clinical Pediatrics.* Edition 6. New York, McGraw-Hill Book Company, 1974.

Wernick, Robert, *The Family.* New York, Time-Life Books, 1974.

Williams, Sue Rodwell, *Nutrition and Diet Therapy.* Edition 3. St. Louis, The C. V. Mosby Company, 1977.

Wright, Joan, "Deaf But Not Mute." *American Journal of Nursing,* 76:795-799, May 1976.

Yoder, Beverly A., "Patching Babies' Eyes for Phototherapy." *American Journal of Nursing,* 75:266, February 1975.

Zahourek, Rothlyn and Jensen, Joseph S., "Grieving and the Loss of the Newborn." *American Journal of Nursing,* 73:836-839, May 1973.